CW01304077

Pediatric Ultrasound

For Elsevier:

Senior Commissioning Editor: Sarena Wolfaard
Project Development Manager: Mairi McCubbin
Project Manager: Derek Robertson
Designer: Judith Wright
Illustrations Manager: Bruce Hogarth

Pediatric Ultrasound
How, Why and When

Rose de Bruyn MBBCh DMRD FRCR

Consultant Pediatric Radiologist,
Department of Radiology,
Great Ormond Street Hospital For Children NHS Trust, London

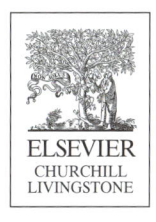

ELSEVIER
CHURCHILL
LIVINGSTONE

EDINBURGH LONDON NEW YORK OXFORD PHILADELPHIA ST LOUIS SYDNEY TORONTO 2005

CHURCHILL LIVINGSTONE
An imprint of Elsevier Limited

© 2005, Elsevier Limited. All rights reserved.

The right of Rose de Bruyn to be identified as author of this work has been asserted by her in accordance with the Copyright, Designs and Patents Act 1988.

No part of this publication may be reproduced, stored in a retrieval system, or transmitted in any form or by any means, electronic, mechanical, photocopying, recording or otherwise, without either the prior permission of the publishers or a licence permitting restricted copying in the United Kingdom issued by the Copyright Licensing Agency, 90 Tottenham Court Road, London W1T 4LP. Permissions may be sought directly from Elsevier's Health Sciences Rights Department in Philadelphia, USA: phone: (+1) 215 238 7869, fax: (+1) 215 238 2239, e-mail: healthpermissions@elsevier.com. You may also complete your request on-line via the Elsevier Science homepage (http://www.elsevier.com), by selecting 'Customer Support' and then 'Obtaining Permissions'.

First published 2005

ISBN 0 443 07275 2

BRITISH LIBRARY CATALOGUING IN PUBLICATION DATA
A catalogue record for this book is available from the British Library

LIBRARY OF CONGRESS CATALOGING IN PUBLICATION DATA
A catalog record for this book is available from the Library of Congress

NOTICE
Medical knowledge is constantly changing. Standard safety precautions must be followed, but as new research and clinical experience broaden our knowledge, changes in treatment and drug therapy may become necessary or appropriate. Readers are advised to check the most current product information provided by the manufacturer of each drug to be administered to verify the recommended dose, the method and duration of administration, and contraindications. It is the responsibility of the practitioner, relying on experience and knowledge of the patient, to determine dosages and the best treatment for each individual patient. Neither the Publisher nor the author assumes any liability for any injury and/or damage to persons or property arising from this publication.

The Publisher

The Publisher's policy is to use **paper manufactured from sustainable forests**

Printed in China

Contents

Contributors vii

Preface ix

1. General issues of methods and equipment 1
   Rose de Bruyn
2. Prenatal sonographic diagnosis of congenital anomalies 15
   Eva Pajkrt, Lyn S. Chitty
3. The urinary tract 39
   Rose de Bruyn
4. The adrenal glands 113
   Rose de Bruyn
5. The liver, spleen and pancreas 131
   Rose de Bruyn
6. The abdomen and bowel 181
   Rose de Bruyn
7. The female reproductive system 207
   Rose de Bruyn
8. The scrotum and testes 235
   Rose de Bruyn
9. The head, neck and spine 251
   Rose de Bruyn
10. The musculoskeletal system 301
    Rose de Bruyn
11. Pediatric interventional ultrasound 321
    Derek J. Roebuck
12. The chest 341
    Rose de Bruyn

Recommended reading 353

Glossary 355

Index 361

Contributors

Lyn S. Chitty BSc PhD MRCOG
Consultant and Senior Lecturer in Genetics and Fetal Medicine, Institute of Child Health and University College London Hospitals NHS Trust, London

Rose de Bruyn MBBCh DMRD FRCR
Consultant Pediatric Radiologist, Department of Radiology, Great Ormond Street Hospital For Children NHS Trust, London

Eva Pajkrt MD PhD
Clinical Fellow in Fetal and Maternal Medicine, Fetal Medicine Unit, Elizabeth Garrett Anderson and Obstetric Hospital, London

Derek J. Roebuck FRCR FRANZCR FHKCR
Consultant Interventional Radiologist, Great Ormond Street Hospital, London

Preface

Ultrasound is one of the most widely used imaging modalities in pediatric radiology and is set to continue to grow and develop as computing and equipment improves and new applications become available. Children are ideally suited to ultrasound, since their low levels of body fat contribute to ultrasound images of exquisite detail.

This book is intended as a practical starting point for radiologists, sonographers and other medical healthcare professionals undertaking ultrasound examinations in children, providing all necessary normative charts and guidelines on examining techniques. The book is not a comprehensive text on all the many different pathologies likely to be encountered in children, but it is intended to highlight the strengths and weaknesses of ultrasound in the important conditions. The aim is to provide the sonographer with a framework to use in diagnosis, so that the maximum amount of information can be gained from the ultrasound.

It is assumed that the sonographer has a basic understanding of how to operate an ultrasound system, together with a fundamental clinical ultrasound training. The intention is to provide an approach to ultrasound examinations and to emphasize the real value of ultrasound and its place in the broader perspective of the imaging modalities available.

Clinical expectations of the diagnostic ability of ultrasound are exceedingly high in pediatrics. The sonographer must strive for a good understanding of what is achievable and for excellence in technique. Working with children can be one of the most challenging and rewarding experiences.

The author gratefully acknowledges the help, stimulation and advice of all her colleagues and sonographers in the ultrasound department at Great Ormond Street Hospital for Children NHS Trust. Also thanks to Michelle Le Maire for her patience, encouragement and invaluable help in preparing the manuscript. This book is for all the sick children.

R.d.B.
London, 2005

Chapter 1

General issues of methods and equipment

CHAPTER CONTENTS

The appointment and appointment letter 1
The waiting area 2
The examination 3
Choosing equipment 5
Use of Doppler in pediatrics 7
Avoidance of occupational injury 8
Image recording and storage 8
   Analogue images 9
   Digital images 9
New applications of ultrasound relevant to pediatrics 10
Safety of ultrasound 12

Providing an ultrasound service for children requires a holistic approach influenced by a variety of considerations. It must not be forgotten that diagnostic examinations in children can be very stressful both for the parents and for the child. Anxiety about whether the child will be cooperative, the findings of the test and the experience of being in a strange clinical environment must not be underestimated, and no effort should be spared to make the experience a positive one.

Contributing to the success of the examination will be the provision of adequate preparatory information, a child friendly waiting area and an ultrasound room that has familiar objects and that does not intimidate or frighten the child. Such an ambience will help to ensure that the child and parents are relaxed, friendly and ready for the examination.

THE APPOINTMENT AND APPOINTMENT LETTER

It is generally good practice to provide the patient with an appointment letter, as there are a number of examinations that require specific preparation. In addition, an attached information leaflet in a format of frequently asked questions and answers is extremely useful. Questions such as:

- What is an ultrasound scan?
- Why does my child need an ultrasound scan?
- What does the ultrasound scan involve?
- Are there any risks?
- What happens before the scan?
- What happens after the scan?

can be addressed and the answers can put the parents' minds at rest. A contact telephone number on the leaflet is also useful in case the parents have any other concerns and want to speak to a member of the ultrasound team.

The appointment letter should clearly state:

- the appointment date
- the time of the scan (including the time at which the patient should arrive in the department, which may be some time before the scan takes place)
- which examination has been booked
- the department in which the scan will take place.

Preparation

Specific preparation for different scans should be worded simply but clearly. Examples are as follows.

- *For ultrasound scans of the gallbladder/liver*—'Please ensure that your son/daughter does not have anything to eat or drink for at least 4–6 hours before the scan appointment time. If your child is a baby then the scan should be timed for just before a feed.'
- *For renal ultrasounds*—'Please ensure that your son/daughter arrives in the department with a FULL BLADDER. If your child is still in nappies, please ensure that they have a bottle of milk or clear fluid prior to the examination.'
- *For pelvic/ovarian ultrasound scans*
  —'Please ensure that your son/daughter arrives in the department with a FULL BLADDER. If your child is still in nappies, please ensure that they have a bottle of milk or clear fluid prior to the examination.'
  —'If your son/daughter is aged 6–11 years they should drink at least 1 pint of water 1 hour prior to the appointment time.'
  —'If your son/daughter is aged 12–16 years they should drink at least 1 1/2 pints of water 1 hour prior to the appointment time.'
- 'This examination involves the use of a sound beam to form pictures of some of the organs within the body to help your doctor. The examination normally takes about 30 minutes and does not hurt.'

All renal tract examinations should be on a well-hydrated child with a full bladder so as to:

- demonstrate dilated lower ureters, which otherwise may be missed
- perform a pre- and post-micturition view which is standard for all.

Infants who are to undergo examinations of the gallbladder and biliary tree should be fasted so that they are scanned just before their next feed, after a 3–4-hour fast. Children should be booked first thing in the morning after an overnight fast, otherwise a minimum 6-hour fast is required.

All children who undergo pelvic examinations should have a full bladder when scanned.

Endovaginal and endorectal scanning are not practiced routinely in children.

If a child is to have multiple examinations it is best to make ultrasound the first examination. Cystography requires bladder catheterization which is invasive and may render the child upset and crying during a later ultrasound examination. Also, studies involving nuclear medicine or intravenous urography generally require an injection, which may also upset the child and make him or her anxious and less cooperative for a later scan. After the injection of a radioisotope the child will also be radioactive. Admittedly the dose is small, but this is an unnecessary radiation exposure for the sonographer. In addition, if a young child voids radioactive urine while being examined, the ultrasound examining couch and equipment may become contaminated, delaying further examinations.

THE WAITING AREA

This is one of the most important areas of the department, and every age range should be catered for. There should be soft play areas for the infants, interesting activities for the children and a games area for the adolescents. A well-designed space where the child can wait and be entertained happily is essential (Fig. 1.1). The availability of Play Specialists, who can explain the examination to the child in a simple way with toys, is extremely helpful. Don't forget that parents are often very anxious about the impending examination, and if the child is bored and unhappy then stress levels will rise and often boil over into anger which may be directed at you the sonographer. Always try to perform the examination on time and do not keep a

GENERAL ISSUES 3

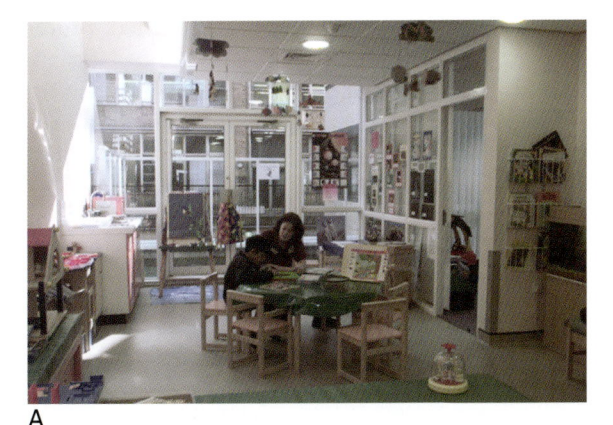

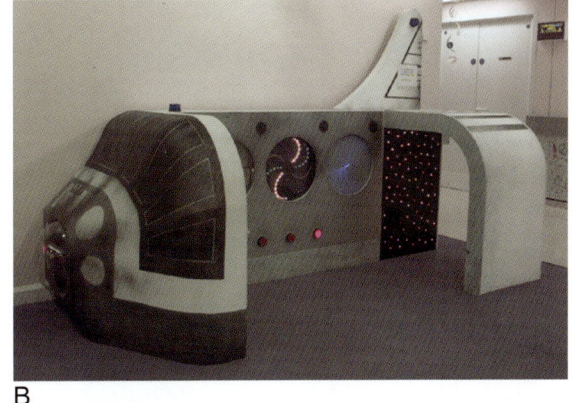

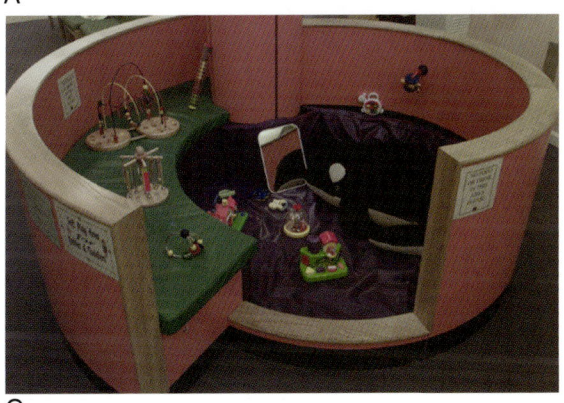

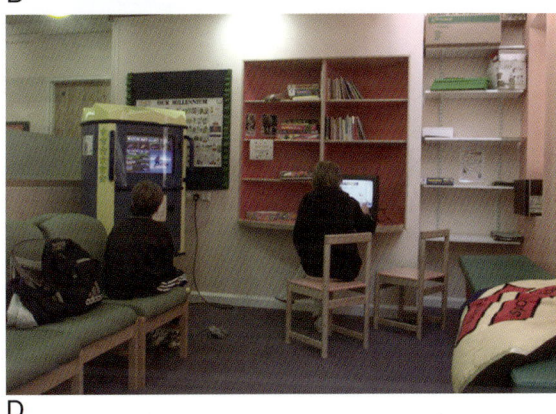

Figure 1.1 Examples of play areas. (A) A well-designed waiting area is an important part of any department undertaking investigations on children. This is an interactive area of the department for young children where they can draw, paint and play with many different types of toys. There are books available on the wall with mobiles on the ceiling. A play specialist to explain the examinations to children in a friendly and gentle way helps alleviate anxiety and fear. The area is light and welcoming with familiar objects. (B) Interactive areas are particularly good to keep children entertained. This space station is designed for children with special needs so that they are attracted by lights and water features. The tail of the space station allows access for children in wheelchairs. (C) All age ranges should be catered for. This is a soft play area for babies where they can fall and not be hurt. (D) This is an area designated for older children. There is a television, a playstation, books and activities for the older child.

child or parents waiting. If there is a delay, take the time to explain this to the parents and give an acceptable reason. Remember often parents have taken time off work and made provision for child care, so a lot of effort will have been made to get to the appointment on time. Having a box of broken toys in the corner is really not adequate, and a small investment in a television playing videos or a games console will make a world of difference. Access to a drinking water fountain is extremely useful, and easy access to a toilet will save time for the post-micturition views.

THE EXAMINATION

The ultrasound area

The ultrasound area also needs to be child friendly and welcoming (Fig. 1.2). Familiar and recognizable cartoon characters at the child's eye level, mobiles on the ceiling, and musical toys are very good for distraction of the younger infant. A television, placed above the examination couch, playing videos has proved to be one of the most successful features of our department. Also, blowing bubbles is a very effective distraction device.

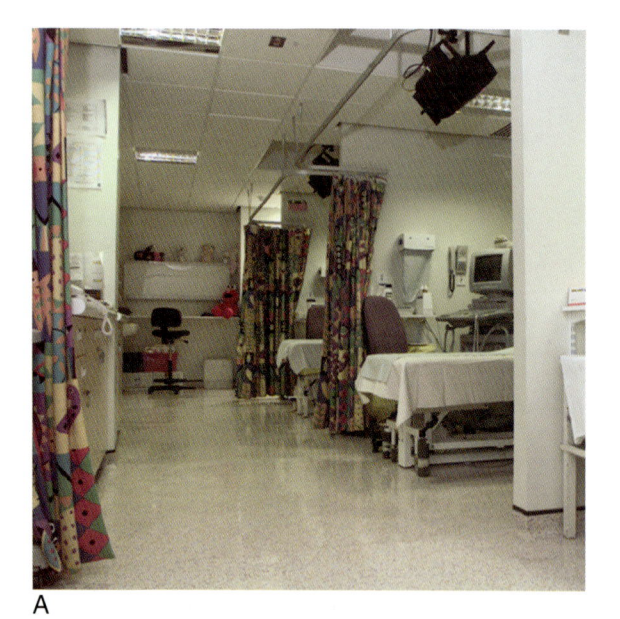

Always have a ready supply of soothers (dummies) available for hungry, restless infants. If young babies are too hungry the examination will be very difficult, so it is generally best to wait until they have been fed and are calmer. Diapers (nappies) should be available for infants.

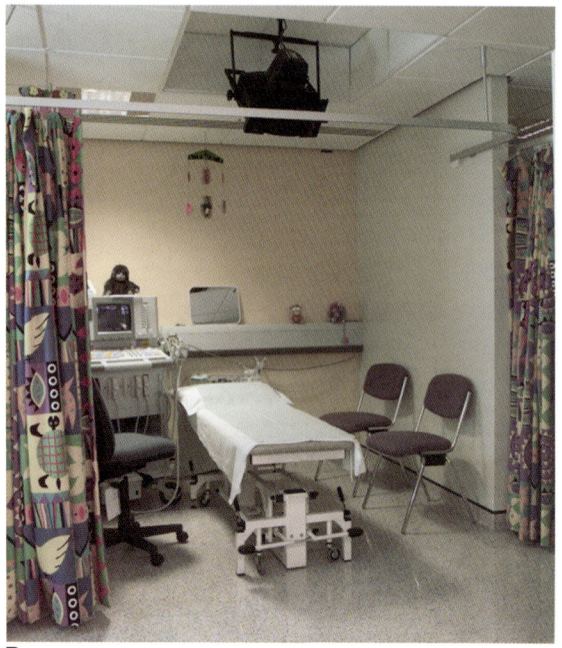

It is considerate to warm the coupling gel. Gel warmers can be obtained at a small cost, and cold gel is one of the major complaints from children. Some ultrasound gel can cause irritation and stinging of the eyes so make sure to check before applying it for eye examinations. Transducers should be cleaned after each patient so as not to promote cross-infection.

Temperature control of the examination area is also very important. Modern ultrasound machines and computer equipment cannot be in an environment that is too hot. By contrast, newborn infants need to be kept warm, as they lose heat and become cold very quickly when exposed for the examination.

Proper lighting should include dimmer switches and non-glare ceiling lighting for the monitors. Lights that cause reflections on the ultrasound screens are not suitable.

The ultrasound area needs to be large enough to accommodate parents, siblings and buggies. In addition, patients on trolleys need access, and it is best if the ultrasound couch can be temporarily removed. Wash facilities and a toilet large enough for wheelchair access should ideally be included in the ultrasound area. In addition a dedicated mother and baby room for infant feeding and changing is essential for any pediatric environment.

Protocols for the department are good practice when undertaking examinations. They provide a common standard for the different sonographers. In any case of litigation the demonstration of up-to-date and regularly reviewed departmental protocols is essential.

Figure 1.2 The ultrasound room. (A) This ultrasound area has been designed with a predominantly open plan feel, with brightly colored curtains screening the front of the bays. There is wide access for beds, buggies and wheelchairs. (B) An individual examining bay with lots of toys to entertain the child and mobiles on the ceiling. Video entertainment on a television above the couch has proved highly successful in distracting the child. For the sonographer the bed is fully adjustable and the examining chair can also be moved to different heights. The whole atmosphere is warm, friendly and non-threatening.

Examining the child

Children are rarely sedated for examinations. However, if a child is to be sedated for another examination such as a CT scan, it is very helpful for the ultrasound examination to be done around the same time. Newborns cannot be scanned when they are extremely hungry and crying, so it is best to ensure that they are fed just prior to the ultrasound so that they are quiet and sleepy.

If children are reluctant to be scanned while lying supine, be adventurous and accommodating for the scanning position (Fig. 1.3). Sit them on mother's lap, get her to lie down on the couch with the child on her tummy, but don't give up without a good attempt. Children do not need to be undressed; removing clothes makes them unhappy and vulnerable. Usually all that is required is to pull up tops and undo trousers or lower garments.

Certificates and/or stickers to mark a successful examination are generally important rewards. Box 1.1 provides a summary of some aspects of good practice in carrying out examinations.

CHOOSING EQUIPMENT

When choosing a machine for dedicated pediatric use, the following aspects of the service need to be considered:

> **Box 1.1 The Optimum Pediatric Examination**
>
> - Ensure the examination request form contains sufficient information for you to be able to perform an adequate scan
> - Before starting the examination decide what you hope to achieve from the scan. Know what you are looking for and review the reports and/or any prior examinations beforehand
> - Use the correct transducers
> - Perform the examination quickly. Younger children only give you a small window of opportunity and goodwill
> - Call someone to help sooner rather than later
> - Rarely, if ever, do children need to be sedated. Have adequate toys available for distraction and get parents to help immobilize the child
> - Always perform a full and thorough examination in children. Never just look at a single system, e.g. renal tract. Congenital anomalies often involve multiple systems. Pathology is missed because it is not looked for

- the age range of the patients to be scanned—from babies to adolescents (i.e. adult size)
- the intended workload and types of examinations to be undertaken—for example, abdominal, cranial, musculoskeletal or interventional.

The biggest mistake made when choosing equipment is generally to provide too few transducers to be able to scan this very wide age range and undertake the variety of types of examination. Often equipment is bought for both adult and pediatric use and a high quality machine is purchased with an insufficient number of transducers. This is false economy, and it would be better to buy a cheaper machine.

Probes

The commonest ultrasound examination in children is the abdominal scan, so once again a good range of transducers is needed. Curved arrays are undoubtedly best and should be in a frequency range suitable for newborns to adolescents, i.e. 7.5 to 3.5 MHz. A minimum of two probes is required (Fig. 1.4).

For neck, eye, musculoskeletal, and soft tissue lumps and bumps, a high frequency linear transducer is needed such as a 15L8. This is an often neglected but essential probe. Cranial scanning can generally be performed using a curved array but sometimes, when the fontanelle is small and access limited, the preference is for a small footprint vector transducer to enable better intracranial views through the anterior fontanelle. For ocular scanning a small footprint, high frequency probe is required.

Machine capabilities

The first requirement of the equipment must be to produce ultrasound images safely and of the highest quality. Generally it is false economy to invest in a cheap machine for pediatrics, as the image quality, transducer availability and Doppler sensitivity is inferior. The following are features to look for in a piece of equipment for pediatric scanning, where the patient is often a moving target and the sonographer has only a short period in which to do the examination:

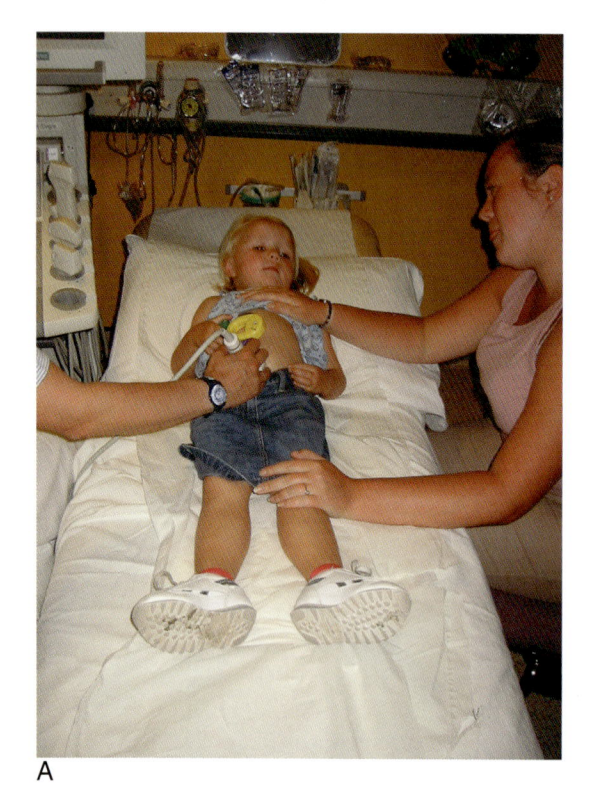

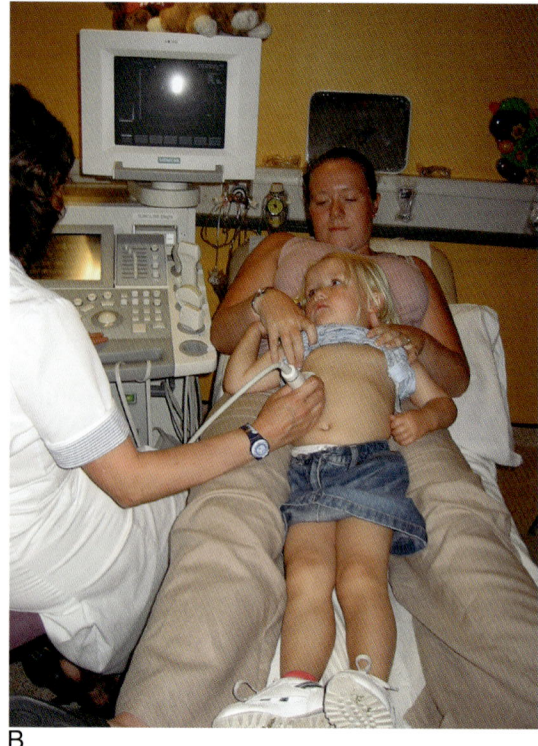

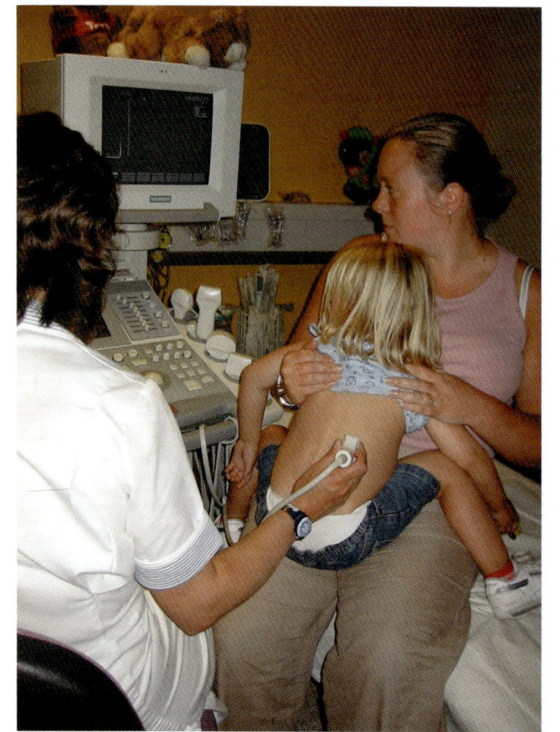

Figure 1.3 Scanning positions. (A) Parents are very good at helping to immobilize children by gently holding the legs and body and distracting their attention. (B) Get parents to lie on the couch with their children. (C) Sit a child on the parent's lap to scan the back.

GENERAL ISSUES

- ergonomically sound, well-positioned and accessible function keys
- ease of use—programmable presets for the range of investigations help save time during the examination and will also help produce images of diagnostic quality
- probes—ability to connect several probes simultaneously, or an easy switching mechanism; change of seating position to enable probe transfer is not desirable
- patient data—patient name and date of examination should be standard
- variable focus and number of focal zones
- freeze frame with excellent static image quality
- cine replay—essential for moving children; assess length and ease of replay
- magnification and zoom facility—essential for small structures; assess ease of use
- labeling—this needs to be achieved quickly; body markers are generally too time consuming
- Doppler capability—pediatric vascular structures are small, and Doppler of the highest sensitivity is essential; programmable presets should be the norm
- simultaneous color and pulse Doppler display—ability to change quickly between color power Doppler (color 'Doppler energy') and color Doppler is extremely useful
- measuring capabilities—measuring is an essential part of pediatric practice; however, the precision is less critical than in obstetric scanning, for example. Generally any delay in being able to perform a measurement prolongs the examination for the child. Caliper measurements are best done by one hand. Measurement packages, for example hip angles, should be standard
- portability—examinations are often required in distant locations, and equipment needs to be readily portable and small enough to fit into intensive care and bedside scenarios. Machines used for portable examinations should be lightweight and robust with moveable monitors and control panels
- DICOM compliance—new equipment should now all be compliant with Digital Image Communications in Medicine standards
- a good relationship with the manufacturer—essential for a reliable 24-hour service and on-site maintenance. New equipment should ideally have remote diagnostics.

USE OF DOPPLER IN PEDIATRICS

Doppler is an integral part of any ultrasound examination in children. Nowadays equipment without the Doppler capability should not even be considered for routine pediatric practice. Likewise, the sonographer should expect to be using and be familiar with Doppler controls in most examinations (Box 1.2).

Power Doppler (sometimes known as Doppler energy) is extremely useful in children, as it gives a quick overview. Power Doppler recognizes moving red cells but gives no information as to whether flow is arterial or venous. It is not angle dependent and is very sensitive. If a child is very restless and agitated, making a conventional study difficult, turning to the power application may allow simple questions, such as the presence of blood flow to an area, to be answered very quickly. It also quickly provides a very useful sketch of the layout of blood vessels before using the color flow imaging.

Peripheral vascular studies are often requested in children for suspected occlusion of vessels from catheters. When performing these studies it is always wise to start off with the vessel on the 'good' side so as to standardize the controls and use the vessel as a reference. Comparison can then be made with the limb suspected of having pathology.

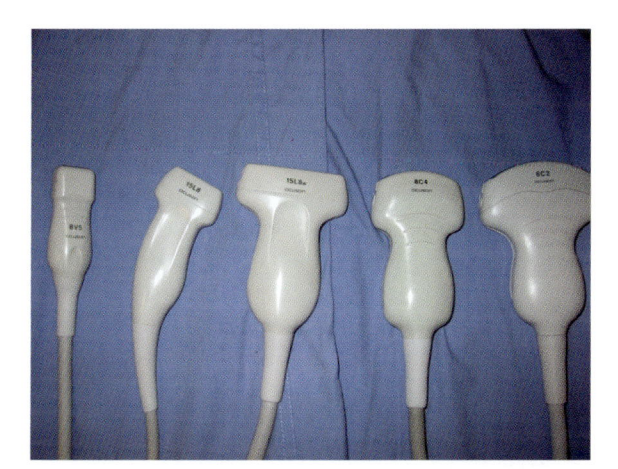

Figure 1.4 A good range of transducers is needed for the wide range of pediatric examinations.

8 PEDIATRIC ULTRASOUND

> **Box 1.2 Tips for Doppler studies in children**
>
> - The examination needs to be quick—a prolonged procedure results in a bored, restless and unhappy child and an unsuccessful examination
> - Have presets installed for all examinations to help minimize use of the Doppler controls and optimize the Doppler capabilities of the equipment
> - When examining limbs, examine the normal limb first so that the settings are optimized. This is particularly important in neonates with suspected vascular occlusion and where vessels are small
> - Use the correct transducer within the appropriate frequency range to obtain adequate penetration. The higher the frequency the higher the sensitivity. Using a lower frequency will improve the frame rate if too slow
> - Magnify the image
> - Doppler receiver gain should be set so that noise is just visible in the background. Set it too low and flow will be missed
> - Identify a vessel with color Doppler and then place the correct size of gate for adequate spectral sampling. The gate must be positioned in the center of flow parallel to the vessel walls. Slow flow will be difficult to detect if the gate is too large
> - Ensure the beam steering is optimally set for the angle of incidence. The angle should be < 60° for Doppler studies
> - Keep the color box size (width) to the minimum. A large box will slow the frame rate unacceptably in children
> - Reducing the pulse repetition frequency (PRF) will increase sensitivity at the cost of reduced frame rate
> - Adjust the baseline and sweep speed so that spectral information is optimally displayed

There are a number of areas where Doppler examinations are an essential part of the standard examination. For example, all examinations of the liver, biliary tree and portal system require a Doppler examination both to show the patency and direction of flow in the hepatic vasculature and to help differentiate normal anatomy in the porta hepatis. Doppler should always be used in renal transplantation, in particular in the immediate post-transplantation period and when looking for arteriovenous shunts in the kidney. Vascular anomalies are common in children. In superficial skin hemangiomas Doppler can help to assess the caliber and flow in the vasculature and whether the hemangioma is suitable for treatment with sclerosant or embolization.

AVOIDANCE OF OCCUPATIONAL INJURY

Repetitive strain injury is well recognized in sonographers, and it is incumbent on all departments to provide a good working environment for staff. General principles include the following.

- The operator's chair should be completely adjustable so that the back-rest and chair height can be altered. There should be lumbar support and a foot rest.
- The examination couches need to be adjustable so that they can be raised or lowered. This is also particularly useful for children in wheelchairs.
- Equipment should be ergonomically sound with an adjustable keypad. Elbows and wrists should be relaxed and not in awkward positions for scanning.
- Monitors should be on a swivel and be at eye level with no light reflection or glare.
- Every effort must be made to schedule patients appropriately so that examinations are performed adequately and not rushed. Sonographers should have frequent breaks during the scanning day.

IMAGE RECORDING AND STORAGE

There are many ways of storing images. The range of analogue devices includes thermal printers, videoprinters, multiformat and laser imagers. All vary in price and quality of image storage.

Analogue images

Hard copy analogue images have major disadvantages compared with electronic archives in this digital age:

- An analogue image is a static image which is stored on paper, film or videotape using a printer, multiformat or laser imagers.
- These hard copies then have to be stored either in X-ray packets or on videos and require a large amount of storage space. If these packets or videos are lost the ability to review images and examinations is also lost.
- Most ultrasound systems do not have an archive, which makes review of previous examinations difficult. An archive is of particular value for accurate reporting of examinations and comparison. This is not possible if hard copy films are constantly lost or mislaid.
- Images are only taken when pathology is recognized, and there is no ability to fully review the examination. There is no potential to re-measure the Doppler calculations. Ultrasound is a dynamic examination which is not fully represented in static images, and they should never be used to make a diagnosis in isolation.
- Static images are used for clinico-radiological meetings and for teaching and training. They may also be required for medicolegal reasons. Electronic archiving reduces film costs.
- The image quality on hard copy is extremely variable and affected by many parameters such as the camera settings and even image degradation in time if paper is used.
- Hard copy images cannot be viewed by several observers simultaneously.

Digital images

Box 1.3 gives a short glossary of acronyms which may be encountered in the field of medical digital imagery.

> **Box 1.3 Acronyms relating to digital imagery**
>
> DICOM: Digital Image Communications in Medicine
> DIN: digital imaging network
> EPI: electronic patient information
> HIS: hospital information index system
> IMACS: information management and communications systems
> LAN: local area network
> PACS: picture archiving and communication system
> PIMS: patient information management system
> RIS: radiology information system

PACS

In this new millennium of computers and the internet, there is no doubt that a picture archiving and communication system (PACS) is the system of the future and should be seriously considered for the present. There are major advantages to installing one of these systems, which in the long run far outweigh the short term expenditure.

Characteristics of PACS, in which images are digitally acquired and stored, are as follows.

- Digital storage means no lost examinations and no need for large physical storage spaces. In addition, time need not be wasted in looking for lost packets and examinations.
- Archiving allows immediate access to current and previous examinations, and this allows more accurate reporting.
- Dynamic clip replay has been a feature reserved for cardiac work but is exceptionally useful in general ultrasound, in particular for demonstration to clinicians and review of previous studies. It is extremely useful when reviewing Doppler studies and difficult examinations.
- The ability to demonstrate examinations dynamically improves clinical meetings as well as teaching and training.
- Records of examinations can be accessed via the internet quickly and easily with no loss in image quality and with simultaneous linkage to a hard

copy device. Images can be transmitted to clinical meetings, outpatient clinics and homes.

Some systems incorporate a reporting package so that there can be simultaneous display of the ultrasound report and image.

Digital images can be stored in a number of ways:

- on board the ultrasound device, such as on the integrated hard disk; they can also be stored on a magneto-optical disk drive
- on external devices such as a single PC workstation with a magneto-optical drive or on networked PCs. The best form of storage is on a PACS.

Digital storage is virtually 'lossless', so that image quality remains the same as when acquired. Images can be acquired and reviewed much more quickly than with conventional systems. Long-term storage is stable, and space requirements are very small. Images can be indexed and accessed from a database and can be communicated for education and conferencing.

Information to be stored includes:

- patient demographics, which can be barcoded and put into work lists; static images and dynamic clips for vessel flow dynamics, organ movement and contrast agents
- Doppler waveforms so that measurements and calculations can be performed
- patient reports transferable to a RIS and retrievable instantly with the examination.

Data may be transferred from the ultrasound device to the PACS. It may be captured on the hard disk and then sent as a batch or it may be sent continuously at the moment of capture. For portable examinations it may be captured to the system hard disk and then downloaded upon return to the department. Dynamic clips are extremely useful for review of the examination and these can be captured as well as still images. Dynamic clip data retains physiological information such as vascular involvement, flow dynamics, musculoskeletal dynamics and ultrasound contrast with phases of intensity. It provides measurable volume data and baseline data for 3D reconstruction.

Special features of an ultrasound PACS system should include color monitors, good monitor resolution, and capability to archive static images, dynamic clips, Doppler waveforms and measurements and calculations. The ultrasound machine should form the foundation for digital archiving. Digital storage in a central archive allows instant access to the complete patient record. It facilitates indexing and reporting, the management of referrals, and retrospective comparison.

Teleradiology, that is the transfer of images from one institution to another, is one of the applications of PACS. This improves radiologist efficiency and allows multiple hospitals to have access to an archive.

Disadvantages PACS systems are very expensive; however, the rapid development of computer capabilities makes PACS increasingly attractive. New PACS systems must be upgradable to keep up with these rapid advances. Old ultrasound machines with analogue images need to be converted to DICOM standard before they can be connected to a PACS. Generally speaking there is no onboard dynamic clip storage with older pieces of equipment. Dynamic clips are large files, so that the demands on a large integrated departmental PACS system become great. Ultrasound departments may need a separate archive for storage of such clips to be feasible. Clipstores are not currently used in general ultrasound practice; however, in teaching departments and for review they are extremely valuable. Currently the monitors are large and take up a lot of space. Flat screen monitors are available and take up less space but are expensive and generally have poorer image resolution. Image compression may affect the image quality.

NEW APPLICATIONS OF ULTRASOUND RELEVANT TO PEDIATRICS

New clinical applications of ultrasound are continually being introduced. The following are some of the more promising and useful in pediatric practice.[1,2]

Tissue harmonic imaging

Tissue harmonic imaging (THI) is a gray scale imaging technique that uses information from harmonic signals generated by non-linear propagation of a sound wave as it passes through tissue. Conventional ultrasound transmits and receives at the same frequency. In THI a low transmit frequency is used and the second harmonic signal is used to form the image using filters. This gray scale technique was originally marketed to be used on the technically difficult obese patient. It is also particularly useful in focal liver lesions. It increases diagnostic confidence in differentiating cystic from solid lesions and certainly improves definition, particularly in the upper abdomen.

Surprisingly, this application can be used in children even though they are not generally obese. We have used it to great effect when examining kidneys, particularly to demonstrate renal scarring. In our experience it enhances the cystic areas where the calyces are dilated and improves visualization of cortical thinning (Fig. 1.5).[3-5]

Extended field of view ultrasound

In early ultrasound scanning the use of articulated arms effectively allowed extended field of view images to be produced. This was lost when real time scanning was introduced. With technological advances in computing, high resolution extended field of view images both in gray scale and Doppler can now be performed. In pediatric practice this new technology is extremely useful, in particular for examination of the neonatal spine, musculoskeletal examinations and examination of abdominal masses, for producing a more accurate overview of pathology and also for measurement (see images in Ch. 9). This technique allows better visualization of anatomical relationships of lesions and is an excellent demonstration and teaching aid. The image needs to appear dynamically during the scan, with no delay while it is computed. This is not available on all pieces of equipment. Linear array transducers are particularly well suited, but curvilinear probes can also be used.[6,7]

Three-dimensional ultrasound

3D ultrasound has been introduced relatively recently into the ultrasound armamentarium. It relies on high quality 2D data as a basis for the reconstruction of images. In addition, advances in

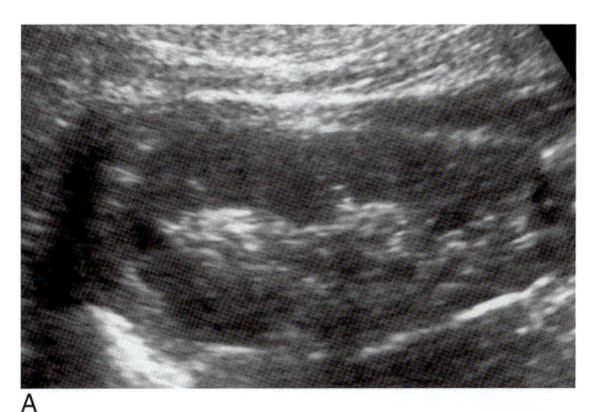

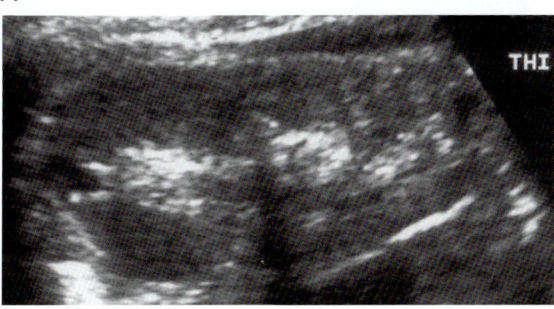

Figure 1.5 Tissue harmonic imaging. (A) Conventional longitudinal sonogram of the kidney. On this image there is an area of cortical thinning predominantly affecting the upper pole. (B) Longitudinal sonogram of the same kidney using harmonic imaging. In the upper pole there is a dilated calyx which extends almost to the edge of the cortex. This child had renal damage due to vesicoureteric reflux and infection. Harmonic imaging is particularly useful in children when trying to enhance contrast so that echo-poor structures stand out. This dilated calyx was seen much better on the harmonic settings.

computing power have resulted in the production of real time 3D ultrasound. Its clinical application in pediatrics is not well established, although it is particularly useful when examining the posterior vertebral elements of the neonatal spine. It has been used in the assessment of the fetal face to supplement 2D images. The undoubtedly huge value of 3D ultrasound will lie in accurate volumetric measurements of tumors, which can be used as a quick non-invasive examination for follow-up after treatment.

Contrast agents

To date contrast agents have not been widely used in clinical pediatric practice apart from a small application in voiding urosonography. Contrast agents are not licensed for use in children in some European countries.

Voiding urosonography is a technique identical to a conventional micturating cystourethrogram where the bladder is catheterized. Ultrasound contrast agents are then instilled into the bladder and show up as echogenic 'microbubbles'. The identification of microbubbles within the pelvicalyceal systems indicates vesicoureteric reflux (VUR). The original authors claim that the technique has a higher detection rate for VUR than conventional contrast cystography. The major advantage of using ultrasound is that there is no radiation. However, to date the disadvantages probably still outweigh the advantages. The patients still need to be catheterized, which is an invasive procedure. In boys the urethra is not shown. The number of contrast cystograms is generally on the decrease, and pediatric radiologists are moving away from this invasive investigation. So while it is an attractive alternative, it is unlikely to gain universal acceptance.[8]

SAFETY OF ULTRASOUND

Ultrasound examinations are one of the commonest examinations undertaken in children. For many years now ultrasound has enjoyed widespread use as a safe and effective diagnostic clinical tool. With the introduction of new techniques in ultrasound, such as contrast agents and non-linear harmonic imaging, the potential for biological effects may also be increased. It is incumbent upon the operator to be aware of the hazards associated with the use of ultrasound. Ultrasound societies have been responsible for producing policy statements on the safety of diagnostic ultrasound, and the sonographer should be familiar with these. The trend has been to shift the responsibility of risk assessment from the regulatory authority to the user. An excellent text on the safe use of ultrasound in medical diagnosis is available from the British Medical Ultrasound Society.[9] The American Institute of Ultrasound in Medicine (AIUM) and the World Federation for Ultrasound in Medicine and Biology (WFUMB) have both published policy statements on the safe use of ultrasound.

Guidelines for the safe use of ultrasound equipment adapted from the British Medical Ultrasound Society specifically for pediatric examinations are as follows.

- Ultrasound examinations for medical diagnosis should have a requesting physician. Always have a proper request form and try not to perform unnecessary examinations on children even if no radiation is involved.
- The examination should be undertaken by operators fully trained in the use of the equipment and its hazards. One of the greatest hazards in pediatric ultrasound is a poorly trained operator.
- Operators should understand the influence of the machine control mode and probe frequency on the thermal and cavitation hazards.
- Power settings—machines should be set up so that the default setting of the acoustic output is low.
- Examination should be kept as short as possible in order to come to a diagnosis. This is particularly important in infants and children.
- Probes should not be held in a stationary position unnecessarily.
- Sensitive tissues—particular care should be taken to reduce the risk of thermal hazard in examinations of the eye and head, brain and spine of an infant or fetus.
- Doppler—the use of spectral pulse Doppler or color Doppler with a narrow write zoom bar is not recommended for eye, intracranial or spinal investigations.
- In eye and intracranial examinations the thermal index should be as low as possible. In particular, transcranial ultrasound investigations may require a higher acoustic output. The eye is particularly vulnerable to thermal hazards at any age as the lens and contents of the eye have no cooling blood supply.[9–13]

SUMMARY

Ultrasound is one of the most important and widely used imaging techniques available for investigating children today. Providing a suitable child friendly environment, choosing the right equipment and being properly trained is essential to successful examinations. With some care and forethought about the needs of the parents and child, pediatric ultrasound can be extremely rewarding and fun.

References

1. Whittingham TA. New and future directions in ultrasonic imaging. Br J Radiol 1997; 70:S119–132.
2. Whittingham TA. An overview of digital technology in ultrasonic imaging. Eur Radiol 1999; 9(suppl 3): S307–311.
3. Desser TS, Jeffrey RB. Tissue harmonic imaging techniques: physical principles and clinical applications. Semin Ultrasound CT MR 2001; 22(suppl 1):1–10.
4. Shapiro RS, Wagreich J, Parsons RB, et al. Tissue harmonic imaging sonography: evaluation of image quality compared with conventional sonography. AJR Am J Roentgenol 1998; 171:1203–1206.
5. Whittingham TA. Tissue harmonic imaging. Eur Radiol 1999; 9(suppl 3):S323–326.
6. Barberie J, Wong AD, Cooperberg PL, et al. US extended field of view sonography in musculoskeletal disorders. AJR Am J Roentgenol 1998; 171:751–757.
7. Cooperberg PL, Barberie J, Wong AD, et al. Extended field of view ultrasound. Semin Ultrasound CT MR 2001; 22:65–77.
8. Darge K, Troeger J, Duetting T, et al. Reflux in young patients: comparison of voiding US of the bladder and retrovesical space with echo enhancement versus voiding cystourethography for diagnosis. Radiology 1999; 210:201–207.
9. ter Haar G, Duck FA, eds. The safe use of ultrasound in medical diagnosis. London: BMUS/BIR; 2000.
10. American Institute of Ultrasound in Medicine. Bioeffects and safety of diagnostic ultrasound. 11200 Rockville Pike, Suite 205, Rockville, Maryland 20852–3139, USA: AIUM; 1993.
11. Herman BA, Harris GR. Theoretical study of steady-state temperature rise within the eye due to ultrasound insonation. IEEE Transactions on Ultrasonics, Ferroelectrics and Frequency Control 1999; 46:1566–1574.
12. Jago JR, Henderson J, Whittingham TA, et al. A comparison of AUIM/NEMA thermal indices with calculated temperature rises for a simple third trimester pregnancy tissue model. Ultrasound Med Biol 1998; 25:623–628.
13. World Federation for Ultrasound in Medicine and Biology. Conclusions and recommendations on thermal and non-thermal mechanisms for biological effects. Ultrasound Med Biol 1998; 24(suppl 1): xv–xvi.

Chapter 2

Prenatal sonographic diagnosis of congenital anomalies

Eva Pajkrt and Lyn S. Chitty

CHAPTER CONTENTS

Routine ultrasound screening for fetal
    malformation 15
    The routine fetal anomaly scan 18
Abnormalities in different systems 22
    Cranial and spinal abnormalities 22
    Cardiac abnormalities 25
    Pulmonary abnormalities 26
    Gastrointestinal abnormalities 28
    Urinary tract abnormalities 28
    Skeletal abnormalities 33
Hydrops 34

Fetal ultrasound is now an established part of standard obstetric care in many countries. It can be performed in early gestation and in the first, second and third trimester (Table 2.1), as part of routine obstetric care, or as a targeted investigation in women at increased risk for a particular problem (Box 2.1). In many countries fetal ultrasound is offered routinely both in the first trimester of pregnancy to establish the gestation and viability and again later (around 20 weeks) to examine the anatomy in more detail. Scanning earlier and later in pregnancy in most units tends to be performed on clinical indication rather than routinely. In this chapter we will confine further discussion to the use of fetal ultrasound for the detection of congenital abnormalities and genetic syndromes in the first and second trimesters of pregnancy. All anatomical systems will be described, but the focus will be on those areas that present for postnatal ultrasonography.

ROUTINE ULTRASOUND SCREENING FOR FETAL MALFORMATION

As congenital anomalies occur in 2–3% of all infants, detection, treatment and prevention of congenital anomalies are considered important goals of prenatal care. Routine screening for fetal structural anomalies has the potential to reduce perinatal mortality by elective termination of pregnancies complicated by serious congenital anomalies, to reduce morbidity by intrauterine treatment and to optimize management of delivery and early neonatal treatment. The ability of the ultrasound

Table 2.1 Use of obstetric ultrasound at different gestational ages

Use	4–10	11–14	18–24	> 24
Viability	y	y	y	y
Estimation of age	y	y	y	n
Diagnosis of multiple pregnancy	y	y	y	n
Chorionicity	y	y	y	n
Anomaly scan	n	y	y	(y)
Growth (± Doppler)	n	n	n	y
Screening Dopplers	n	n	y	n
Down syndrome screening	n	Nuchal translucency	Markers	n
Cervical competence	n	n	y	(y)
Placental localization	n	n	n	y

Columns show Gestational age in weeks.

examination to detect fetal structural anomalies is central to the consideration of its clinical value, especially for anomalies detected before 24 weeks' gestation.

Box 2.1 Indications for detailed anomaly scanning

Family or medical history
Previous abnormal child
Family history of abnormality / genetic condition
Maternal diabetes
Maternal epilepsy
Maternal medication (anti-epileptic, warfarin, lithium)
Maternal recreational drug use
ICSI pregnancy

Risk factors developing in pregnancy
Increased nuchal translucency on 10–14 week scan
Raised maternal serum alfa-fetoprotein
Abnormality detected on routine scanning
Multiple pregnancy
Oligo- or polyhydramnios
Small or large for gestation age

ICSI, intracytoplasmic sperm injection

Despite the potential advantages of prenatal ultrasound examination, there is still much controversy about the value of ultrasound for routine fetal malformation screening. Studies report a considerable variation in the sensitivity, ranging from 20.7% to 82.4% in the first trimester (Table 2.2)[1-6] and from 16.6% to 84.3% in the second trimester (Table 2.3).[7-23] When interpreting this data it is important to differentiate between studies examining the use of routine fetal ultrasound as opposed to ultrasound used in a high risk population where the investigation is targeted and detection rates are higher.[24] Furthermore, the sensitivity of ultrasound screening varies according to the nature and severity of the malformation, the gestational age of the fetus, equipment used, fetal position, maternal body mass index and the experience of the ultrasonographer. Many of the studies reported (Tables 2.2 and 2.3) do not define these variables well. Finally, it must be remembered that the spectrum of abnormalities seen using prenatal ultrasound varies considerably from that seen postnatally. The prenatal sonographer will detect many lethal abnormalities (anencephaly, severe uropathies causing oligohydramnios and pulmonary hypoplasia, or complex cardiac anomalies) as well as anomalies that will be clinically silent in the newborn period and beyond (many renal anomalies, cystic lung lesions, or mild ventriculomegaly). The latter pose a difficult problem in defining optimum clinical management.

Table 2.2 Summary of studies reporting the detection of fetal abnormalities before 14 weeks using routine ultrasound

Study	Period	Number of fetuses	Method	Prevalence of abnormalities (%)	Sensitivity (%) before 14 weeks	Specificity (%) before 14 weeks	Sensitivity (%) before 24 weeks	Specificity (%) before 24 weeks
Hernádi & Töröcsik[1]	1992–1995	3991	TVS	1.4	40.8	99.6	59.2	?
D'Ottavio et al[a2]	1991–1996	3514	TVS	2.9	40.2	98.8	90.2	98.0
Economides et al[3]	Unspecified	1632	TAS/TVS	1.0	78.6	99.0	82.3	99.0
Whitlow et al[4]	Unspecified	6643	TAS/TVS	1.4	58.7	99.9	81.0	?
Carvalho et al[5]	1995–unspec.	2853	TAS	4.6	22.3	?	60.8	?
Drysdale et al[6]	1998–1999	960	TAS	3.0	20.7	99.9	86.2	96.6

[a]Detection rate before 15 weeks instead of 14.
TAS, transabdominal sonography; TVS, transvaginal sonography.

Table 2.3 Summary of studies reporting the detection of abnormalities before 24 weeks using routine ultrasound

Study	Period	Number of fetuses	Prevalence of abnormalities (%)	Sensitivity (%)	Specificity (%)
Rosendahl and Kivinen[7]	1980–1988	9012	1.0	39.4	99.9
Saari-Kemppainen et al[a8]	1986–1987	4073	0.4	36.0/76.9[b]	99.8
Chitty et al[9]	1988–1989	8785	1.5	74.4	99.9
Levi et al[10]	1984–1989	15654	2.3	21.0	100
Shirley et al[11]	1989–1990	6412	1.4	60.7	99.9
Luck[12]	1988–1991	8844	1.9	84.3	99.9
Ewigman et al[a13]	1987–1991	7685	2.5	16.6	?
Levi et al[14]	1990–1992	9392	2.5	44.5	99.9
Papp et al[15]	1988–1990	51675	2.3	63.9	100.0
Anderson et al[16]	1991–1993	7880	1.8	58.3	?
Geerts et al[a17]	1991–1992	496	2.8	55.5	?
Boyd et al[18]	1991–1996	33376	2.2	54.6	99.5
Schwärzler et al[19]	1997–1998	1206	0.6	71.4	?
Smith and Hau[20]	1989–1994	246481	1.1	53.0	?
Eurenius et al[21]	1990–1992	8324	1.7	22.1	99.8
Grandjean et al[22]	1990–1993	170800	2.2	41.1	?
Wong et al[23]	1993–1998	12169	1.4	72.8	?

[a]Data include ultrasound screened group only.
[b]City Hospital / University Hospital.

The routine fetal anomaly scan

The Royal College of Obstetricians and Gynaecologists (RCOG) has issued guidelines for standards that should be applied for routine fetal anomaly scanning at 20 weeks' gestation (Table 2.4).

The head is examined in the axial plane, and the skull shape and mineralization are checked. Measurements of the circumference (HC) and the width of the anterior horns and posterior horns of the lateral ventricles should be performed at the level of the cavum septum pellucidum and the third ventricle (Fig. 2.1A). The sub-occipitobregmatic view will demonstrate the posterior fossa with the cerebellum and cisterna magna (Fig. 2.1B).

The thorax is examined both in the longitudinal and axial planes. In the longitudinal view the hemidiaphragms can be identified, with the stomach lying below the diaphragm and the heart above (Fig. 2.2). In the axial plane the four-chamber view of the heart can be examined and should occupy one third of the fetal chest (Fig. 2.3).

The abdomen is examined in the axial plane at the level of the stomach and the portal sinus of the liver for its shape and contents, and the circumference (AC) is measured at this level. A baseline AC measurement should be obtained in case growth failure is suspected later in pregnancy. The abdominal cord insertion is examined to exclude anterior abdominal wall defects. The kidneys (Fig. 2.4) and bladder are identified. The anteroposterior (AP) diameter of the renal pelvis should be measured and should normally be less than 5 mm. The perivesical arteries can be identified running around the bladder.

The spine should at the very least be examined in the sagittal and axial planes and, if possible, in the coronal plane (Fig. 2.5). In the axial plane the three ossification centers should be identified, with their skin covering, and should be seen to widen in the cervical region and narrow at the sacrum. In the sagittal plane (Fig. 2.5A) the normal curvature of the spine can be seen, with the upward sweep of

Table 2.4 The routine fetal anomaly scan

Structure	Features examined	
	Routine anomaly scan	Extended views
Head	Skull shape	
	Ventricles, cerebellum, cavum septum pellucidum	
	Measure circumference and diameter	
Face		Lips, nose
Neck	Observe and measure nuchal fold	
Spine	Longitudinal and transverse views	
Heart	Four-chamber view	Left and right outflow tracts, aortic arch
Thorax	Diaphragm	
Abdomen	Stomach	
	Cord insertion	
	Kidneys and bladder	
	Measure diameter	
Limbs	Three long bones in each limb	Count fingers and toes
	Orientation of hands and feet	
	Measure femur length	

From Guidelines for a routine fetal anomaly scan. London: Royal College of Obstetricians and Gynaecologists; 1997, 2001.

the sacrum. Again the skin covering should be identified and the alignment of the laminae and vertebral bodies should be identified. In the coronal plane (Fig. 2.5B) the alignment of the transverse processes and laminae give a railway track appearance of the spine, which widens at the head and narrows towards the sacrum. In this view the alignment of the ribs can also be seen. With increasing resolution of modern ultrasound machines the spinal cord and cauda equina can be demonstrated (Fig. 2.5C).

The presence of three bones in each limb as well as hands and feet should be confirmed, although there is no expectation that fingers and toes should be counted at a routine scan. The femur length is measured, as again this gives a good baseline measurement for later comparison when growth restriction may occur. It also enables early detection of many major skeletal dysplasias.

If time and resources exist, the fetal face should be examined to check the integrity of lips and nose, orbits, lens, and symmetry of the face. Anomalies of the palate are difficult to see, because of shadowing from surrounding bony structures. Examination of the fetal profile can be useful in the detection of micrognathia.

Finally, fetal gender can be examined and, when requested, revealed to the parents. Using this protocol around 80–85% of severely handicapping or lethal abnormalities and varying proportions of other anomalies should be detected (Table 2.5).

Ultrasound markers of fetal aneuploidy

One group of cases that may not present to the postnatal sonographer are those associated with major chromosomal anomalies, since many of these conditions are lethal. In view of the high incidence (around 14%) of chromosomal disorders in structurally abnormal and growth retarded fetuses, karyotyping is discussed in most cases following the detection of most major and some minor anomalies or so called soft markers (Table 2.6). This is particularly recommended when more than one abnormality or marker is seen, as the incidence of aneuploidy increases from less than 2% in fetuses with isolated defects to 29% in those with multiple anomalies.[25]

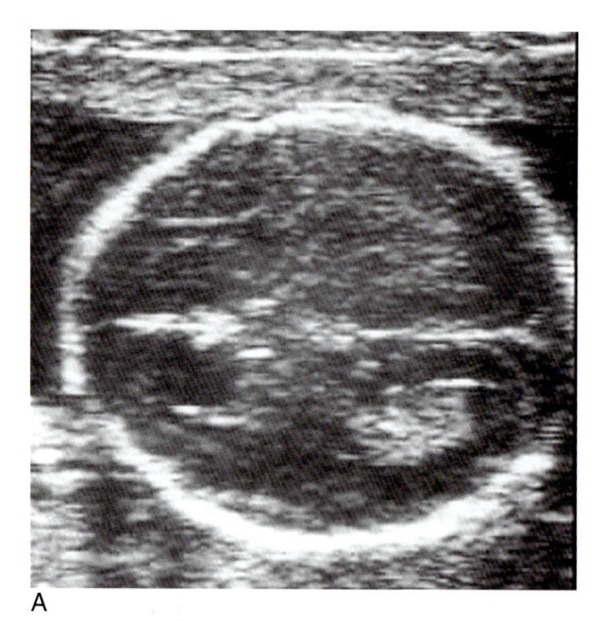

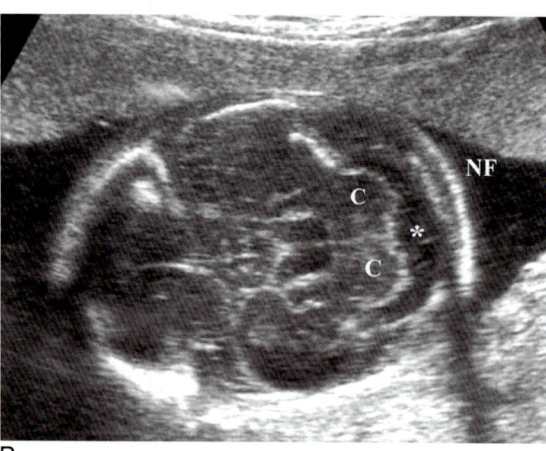

Figure 2.1 Axial views of the fetal head demonstrating (A) the view used to measure the head circumference, showing the anterior and posterior horns of the lateral cerebral ventricles, together with the cavum septum pellucidum. (B) The cerebellum (C), cisterna magna (*) and nuchal fold (NF) are seen in a slightly lower plane.

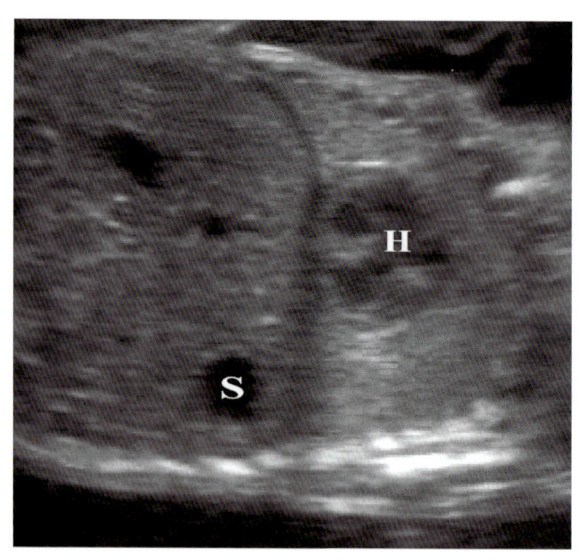

Figure 2.2 Longitudinal view through the fetal thorax in which the stomach (S) can be seen lying below and the heart (H) lying above the diaphragm.

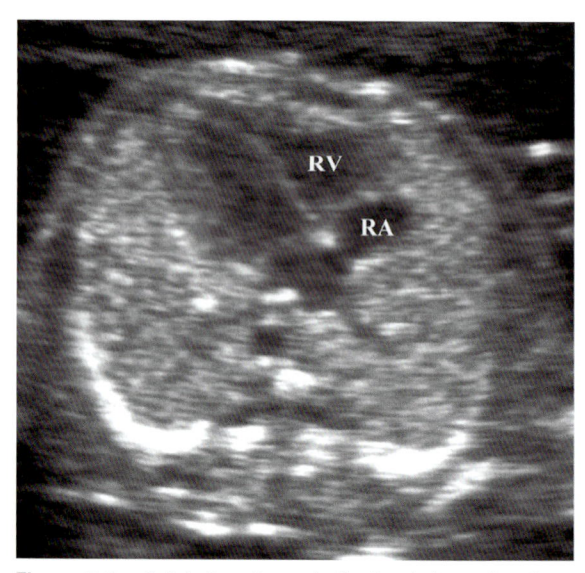

Figure 2.3 Axial view through the fetal chest showing the orientation and four chambers of the heart. The right side lies anterior (RA, right atrium; RV, right ventricle).

Fetal Doppler

Intrauterine growth restriction (IUGR) occurs in 5–10% of all pregnancies and increases the risk of hypoxemia and acidemia, possibly resulting in perinatal death or significant morbidity in adult life.[26] Fetal weight can be estimated using a formula incorporating a combination of sonographic fetal measurements, usually HC, AC and femur length. A fetus with a weight below the 10th centile is defined as small for gestational age, but not necessarily growth restricted. The use of fetal and maternal Doppler has helped in making the prenatal distinction between constitutionally small fetuses,

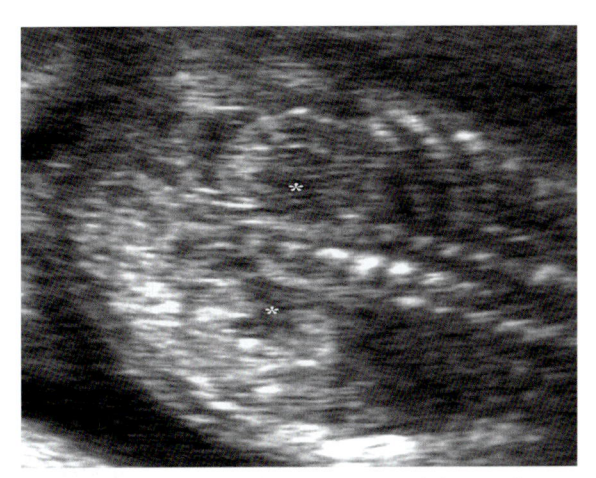

Figure 2.4 Ultrasound image at 19 weeks' gestation showing normal fetal kidneys in the coronal plane. Note the renal pelvis (*).

those that are small because of an underlying genetic etiology and those where placental insufficiency (IUGR) is the cause. The interpretation of the hemodynamic changes in various fetal arterial and venous waveforms demonstrated by Doppler ultrasound make it possible to focus on the fetoplacental circulation and to evaluate the condition of the growth-restricted fetus.

The umbilical artery was the first vessel to be evaluated by Doppler velocimetry. In normal fetuses a progressive rise in the end-diastolic velocity and subsequent decrease in pulsatility index can be demonstrated with advancing gestation. In IUGR fetuses an increase in pulsatility index can occur. With progressive deterioration of the fetoplacental circulation the umbilical artery waveform will change, showing absent or reversed end-diastolic blood flow. Growth restricted fetuses with abnormal umbilical waveforms often have a poorer perinatal outcome than those with normal waveforms.[27]

There is a direct correlation between umbilical artery Doppler and changes in the diastolic and mean blood flow velocity in the middle cerebral artery (MCA). During fetal hypoxia a pathophysiological adaptation occurs which results in preferential perfusion of vital organs. In the fetal brain this results in decrease in pulsatility index in the MCA as a direct consequence of vasodilation,[28] also referred to as redistribution or the 'brain-sparing effect'.

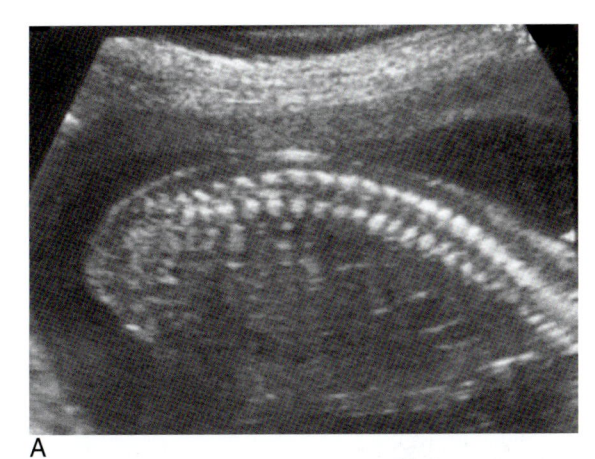

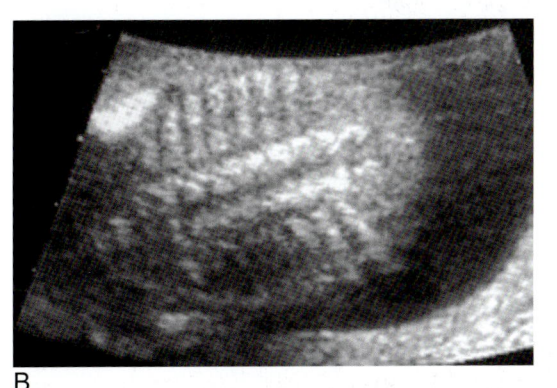

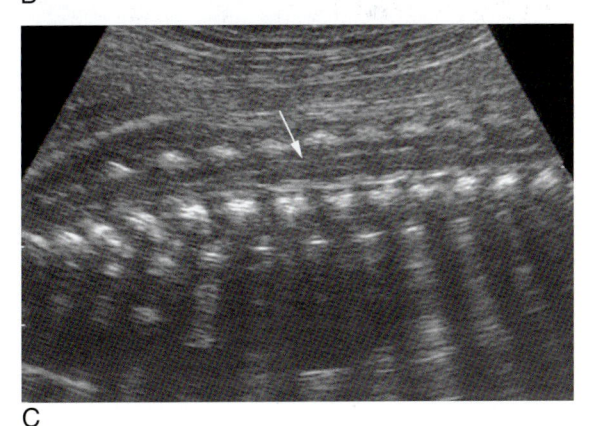

Figure 2.5 Standard views of the spine which should be examined in the axial, (A) sagittal and (B) coronal planes. (C) The spinal cord and cauda equinae (arrow) can often be seen using modern ultrasound equipment.

Besides the brain, the myocardium is also spared (the 'heart-sparing effect'), leading to abnormal velocimetry of the aorta and inferior vena cava.[29] Doppler velocimetry has been applied to a variety

Table 2.5 Rate of detection (%) of fetal abnormalities before 24 weeks' gestation, using different screening protocols

	Screening protocol		
	Second trimester	First trimester	Indication based
Anencephaly	99	100	94
Spina bifida	90		77
Central nervous system	75		45
Thoracic	66		36
Cardiac	25		7
Anterior abdominal wall defects	90		100
Intestinal obstruction	35		8
Major urinary tract	70		49
Musculoskeletal	50		8

Data derived from review of literature.

of other fetal arteries and veins. Recent studies provide evidence that increased pulsatility index in the ductus venosus seems to be closely related to the presence of metabolic acidemia.[30,31] These studies furthermore provide evidence that IUGR fetuses develop changes in Doppler velocimetry in a time-dependent, progressive sequence. Increase in umbilical artery pulsatility index occurs first followed by a decrease in MCA pulsatility index. When the fetus becomes further hypoxic this will lead to Doppler changes in ductus venosus and aortic flow. The clinical utility of these Doppler changes in optimal timing of delivery in IUGR fetuses remains to be established.

On the maternal side of the fetal circulation the flow in the uterine arteries is used as a screening tool, at 24 weeks of gestation, for placental insufficiency likely to result in pre-eclampsia or IUGR.[32] Abnormal changes in the uterine artery waveform are characterized by increased impedance indices and 'notches' in the waveform. Patients displaying abnormal uterine artery waveforms should be seen at regular intervals for monitoring of maternal wellbeing and fetal growth.

Beside its usefulness in IUGR fetuses, assessment of Doppler changes in the MCA is becoming an accepted non-invasive method for diagnosis of fetal anemia in red blood cell alloimmunized pregnancies. Among fetuses at risk for immunological hydrops, 25% will need intrauterine transfusions. Up to 40% of the remaining group will develop mild to moderate anemia and hyperbilirubinemia postnatally, requiring phototherapy. In uncomplicated pregnancies the blood velocity in the cerebral vessels increases with advancing gestation. An increased MCA peak systolic velocity above 1.5 multiples of the median will identify 88% of those fetuses requiring intrauterine transfusion.[33]

ABNORMALITIES IN DIFFERENT SYSTEMS

Cranial and spinal abnormalities

Many intracranial abnormalities are detectable at the time of the routine 20-week scan. One of the most common findings is that of choroid plexus cysts (CPCs), which occur in 1–2% of all fetuses. These can be uni- or bilateral, single or multiple (Fig. 2.6). More than 95% resolve spontaneously before 26 weeks' gestation. When seen with other soft markers, sonographic abnormalities or other risk factors for aneuploidy, such as maternal age ≥ 36 years or positive maternal serum screening, they may be associated with trisomy 18. They are not associated with any other adverse outcome. In the vast majority of cases CPCs are a benign transient finding with no clinical significance.[34] Other major abnormalities such as holoprosencephaly, anencephaly and posterior fossa cysts (Fig. 2.7) may be detected at the time of a routine first or second

Table 2.6 Sonographic findings in common chromosome anomalies

	Trisomy 21	Trisomy 18	Trisomy 13	Turner	Triploidy
Major abnormalities					
Holoprosencephaly	–	–	+	–	–
Microcephaly	–	+	+	–	–
Posterior fossa cyst	–	+	–	–	–
Neural tube defect	–	+	–	–	–
Cystic hygroma	+	–	–	+	–
Diaphragmatic hernia	–	+	(+)	–	–
Cardiac abnormality	+ (AVSD)	+	+	+ (coarctation)	+
Omphalocele	–	+	(+)	–	–
Duodenal atresia	+	–	–	–	–
Renal abnormalities	(+)	+	+	+	–
Radial aplasia	–	+	(+)	–	–
Hydrops	+	–	–	+	–
IUGR	(+)	+	+	–	+
'Minor' abnormalities/markers					
Mild ventriculomegaly	+	+	(+)	–	(+)
Choroid plexus cysts	–	+	–	–	–
Strawberry skull	–	+	–	–	–
Facial cleft	–	unilateral	midline/bilateral	–	–
Micrognathia	–	+	(+)	–	(+)
Nuchal edema (> 6 mm)	+	(+)	(+)	+	–
Nuchal translucency	+	+	+	+	+
Echogenic cardiac focus	(+)	–	(+)	–	–
Mild renal pelvic dilation	+	(+)	–	–	–
Clenched fist / overlapping fingers	–	+	–	–	–
Talipes	–	+	(+)	–	–
Rocker-bottom feet	–	+	(+)	–	–
Short femur/humerus	+	–	–	+	–
Sandal gap	+	–	–	–	–
Clinodactyly	+	–	–	–	–
Polydactyly	–	–	+	–	–
Echogenic bowel	+	–	–	–	–

+, common association; (+), less common; –, rare.
AVSD, atrioventricular septal defect; IUGR, intrauterine growth restriction.

trimester scan. However, unfortunately, many of the sonographic signs associated with other intracerebral anomalies develop later in pregnancy and are thus less amenable to detection in the second trimester. These include many, but not all, cases of hydrocephaly, microcephaly, agenesis of the corpus callosum, arachnoid cysts (Fig. 2.8) and tumors. Many intracerebral abnormalities will therefore only be detected if the scan is initiated because of a clinical indication later in pregnancy,[10] whereas detection of anomalies such as anencephaly approaches 100% in the first[35] and second trimesters (see Tables 2.2 and 2.3).

One of the most common serious congenital anomalies is open neural tube defect (Fig. 2.9). Open spina bifida can be identified by examination in all three planes (Fig. 2.5), sometimes just by loss of alignment of the vertebral bodies and absence of skin covering, but in more severe cases by identification of gross kyphoscoliosis. The diagnosis can

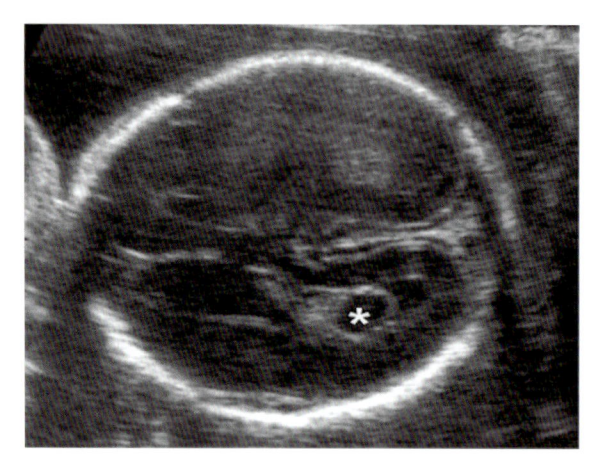

Figure 2.6 Unilateral choroid plexus cyst (*).

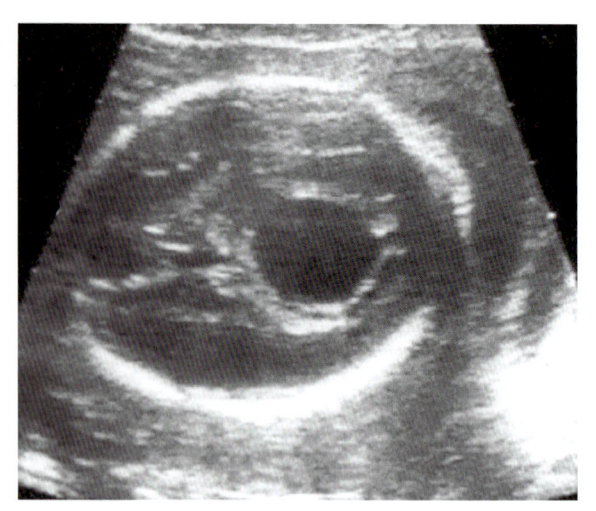

Figure 2.8 A fetal head showing a single large arachnoid cyst.

be particularly difficult if the fetus is in the breech position, and low sacral lesions are readily overlooked. Identification of the cranial signs associated with spina bifida has resulted in a significant improvement in the diagnosis of this lesion, as the head is readily examined. In the presence of spina bifida the skull has a lemon shape in 98% of cases when scanned before 24 weeks, whilst the cerebellum is banana shaped in 72% (Fig. 2.10).[36] These signs are also seen in 1% of normal fetuses.[37] Ultrasonographic detection of open neural tube defects compares favorably with maternal serum alfa-fetoprotein (MSAFP) measurements, which can identify around 80% of fetuses with spina bifida.

Examination of the fetal spine will result in the detection of other less common anomalies—for example, hemivertebrae (Fig. 2.11). Identification of one anomaly must alert the sonographer to the presence of an underlying syndrome or association. For example, hemivertebrae may be seen as part of the VACTERL spectrum, so that a detailed exami-

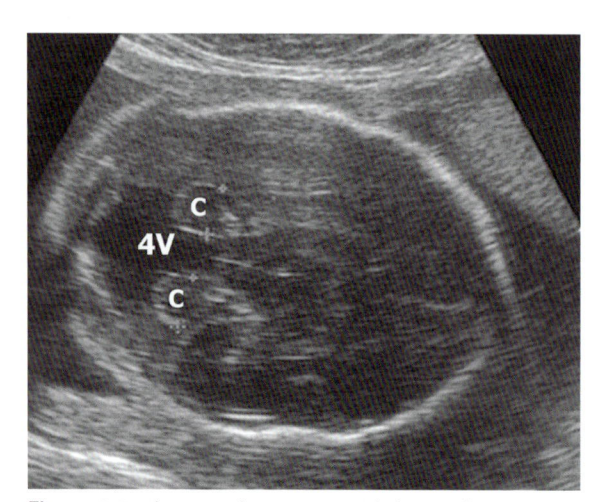

Figure 2.7 Image taken at 19 weeks' gestation showing a Dandy–Walker malformation. The cerebellar vermis is absent, the cerebellar hemispheres (C) separated, and a dilated fourth ventricle (4V) occupies the posterior fossa.

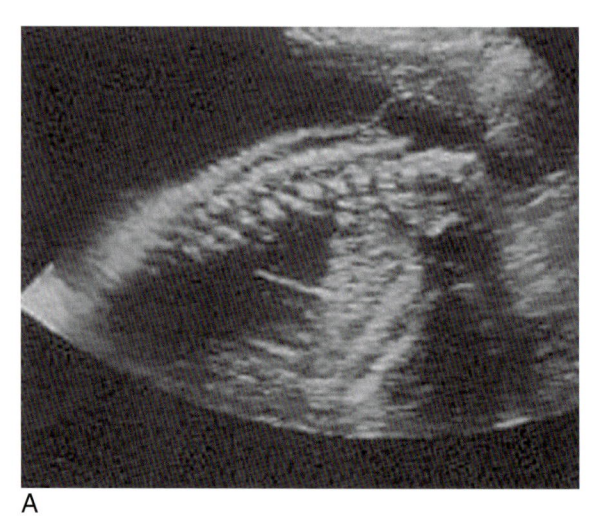

A
Figure 2.9 Spina bifida: (A) sagittal,

PRENATAL SONOGRAPHIC DIAGNOSIS OF CONGENITAL ANOMALIES 25

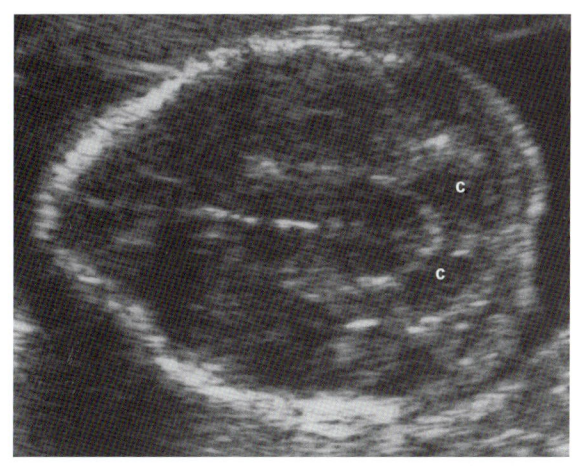

Figure 2.10 Axial view through the head in a fetus at 20 weeks' gestation showing the typical lemon-shaped head with scalloping of the frontal bones and banana-shaped cerebellum (c) in the posterior fossa.

Cardiac abnormalities

Cardiac abnormalities are among the more common congenital abnormalities, occurring in about 1 in every 120 births. About half of these are likely to be life threatening, and about 50% of these may be detected at the time of the routine scan examination of the four-chamber view of the fetal heart at 20 weeks.[38] This view (Fig. 2.3) will only identify significant abnormalities of chamber size and valves and not abnormalities of the outflow tracts of the great arteries. To increase the sensitivity of

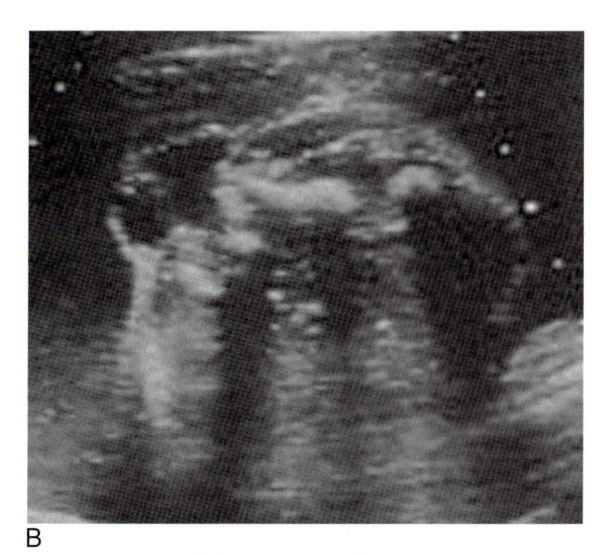

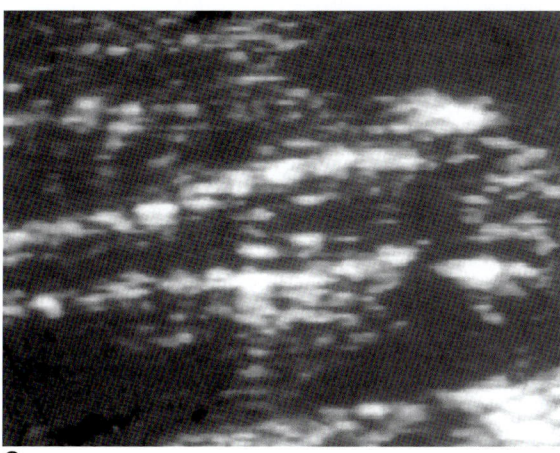

Figure 2.9, cont'd (B) axial and (C) coronal views of the spine in a fetus with lumbar spina bifida, demonstrating the meningocele and splaying of the ossification centers.

nation of arms and kidneys should be made following the unexpected detection of any spinal lesion. A short spine may be part of the caudal regression spectrum seen more commonly in pregnancies of diabetic mothers, but can sometimes be identified prenatally in fetuses with cloacal anomalies. Abnormalities of the fetal spine are also commonly seen in association with a variety of skeletal dysplasias, for example, the extra calcification in some of the chondrodysplasia punctata or the hypomineralization seen in achondrogenesis.

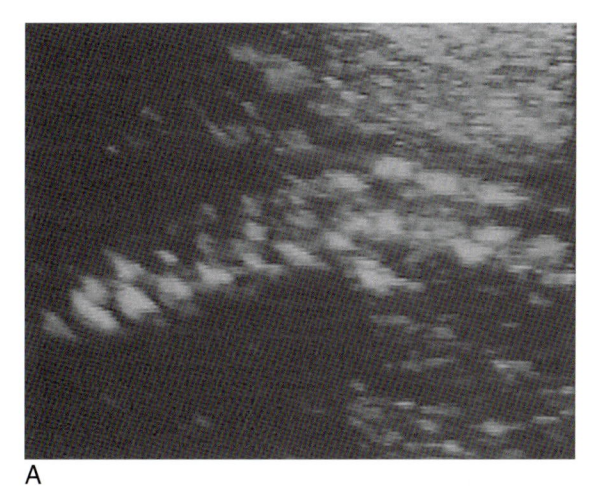

Figure 2.11 Hemivertebra: (A) sagittal and

Continued

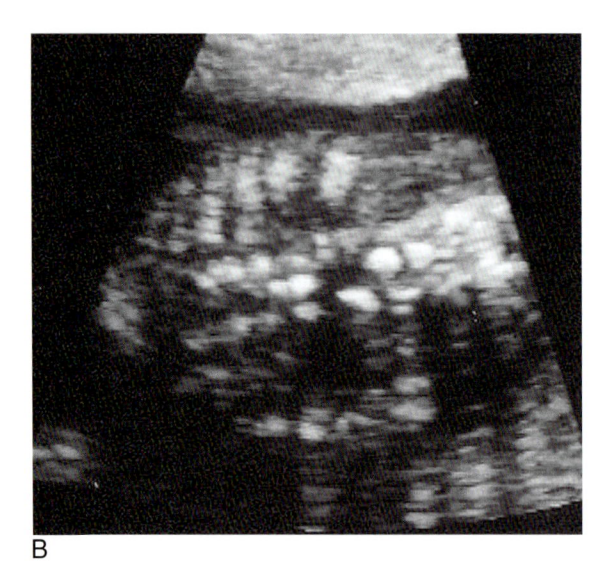

Figure 2.11, cont'd (B) coronal views of a fetal spine at around 20 weeks' gestation demonstrating the appearance of the spine in the presence of a single hemivertebra. It was the unusual angulation of the spine that alerted the sonographer to look more closely when performing a routine 20-week scan.

ultrasound for the detection of cardiac anomalies the cardiovascular examination should include the heart and great vessels, as well as the evaluation of the arrangement of the intrathoracic and intra-abdominal organs.

Recent guidelines from the Royal College of Obstetricians and Gynaecologists suggest that examination of the four-chamber view of the heart at a routine anomaly scan is mandatory. Where resources allow choices, visualization of the outflow tract should be included with the potential to increase the detection rate of cardiac anomalies to around 75%.[5,39]

Another strategy to screen for congenital heart defects might be by measurement of fetal nuchal translucency thickness at the first trimester scan. If all patients with a nuchal translucency above the 95th centile for gestational age were to be offered a fetal cardiac scan at 20 weeks, potentially 56% of the major anomalies of the heart and great arteries could be detected.[40]

Prenatal diagnosis of congenital heart defects is important as it potentially alters the neonatal short-term and long-term outcome. Correct prenatal identification of hypoplastic left heart syndrome and transposition of the great arteries seem to reduce neonatal mortality and morbidity compared with diagnosis in the neonatal period, but has to be further evaluated.[41,42] Therefore, when a congenital cardiac anomaly is suspected the patient should be referred to a center specializing in fetal echocardiography, as addition of color Doppler will complete the real time examination of the fetal heart and enable refinement of the diagnosis. It has been suggested that, in the near future, real time three-dimensional fetal echocardiography might become the instrument of choice to diagnose fetal cardiac anomalies.

Pulmonary abnormalities

Pulmonary abnormalities should be suspected when the position or orientation of the heart is shifted, or when cystic masses are seen in the thorax. Probably the most common abnormality of the respiratory system seen in the prenatal period is a congenital diaphragmatic hernia (CDH), which occurs in about 1 in 2000–5000 births. This can be diagnosed at 20 weeks; however, many cases are diagnosed later in pregnancy when a scan is initiated because of the associated polyhydramnios. Classic signs include a shift of the mediastinum to the right with a cystic lesion (the stomach) occupying the left side of the chest in a left-sided CDH. Confirmation of this diagnosis is achieved by failure to identify the stomach in the abdomen, the observation of bowel peristalsis in the chest or of paradoxical visceral movement with fetal breathing movements. Right-sided CDH may be more difficult to diagnose as in this situation it would usually be the liver that is herniated into the chest and this has the same echogenicity as lung. Diagnosis in this situation depends upon the identification of mediastinal shift with loss of visualization of the right hemidiaphragm, with a distorted intra-abdominal course for the intrahepatic vein.

The main differential diagnosis for CDH is congenital cystic adenomatoid malformation of the lung (CCAML). This lesion can be either macrocystic (Fig. 2.12) or microcystic (Fig. 2.13), where the differential diagnosis includes pulmonary sequestration. Up to 15% of cases have bilateral lung involvement. Accurate prediction of outcome can be difficult at the first scan. This is because

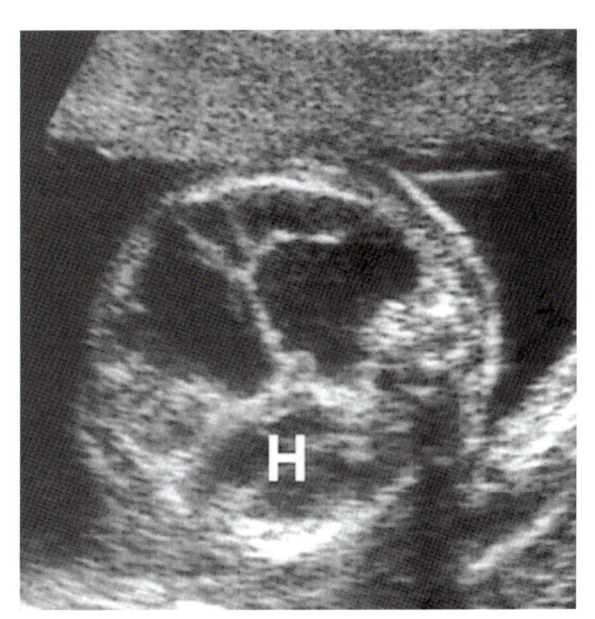

PRENATAL SONOGRAPHIC DIAGNOSIS OF CONGENITAL ANOMALIES

Figure 2.12 Axial view of a fetus with a macrocystic adenomatoid malformation of the right lung, causing compression of the heart (H) and significant mediastinal shift. This fetus required aspiration and shunting of the major cysts, which enabled resolution of the early onset hydrops. Urgent pneumonectomy was required because of neonatal respiratory compromise.

spontaneous in-utero improvement can occur and has been observed. Deterioration only occurs in a small number of fetuses with CCAML, who may develop polyhydramnios and fetal hydrops. Both of these signs carry a poor prognosis, particularly if

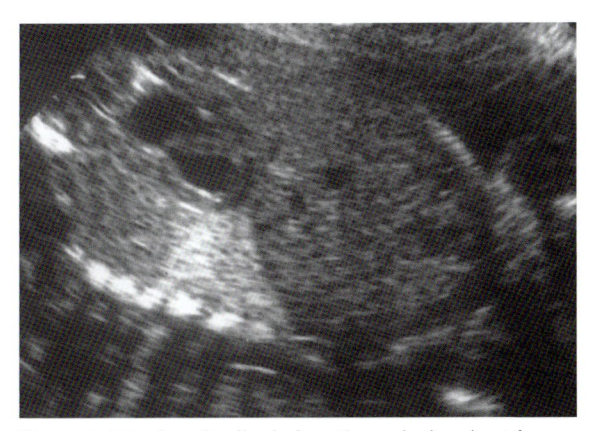

Figure 2.13 Longitudinal view through the chest in a fetus with microcystic adenomatoid malformation of the lower lobe of the left lung. The lesion causes a mediastinal shift pushing the heart to the right.

evident at the initial presentation in the second trimester. Mediastinal shift may be less reliable as a prognostic indicator in the second trimester, as this often improves with increasing gestation. In all cases early consultation with neonatal and pediatric surgical staff is helpful for parents.

Serial scans will detect those lesions that progress in size and display adverse prognostic features and may enable early consideration of intervention. In macrocystic CCAML with single or multiple large cysts (Fig. 2.12) and associated hydrops or polyhydramnios, improvement has been reported following decompression of the cysts or the insertion of a shunt. Intrauterine surgery to remove these lesions has also been reported. In those fetuses where the lesion persists or increases in size with mediastinal shift in the third trimester, delivery in a center with neonatal intensive care and surgical facilities should be considered, as early intervention may be required. Where prenatal improvement or resolution has occurred, careful postnatal radiography with computerized tomography is recommended, as in many cases plain X-rays do not demonstrate the lesion. However, management decisions in many cases are difficult because most neonates are asymptomatic, and there is much debate as to whether surgical excision is warranted. This is currently a subject of a multicenter long term follow-up study.

The differentiation between microcystic CCAML and bronchopulmonary sequestration (BPS) in the fetus can be difficult. Demonstration of an independent blood supply on ultrasound is a useful marker for the diagnosis of BPS. These lesions can occur above (Fig. 2.14) or below (Fig. 2.15) the diaphragm and must be considered in the differential diagnosis of an echogenic mass within the abdomen. Although most are unilateral and include only a part of the lung, bilateral cases have been reported, but care must be taken to exclude laryngeal or tracheal atresia before making this diagnosis. The sequestrated lobe is variable in size, and its most common location is between the lower lobe and the diaphragm.

In the absence of hydrops, the outlook for a fetus with an isolated sequestration is generally good, and spontaneous resolution has been reported. Once the diagnosis is made and other

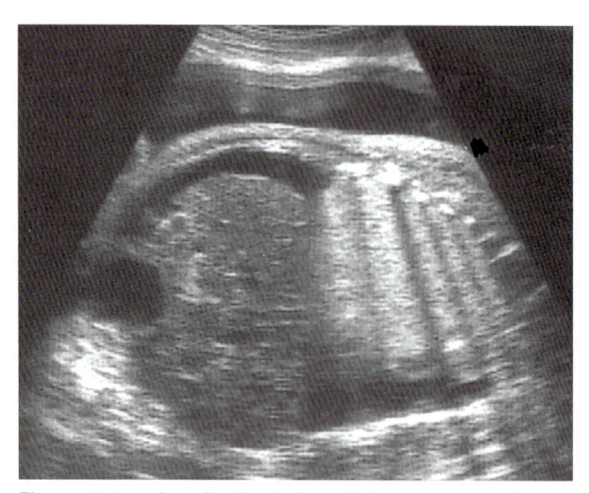

Figure 2.14 Longitudinal view of the thorax in a fetus that presented with polyhydramnios and hydrops at 34 weeks' gestation. Note the large sequestrated lobe of lung associated with pleural effusions and skin edema. The neonate died shortly after birth, as ventilation could not be established. Postmortem examination confirmed the diagnosis and demonstrated associated pulmonary hypoplasia.

anomalies have been excluded, fetal surveillance by serial ultrasound should be instigated.

For lesions that are large and where the mediastinal shift is significant in the third trimester, delivery in a center with neonatal intensive care and surgical facilities is advised, as respiratory support and early surgery may be required. Parents should be offered the opportunity to consult with a pediatric surgeon to discuss postnatal management.

Gastrointestinal abnormalities

The routine examination in the fetus should include examination of the abdominal shape and content at the level of the stomach, as well as the cord insertion. If this is done then anterior abdominal wall defects, gastroschisis and exomphalos are readily seen, with detection rates approaching 100% (Table 2.5). On the other hand, intestinal obstruction or atresia is less amenable to diagnosis in the second trimester because the classical signs of the dilated stomach or proximal loops of small bowel do not appear until later in pregnancy. These abnormalities are more likely to be detected in the third trimester when a scan is performed because of polyhydramnios. Isolated esophageal atresia may be diagnosed in early pregnancy if there is persistent failure to visualize the stomach bubble. If this diagnosis is suspected then detailed examination of the spine (looking for hemivertebrae) and arms (for radial defects) is warranted in view of the association with VACTERL. However, in 95% of cases of esophageal atresia there is a coexistent fistula to the trachea (tracheoesophageal fistula) through which the stomach can fill. Intra-abdominal cystic structures are occasionally seen but the precise origin of these is usually impossible to define prenatally. Etiologies include mesenteric, choledochal, retroperitoneal, bowel duplication or, most commonly in female fetuses, ovarian cysts, and spontaneous resolution is common. Care must be taken to ensure the cyst is not associated with renal pathology. In some fetuses the bowel may appear 'bright', or echogenic (Fig. 2.16). This frequently resolves spontaneously but there is an association with aneuploidy, growth retardation, congenital infection or cystic fibrosis. In the latter case, progression to meconium peritonitis has been reported.

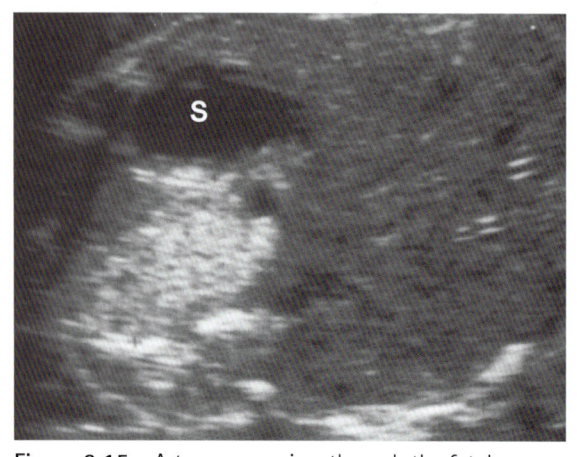

Figure 2.15 A transverse view through the fetal abdomen demonstrating the echogenic area lying behind the stomach (S). Postnatal ultrasound-guided biopsy confirmed the prenatal diagnosis of pulmonary sequestration. The lesion spontaneously decreased in size without surgical intervention.

Urinary tract abnormalities

Fetal kidneys can be identified from around 12 weeks' gestation, and the bladder is seen in 80% of

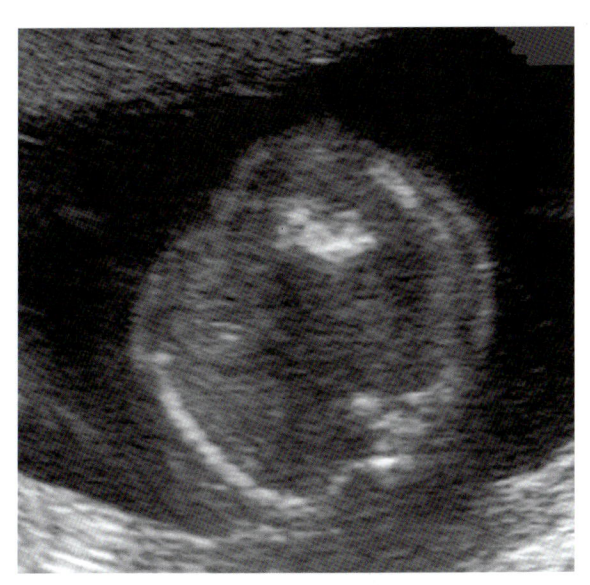

Figure 2.16 A transverse view taken at 20 weeks' gestation of a fetus with hyperechogenic bowel.

fetuses from 11 weeks onwards. Abnormalities of the urinary tract account for about 15% of all abnormalities diagnosed prenatally. However, evaluation of the efficacy of routine ultrasound screening for fetal urinary tract abnormalities is difficult. Although neonates with severe bilateral abnormalities of the urinary tract such as bilateral renal agenesis or dysplasia or urethral atresia are likely to present with clinical problems in the newborn period, the majority of renal problems are clinically silent. Accurate assessment of the sensitivity of any prenatal screening program would require detailed, long term follow-up of neonates in order to achieve more complete ascertainment. Even routine evaluation of the neonatal tract using ultrasound shortly after birth would be unlikely to determine the true incidence of problems, as this has been shown to have a relatively high false negative and false positive rate. Review of routine ultrasound programs demonstrates that they appear to be quite effective in detecting bilateral lesions but less good for the detection of renal dysplasia and obstructive uropathies (Table 2.7).[9,10,14,20,43] Whilst severe bilateral anomalies have clear prognostic implications for a fetus, many unilateral lesions or less severe bilateral lesions carry uncertain clinical significance.

A wide variety of renal abnormalities can be identified, and these can be broadly separated into obstructive and dysplastic lesions. The most common renal anomaly seen is mild dilation of the fetal renal pelvis (Fig. 2.17), which can be uni- or bilateral. It has an association with aneuploidy, particularly when seen with other abnormalities or in a woman with other risk factors (raised maternal age or positive Down syndrome screening).[44] It is also associated with a pathological outcome but only in a very small percentage of cases.

In a large series of cases in a multicenter study seen at the time of a routine scan only 4% of the 700 babies identified with mild upper tract dilation in the second trimester required surgical intervention in childhood. More than half had a normal postnatal renal ultrasound scan, and of those with an abnormal scan the majority required no intervention. The main prenatal prognostic factor identified was an AP diameter of the pelvis of 10 mm or greater in the third trimester.

Table 2.7 Gestational age for the diagnosis of common severe renal anomalies at the time of routine anomaly scanning[9,10,14,20,43]

	Number detected at various gestational ages		
	< 24 weeks	> 24 weeks	Not detected
Obstructive uropathies	28 (17%)	104 (63%)	32 (20%)
Bilateral renal agenesis	35 (37%)	41 (43%)	19 (20%)
Bilateral renal dysplasia	19 (50%)	14 (37%)	5 (13%)

Data derived from review of literature.

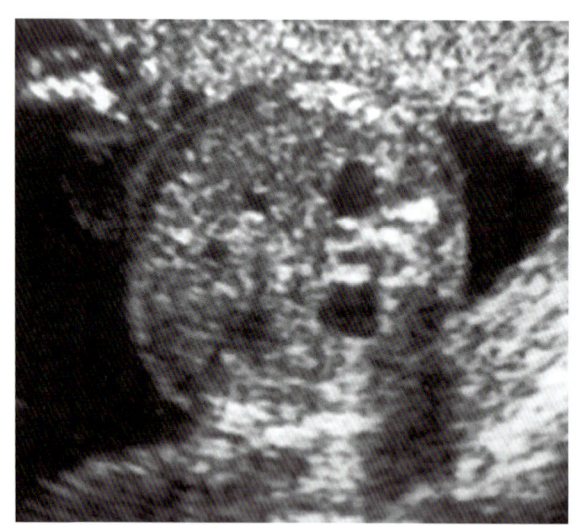

Figure 2.17 Mild bilateral dilation of the fetal renal pelvis seen in the transverse plane.

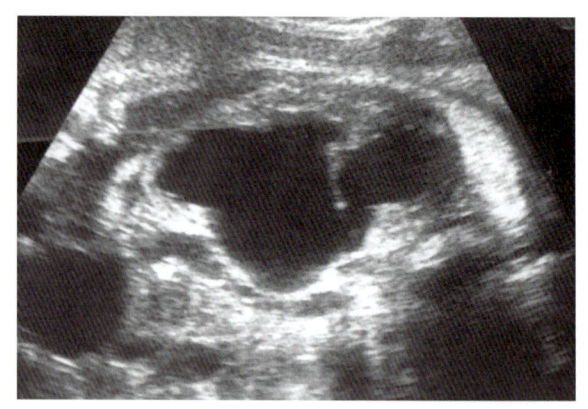

Figure 2.18 The classical appearance of pelviureteric junction obstruction seen in the longitudinal plane.

There is still much debate as to the significance of mild dilation of the fetal renal pelvis and to the extent to which this should be investigated in the neonatal period.[44] There are those who advocate an ultrasound scan and micturating cystourethrogram for all cases because some studies have shown a high incidence of vesicoureteric reflux in neonates presenting with prenatal pelvic dilation. However, the population detected prenatally differs from that presenting clinically in infancy, with significantly more males than females observed in the prenatal population. In general, these neonates are asymptomatic, and some suggest that the dilation is physiological with no significant pathological implications in cases where dilation resolves or remains less than 10 mm.

More significant degrees of upper tract dilation can indicate pelviureteric junction obstruction (Fig. 2.18) or duplex systems (Fig. 2.19A); the diagnosis in the latter case can often be confirmed following detection of an ureterocele in the bladder (Fig. 2.19B). Upper tract dilation seen in association with ureteric dilation should suggest vesicoureteric junction obstruction or reflux (Fig. 2.20), but early outflow obstruction must be considered. When seen with a persistently enlarged bladder or a thick-walled bladder, outflow obstruction (Fig. 2.21) should be considered, particularly in male fetuses where the etiology is most commonly posterior urethral valves. In this situation the prognosis is poor if the liquor volume is reduced in mid-trimester. However, in cases where the liquor volume remains within normal limits the outcome is difficult to predict, and reflux with megaureters must be considered in the differential diagnosis.[45] Cloacal anomalies or megacystis microcolon are more likely in female fetuses with suspected outflow obstruction. In the former, abnormalities of the spine or genital tract may give a clue to the etiology.[46] Megacystis microcolon presents with normal or increased liquor and a significantly dilated bladder. As this is inherited in an

A

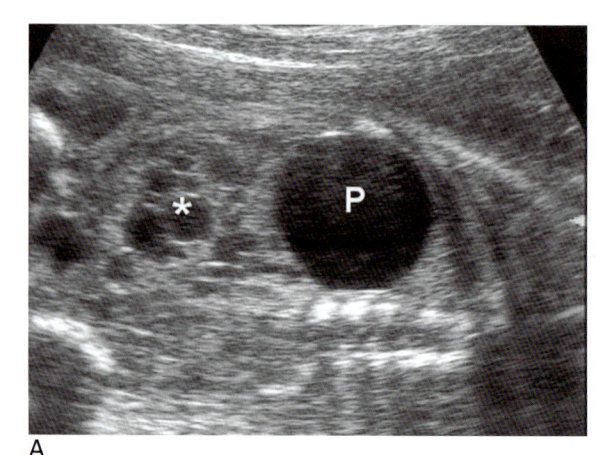

Figure 2.19 A duplex kidney (A) with a dilated upper pole (P) and multicystic lower pole (*). The diagnosis was clear in this case, with

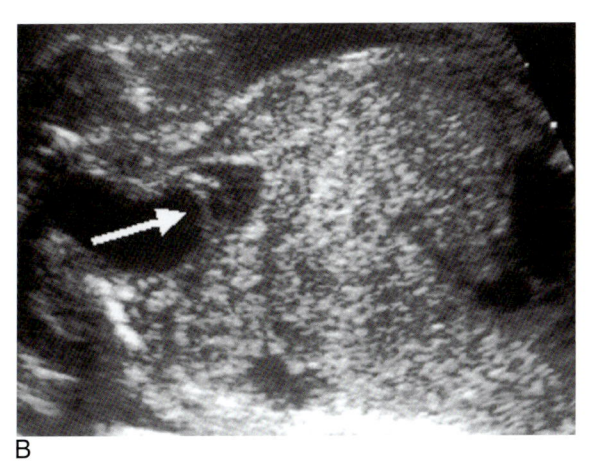

Figure 2.19, cont'd (B) an associated ureterocele (arrow) seen in the bladder.

autosomal recessive fashion, it is important to make a definitive diagnosis after delivery.

Failure to identify the bladder suggests either that there is severe intrauterine growth restriction or renal agenesis. In both cases liquor volume should be reduced or absent. The use of fetal and uterine artery Doppler can be of use in these situations.[47] Failure to identify the renal arteries with color Doppler implies a diagnosis of renal agenesis. It is also useful to visualize the perivesical arteries to delineate the bladder. Even in severe IUGR the bladder will usually contain a little urine. When the bladder is not identified in the presence of normal liquor volume a diagnosis of bladder exstrophy

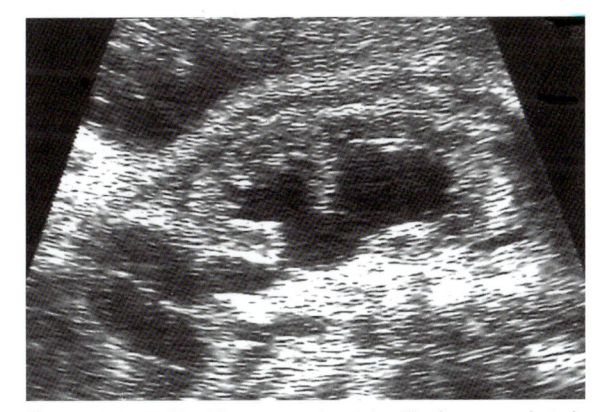

Figure 2.20 Significant renal pelvic dilation associated with a dilated ureter in a fetus where postnatal investigations showed severe vesicoureteric reflux.

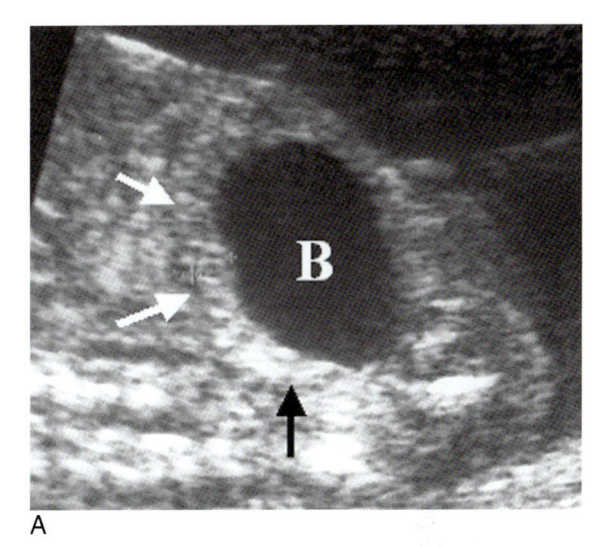

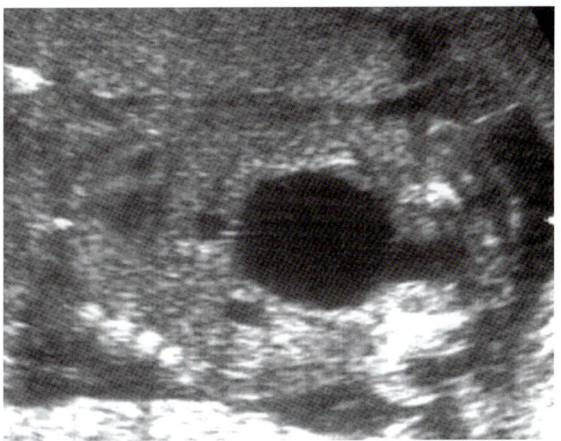

Figure 2.21 (A) A thickened bladder (B) wall (arrow) seen in association with upper tract dilation in a fetus with outflow obstruction. (B) When seen with the typical keyhole appearance of the dilated posterior urethra in a male fetus, this indicates a diagnosis of posterior urethral valves.

should be considered.[47] In this situation ambiguity of the genitalia can sometimes be observed.

Varying degrees of renal dysplasia can be identified in the prenatal period, often at the time of a routine scan, but in some cases detection does not occur until late in pregnancy when the liquor volume reduces (Table 2.7). The classical appearance of the multicystic dysplastic kidney (Fig. 2.22A) usually carries a good prognosis if unilateral. The use of color Doppler will often show absence of

32 PEDIATRIC ULTRASOUND

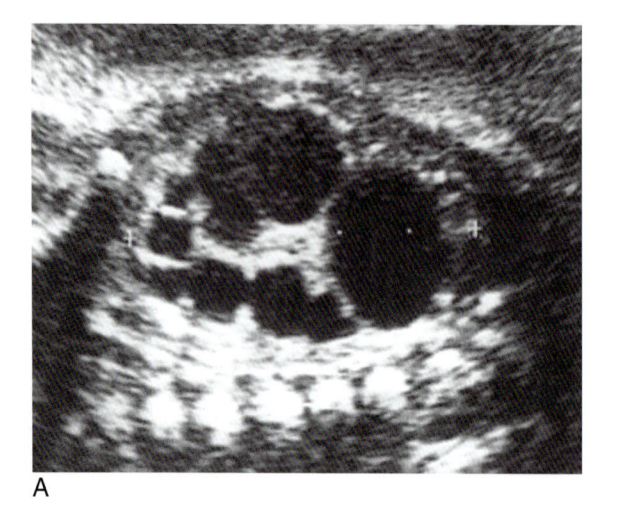

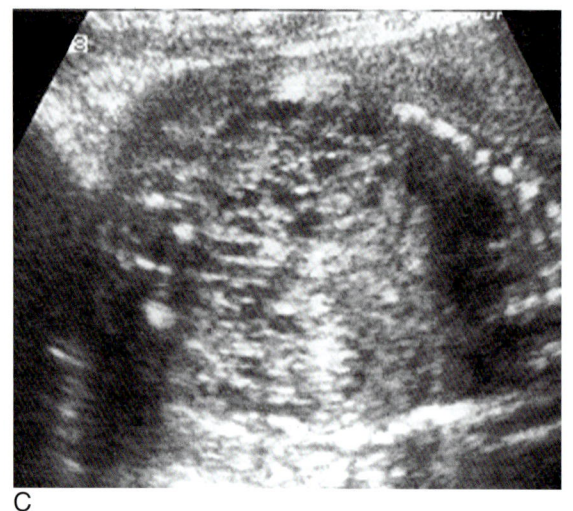

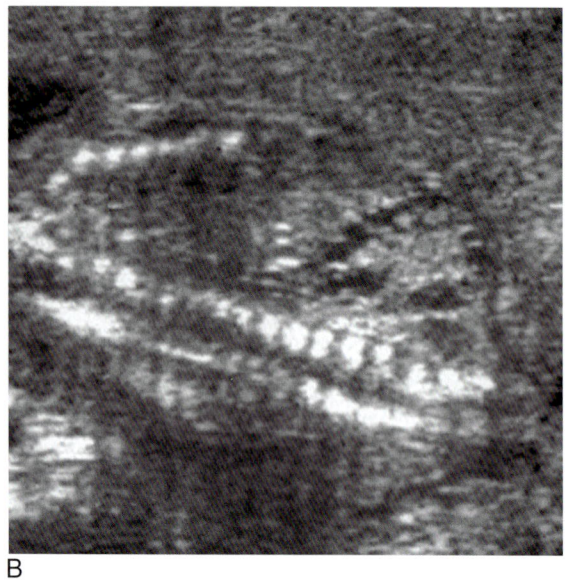

Figure 2.22 (A) The classical appearance of a multicystic dysplastic kidney seen in the axial plane. (B) Occasionally only a rim of cysts can be seen. (C) When bilateral there is a significant association with aneuploidy and genetic syndromes.

flow to the abnormal side. In the majority of cases the multicystic kidney will tend to reduce in size before birth, with contralateral hypertrophy of the normal kidney. Sometimes only a rim of peripherally situated cysts is seen (Fig. 2.22B). When the abnormality is bilateral (Fig. 2.22C) the prognosis is poor and there is a higher association with aneuploidy and other genetic syndromes. Occasionally small unilateral dysplastic kidneys may be detected prenatally, again associated with hypertrophy of the contralateral normal kidney. Postnatal imaging in these cases often fails to identify any renal mass on the abnormal side. This may well reflect the complete involution of the abnormal kidney.

One other less common, but potentially serious renal problem seen in the fetus is that of echogenic kidneys (Figs 2.23 and 2.24). The term 'echogenic kidneys' (hyperechogenic or hyperechoic or bright) is used to describe a heterogeneous group of conditions characterized by renal echogenicity greater than that of the liver or the spleen. Renal echogenicity in the fetal period has many causes, some of which are relatively benign, but others may reflect a more serious underlying renal disease (Table 2.8).[48] It must be remembered at all times that while ultrasound is sensitive in detecting echogenic kidneys, it is generally non-specific, and the ultimate diagnosis will depend on the clinical and family history, presentation, laboratory tests and further imaging studies and/or histology. Definitive diagnosis before delivery is seldom made unless there is a positive family history or other sonographic findings that

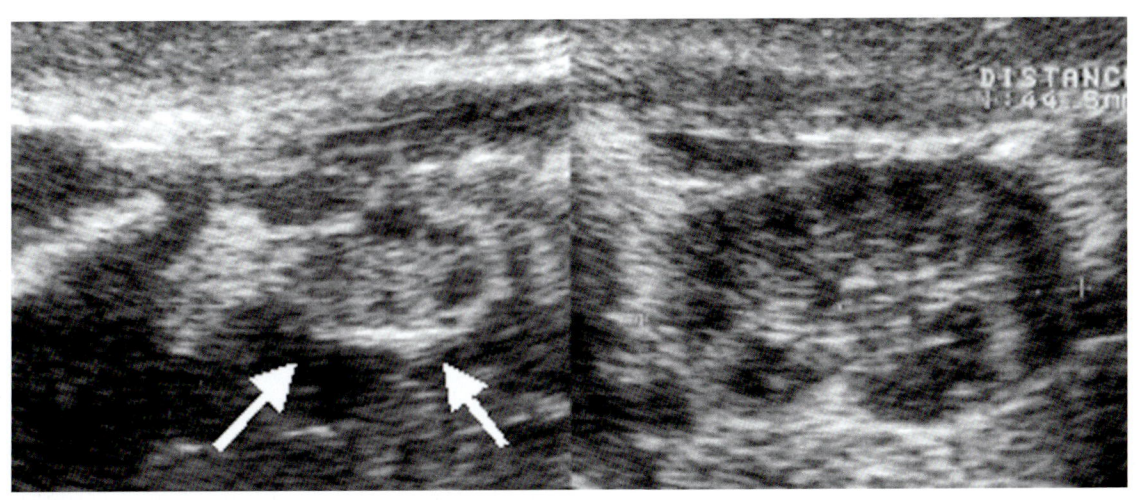

Figure 2.23 A small, slightly echogenic kidney (arrows) seen with the normal contralateral one in the longitudinal plane.

indicate an underlying genetic syndrome (e.g. an encephalocele in Meckel Gruber syndrome). If a pregnancy is terminated or results in perinatal death, the family should be strongly advised to consent to a detailed perinatal postmortem in order to obtain histology to define the diagnosis and recurrence risks for future pregnancies.

In summary, fetal renal anomalies are common and the etiology varied. Aneuploidy should always be considered, particularly when there are other risk factors or sonographic abnormalities. There is also a strong association with many other syndromes (Table 2.9), most commonly VATER syndrome.[49] A detailed fetal anatomical examination should be carried out, paying particular attention to the fetal spine and arms, in the presence of any renal lesion in order to exclude the possibility of associated pathology. Patients are best seen in a combined fetal medicine and pediatric urology clinic, as prognosis is often difficult to define for a fetus with a significant renal lesion and parents find discussion with the pediatric team helpful.

Skeletal abnormalities

Visualization of the fetal long bones at the time of the routine scan is usually achieved, and the measurement of the femur is a standard part of the examination. Many of the lethal skeletal dysplasias have severe limb shortening which is evident early in pregnancy, making these conditions amenable to detection with routine ultrasound. However, examination of the hands and feet may be more difficult because there are often time constraints which prevent detailed examination of the extremities, resulting in relatively poor detection rates for abnormalities such as talipes and limb reduction deformities in the unselected population. However, in a high risk situation where there is a suspicion of abnormality or past history,

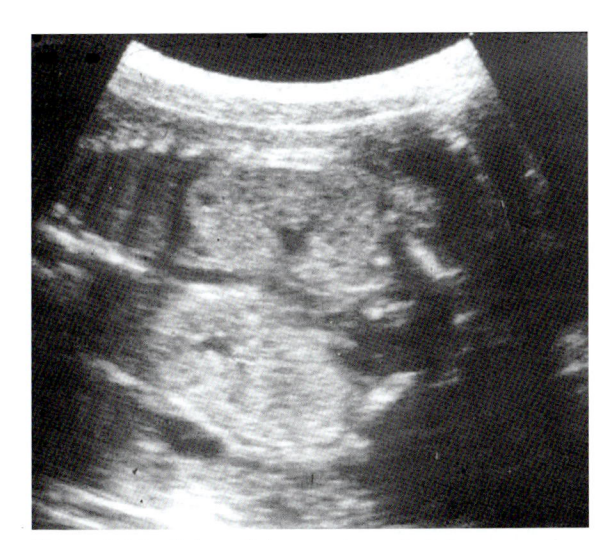

Figure 2.24 Enlarged, hyperechogenic kidneys seen in the longitudinal view in a fetus in which a diagnosis of autosomal recessive polycystic kidney disease was made following histological examination of the liver and kidneys at postmortem examination.

Table 2.8 Conditions that may be seen in the presence of hyperechogenic kidneys

	Liquor	Renal cysts	RPD	Macrosomy	Other anomalies	Gene locus	Inheritance
ARPKD	N/oligo	–	–	–	–	6p	AR
ADPKD	N/oligo	(+)	–	–	–	16p 4q	AD
Beckwith–Wiedemann	N/poly	–	+/–	+	Macroglossia, omphalocele, hemihypertrophy, visceromegaly	11p	Disomy Sporadic
Perlman	N/oligo	–	+/–	+	Ascites, cardiac, CDH, genital	Nk	AR
Simpson–Golabi–Behmel	?	?	?	+	Polydactyly, DDH, cardiac, genital, vertebral, visceromegaly	Xq	X-linked
Trisomy 13	Oligo	–	+/–	–	Intracranial, cardiac, polydactyly, IUGR, facial cleft		Sporadic
Meckel–Gruber	Oligo	–	–	–	Encephalocele, anencephaly, cardiac, polydactyly, facial cleft	17q 11q	AR
Obstruction	N/oligo	–	+	–	–		Sporadic
Nephrocalcinosis	N	–	–	–	–		Sporadic
Finnish congenital nephrosis	N	–	+/–	–	Very high MSAFP, edema, ascites, hydropic placenta	NPHS1 mutation	AR

AD, autosomal dominant; ADPKD, autosomal dominant polycystic kidney disease; AR, autosomal recessive; ARPKD, autosomal recessive polycystic kidney disease; CDH, congenital diaphragmatic hernia; IUGR, intrauterine growth retardation; MSAFP, maternal serum alfa-fetoprotein; N, normal; RPD, renal pelvic dilation.

detection of these abnormalities is significantly improved.

HYDROPS

Fetal hydrops is defined as accumulation of serous fluid in fetal tissues and/or body cavities. The fetus can have subcutaneous edema, ascites, hydrothorax and pericardial effusion. The umbilical cord and placenta can both be edematous and the amount of amniotic fluid is often increased. If there is evidence of fetomaternal blood group incompatibility and maternal hemolytic antibodies, fetal hydrops is defined as immune hydrops. Otherwise, the condition is called non-immune hydrops and this is usually the end stage of a wide variety of cardiovascular, pulmonary, renal, gastrointestinal, hepatic, neoplastic, chromosomal, genetic metabolic, hematologic or infectious disorders or the result of twin-to-twin transfusion syndrome (Box 2.2).[50]

Over 80 conditions are now associated with hydrops, cardiovascular disorders being the most frequent. The very varied etiologies of fetal hydrops means that the use of targeted diagnostic tests is limited and the underlying etiology of this condition often remains unknown. Even with improved ultrasound technology, fetal echocardiography, color Doppler and invasive fetal testing such as amniocentesis and fetal blood sampling,

Table 2.9 Some common syndromes detectable by prenatal ultrasound[a]

Primary sonographic sign	Syndrome	Associated detectable findings
Abnormal skull shape	Spina bifida	Hydrocephaly, spinal dysraphism
	Aperts	Mitten hands and feet
	Thanatophoric dysplasia	Very short limbs, short ribs
Abnormal skull mineralization	Osteogenesis imperfecta IIa, b, c	Short bent limbs
	Achondrogenesis	Short limbs, unossified vertebral bodies
Posterior fossa cyst	Joubert	Polydactyly, renal anomalies
	Meckel–Gruber syndrome	Large bright kidneys, polydactyly
Encephalocele	Meckel-Gruber syndrome	Cystic kidneys, polydactyly
Nuchal fold / cystic hygroma	Noonans	Short femora, cardiac abnormality, pleural effusion
	Smith-Lemli-Opitz	Microcephaly ± CNS anomaly, ambiguous genitalia, short femora, polydactyly
	Fryns	IUGR, diaphragmatic hernia
Cardiac abnormalities	CHARGE association	IUGR, renal anomalies, polyhydramnios
	Noonans	Short femora, nuchal edema, late onset pleural effusions
	Holt–Oram	Radial dysplasia, positive family history
Diaphragmatic hernia	Fryns	Nuchal edema, cataracts, contractures, micrognathia, CNS abnormalities, IUGR
	Pallister–Killian (tetrosomy 12p)	Nuchal edema, IUGR, rocker bottom feet, polydactyly
Omphalocele	Beckwith–Wiedemann	Echogenic kidneys, overgrowth, polyhydramnios, macroglossia
	Many skeletal dysplasias	Short limbs
Radial dysplasia	Thrombocytopenia absent radius	Normal thumbs, cardiac abnormalities, bowed limbs
	Holt–Oram	Cardiac abnormalities, positive family history
	Cornelia de Lange	IUGR, microcephaly, small hands and feet
	Nager acrofacial dysostosis	Micrognathia, microcephaly, IUGR
	VA(C)TER(L)	Vertebral, (cardiac), renal, (other limb) anomalies, esophageal atresia
Short femora	Multiple associations, including skeletal dysplasias and other genetic syndromes	
Bent femora	Caudal regression	Short spine, renal anomalies
	Multiple associations with many skeletal deformities	
Ambiguous genitalia	Smith-Lemli-Opitz	Cardiac anomalies, short limbs, polydactyly
	Campomelic dysplasia	Short bent femora, bent tibia and fibula, cardiac anomaly

[a] For association with aneuploidy see Table 2.6, and with renal echogenicity see Table 2.8.
CHARGE, coloboma, heart disease, atresia of the choanae, retarded growth and mental development, genital anomalies, and ear malformations and hearing loss; VACTERL, VATER plus cardiovascular and limb defects; VATER, vertebral defects, anal atresia, tracheo-esophageal fistula and/or esophageal atresia, radial dysplasia, renal defects.

> **Box 2.2 Most common causes of fetal non-immune hydrops**
>
> Cardiovascular disorders
>   Cardiac malformations
>   Tachycardia/bradycardia
>   Cardiomyopathy
>   Myocarditis
>   Myocardial infarction
>   Cardiac tumors
>   Arteriovenous shunt
> Chromosomal anomalies
>   Turner syndrome
>   Down syndrome
> Thoracic anomalies
>   Diaphragmatic hernia
>   Pulmonary sequestration
>   Cystic adenomatoid malformation of the lung
> Anemia
>   Fetomaternal transfusion
>   Alfa-thalassemia
>   G-6-PD deficiency
> Maternal infection
>   Parvovirus B 19
>   Cytomegalovirus
>   Toxoplasmosis
>   Rubella
>   Syphilis
>   Varicella
> Monochorionic twin pregnancies
>   Twin-to-twin transfusion syndrome
>   Acardiac twin malformation
> Other conditions
>   Skeletal dysplasias
>   Genetic syndromes
>   Metabolic disease
>   Tumors

the perinatal mortality rate of fetal hydrops remains as high as 85%.[51]

SUMMARY

Fetal anomaly scanning is now part of routine obstetric care in many parts of the developed world. Detection of one anomaly should stimulate a detailed examination of the rest of the fetus in order to exclude the possibility of underlying genetic syndromes. Aneuploidy is common in malformed fetuses, and karyotyping should be discussed in most cases (Table 2.6). In the euploid fetus with multiple abnormalities, an underlying genetic syndrome must be considered (Table 2.9). Recognition of the associations may help target investigations, aiding accurate diagnosis and counseling of parents. This aspect of prenatal ultrasound is becoming increasingly relevant as more genes are mapped.

In ongoing pregnancies a team approach to management is helpful; parents should be offered consultation with the relevant pediatric or genetic specialists, and delivery should be planned as appropriate to facilitate postnatal investigations and management.

Where termination of pregnancy is an option, a pediatric or genetic consultation may also be advantageous, as this will often enable a more objective discussion of prognosis and possible management options.

Where the diagnosis is unclear, an MRI scan can sometimes help define the problem, particularly with intracranial lesions. The opinion of a radiologist with appropriate neonatal and pediatric skills can also be useful.

The use of prenatal ultrasound has significantly changed many aspects of neonatal and pediatric practice. Prognosis has improved for lesions such as gastroschisis and congenital diaphragmatic hernia where urgent expert neonatal care is essential. It has, however, presented pediatricians with difficult management dilemmas as they are now faced with a population of infants who are asymptomatic but have an 'abnormality', the clinical significance of which is unclear in many, if not most, cases. There is an obvious need for long-term observational studies to define the natural history of many of these 'abnormalities' to aid both prenatal counseling of parents and to inform postnatal management decisions.

References

1. Hernádi L, Töröcsik M. Screening for fetal anomalies in the 12th week of pregnancy by transvaginal sonography in an unselected population. Prenat Diagn 1997; 17:753–759.
2. D'Ottavio G, Meir YJ, Rustico MA, et al. Screening for fetal anomalies by ultrasound at 14 and 21 weeks. Ultrasound Obstet Gynecol 1997; 10:375–380.
3. Economides DL, Braithwaite JM. First trimester ultrasonographic diagnosis of fetal structural abnormalities in a low risk population. Br J Obstet Gynaecol 1998; 105:53–57.
4. Whitlow BJ, Chatzipapas IK, Lazanakis ML, et al. The value of sonography in early pregnancy for the detection of fetal abnormalities in an unselected population. Br J Obstet Gynaecol 1999; 106:929–936
5. Carvalho MBH, Brizot ML, Lopes LM, et al. Detection of fetal structural abnormalities at the 11–14 week ultrasound scan. Prenat Diagn 2002; 22:1–4.
6. Drysdale K, Ridley D, Walker K, et al. First-trimester pregnancy scanning as a screening tool for high-risk and abnormal pregnancies in a district general hospital setting. J Obstet Gynaecol 2002; 22:159–165.
7. Rosendahl H, Kivinen S. Antenatal detection of congenital malformations by routine ultrasonography. Obstet Gynecol 1989; 73:947–951.
8. Saari-Kemppainen A, Karjalainen O, Ylöstalo P, et al. Ultrasound screening and perinatal mortality: controlled trial of systematic one-stage screening in pregnancy. Lancet 1990; 336:387–391.
9. Chitty LS, Hunt GH, Moore J, et al. Effectiveness of routine ultrasonography in detecting fetal structural abnormalities in a low risk population. BMJ 1991; 303:1165–1169.
10. Levi S, Hyjazi Y, Schaaps J-P, et al. Sensitivity and specificity of routine antenatal screening for congenital anomalies by ultrasound: The Belgian Multicentric Study. Ultrasound Obstet Gynecol 1991; 1:102–110.
11. Shirley IM, Bottomley F, Robinson VP. Routine radiographer screening for fetal abnormalities by ultrasound in an unselected low risk population. Br J Radiol 1992; 65:564–569.
12. Luck CA. Value of routine ultrasound scanning at 19 weeks: a four year study of 8849 deliveries. BMJ 1992; 304:1474–1478.
13. Ewigman BG, Crane JP, Frigoleto FD, et al. Effect of prenatal ultrasound screening on perinatal outcome. N Engl J Med 1993; 329:821–827.
14. Levi S, Schaaps J-P, De Havay P, et al. End-result of routine ultrasound screening for congenital anomalies: The Belgian Multicentric Study 1984–1992. Ultrasound Obstet Gynecol 1995; 5:366–371.
15. Papp Z, Tóth-Pal E, Papp CS, et al. Impact of prenatal mid-trimester screening on the prevalence of fetal structural anomalies: a prospective epidemiological study. Ultrasound Obstet Gynecol 1995; 6:320–326.
16. Anderson N, Boswell O, Duff G. Prenatal sonography for the detection of fetal anomalies: results of a prospective study and comparison with prior series. ARJ 1995; 165:943–950.
17. Geerts LTGM, Brand EJ, Theron GB. Routine obstetric ultrasound examinations in South Africa: cost and effect on perinatal outcome–a prospective randomised controlled trial. Br J Obstet Gynaecol 1996; 103:501–507.
18. Boyd PA, Chamberlain P, Hicks NR. 6-year experience of prenatal diagnosis in an unselected population in Oxford, UK. Lancet 1998; 352:1577–1581.
19. Schwärzler P, Senat MV, Holden D, et al. Feasibility of the second-trimester fetal ultrasound examination in an unselected population at 18, 20 or 22 weeks of pregnancy: a randomized trial. Ultrasound Obstet Gynecol 1999; 14:92–97.
20. Smith NC, Hau C. A six year study of the antenatal detection of fetal abnormality in six Scottish health boards. Br J Obstet Gynaecol 1999; 106:206–212.
21. Eurenius K, Axelsson O, Cnattingius S, et al. Second trimester ultrasound screening performed by midwives; sensitivity for detection of fetal anomalies. Acta Obstet Gynecol Scand 1999; 78:98–104.
22. Grandjean H, Larroque D, Levi S, et al. The performance of routine ultrasonographic screening of pregnancies in the Eurofetus Study. Am J Obstet Gynecol 1999; 181:446–454.
23. Wong SF, Chan FY, Cincotta RB, et al. Routine ultrasound screening in diabetic pregnancies. Ultrasound Obstet Gynecol 2002; 19:171–176.
24. Sabbagha RE, Sheikh Z, Tamura RK. Predictive value, sensitivity, and specificity of ultrasonic targeted imaging for fetal anomalies in gravid women at high risk for birth defects. Am J Obstet Gynecol 1985; 12:822–827.
25. Nicolaides KH, Snijders RJM, Gosden CM, et al. Ultrasonographically detectable markers of fetal chromosomal abnormalities. Lancet 1992; 340:704–707.
26. Barker DJ, Gluckman PD, Godfrey KM, et al. Fetal nutrition and cardiovascular disease in adult life. Lancet 1993; 341:938–941.
27. Karsdorp VHM, van Vugt JMG, van Geijn HP. Clinical significance of absent or reversed end diastolic velocity waveforms in umbilical artery. Lancet 1994; 344:1664–1668.

28. Mari G, Deter RL. Middle cerebral artery flow velocity waveforms in normal and small-for-gestational-age fetuses. Am J Obstet Gynecol 1992; 166:1262–1270.
29. Baschat AA, Gembruch U, Reiss I, et al. Demonstration of fetal coronary blood flow by Doppler ultrasound in relation to arterial and venous flow velocity waveforms and perinatal outcome–the 'heart-sparing effect'. Ultrasound Obstet Gynecol 1997; 9:162–172.
30. Hecher K, Bilardo CM, Stigter RH, et al. Monitoring of fetuses with intrauterine growth restriction: a longitudinal study. Ultrasound Obstet Gynecol 2001; 18:564–570.
31. Ferrazzi E, Bozzo M, Rigano S, et al. Temporal sequence of abnormal Doppler changes in the peripheral and central circulatory systems of the severely growth-restricted fetus. Ultrasound Obstet Gynecol 2002; 19:140–146.
32. Bower S, Schuchter K, Campbell S. Doppler ultrasound screening as part of routine antenatal scanning: prediction of pre-eclampsia and intrauterine growth retardation. Br J Obstet Gynaecol 1993; 100:989–994.
33. Zimmermann R, Durig P, Carpenter RJ, et al. Longitudinal measurement of peak systolic velocity in the fetal middle cerebral artery for monitoring pregnancies complicated by red cell alloimmunisation: a prospective multicentre trial with intention-to-treat. Br J Obstet Gynaecol 2002; 109:746–752.
34. Chitty LS, Chudleigh P, Wright E, et al. The significance of choroid plexus cysts in an unselected population: The results of a multicentre study. Ultrasound Obstet Gynecol 1998; 12:391–397.
35. Johnson SP, Sebire NJ, Snijders RJM, et al. Ultrasound screening for anencephaly at 10–14 weeks of gestation. Ultrasound Obstet Gynecol 1997; 9:14–16.
36. Van den Hof MC, Nicolaides KH, Campbell J, et al. Evaluation of the lemon and banana signs in one hundred thirty fetuses with open spina bifida. Am J Obstet Gynecol 1990; 162:322–327.
37. Campbell J, Gilbert WM, Nicolaides KH, et al. Ultrasound screening for spina bifida: cranial and cerebellar signs in a high-risk population. Obstet Gynecol 1987; 70:247–250.
38. Tegnander E, Eik-Nes SH, Johansen OJ, et al. Prenatal detection of heart defects at the routine fetal examination at 18 weeks in a non-selected population. Ultrasound Obstet Gynecol 1995; 5:372–380.
39. Carvalho JS, Mavrides E, Shinebourne EA, et al. Improving the effectiveness of routine prenatal screening for major congenital heart defects. Heart 2002; 88:387–391.
40. Hyett J, Perdu M, Sharland G, et al. Using fetal nuchal translucency to screen for major congenital cardiac defects at 10-14 weeks of gestation: population based cohort study. BMJ 1999; 318:81–85.
41. Kumar RK, Newburger JW, Gauvreau K, et al. Comparison of outcome when hypoplastic left heart syndrome and transposition of the great arteries are diagnosed prenatally versus when diagnosis of these two conditions is made only postnatally. Am J Cardiol 1999; 83:1649–1653.
42. Bonnet D, Coltri A, Butera G, et al. Detection of transposition of the great arteries in fetuses reduces neonatal morbidity and mortality. Circulation 1999; 99:916–918.
43. Crane JP, LeFevre MI, Winborn RC, et al. A randomized trial of prenatal ultrasonographic screening impact on the detection, management, and outcome of anomalous fetuses. The RADIUS Study Group. Am J Obstet Gynecol 1994; 171:392–399.
44. Chudleigh P, Chitty LS, Campbell S, et al. The association of aneuploidy and mild fetal pyelectasis in an unselected population: the results of a multicentre study. Ultrasound Obstet Gynecol 2001; 17:197–202.
45. McHugo J, Whittle M. Enlarged fetal bladders: aetiology, management and outcome. Prenat Diagn 2001: 21:958–963.
46. Warne S, Chitty LS, Wilcox DT. Prenatal diagnosis of cloacal anomalies. Br J Urol Int 2002; 89:78–81.
47. Wilcox DT, Chitty LS. Non-visualisation of the fetal bladder: Aetiology and management. Prenat Diagn 2001; 21:977–983.
48. Winyard P, Chitty LS. Dysplastic and polycystic kidneys: diagnosis, associations and management. Prenat Diagn 2001; 21:924–935.
49. Wellesley D, Howe DT. Fetal renal anomalies and genetic syndromes. Prenat Diagn 2001; 21:992–1003.
50. Machin GA. Hydrops revisited: literature review of 1414 cases published in the 1980s. Am J Med Genet 1989; 34:366–390.
51. McCoy MC, Katz VL, Gould N, et al. Non-immune hydrops after 20 weeks' gestation: review of 10 years' experience with suggestions for management. Obstet Gynecol 1995; 85:578–582.

Chapter 3

The urinary tract

CHAPTER CONTENTS

Embryology 39
Urinary tract anomalies 41
   Anomalies of the upper urinary tract 41
   Anomalies of the lower urinary tract 43
Ultrasound preparation and technique 47
   Normal ultrasound appearances 47
Postnatal investigation of prenatally diagnosed urological abnormalities 52
   Normal postnatal scan following prenatal detection of renal pelvic dilation 53
   Unilateral renal pelvic dilation 55
   Bilateral renal pelvic dilation 56
   Megaureter 56
   Multicystic kidney 57
   Posterior urethral valves 59
   The duplex kidney 63
   Guidelines for referral 65
Urinary tract infection 65
   Imaging urinary tract infections 65
   Imaging protocol for urinary tract infection 68
   Unusual infections 69
Cystic kidneys 70
   Genetic disease 72
   Non-genetic disease 78
The 'bright' kidney 79
   The neonate 80
   The older child 83
Renal calculi and nephrocalcinosis 84
   Renal calculi 84
   Nephrocalcinosis 86

Hypertension in children 89
   Imaging 90
Renal trauma 94
Renal transplantation in children 94
Tumors of the kidney 102
   Wilms tumor 103
   Other renal tumors of childhood 106
   Rhabdomyosarcoma 109

EMBRYOLOGY

In the human fetus the development of the urinary system is intimately related to that of the genital system, so much so that ducts from the early urinary system go on to be incorporated into the male genital system. This intimate developmental relationship explains why some of the congenital anomalies affect both systems.

Three sets of excretory organs develop in a human embryo in a cranial to caudal progression (Fig. 3.1):

- pronephroi—rudimentary and non-functional
- mesonephroi—well developed and function briefly
- metanephroi—become the permanent kidneys.

Mesonephroi These are the interim kidneys until the permanent kidneys develop. The mesonephric ducts open into the cloaca. Medial to the two mesonephroi are the developing gonads; after the mesonephroi degenerate, the tubules become incorporated into the male genital system. They disappear in the female. The mesonephric ducts or

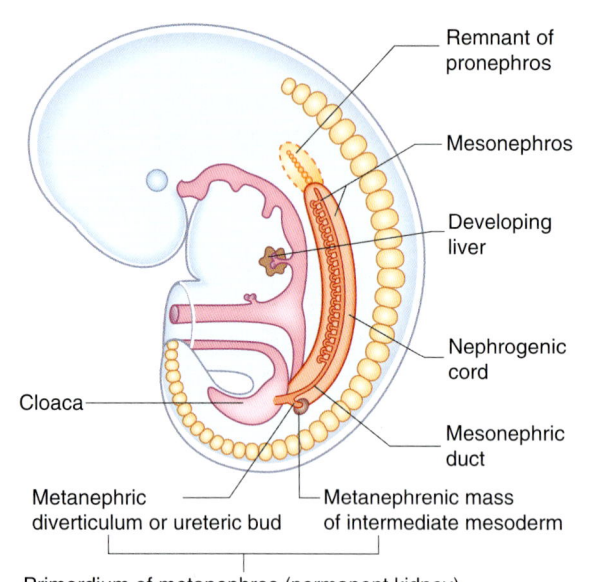

Wolffian ducts have several adult derivatives in the male.

Metanephroi These are the permanent kidneys and begin to develop in the fifth week. They develop from two sources:

- The ureteric bud is an outgrowth from the mesonephric duct close to its entry into the fetal cloaca. The ureteric bud goes on to develop the ureter, renal pelvis, calices and collecting tubules. The collecting tubules undergo repeated branching which induces clusters of mesenchymal cells in the metanephric mass of mesoderm. These go on to form the metanephric tubules which ultimately progress to form the nephron (Fig. 3.2).
- The metanephric mass of intermediate mesoderm. The nephron is derived from the metanephric mass.

The fetal kidneys are subdivided into lobes which give it the characteristic fetal lobulation.

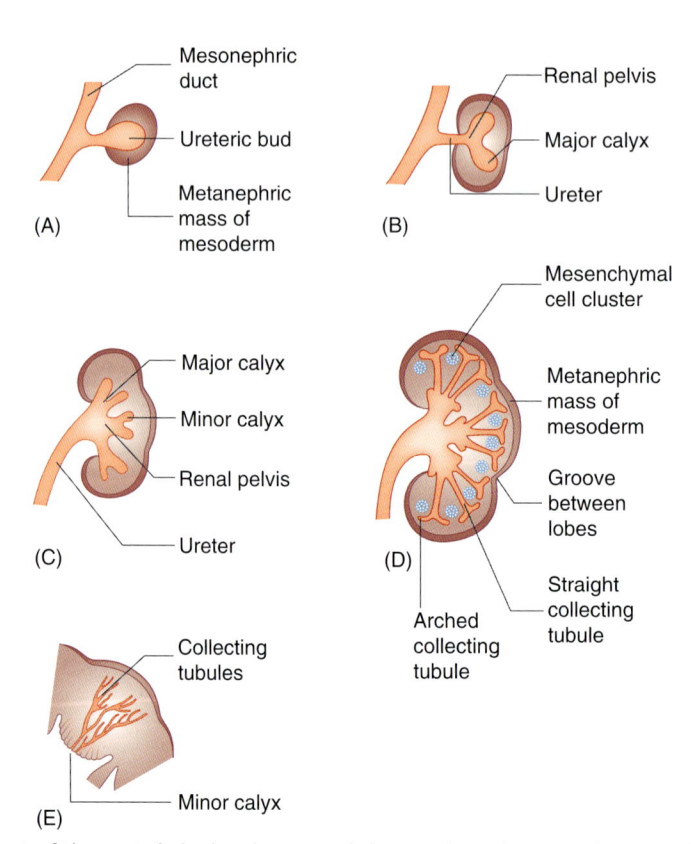

Figure 3.1 Development of the kidney in early fetal life. Notice the developing ureteric bud arising close to the cloaca from the mesonephric duct.

Figure 3.2 Development of the ureteric bud and metanephric mass into the parenchyma and collecting system of the kidney.

THE URINARY TRACT

This disappears during infancy as the nephrons increase and grow.

Initially the permanent kidneys lie close to each other in the pelvis. As the abdomen grows, the kidneys move cranially (towards the head) and gradually move further apart. Eventually they come to lie in the retroperitoneum on the posterior abdominal wall. As they ascend from the pelvis they receive a higher and higher blood supply so that eventually they receive blood supplied from the aorta. This also accounts for the multiple renal arteries which often supply the kidneys. When they come into contact with the adrenal gland the ascent stops (Fig. 3.3).

Figure 3.4 is a schematic diagram of some of the more common anomalies of the urinary system. Renal anomalies occur in some 3–4% of newborn infants and are usually those of number of kidneys, rotation and position.

URINARY TRACT ANOMALIES

Anomalies of the upper urinary tract

Renal agenesis

Unilateral renal agenesis is relatively common, occurring in about 1 in 1000 newborn infants. Some cases may, in fact, be as a result of an involuted multicystic kidney in later life. Males are more affected than females, and the left is more commonly the one that is absent. The contralateral kidney usually undergoes compensatory hypertrophy. Unilateral renal agenesis should be suspected in infants with a single umbilical artery (Fig. 3.5).

Bilateral renal agenesis Bilateral renal agenesis is incompatible with life. Prenatally it is associated with oligohydramnios because no urine is formed. These infants have characteristic facial appearances with low set ears, wide set eyes, flat and broad noses and a receding chin. Most die shortly after birth.

Abnormalities of position

Abnormal rotation of the kidneys is often associated with ectopia, that is abnormal position of the kidneys. A malrotated ectopic kidney is more susceptible to developing urological complications and to trauma.

Ectopic kidneys One or both kidneys may be in an abnormal position if they fail to progress along their normal migratory path. Most kidneys are located in the pelvis, in which case they may fuse to form a pancake kidney. Ectopic kidneys may present as a mass, and some have been inadvertently removed. Occasionally a kidney may continue to migrate cranially, in which case it may be

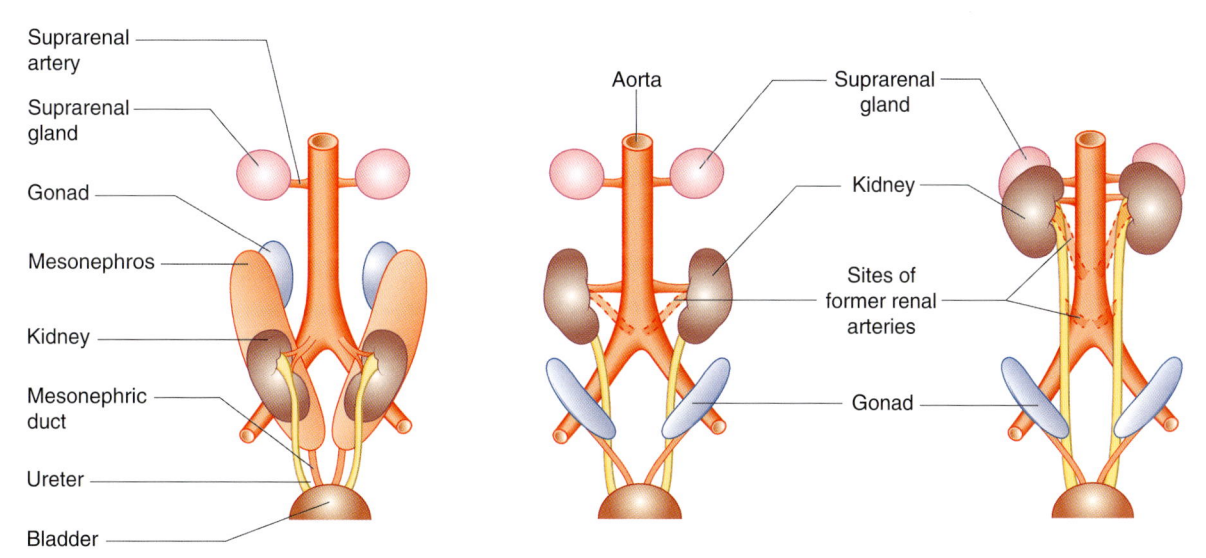

Figure 3.3 Ventral views of the ascent of the kidneys during intrauterine life from the pelvis to their normal position in the abdomen.

42   PEDIATRIC ULTRASOUND

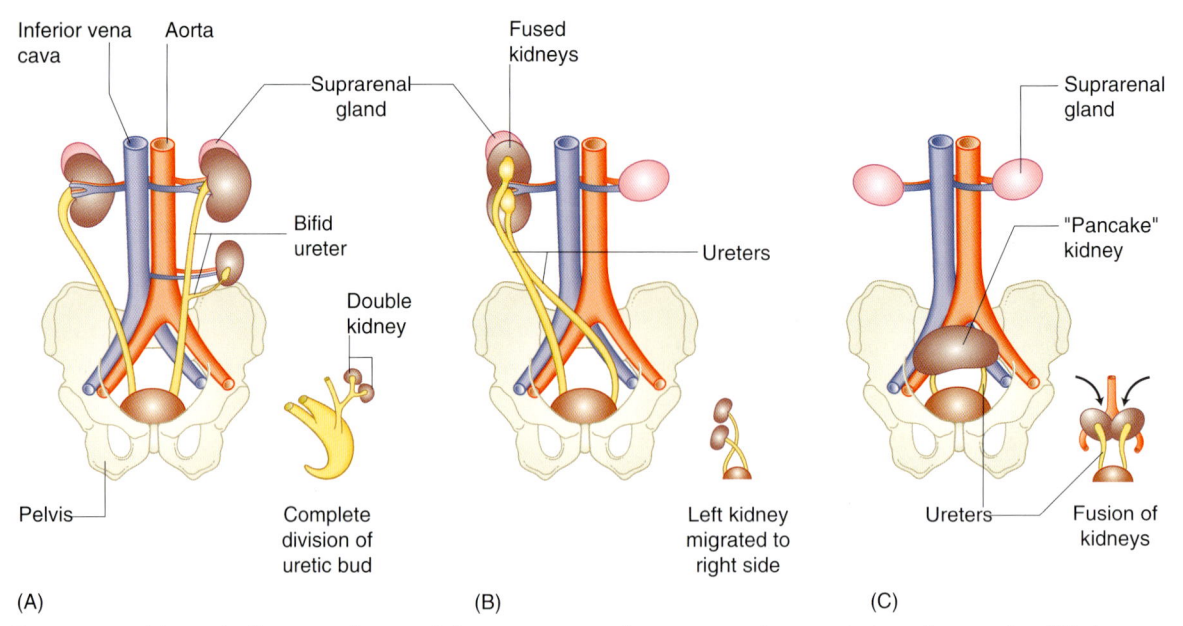

Figure 3.4 Schematic diagrams of some of the more commonly encountered congenital renal anomalies. (A) shows a rotated kidney and bifid ureter. (B) shows a crossed-fused ectopic kidney, and (C) shows a pelvic pancake kidney.

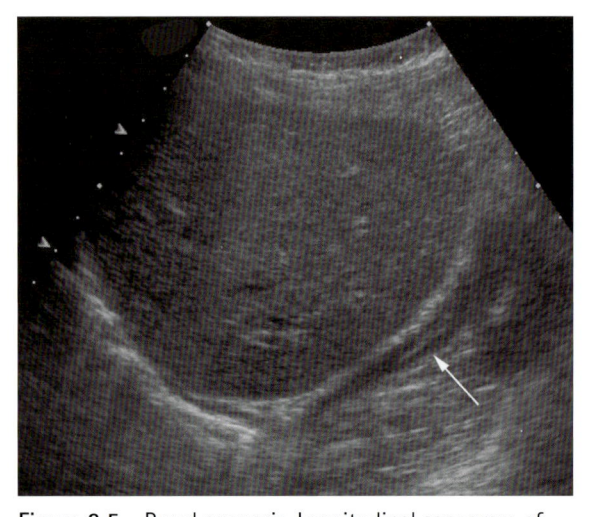

Figure 3.5 Renal agenesis. Longitudinal sonogram of the right flank showing the liver and the linear hypoechoic psoas muscle. Note that there is no kidney. The psoas muscle is a very valuable landmark when searching for absent kidneys, and the flank down to the pelvis and behind the bladder should be examined.

found in the chest. Ectopic kidneys receive their blood supply from blood vessels near them (for example iliac arteries if they lie in the pelvis) and are often supplied by multiple vessels (Fig. 3.6).

Horseshoe kidneys In about 1 in 500 the poles, usually the lower poles, of the kidneys are fused. There is a higher incidence in Turner syndrome. Normal ascent of the horseshoe kidney is prevented by the inferior mesenteric artery.

Crossed-fused ectopia When one kidney is displaced across the midline and fused inferiorly to another normally positioned kidney this is termed cross-fused ectopia. The lower (i.e. displaced) kidney's ureter enters the bladder normally on the contralateral side. These kidneys are prone to develop obstructive uropathy, and there is also an increased incidence of VUR. Crossed-fused ectopia and single kidneys are the renal anomalies most commonly associated with the VACTERL syndrome (Fig. 3.7).

THE URINARY TRACT   43

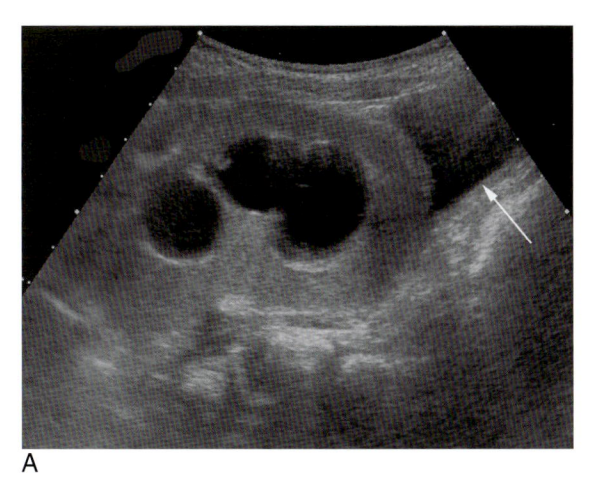

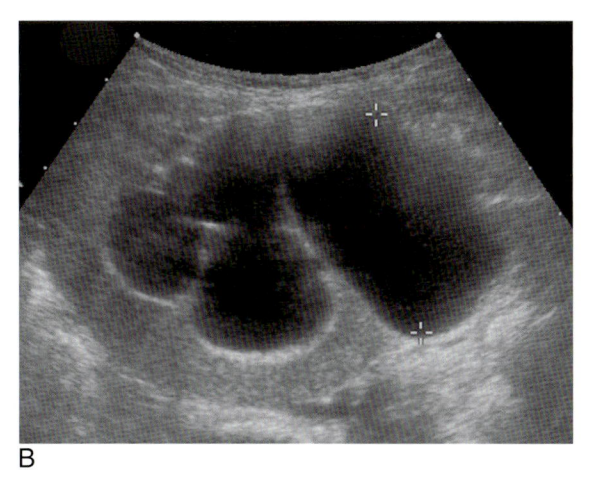

Figure 3.6 Ectopic kidney. (A) Longitudinal sonogram of the pelvis showing the bladder (arrow) and pelvic kidney. The ectopic kidney is lying just above the bladder, and the calices and renal pelvis are dilated. (B) Transverse sonogram at the hilum of the ectopic kidney showing the dilated calices and renal pelvis (between calipers). Ectopic kidneys have a higher incidence of complications such as vesicoureteric reflux and pelviureteric junction obstruction.

Bifid ureter

A bifid ureter results from a duplication of the ureter. This may be only a bifid renal pelvis in which case it is a variation of normality. The two ureters may fuse anywhere along their course. Rarely yo-yo reflux may occur where ureteroureteral (reflux from one upper ureter into the other) occurs.

Duplex kidneys

Duplex kidneys occur when two ureteric buds from the bladder present to the mesoderm. The ureter from the upper moiety of the kidney migrates more caudally than the lower ureter so that eventually its orifice in the bladder comes to lie below the lower moiety ureter. When the two ureteric orifices lie close together, there are generally no complications. However, when they are ectopic, i.e. not in the normal location, then complications occur. The upper moiety orifice may be associated with an obstructing ureterocele in the bladder, and in girls it may even open ectopically in the vagina. The lower moiety ureter has a shorter and more vertical intravesical course and thus the lower moiety may have vesicoureteric reflux. There is also a higher incidence of pelviureteric junction obstruction in the lower moiety.

Anomalies of the lower urinary tract

Anomalies of the distal ureter

Primary megaureter   Megaureter is a general term used to describe the presence of a dilated

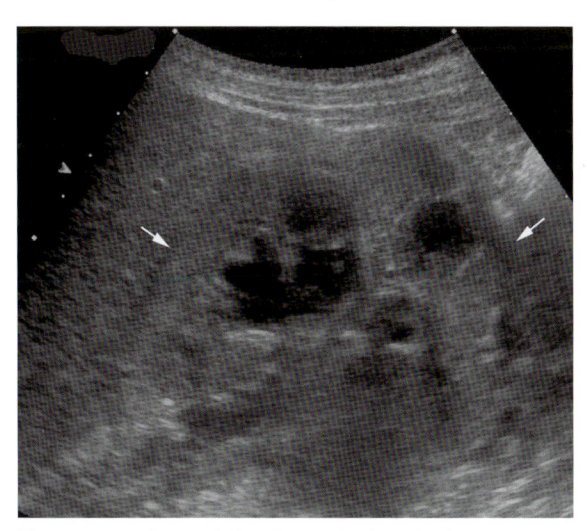

Figure 3.7   Crossed-fused ectopia. Longitudinal sonogram of a crossed-fused ectopic kidney. Note the renal bulk is larger than normal with an unusual contour of the two renal moieties, which are joined (arrows). This anomaly should be suspected when a single renal mass with two large collecting systems and an absent kidney on the contralateral side is found.

ureter with or without associated dilation of the upper collecting system. The diameter of the normal ureter in children is rarely more than 5 mm,[1] and if a ureter is detected on ultrasound it is generally considered to be abnormal. The term primary megaureter includes all abnormalities related to a congenital alteration at the vesicoureteric junction (VUJ), which may be obstructed, refluxing, or non-refluxing non-obstructed.

Typically there is a short, narrowed non-peristaltic section of ureter next to the bladder which inserts into the normal position. The normal ureter proximal to this segment dilates. The cause is unknown. A refluxing megaureter is due to a short or absent intravesical ureter or an abnormality of the VUJ.

Secondary megaureter occurs as a result of some other abnormality involving the bladder or urethra, such as urethral obstructions, for example posterior urethral valves (PUV), or bladder abnormalities, for example neuropathic bladders.

Nowadays most infants are detected prenatally, and all will require cystography to exclude secondary causes and VUR.

Ectopic ureter An ectopic ureter refers to the abnormal insertion of the ureter into the bladder. This is related to the abnormal intrauterine development of the ureteric bud where it fails to separate from the mesonephric duct (Wolffian duct) and is carried caudally. In males it may empty into the posterior urethra, lower bladder, seminal vesicle or ejaculatory duct. In females it may insert into the lower bladder, urethra, vestibule or vagina. The most important feature that differentiates ectopic ureters in girls and boys is that girls become incontinent whereas boys remain continent. A history of 24-hour wetting in a girl is highly suggestive of an ectopic ureter. Ectopic ureters are most commonly associated with ureteral duplication so that the upper moiety ureter inserts below and medial to its normal location and to that of the lower moiety ureter. For this reason it is frequently associated with ureterocele. Ectopic ureters can also drain a single kidney. They are associated with dysplasia of the draining moiety, most commonly the upper moiety.

Ureterocele Ureteroceles are cystic dilations of the intravesical segments of the ureter and may be associated with either single or duplex ureters. The wall is composed of bladder and ureteral epithelium. A ureterocele may be small or fill the whole bladder and even prolapse out of the urethra. When they are large and fill the bladder they may obstruct the contralateral ureter and may be missed on ultrasound. They may be simple or ectopic. A simple ureterocele refers to a normal position in the bladder with a stenosis of the ureteral orifice. This is more common in adults and is thought to be related to infection.

On ultrasound the ureterocele appears as a cystic structure with a thin membrane within the bladder almost always associated with a dilated ureter. If large enough it will obstruct the bladder, and in boys may even be mistaken for PUV with an irregular trabeculated bladder wall (Fig. 3.8). In nearly three quarters of pediatric patients an ectopic ureterocele is associated with a duplex collecting system and is the distal portion of the upper moiety ureter. The upper moiety is usually obstructed by the ureterocele. Due to the stasis of urine, urinary tract infections and stones in the ureterocele may occur. VUR may be associated with the lower moiety duplex because of the shorter and more vertical intravesical course of the ureter, as mentioned previously.

Primary vesicoureteric reflux (VUR) Vesicoureteric reflux is the flow of urine from the bladder into the ureter and upper collecting system. It may be isolated but is commonly associated with other abnormalities, in particular bladder and bladder outflow obstructions. There is also a known association with duplex systems and multicystic kidneys, and it is known to be a familial condition. Table 3.1 gives definitions of grades of VUR.

Cystography, that is the catheterization of the bladder and the instillation of radiographic contrast (the conventional method), radioisotope or ultrasound contrast agents is the only method of directly detecting VUR.

Anomalies of the bladder

Bladder agenesis is extremely rare, and most affected infants are stillborn.

Urachal abnormalities The urachus is situated in the midline superficially and just anterior to the peritoneum in the space of Retzius. It extends from the dome of the bladder to the umbilicus. It is obliterated before birth but in some it may persist as a cyst or sinus which is a result of failure of closure.

THE URINARY TRACT

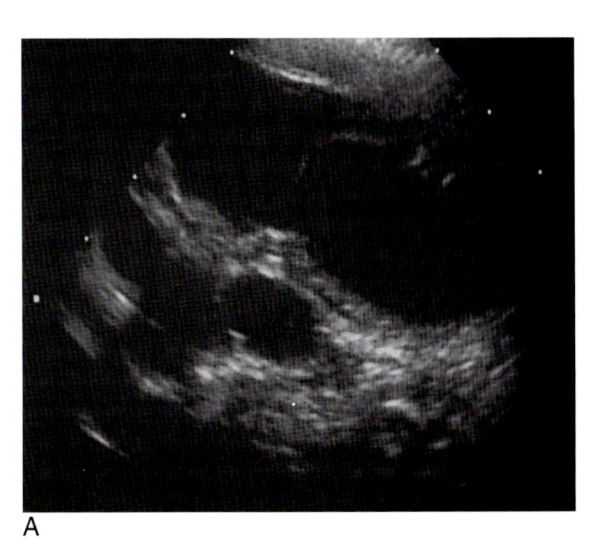

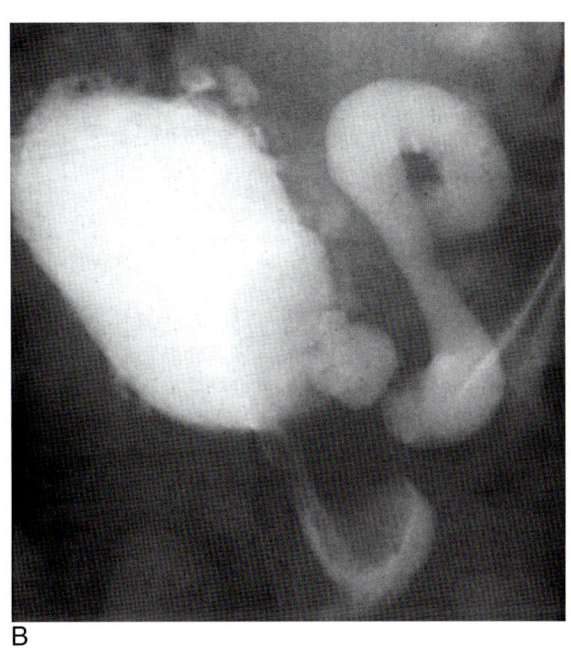

Figure 3.8 Ureterocele mimicking posterior urethral valves. (A) Longitudinal sonogram of the bladder in a male infant showing the thin wall of the ureterocele and a large full bladder. (B) Cystogram on the same infant showing the filling defect of the ureterocele obstructing the bladder outlet. The bladder wall is trabeculated as one might expect to see in posterior urethral valves (PUV). This infant was mistakenly thought to have PUV prenatally.

This is associated with obstruction to the lower urinary tract or ventral abdominal wall defects. It may be diagnosed in the neonate as urine leaking from the umbilicus. A urachal cyst forms when the umbilical and bladder section of the lumen close leaving fluid in the intervening portion. This looks like a midline cyst on ultrasound and may present clinically because of infection or bleeding.

Bladder duplication This is also an extremely rare anomaly. It may occur in the sagittal or coronal plane, most commonly sagittal, with two bladders lying side by side. Each bladder receives the ureter of the ipsilateral kidney and is drained by its own urethra. Associated congenital anomalies are duplication of the external genitalia and lower GI tract together with spinal duplication.

Table 3.1 Grades of vesicoureteric reflux based on guidelines of the International Reflux Study Committee[21]

Grade	Characteristics
I	Ureter only
II	Ureter, pelvis and calices; no dilation; normal caliceal fornices
III	Mild or moderate dilation or tortuosity of the ureter and moderate dilation of the renal pelvis; no or slight blunting of the fornices
IV	Moderate dilation or tortuosity of the ureter and moderate dilation of the renal pelvis and calices; complete obliteration of the sharp angle of the fornices but maintenance of the papillary impressions in the majority of calices
V	Gross dilation and tortuosity of the ureter; gross dilation of the renal pelvis and calices; papillary impressions are no longer visible in the majority of the calices

Bladder diverticulae Large congenital bladder diverticulae are found in approximately 1.7% of children, almost exclusively boys. They may occur as a periureteric diverticulum classically known as a Hutch diverticulum which is associated with VUR. They are caused by a congenital bladder muscular anomaly. They may be unilateral or bilateral and are not associated with bladder or bladder outflow abnormalities. They are generally diagnosed at cystography when the child is being evaluated for a urinary tract infection or incontinence. They may be quite difficult to appreciate on ultrasound, only appearing as an unusual contour to the bladder. Post-micturition they do not always empty and may in fact enlarge, which will be the clue to the diagnosis. When associated with VUR they are generally excised as they alter the ureteric insertion and VUR will not spontaneously cease.

Prune belly syndrome (Eagle–Barrett syndrome)

The term 'prune belly' refers to the prune-like, wrinkled abdominal wall in these children. It is a syndrome which is associated with other anomalies of the respiratory, gastrointestinal, musculoskeletal and cardiovascular systems. The prune-like appearances of the anterior abdominal wall is thought to be related to intrauterine ascites which stretches the abdominal wall. There are bilateral undescended testes, varying degrees of dysplasia and dilation of the upper urinary tract and a large bladder. It occurs almost exclusively in males.

Cloacal abnormalities

The term cloaca means 'sewer' in Latin. Cloacal malformations refer to the common channel of the urinary, genital and gastrointestinal tracts so that there is a single perineal opening. This anomaly is a result of the failure of these structures to separate and have their own opening onto the perineum. The anterior abdominal wall is intact. Abnormalities of the bladder, uterus, vagina and bony pelvis together with the lower spinal cord are common associations. This only occurs in girls.

Cloacal exstrophy is a different condition where the lower abdominal wall fails to close and the bladder opens onto the anterior abdominal wall. It occurs in both girls and boys.

Urogenital sinus is where the urinary and genital tracts have a common orifice, with the gastrointestinal tract separate, so that there are two orifices: one for the bladder and vagina and one for the anus. The anterior abdominal wall is normal. This only occurs in girls.

Urethral abnormalities

Posterior urethral valves This is the commonest urethral abnormality occurring in boys. There is a thick membrane in the posterior urethra which behaves as a valve so that, while a catheter can be passed into the bladder, the infant is unable to adequately void and empty the bladder. This causes a typical dilation of the posterior urethra, proximal to the obstructing valve (Fig. 3.9).

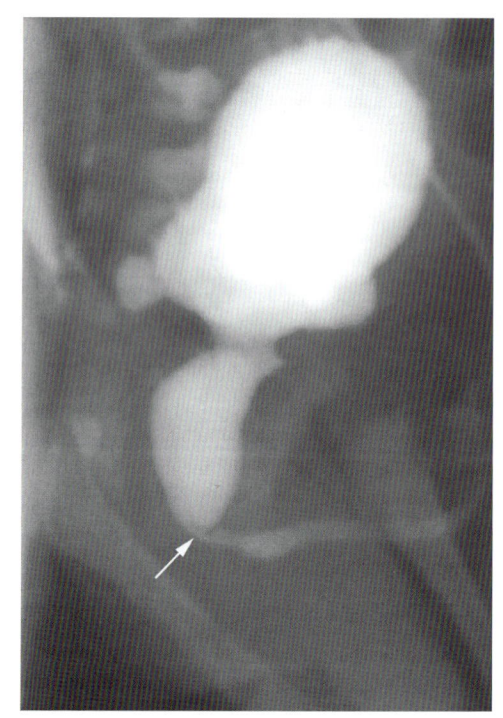

Figure 3.9 Posterior urethral valves on micturating cystourethrogram. Image of the posterior urethra in a male infant while voiding. The posterior urethra is markedly dilated with a sharp transition to the anterior urethra (arrow). The bladder neck appears hypertrophied with a trabeculated bladder wall. These are the typical appearances of posterior urethral valves.

These infants are primarily detected prenatally but a significant number are still seen with a late diagnosis postnatally. Dilation and dysplasia of the upper urinary tract is variable and dependent on when the valve became effective in intrauterine life.

Other urethral abnormalities Anterior urethral valve, urethral duplication, megalourethra and congenital urethral stricture are all rare urethral abnormalities which are generally diagnosed by cystography.

ULTRASOUND PREPARATION AND TECHNIQUE

Ultrasound is the first investigation in all children suspected of having any urinary tract abnormality. The findings of the ultrasound will then direct further investigation, so it is crucial that the sonographer performs a meticulous examination with a properly prepared child.

The anatomical information given by ultrasound is independent of function. Functional information is generally obtained from nuclear medicine studies. Sometimes further anatomical information, particularly of the ureters and calices, is needed, and for this an intravenous urogram (IVU) is performed (Table 3.2 and Fig. 3.10).

Examine the child well hydrated and with a full bladder wherever possible. Failure to have a full bladder could result in the sonographer missing an intermittent pelviureteric junction obstruction, dilated lower ureters, intravesical pathology such as ureteroceles, or pelvic masses, and being unable to assess bladder emptying.

Start with the patient supine and examine the bladder first as the infant may micturate and vital information will be lost.

An overfull bladder may cause a mild fullness of the collecting system, so it is best to start the examination of the full bladder and then get the patient to micturate. After micturition, examine the kidneys. If the kidneys appear dilated with the full bladder then it is generally best to wait at least 15 minutes before examining them again. Establish a local protocol so that the referring nephro-urologists know exactly when (i.e. before or after micturition) and where the renal pelvis is measured. Box 3.1 lists a normal renal ultrasound series.

Doppler evaluation is integral to the examination but particularly important in conditions such as:

- renal transplant assessment (to evaluate blood flow to the kidney and areas of hypo- and hyperperfusion)
- primary non-function of the renal transplant (where it is essential)
- suspected renal vein thrombosis (to evaluate the renal vein and inferior vena cava)
- renal tumor (to evaluate renal vein and IVC for tumor thrombus)
- hypertension (to look at the caliber of the aorta, aneurysmal dilation of the main renal vessels, and particularly to assess the intrarenal spectral trace).

Box 3.2 provides some tips on examination of the urinary tract.

Normal ultrasound appearances

The normal ultrasound appearances in a neonate typically show higher cortical echogenicity than in an older child. Normally the parenchymal echogenicity is equal to or greater than that of the liver and spleen. This can persist for up to 6 months and is thought to be related to the greater volume of glomeruli occupying the renal cortex. The medullary pyramids are prominent, hypoechoic, triangular structures with base on the renal cortex and regularly arranged around the central collecting system. There is an echogenic 'dot' on the base of the triangle which is the arcuate artery passing between the cortex and medulla. This is an easily identifiable structure on dynamic scanning and allows accurate differentiation between caliceal dilation and cysts. The central sinus echoes in a neonate are much less evident than in an adult or older child. Fetal lobulation may still be present (Figs 3.11 and 3.12).

After 6 months the cortex becomes more hypoechoic and appears thicker in relation to the medullae. The central sinus echoes become more prominent with age and body fat. Normally no caliceal dilation is seen. The renal pelvis shows some variation in size, and a transverse pelvic diameter of < 10 mm is considered to be within the normal range. Good hydration of the child

Table 3.2 Renal investigations in children

Investigation	Description	Indication
Micturating cystourethrogram (MCU)	Bladder catheterization. Demonstrates bladder size and shape. VUR if present. Only test which will show urethral abnormalities in boys	Suspected PUV. Thick-walled bladder. Ureteric dilation. UTI in boy < 1 year. Prenatal diagnosis of bilateral renal pelvic dilation
Direct isotope cystogram (DIC)	Bladder catheterization and isotope contrast	First investigation in girls and for follow-up in toddlers who are not potty-trained. Lower radiation dose than IRC
Voiding urosonography	Bladder catheterization and ultrasound contrast	Similar to DIC. Not yet universally accepted
Indirect radioisotope cystogram (IRC)	Dynamic renogram followed by voiding to look for VUR	Follow-up of VUR in older continent children. Gives functional information about kidneys
^{99m}Tc-dimercaptosuccinic acid (DMSA)	Isotope gets fixed in the kidney	To look for scars in the kidney following UTI. To search for functioning renal tissue not seen on US. To assess differential renal function
^{99m}Tc-diethylenetriaminepentaacetate (DTPA)	Dynamic renogram	Assess differential renal function and drainage
^{99m}Tc-mercaptoacetyltriglycine (MAG3)	Isotope taken up by kidney and passed in urine. After 30 min, micturition views to look for VUR (as IRC)	Postoperative evaluation of the collecting system: Indirect cystography. Following renal transplantation. Renography with captopril stimulation for renovascular hypertension
Intravenous urogram (IVU)	Contrast injected intravenously. Series of views of the kidneys and bladder as the contrast passes through the system	To demonstrate caliceal anatomy. In the workup of calculi. To demonstrate ureteric anatomy. Difficult duplex systems

PUV, posterior urethral valves; UTI, urinary tract infection; VUR, vesicoureteral reflux.

and a very full bladder may result in it being more prominent.[1]

When imaging the renal tract it is important to have the child fully hydrated in order to accurately assess any degree of pelvicaliceal dilation. A grading system of hydronephrosis has been proposed:[2]

- Grade 0—no hydronephrosis
- Grade 1—renal pelvis only visualized
- Grade 2—a few but not all calices are identified in addition to the renal pelvis
- Grade 3—all calices are seen
- Grade 4—similar to grade 3 but with parenchymal thinning.

This system should only be used after vesicoureteric reflux has been excluded. The emphasis of this system is on evaluating the intrarenal portion of the pelvicaliceal system rather than unduly

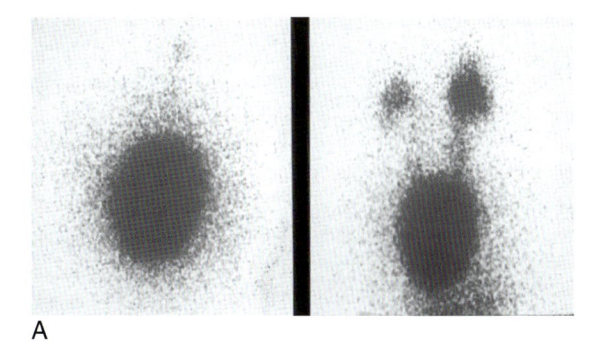

THE URINARY TRACT

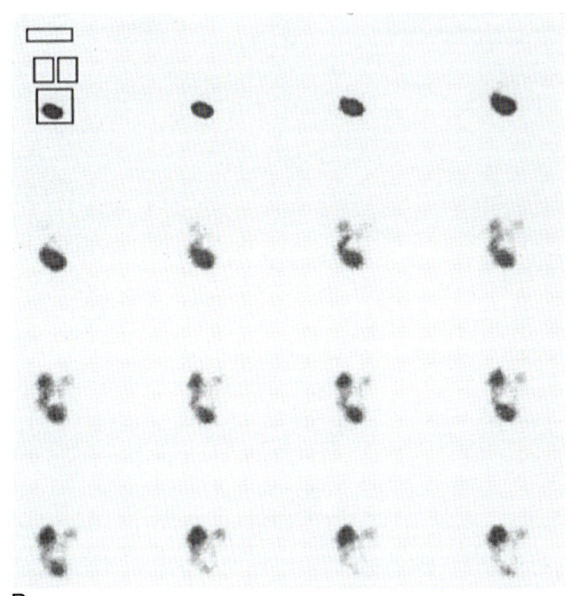

Box 3.1 Normal renal tract ultrasound series

1. Supine longitudinal and transverse full bladder views. Bladder wall measurements away from the trigone
2. Post-micturition supine longitudinal of the right kidney and left kidney comparing the echogenicity with that of the liver and spleen
3. Prone bipolar measurement of maximal length of both kidneys
4. Prone transverse pelvic diameter at the point of maximal width (either intra- or extrarenal). Use Doppler to identify the renal vessels
5. Supine post-micturition longitudinal and transverse views of the bladder and a volume measurement of post-micturition residue if present

Figure 3.10 Nuclear medicine cystography. (A) Direct isotope cystogram (DIC). This form of cystography is used in children who are not potty-trained. The bladder has been catheterized and isotope instilled into it. This example shows bladder filling and bilateral vesicoureteric reflux into the kidneys. (B) MAG3 (see Table 3.2) and indirect radioisotope cystogram (IRC). In this examination a formal MAG3 study is performed. This image shows isotope in the bladder at the end of the examination (top left image). The child is then asked to void, and vesicoureteric reflux is seen into both kidneys (images to bottom right).

Box 3.2 Some tips on examination of the renal tract

- Always start with the bladder
- If the kidneys are tucked underneath the ribs try using deep inspiration or expiration, or ask the child to blow their tummy up like a balloon, i.e. Valsalva
- Dilated ureters in a neonate are best seen in the supine position
- Try scanning the upper ureter by angling the probe 45° medial of the maximum renal length in the prone position
- Bipolar length must be measured prone. Supine renal length measurement may be falsely high because of image magnification
- Bladder wall should be measured away from the trigone as the musculature here is slightly thicker than in the rest of the bladder wall and may give falsely high measurements
- A renal ultrasound examination is incomplete if the bladder has not been examined full and after micturition

emphasizing an extrarenal pelvis. Evidence suggests that caliceal dilation has a poorer prognosis for the kidney, and generally the threshold for further imaging is lower in these children.

Normative charts must be available and used for all examinations (see, for example, Fig. 3.13). The

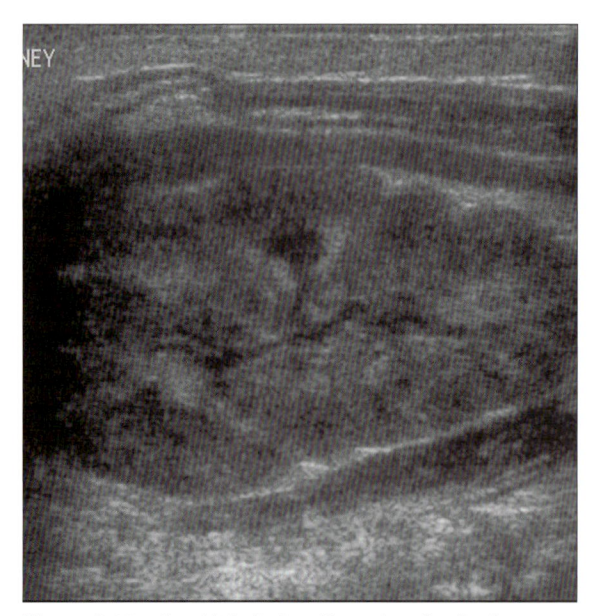

Figure 3.11 Fetal lobulation. Prone longitudinal sonogram of the right kidney in a neonate. The outline of the kidney has regular indentations of fetal lobulation. The indentations occur between the medullae. This appearance must not be mistaken for renal scarring; the latter usually extends over a greater area, and the angle at indentation of the cortex is not so acute.

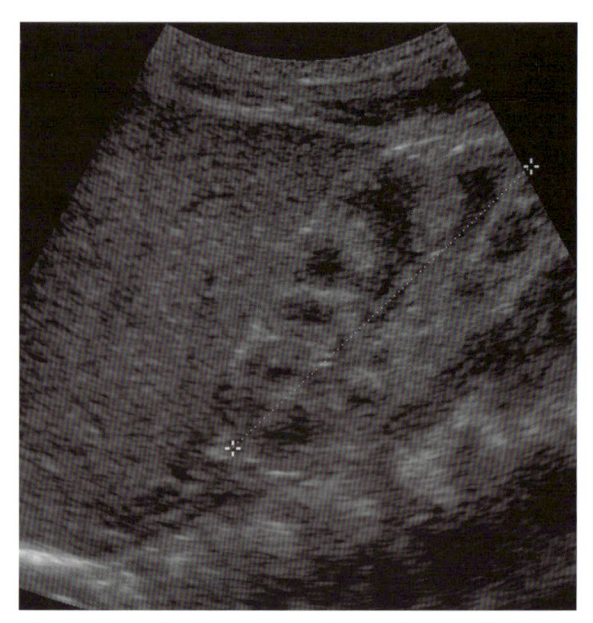

Figure 3.12 Normal neonatal kidney. Longitudinal sonogram of the right kidney in a normal neonate. The parenchyma of the cortex has the same or higher echogenicity as the liver. The cortex is thinner than in the older child and adult and there are very few central sinus echoes. The medullae are triangular in shape and regularly arranged around the central collecting system. The capsule is not visible.

normal renal length relative to age should be quoted in all reports. However, renal patients are often poorly grown and small so that it is our preference to use charts that also allow us to compare weight and height rather than age alone. The length of the kidney is the easiest parameter to assess, but volume has a more accurate correlation with most body size parameters (i.e. weight and height, which is important in children). The renal length in normal term neonates is 3.4–5.0 cm, and the renal volume is 5.7–14.3 cm^3. As a rule of thumb in premature infants use 1 mm renal length per week of gestation in order to assess renal size.[3–5] In children who have had a kidney removed or only have a single functioning kidney, because of a multicystic dysplastic kidney for example, use charts for a single kidney.[6]

The normal bladder wall (Fig. 3.14) when distended (90–100% of capacity) is 0.04–0.27 cm thick and when empty (0–10% of capacity) is 0.16–0.39 cm thick.[7]

In little girls a normal phenomenon occurs of vaginal filling post-micturition (Fig. 3.15). This is occasionally observed in cystography.

Doppler examination

Doppler examination is integral to a full examination of the kidneys. Often children are unable to lie still for a long examination, so it is wise to have manufacturer presets readily accessible on the equipment and good entertainment and distraction for the child. Equipment which incorporates both color energy, spectral and color Doppler is essential in pediatric ultrasound practice, with easy switching between the three and simultaneous display of color and spectral Doppler.

The color Doppler should be used as an adjunct when assessing the renal pelvis and hilar vessels and for a quick overview of the blood flow to a kidney. It is particularly useful in renal transplantation. It should be used in suspected renovascular

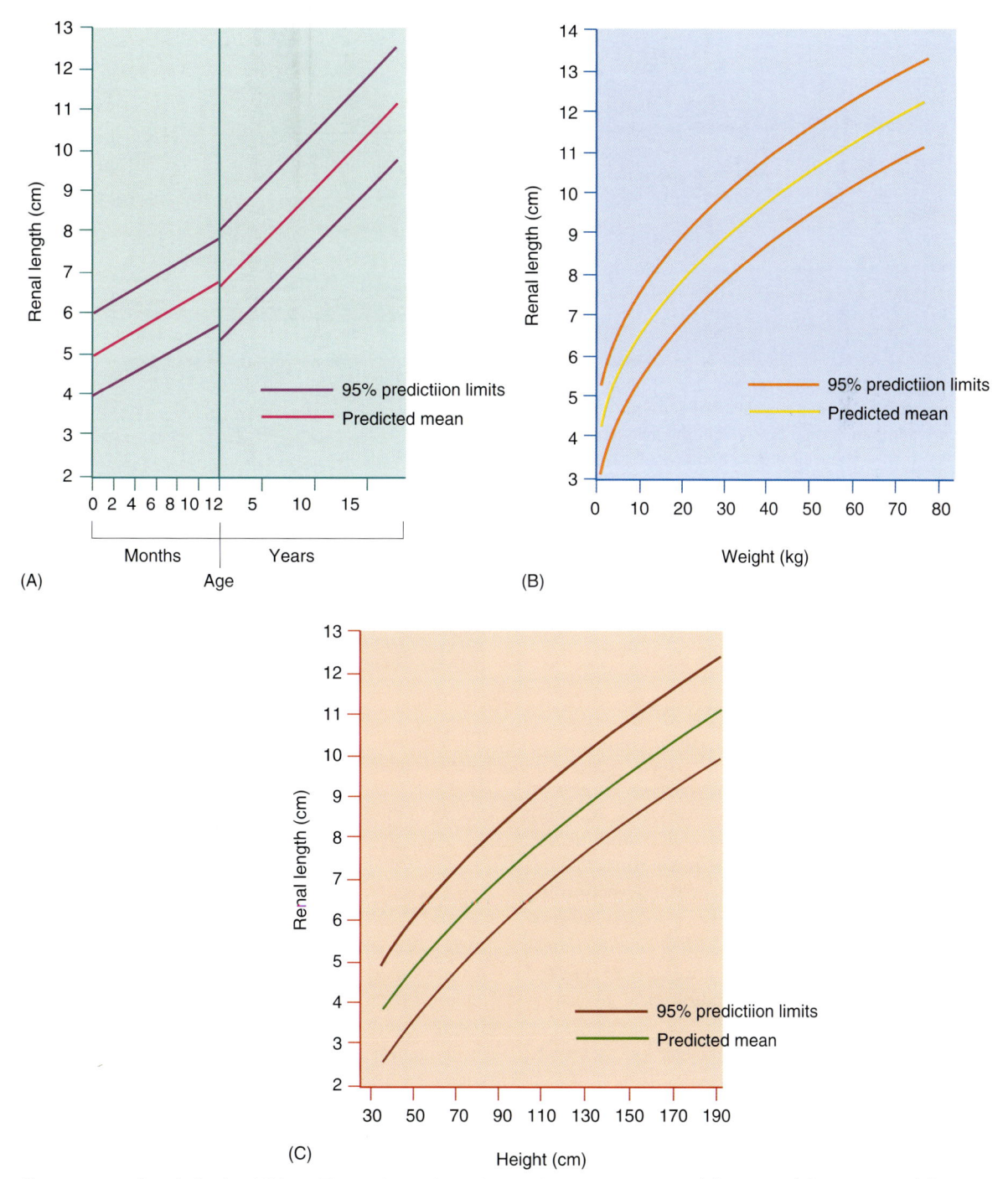

Figure 3.13 Renal size in children. These charts show the maximum renal length (A) for age, (B) for weight, (C) for height. (After Han BK & Babcock DS, *AJR Am J Roentgenol* 1985; 145:611–616.)

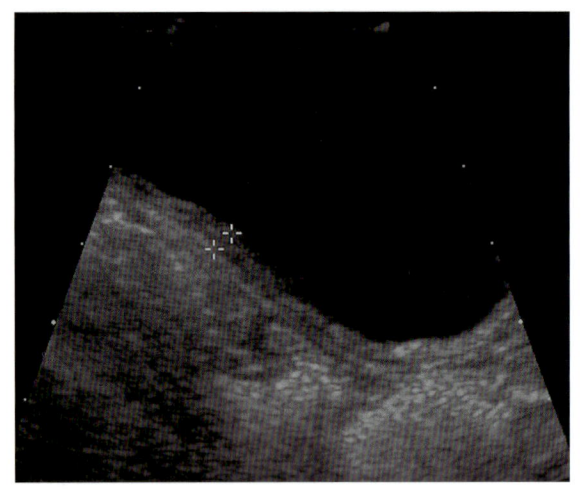

Figure 3.14 Normal bladder wall. Longitudinal sonogram of the normal bladder. Bladder wall measurements should be taken from the echogenic mucosa to the echogenic serosa and away from the trigone (between calipers).

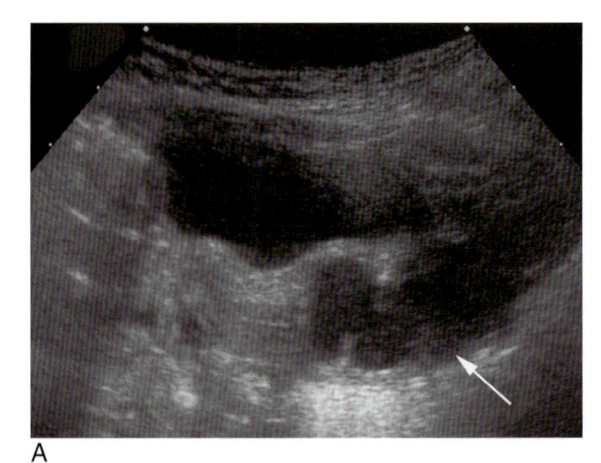

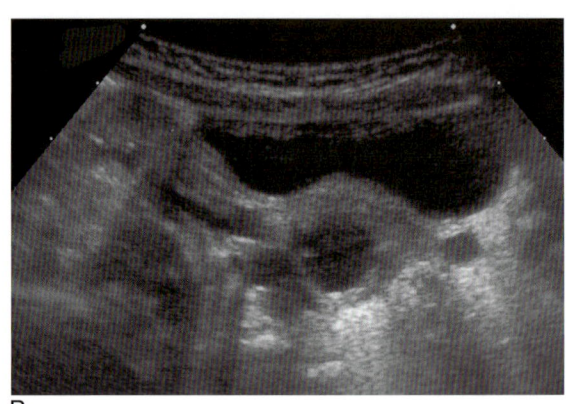

Figure 3.15 Fluid in the vagina. (A) Longitudinal and (B) transverse sonogram of the bladder in a female infant. Fluid in the vagina (arrow) can occur normally in little girls and is occasionally found as an incidental finding in the absence of other pathology.

hypertension both to evaluate the aorta and the kidneys. The appearance of the normal intrarenal Doppler waveform is shown in Figure 3.16 and reflects the low resistance of the renal bed.

POSTNATAL INVESTIGATION OF PRENATALLY DIAGNOSED UROLOGICAL ABNORMALITIES

Since the introduction of routine prenatal scanning and, latterly, more detailed anomaly scanning, the prenatal ultrasonic diagnosis of renal abnormalities is now well established. This prenatal detection has resulted in a whole new group of patients presenting to pediatric urologists in the last decade. These infants are primarily asymptomatic, and are referred for urological opinion and radiological investigation and monitoring (see Ch. 2). Treatment is mainly preventive and relies on close follow-up and timely intervention when necessary.

Accurate postnatal ultrasound in conjunction with knowledge of the prenatal findings is of fundamental importance in these infants and guides further imaging. Practice varies, but it is generally accepted that the first postnatal ultrasound should be when the baby is well hydrated, and this is generally once the mother's milk has come on at around 2–3 days of age. Depending on resources some centers would repeat the ultrasound at 6 weeks to confirm normality. Babies suspected of having posterior urethral valves, duplex systems or complex anomalies, i.e. conditions requiring urgent investigation and treatment, should be referred without waiting.

Infants referred for postnatal follow-up are those who at the 18-week scan have a renal pelvic diameter of 5 mm or more which either enlarges or remains static during pregnancy. Some would also include those with a measure of 8 mm at 8 months. One millimeter per month of gestation is a good rule of thumb.

THE URINARY TRACT

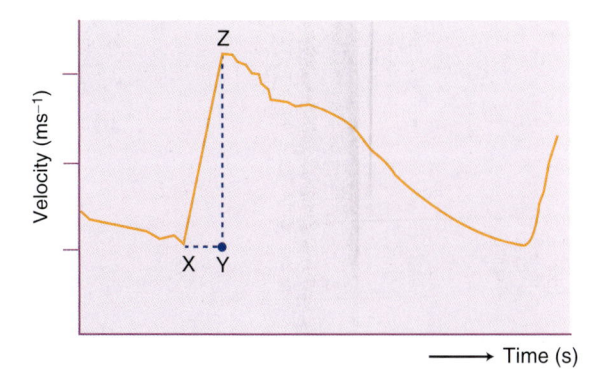

Figure 3.16 Doppler spectral trace. Line diagram demonstrating the normal renal Doppler spectral trace and intrarenal waveform. There is forward flow in systole and diastole, and the systolic upstroke is well-defined and sharp. The acceleration time is defined as $(y-x)$, and the acceleration index is $(z-x)/(y-x)$.

The role of ultrasound postnatally is to:

- confirm the prenatal diagnosis.
- detect infants that may need more urgent investigation.
- provide baseline measurements for long term follow-up.

The differential diagnosis of prenatal hydronephrosis is listed in Box 3.3, and the echogenic or bright kidney will be dealt with later. General concepts for a postnatal imaging protocol are listed in Box 3.4.

Box 3.4 General concepts for postnatal imaging protocol

- Use of antibiotics in all patients is controversial. Some advocate prophylactic trimethoprim at least until VUR has been excluded
- Postnatal ultrasound after 2–3 days when the infant is well hydrated
- Follow-up examination after 6 weeks to confirm the perinatal ultrasound findings
- Urgent urological referral for infants suspected of having PUV or complex duplex systems
- Conventional contrast cystography on dilated ureters, duplex systems and suspected PUV 'thick-walled bladders'
- Functional imaging generally after 3 months (after period of transitional nephrology), usually MAG3 (see Table 3.2)

Normal postnatal scan following prenatal detection of renal pelvic dilation

The commonest abnormality in general obstetric practice is mild renal pelvic dilation which on postnatal ultrasound is found to be normal. This is the largest group of children detected. Thirty percent of these have been shown to have vesicoureteric reflux, and it is for this reason that some centers

---

Box 3.3 Differential diagnosis of prenatal hydronephrosis

Unilateral
- RPD
- VUR
- Megaureter (± VUR)
- MCK (simple)
- Complicated duplex kidney, i.e. obstructed upper moiety with ureterocele and/or refluxing lower moiety

Bilateral
- RPD
- VUR
- Megaureters (± VUR)
- MCK (complicated); cystic dysplastic or dilated (PUJ) kidney on the opposite side;
- Complicated duplex kidneys
- Bladder or outlet pathology, e.g. neurogenic bladder or PUV with bilateral upper tract dilation

MCK, multicystic dysplastic kidney; PUJ, pelviureteric junction; PUV, posterior urethral valves; RPD, renal pelvic dilation; VUR, vesicoureteric reflux.

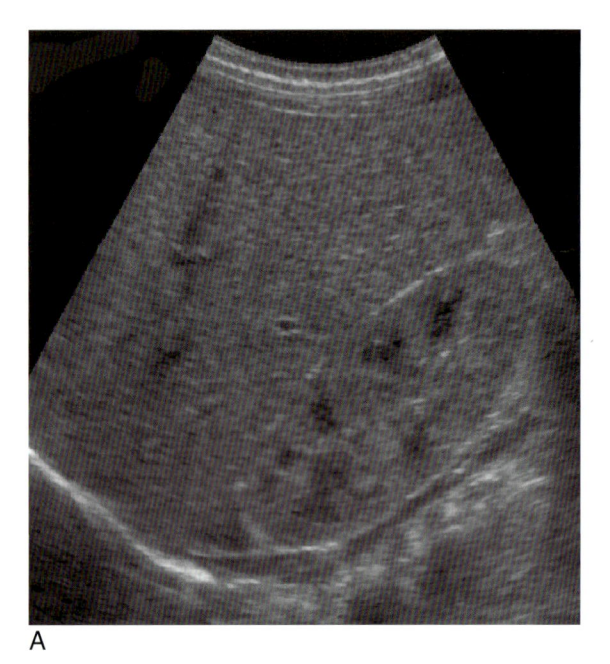

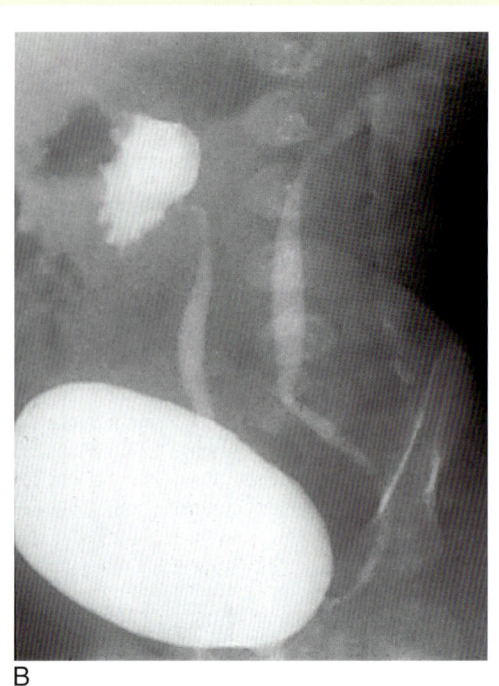

Figure 3.17 Normal kidney and vesicoureteric reflux (VUR). (A) Longitudinal sonogram on an infant showing a normal right kidney. The left kidney also appeared normal with no dilation of the collecting systems. The renal outline and parenchyma appear normal. (B) A micturating cystourethrogram examination performed just after the ultrasound. There is bilateral VUR into the upper tract. It is well recognized that approximately 30% of infants with a prenatal diagnosis of renal pelvic dilation will have a normal scan postnatally and will have VUR.

advocate the routine use of cystography (Fig. 3.17). However, this is controversial as it imposes a large workload on radiology departments, and some argue that there will be too many false negative results because VUR resolves anyway. Long term studies do not exist in this group but it would appear that, while VUR exists, these kidneys are normal and not scarred or dysplastic. However, their potential for renal damage in the presence of infection must be high.

There is another group of patients who have a prenatal diagnosis of hydronephrosis but whose kidneys are not entirely normal on ultrasound, with irregular outlines and areas of cortical thinning, increased echogenicity and dilation of the collecting system (Fig. 3.18). These patients appear to have damaged or dysplastic kidneys in the presence of prenatal VUR and have a different prognosis with a much higher potential for further renal damage should infection occur.[8–13]

Interestingly, this whole group is more common in male infants.[14] Further imaging will depend on management and the postnatal ultrasound examination. Depending on local protocols, in some centers contrast cystography will be performed on these infants. Those with VUR will be placed on antibiotic cover and have a DMSA performed. If, after the normal postnatal ultrasound, no further imaging including a cystogram is undertaken, then it is reasonable for these children to be placed on antibiotic prophylaxis at least for the first year of life while the potential for renal damage is at its highest.

Continuing renal pelvic dilation and/or caliceal dilation postnatally is still the most important finding in suspected VUR, but other indicators such as irregular outlines, small size, loss of the corticomedullary differentiation, any ureteric dilation or an abnormal thick-walled bladder must be carefully looked for. Further investigation is warranted in these high risk infants such as an MCU and DMSA scan.

THE URINARY TRACT 55

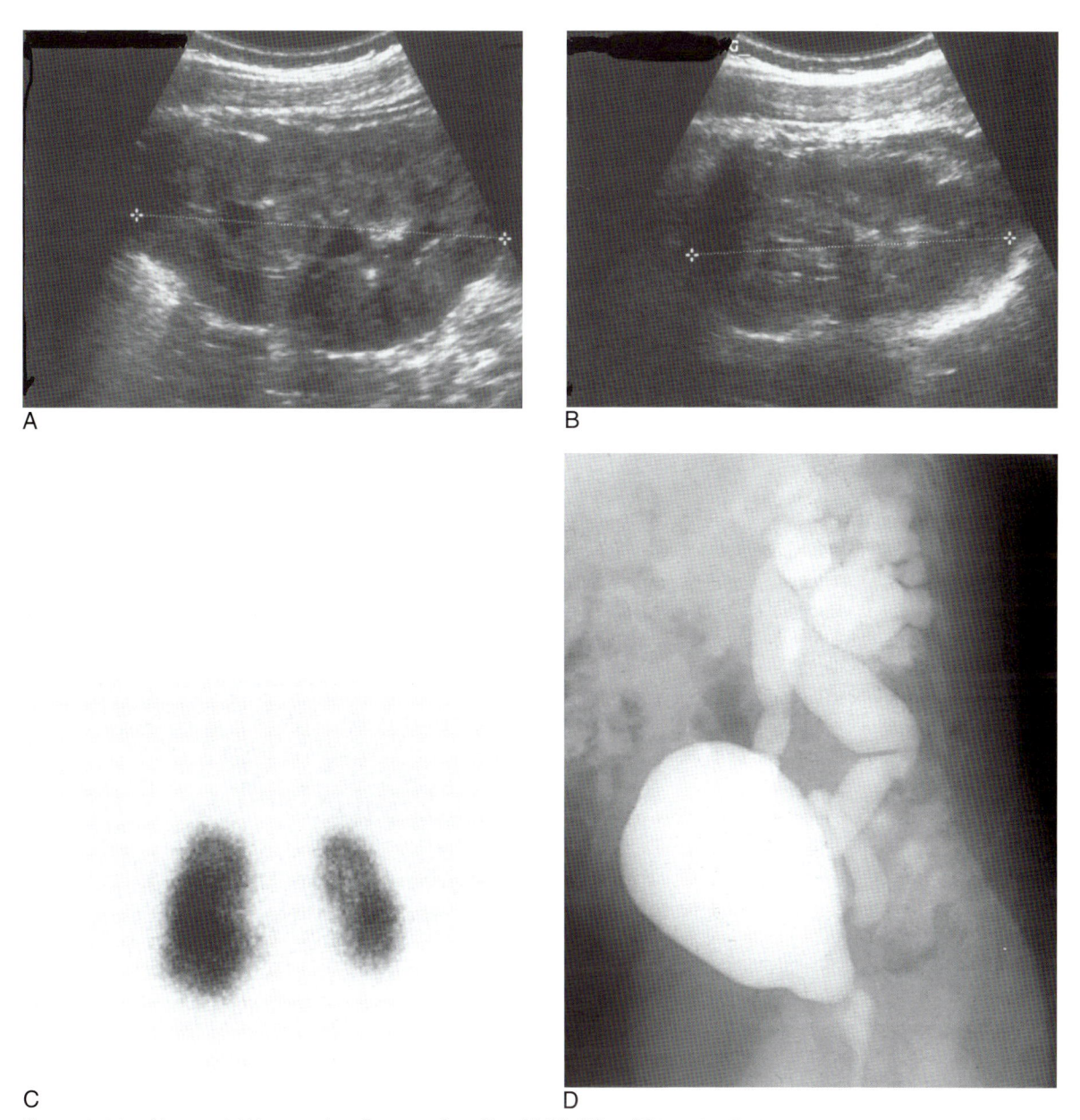

Figure 3.18 Abnormal kidney and vesicoureteric reflux (VUR). (A) & (B) Longitudinal sonogram of left and right kidneys in an infant with prenatally diagnosed renal tract dilation. There is asymmetry in size of the kidneys and abnormal outline. (C) DMSA (see Table 3.2) on the same infant showing the grossly abnormal renal outlines of both kidneys. The right kidney is smaller than the left. (D) There was bilateral VUR at cystography. These antenatally diagnosed infants are a well-defined group and have never had a urinary infection. This is termed fetal reflux nephropathy and they are at greater risk of long term renal damage if infection occurs.

Unilateral renal pelvic dilation

Mild renal pelvic dilation is one of the commonest prenatal diagnoses the sonographer will encounter.

When reporting the examination it should be clearly stated whether there is caliceal dilation and the size of the renal pelvis. Simply calling the dilation a hydronephrosis is not sufficient and poorly describes the state of the collecting system. This is particularly important for monitoring and accurate long term follow-up. Care should be taken not to mistake the renal pelvis for renal vasculature at the hilum, and a quick Doppler to confirm the position of the vasculature is sometimes needed (Fig. 3.19).[15,16]

A renal pelvic diameter of 10 mm or less is generally considered to be within the normal range.[17] Isolated RPD < 10 mm is virtually always benign, and no aggressive investigations should be undertaken. Urologists vary in their opinion but some would even take renal pelvic diameters of < 15 mm to be benign and treat conservatively. Most would not undertake further imaging and would simply follow with ultrasound examinations. However, if there is caliceal dilation (Fig. 3.20) the prognosis for the kidney is generally worse and the threshold for imaging is lower. It is essential that the sonographer is able to recognize caliceal dilation. Caliceal and/or ureteric dilation irrespective of renal pelvis diameter are always significant, and both reflux and obstruction must be excluded. This dilation of the renal pelvis is sometimes called PUJ (pelviureteric junction) obstruction.[18]

All these infants are asymptomatic and are now generally managed conservatively. Documented increase in RPD at follow-up requires further investigation such as MAG3 and referral to a urologist. Box 3.5 gives an imaging protocol for RPD.

Bilateral renal pelvic dilation

Mild RPD may be bilateral. No general agreement on how to manage these patients exists. Postnatal imaging should be the same as that for unilateral RPD. Some centers include a cystogram.

Megaureter

A megaureter simply refers to an enlarged ureter which may or may not reflux. The kidney has good function, and the degrees of caliceal and upper ureteric dilation are less than the degree of lower ureteric dilation. When undertaking the sonogram

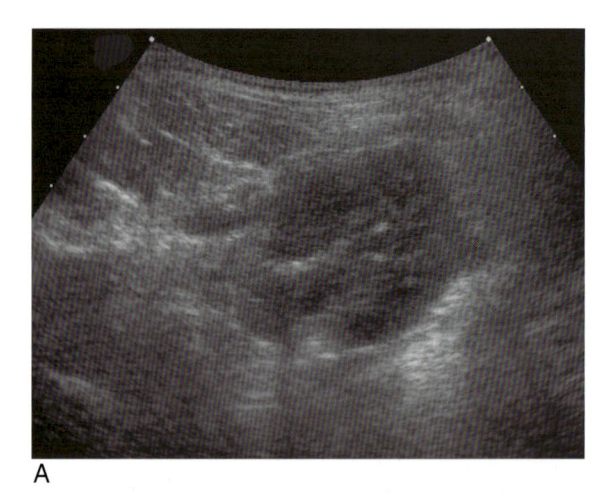

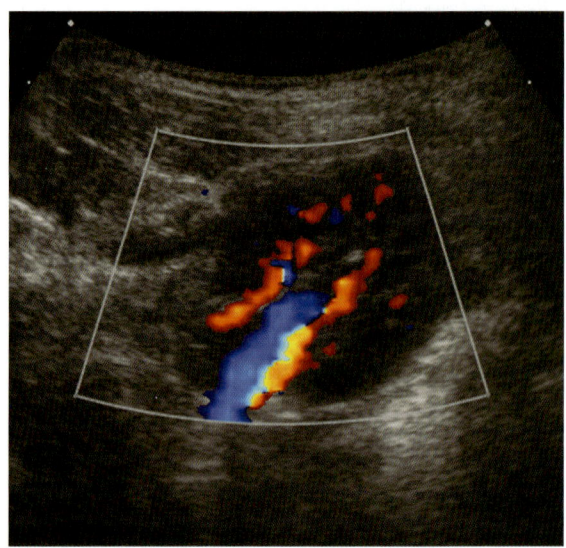

Figure 3.19 Renal pelvic vasculature. (A) Transverse sonogram of the renal pelvis, which appears to be dilated on the gray scale image. (B) Transverse sonogram with color Doppler of the same renal hilum showing that the 'pelvis' is in fact the renal artery and vein. A Doppler of the pelvis is very useful to clearly define the real renal pelvis.

this condition will be suspected when the lower ureter is seen to be markedly dilated, typically tapering down to the vesicoureteric junction (VUJ) in the presence of a relatively normal or mildly dilated upper collecting tract. It is important to ensure on ultrasound that there is not a ureterocele in the

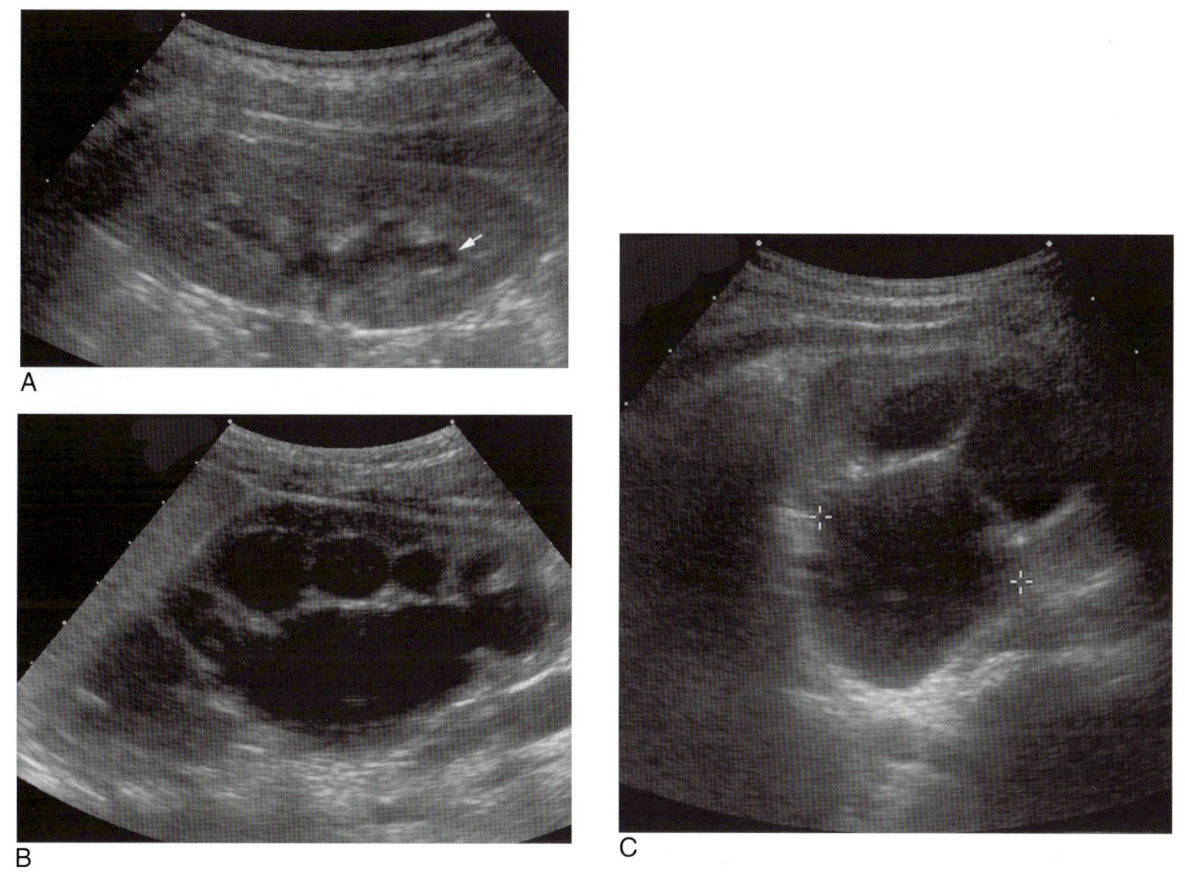

Figure 3.20 Caliceal and renal pelvic dilation. (A) Prone longitudinal scan of the left kidney with mild caliceal dilation (arrow). (B) Supine longitudinal scan of the right kidney showing severe caliceal dilation. (C) Prone transverse scan of the same kidney. The dilated calices and renal pelvis look like 'mickey mouse'. This is the position to measure the dilated renal pelvis (between calipers). It is measured at its widest point in this prone position.

bladder and that the bladder wall appears normal. When unilateral, the investigative protocol is similar to that of renal pelvic dilation with the addition of an MCU because of the dilated ureter and in order to exclude vesicoureteric reflux.

Multicystic kidney (MCK)

This is a non-hereditary cystic kidney which is sometimes otherwise known as multicystic dysplastic kidney (Fig. 3.21). The characteristic feature of a multicystic kidney is the atretic ureter, and there

---

Box 3.5 Imaging protocol for renal pelvic dilation

Unilateral
- Postnatal ultrasound after 2–3 days.
- MAG3 renogram after 2–3 months if RPD > 15 mm.
- No MCU if no dilated ureter

Bilateral
- Same as unilateral but add MCU

MCU, micturating cystourethrogram.

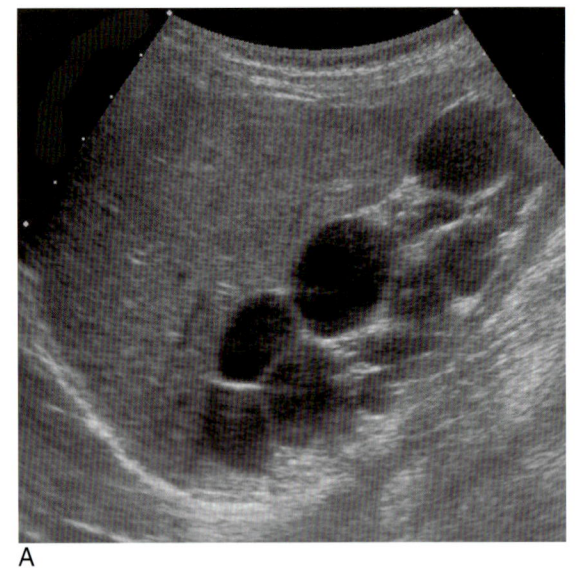

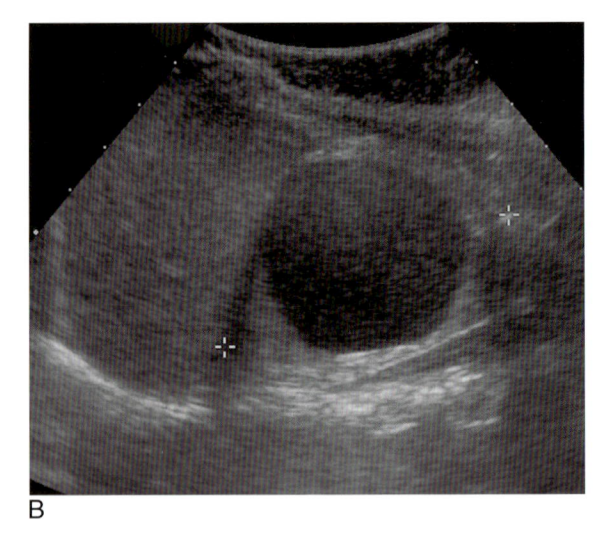

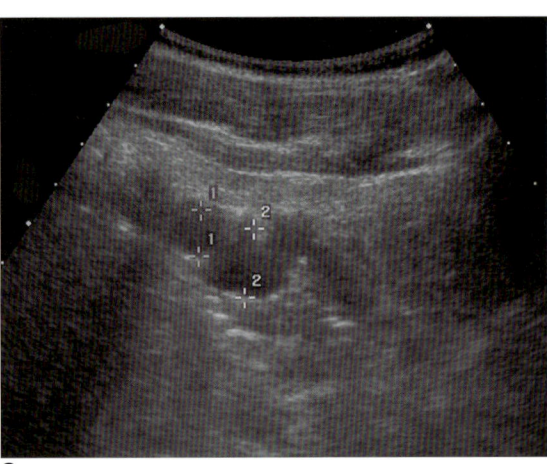

Figure 3.21 Variations in appearance of the multicystic kidney (MCK). (A) Longitudinal sonogram of the right kidney. There are a number of cysts of varying sizes. This is the typical appearance of a MCK. If the renal cortex can be identified then the diagnosis of MCK must be in doubt. (B) Longitudinal sonogram of the right kidney (between calipers). There is a single large cyst. (C) Prone longitudinal sonogram of the left flank. This is a small involuted MCK. Small cysts are measured between calipers. Since prenatal detection, the spectrum of appearances in MCK is wide: from a small single cyst to the large multiple cysts.

is no continuity between the glomerulus and the calices. On functional radionuclide studies they are non-functioning. The condition is more common in males, and the natural history is to involute with time either prenatally or postnatally. Urological opinion varies, and nowadays these kidneys are not removed unless they are causing symptoms or evidence of respiratory embarrassment. There have been reported associations with hypertension and malignancy, although generally these are not used as indications for early removal of the MCK.

Bilateral MCK is incompatible with life. The prognosis for unilateral MCK depends on the function of the contralateral kidney, for which there is a high association with abnormalities, usually PUJ or ureteric stenosis (30%).

Postnatal ultrasound and other imaging

Postnatal ultrasound should confirm the diagnosis of a multicystic kidney and provide a baseline for follow-up. In terms of management and prognosis, they are then divided into two groups. A MCK and normal contralateral kidney is considered to be simple, whereas a MCK with an abnormal contralateral kidney is considered to be complicated. The typical appearance of a MCK is a single large cyst with multiple smaller cysts. However, there is a wide variation in size and appearance of these kidneys. Normally no renal parenchyma should be seen around the edge of the cysts. If parenchyma is seen then the possibility of a large PUJ obstruction causing similar 'cystic' appearances should be considered. Nuclear medicine studies will not discriminate the two, as neither will function, and the prognosis is the same. A small proportion of multicystic kidneys will have a ureterocele in the bladder.

Box 3.6 gives an imaging protocol for MCK. The ultrasound examination should include measurement of the bipolar renal length of the MCK, measurement of the largest cyst and approximate number of cysts within the kidney. Follow-up examinations will therefore be able to assess whether the MCK is involuting. A small number may enlarge.

The contralateral kidney should be carefully examined for dilation of the calices, pelvis or ureter and for increased parenchymal echogenicity which may indicate renal dysplasia (Fig. 3.22).

There is a known association with ipsilateral and contralateral VUR. It is for this reason that cystography was originally advocated. However, it is well recognized that the grades of reflux are low and the contralateral kidney is unlikely to be damaged, so the current role of cystography is controversial.

In some centers a DMSA or MAG3 study is performed in order to document the normality of the contralateral kidney. This is also controversial, and some would only perform these examinations on an abnormal (so called 'complicated') contralateral kidney detected by ultrasound.

Cystic kidneys are discussed further on page 70.

Posterior urethral valves

Posterior urethral valves refers to a condition where quite simply a flap of mucosa obstructs the urethra. The mucosal flap extends from the wall of the urethra to the verumontanum and effectively acts as a 'windsock'. There is a pinhole orifice, so that a urinary catheter can be passed up the urethra but on micturition, the valve balloons so that there is an obstruction to the passage of urine out of the bladder and down the urethra. The clinical presentation is very variable, with the most obstructed systems detected prenatally and the less severely affected in early infancy. The appearances seen on ultrasound are related to a hypertrophy of the bladder wall as it tries to overcome the outflow obstruction. The kidney changes depend on the time of onset of the obstruction in intrauterine life, so that the earlier the onset, the higher the risk of severe consequences to the kidneys such as dysplasia. The later the onset, the more likely the kidneys will be simply hydronephrotic or in older boys may even be normal. Urinomas, or collections of urine around the kidney, develop when a calix ruptures because of the high pressure in the collecting system. This is a protective event for the kidney as it allows the kidney to decompress.

The presence of bilateral hydronephrosis and a full bladder during intrauterine life, associated with oligohydramnios, is the essential criterion for prenatal diagnosis (see Ch. 2). These infants need urgent

---

Box 3.6 Imaging protocol for MCK

Simple
- Postnatal ultrasound after 2–3 days
- No need for prophylactic antibiotics
- Repeat scan at 6 weeks
- DMSA or MAG3 renogram. If any function on these tests, MCK is unlikely. Refer to urologist

Complicated
Contralateral renal pelvic diameter > 15 mm
- Exclude obstruction.
- MAG3 renogram after 2–3 months
- Prophylactic antibiotics

Contralateral renal pelvic diameter < 15 mm with ureteric dilation
- MCUG and, if VUR, then follow as for VUR. If no VUR then follow as for simple kidney

postnatal imaging in order to confirm the diagnosis and allow early treatment of the bladder outflow obstruction. Also these infants have a high risk of developing a urinary tract infection which could further compromise the kidneys and even prove fatal.

Postnatal ultrasound findings may include bilateral hydronephrosis and hydroureters, echogenic cystic dysplastic kidneys, a urinoma where the urine has ruptured out of the kidney from a calix, and a thick-walled bladder (Fig. 3.23).

In suspected PUV a longitudinal ultrasound examination of the perineum using a high frequency linear transducer will be able to demonstrate the thick-walled bladder base and a dilated posterior urethra. This should be done when the infant is voiding so that there is maximal dilation of the posterior urethra (Fig. 3.24). Dilation of the posterior urethra measuring more than 7 mm is abnormal.

The infant suspected of having PUV should have an urgent MCU. Further management is then

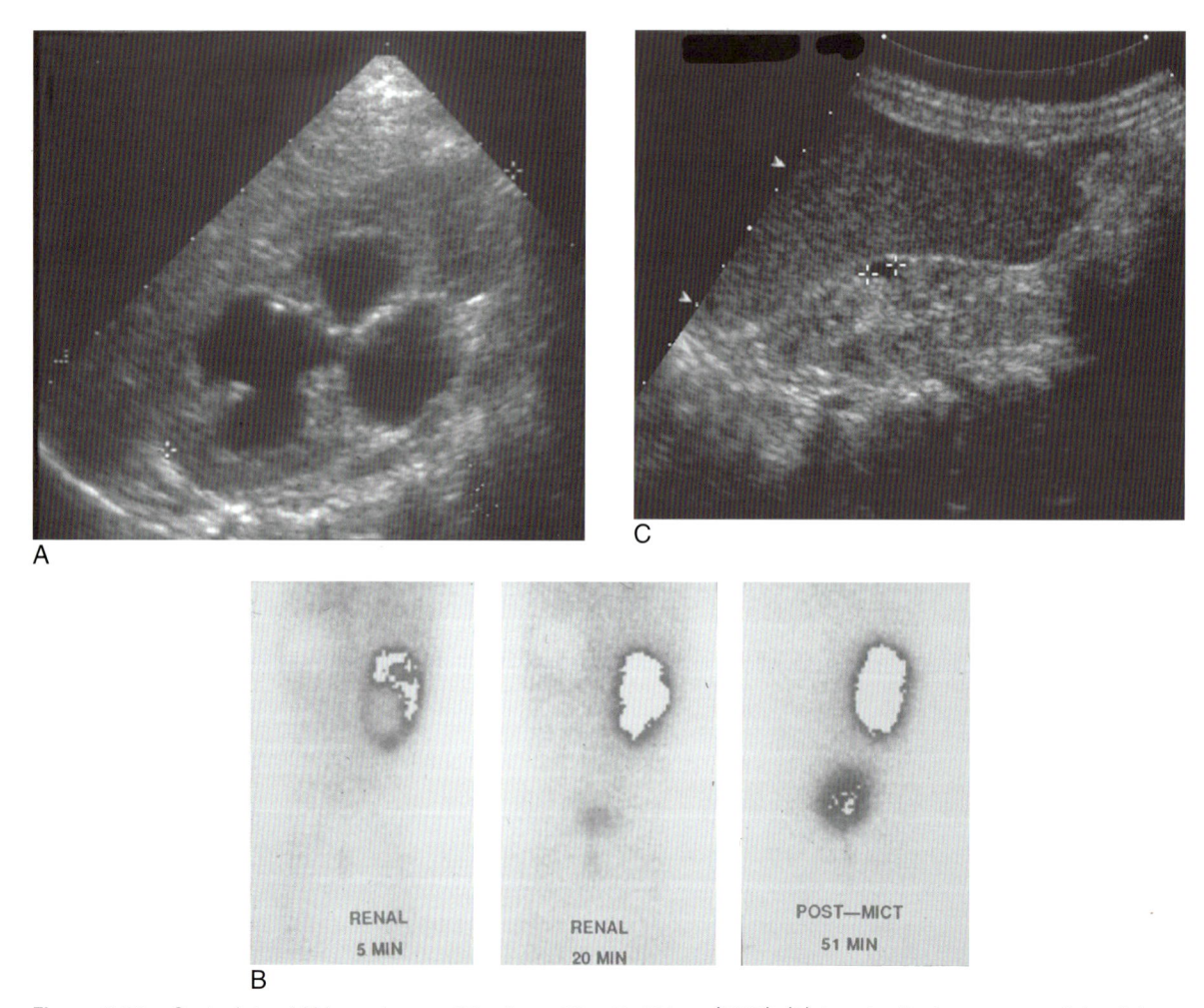

Figure 3.22 Contralateral kidney abnormalities in multicystic kidney (MCK). (A) Longitudinal sonogram of the right kidney showing dilation of the calices. The left kidney was multicystic. (B) This dynamic renogram in the same child demonstrates non-function on the side of the MCK and delayed transit of isotope through the dilated contralateral kidney. PUJ and ureteral stenoses are a well-recognized association with MCK. (C) This is the contralateral kidney in another child with an MCK. It shows a global increase in echogenicity with loss of the corticomedullary differentiation and a small subcortical cyst (between calipers) which is typical of cystic dysplasia.

THE URINARY TRACT 61

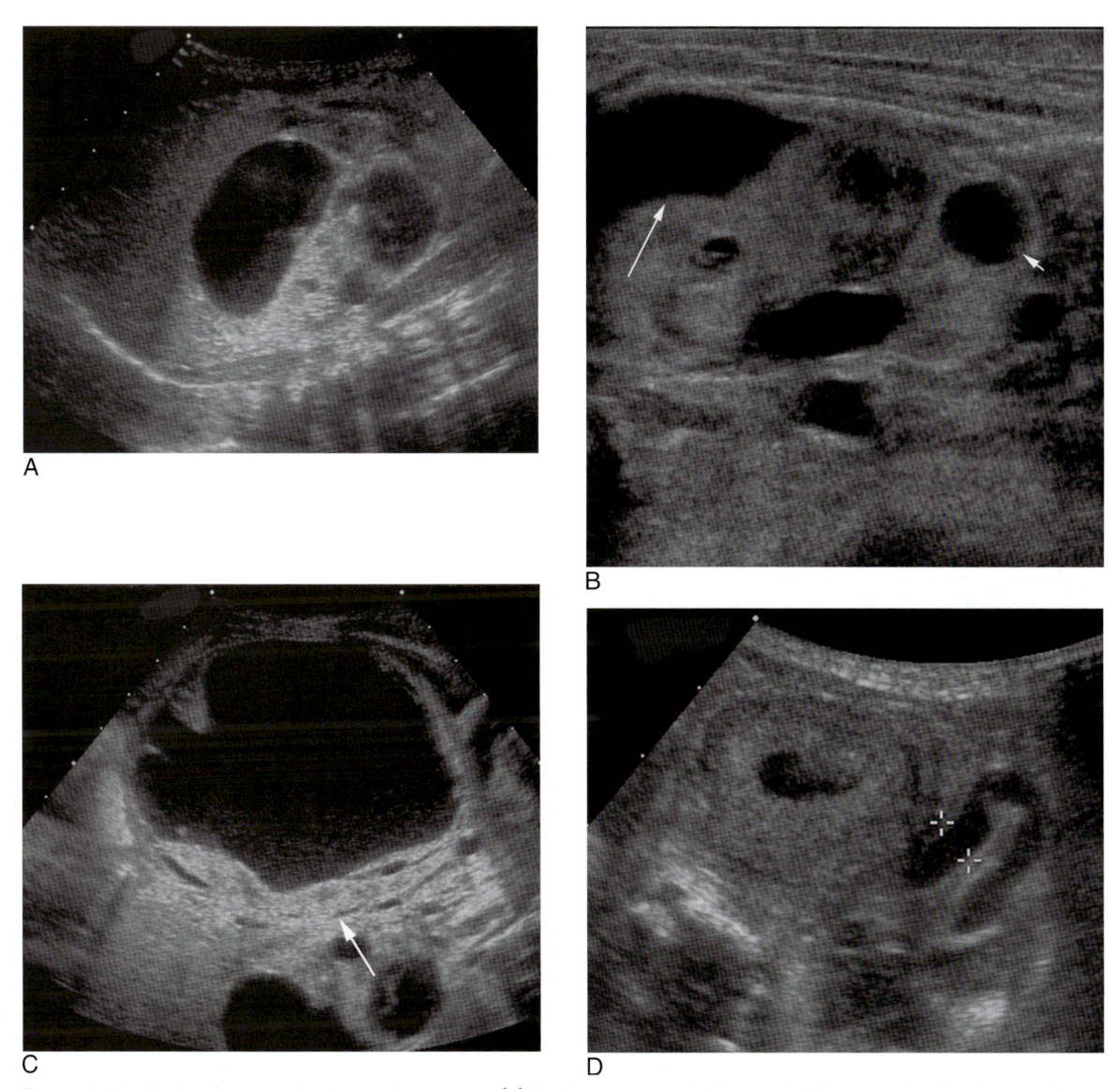

Figure 3.23 Posterior urethral valves and urinomas. (A) Supine sonogram of the right kidney showing two large cystic areas. This infant had a combination of a subcapsular urinoma and cystic dysplastic kidney as seen in posterior urethral valves. The renal cortex is very echogenic. (B) Prone longitudinal scan of the right kidney. The renal parenchyma is echogenic and there is a large cyst (small arrow) and a subcapsular urinoma (long arrow). The renal pelvis is also dilated. (C) Supine longitudinal scan of the contralateral left kidney. There is a large urinoma occupying the flank. The renal parenchyma is compressed posteriorly (arrow). (D) Transverse views of the bladder showing the markedly thickened bladder wall with dilated tortuous lower ureters (between calipers).

Continued

62 PEDIATRIC ULTRASOUND

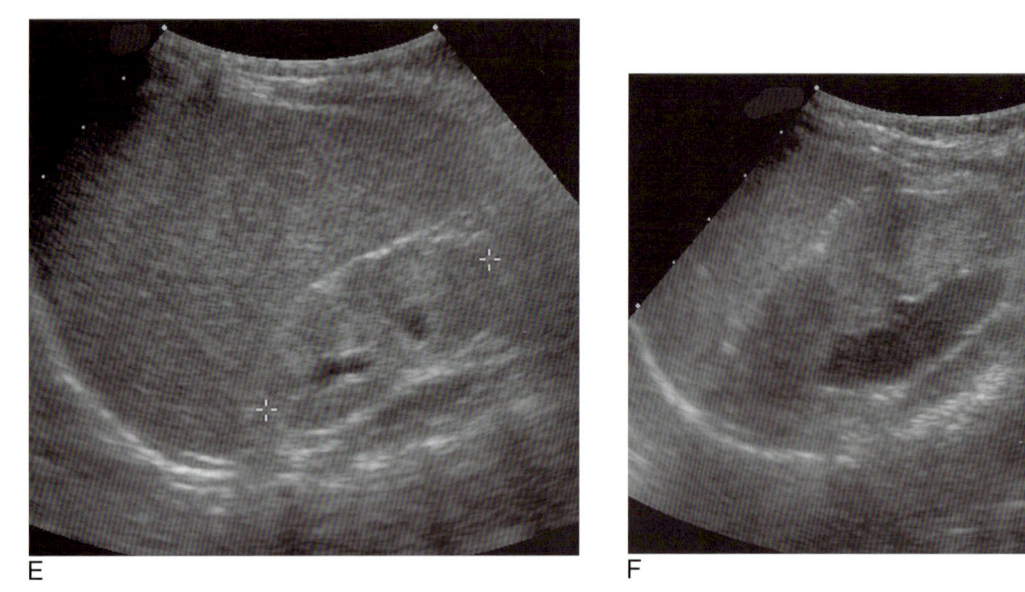

Figure 3.23, cont'd (E) Longitudinal sonogram of the right kidney (between calipers) in the same child 6 months later after relieving the posterior urethral valve obstruction. The right kidney is small but there are no longer cysts or fluid collections. There is only mild fullness of the collecting system. (F) Longitudinal sonogram of the left kidney after 6 months. There is a reasonable amount of renal parenchyma and the renal pelvis is dilated. There is no corticomedullary differentiation in either kidney, indicating that the kidneys are dysplastic.

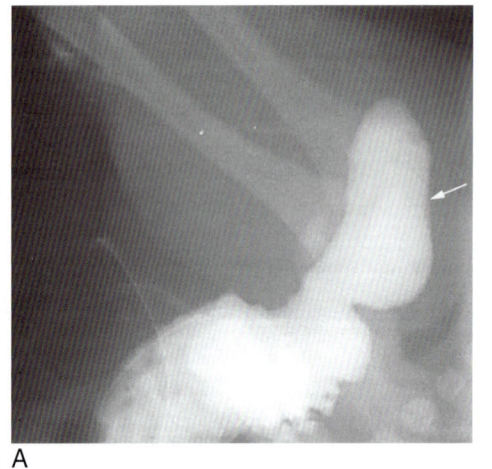

Figure 3.24 Ultrasound demonstration of posterior urethra in posterior urethral valves (PUV). (A) Micturating cystourethrogram on a male infant with PUV. The posterior urethra is markedly dilated (arrow). (B) Longitudinal sonogram of the posterior urethra scanned on the perineum in the same child. These are views with the infant micturating. Notice how the posterior urethra balloons during micturition and there is excellent demonstration of the dilation as seen in PUV.

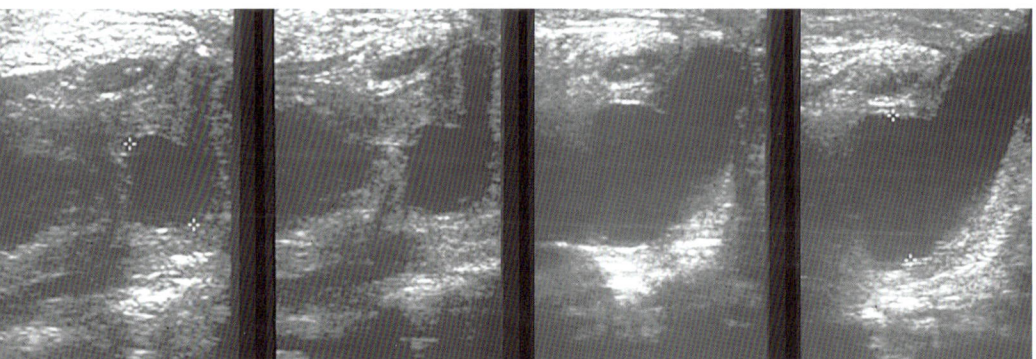

planned, such as valve ablation. Functional imaging is not undertaken immediately.

The duplex kidney

The duplex kidney can be very easy to diagnose but is also one of the most difficult and complex conditions, requiring the use of all imaging modalities. However, ultrasound plays an important diagnostic role, and the sonographer needs to be aware of all the variations in the condition's appearance and clinical presentation (Fig. 3.25). Dilated systems with ureteroceles tend to be detected prenatally, but older children may present with urinary tract infections and girls with constant 24-hour wetting.

Ultrasonically there are a number of features to look for:

- The duplex kidney may be longer than the contralateral kidney. A bifid renal pelvis is considered to be a normal variation (Fig. 3.26).
- The upper moiety obstructs and is associated with either a ureterocele in the bladder or ectopic drainage, for instance into the vagina.

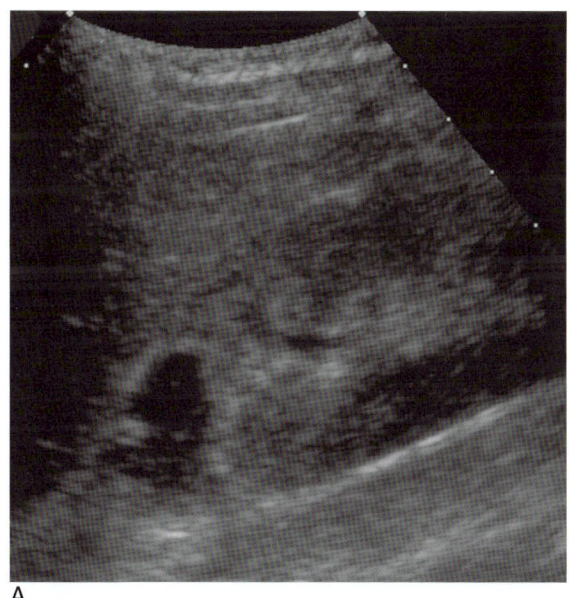

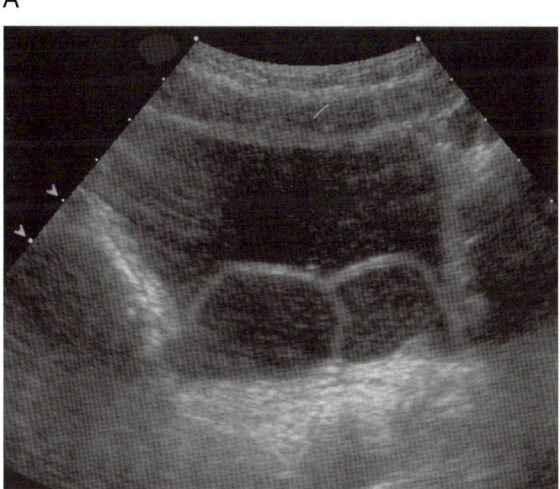

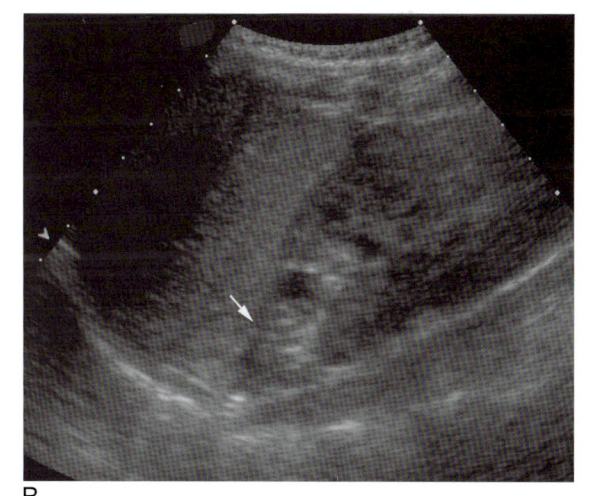

Figure 3.25 Bilateral duplex kidneys. This girl presented at the age of 6 years with a urinary tract infection. (A) Longitudinal sonogram of the right kidney showing a small dilated upper moiety of a duplex with a normal lower pole. (B) Longitudinal sonogram of the left kidney showing a small scarred upper pole with a mildly dilated calix (arrow). (C) Transverse sonogram of the bladder showing the two dilated ureteroceles in the bladder. This patient had small upper moieties which were associated with ureteroceles in the bladder.

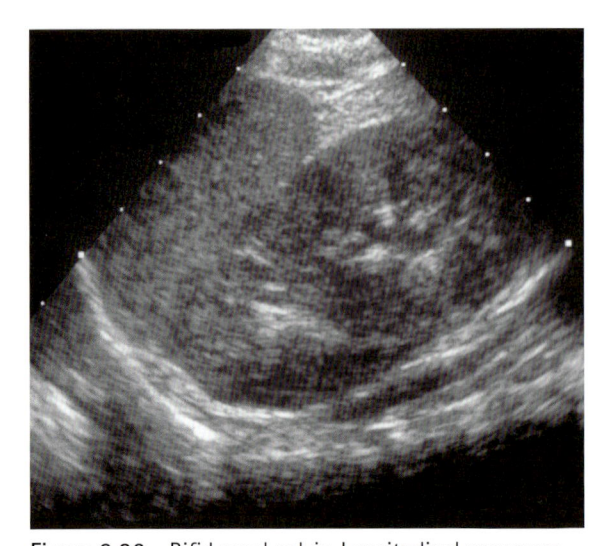

Figure 3.26 Bifid renal pelvis. Longitudinal sonogram of the left kidney. The renal sinus echoes are in two parts with intervening cortex. This is the most reliable appearance of an uncomplicated duplex or bifid renal pelvis. A bifid pelvis is a normal variant. Ultrasound is not always reliable to diagnose uncomplicated duplex systems and bifid renal pelves.

The ureters must be carefully examined in particular in a girl for entry into the vagina. The vagina full of fluid in a suspected duplex situation is an important finding.
- The upper moiety may have small peripheral cortical cysts and evidence of increased echogenicity and dysplasia (Fig. 3.27A).
- In a small cryptic duplex system the only finding may be a dilated ureter from the tiny upper moiety, which is often best detected on the prone views of the kidney as a tubular structure passing anterior to the kidney.
- The lower moiety dilates, which is usually VUR but may be RPD alone (Fig. 3.27B).
- Duplex kidneys are often bilateral.

The ultrasound diagnosis may be extremely difficult if there is a very small draining upper moiety and is easiest when there is dilation of one or both of the moieties in the duplex.

On functional imaging there may be equal function between upper and lower moiety. In some, the upper moiety function may be reduced

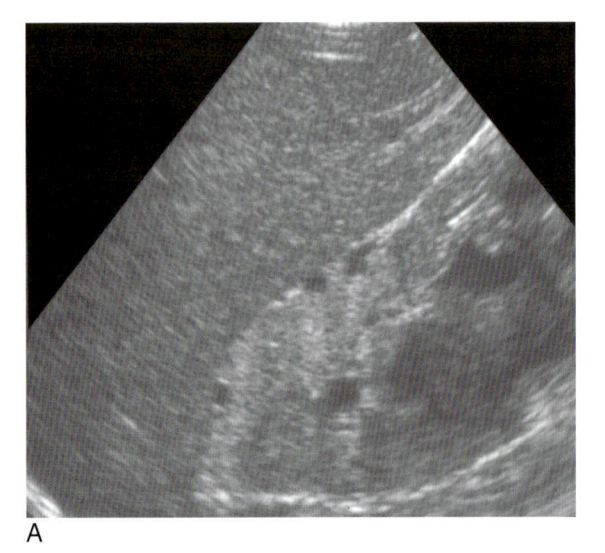

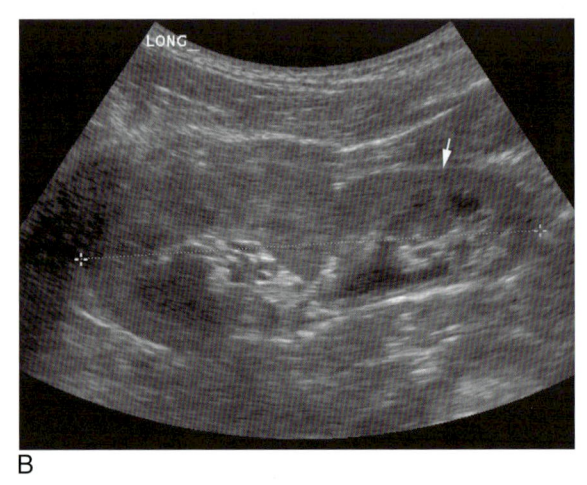

A   B

Figure 3.27 Duplex kidneys showing upper moiety dysplasia and lower moiety scarring. The images show two examples of complications that may occur in a duplex kidney: (A) In this duplex kidney the upper moiety is dysplastic. The ultrasound demonstrates increased echogenicity with loss of the corticomedullary differentiation and small subcortical retention cysts typical of dysplasia. (B) Prone longitudinal sonogram shows a duplex kidney with a normal upper moiety but gross cortical thinning of the lower moiety. Some uroepithelial thickening can also be seen. Thinning of the cortex in the lower moiety of a duplex is associated with vesicoureteric reflux into the lower moiety and renal damage (arrow).

THE URINARY TRACT 65

> **Box 3.7 Investigation of prenatally detected nephrourological abnormalities—general guidelines for referral to Nephrourology**[a]
>
> - Bilateral RPD with renal pelvic diameter > 15 mm and no reflux
> - Non-refluxing megaureters
> - Complicated multicystic dysplastic kidney
> - Dilated solitary kidney
> - Dilated upper or lower moiety of a duplex
> - Increasing RPD
> - Differential renal function < 40%
> - Symptomatic patients, e.g. UTI and pain
>
> [a]That is, all potentially obstructed systems and where surgical intervention may be required.
> RPD, renal pelvic dilation; UTI, urinary tract infection.

by dysplasia or obstruction. Lower moiety function may also be reduced by scarring from VUR. Cystograms must be performed. Nuclear medicine studies such as DMSA and MAG3 (see Table 3.2) are performed to show a differential function and drainage. An intravenous urogram is generally not needed in all duplex systems. However when the ultrasound and nuclear medicine studies do not entirely complement each other, this may then necessitate a carefully performed IVU.

Guidelines for referral

Box 3.7 summarizes indications for referral to Nephrourology.

URINARY TRACT INFECTION

Three percent of girls and 1% of boys have a symptomatic urinary tract infection (UTI) before the age of 11 years. All children should be thoroughly assessed and investigated following their first proven UTI.

Ultrasound is the first line of investigation in any child with a UTI. There are a number of terms related to UTIs with which the sonographer should be familiar:

- Proven urinary tract infection—a bacterial culture > 10^5 colony-forming units of a single organism per milliliter of urine gives a 90% probability of infection. Microscopy will demonstrate pyuria, or white cells in the urine, and organisms may be identified.
- Bacteriuria—the discovery of bacteria in the urine. This is usually incidental and the child is asymptomatic. Treatment will eradicate the bacteria, but recurrence is common. Asymptomatic bacteriuria does not need treatment and it does not cause renal damage.
- Acute pyelonephritis—acute infection involving the renal parenchyma.
- Recurrent urinary tract infection—a treated urinary tract infection but the child then presents with a further bacteriologically proven urinary tract infection.
- Renal abscess or focal nephronia—a focal renal abscess usually complicating acute pyelonephritis.

Imaging urinary tract infections

Broadly speaking, of 100 children presenting with UTIs, approximately 10 will have a dilating structural abnormality and another 10 will have renal abnormalities and changes associated with VUR and will therefore be at potential risk of developing hypertension. The dictum that only children with a proven UTI should be investigated does not hold true in the real world. Many children are sent for sonography with a clinical history (often even just a suspicion) of a UTI, and the high, often routine, workload can result in a complacent sonographer. It is incumbent on every sonographer undertaking these examinations to know what to look for on the ultrasound and perform a meticulous examination. The ultrasound must also be used to detect bladder dysfunction, so that every examination should include post-micturition views and a measurement of the residual bladder volume if there is one.

Structural abnormalities

This category includes all the congenital abnormalities such as pelvic kidneys, cross-fused ectopia, horseshoe kidneys and duplex systems. In particular, any obstructive uropathy and dilation of the collecting system should be sought.

Renal calculi

These are a potent cause of UTI in children. Stones are particularly associated with *Proteus* infections in boys, and any indication on the request form of a *Proteus* infection should immediately alert the sonographer to search for calculi. The report of the ultrasound examination in UTI should always make a specific statement about the presence or absence of renal calculi.

Direct or indirect evidence of vesicoureteric reflux and renal damage caused by infection

Embedded in the medical dogma is that ultrasound is not the gold standard for detecting renal scarring. To some (usually not sonographers) this may be true, but nowhere else in pediatric ultrasound is the diagnosis more reliant on the experience and expertise of the sonographer. While sonography may not be the investigation to detect renal scarring, it can go a long way towards making the diagnosis provided the sonographer is alert and knows what to look for.

Focal nephronia and renal abscess

Focal nephronia is the term used to describe the stage before a localized abscess in the kidney parenchyma has formed, and its appearance on ultrasound depends on the stage of its evolution and treatment. Early in the infective process where there is severe focal inflammation in the parenchyma, the kidney may simply appear swollen and enlarged compared with the normal kidney, sometimes with one particular pole being involved. The area usually has a lower reflectivity, is solid and ill-defined and may even be mistaken for a renal tumor. Later, often after no or inadequate treatment with antibiotics, the central area will liquefy and become necrotic and develop into a full blown abscess. Ultimately the area will become cystic and appear as a thick-walled simple cyst which will resolve over a number of months. If large, an abscess may even rupture out of the renal capsule or into the collecting system, producing a pyonephrosis. Small abscesses can be successfully treated with antibiotics but larger ones will need percutaneous drainage.

Often the clue to the diagnosis is in the clinical history of a preceding infection which has resulted in this bloodborne infection reaching the kidney.

Ultrasound examination

Features to look for in the kidneys are the following.

- Dilation of the collecting system is still the most easily and reliably detected abnormality in VUR. Uroepithelial thickening of the renal pelvis or of the lower ureter is often seen in association with the dilation but is non-specific.
- Any dilation of the ureter should be considered to be abnormal in these children.
- Increasing dilation of the upper tract collecting system post-micturition may give indirect evidence of existing VUR.
- Accurate bipolar prone lengths of both kidneys must be stated in the report, and comparative normal renal lengths from charts should be given. Renal scarring is predominantly polar in position. A difference of 10% in renal length can be accepted in children, after which the kidneys should be further imaged using a DMSA scan. The discrepancy in renal length may be related to polar cortical loss which may not be obvious or detected on the ultrasound.
- Evaluation of the renal cortical thickness is a good but often subtle finding. Careful evaluation of the thickness of the renal cortex must be made, comparing the distance from the edge of the renal capsule in relation to the central collecting system around the whole perimeter of the kidney in both the longitudinal and transverse planes (Fig. 3.28).
- An irregular outline with long, smooth areas of cortical thinning. Fetal lobulation must not be mistaken for focal cortical damage. The indentations from fetal lobulation are sharper, shorter and occur between the medullae.

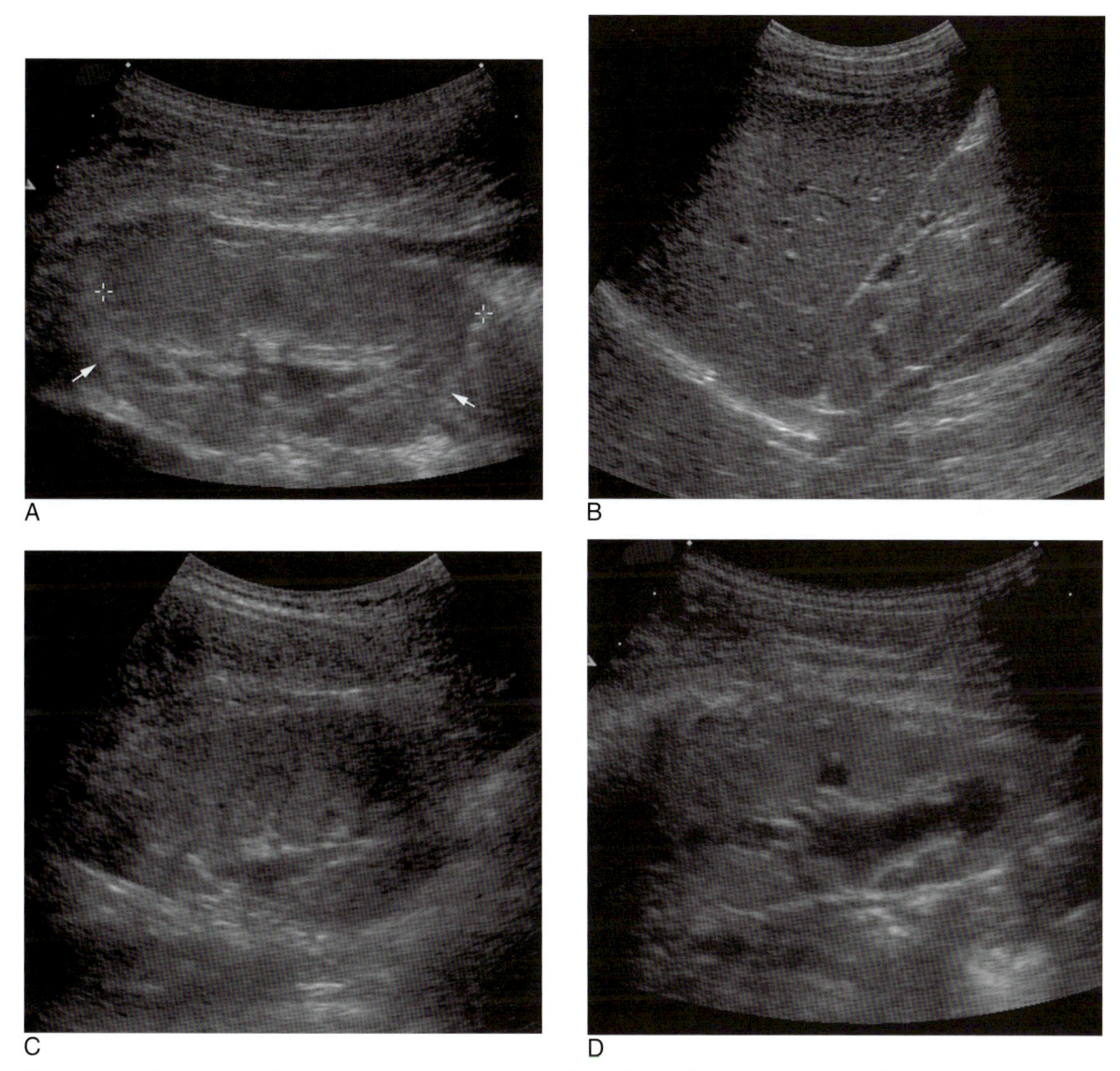

Figure 3.28 Examples of kidneys with cortical thinning. (A) Longitudinal sonogram of the right kidney (between calipers). There is cortical thinning and this is predominantly polar (arrows). Cortical thinning can be diagnosed on ultrasound by comparing the relationship of the central sinus echoes and the edge of the cortex. (B) & (C) Supine and longitudinal scan of the right kidney. There is cortical thinning anteriorly, seen best on the supine view. On the prone view the cortical thinning is also affecting the poles of the kidney. (D) Longitudinal sonogram of the left kidney showing that the whole kidney is globally small with dilation of the calices. When the kidney becomes small and scarred there is an increase in echogenicity. When differentiating small kidneys it is important to assess whether they appear scarred or just small. Subtle pointers include irregular outline, corticomedullary loss, collecting system dilation and uroepithelial thickening.

- Increase in echogenicity with loss of corticomedullary differentiation. This is a later finding in the progression of reflux nephropathy, and the kidneys tend to be smaller at this stage and the cortical outline irregular.
- Focal or diffuse caliceal dilation associated with cortical thinning. Focal caliceal dilation which extends up to the edge of the renal cortex is abnormal (see Fig 3.28D). Harmonic imaging is very useful for enhancing the edges and increasing the contrast between parenchyma and dilated calix. If available it should be used as an adjunct when trying to confirm the diagnosis.
- Small echogenic damaged kidney with an irregular outline. This is the last and end-stage of reflux nephropathy. It is to be hoped that all sonographers will be able to detect this.

In addition to the kidneys, the bladder must be carefully examined with regard to the bladder wall thickness, contour or diverticulae, and all children must have a post-micturition residue assessed.

Imaging protocol for urinary tract infection

The imaging protocols for investigating a child with UTI are extremely controversial, and the following serves to provide a guideline which limits invasive procedures and excessive investigation. UTI investigation has generated a massive workload for Radiology departments and exposed large numbers of children to significant radiation without much evidence of benefit. Among pediatric radiologists there has been a swing away from invasive cystography to demonstrate VUR. In Sweden children over 2 years old with simple UTIs are not referred for further imaging procedures unless there is an additional risk factor such as recurrent UTI or evidence of upper tract involvement. The prevalence of renal scarring is low in Sweden, and this is thought to be related to the excellent facilities for early diagnosis and treatment of UTIs.[19-21]

Imaging first proven urinary tract infection

The protocol for imaging a first UTI depends on the age of the child. The reason for this is that the natural history of VUR is to resolve and disappear in the older the child, so that cystography is likely to be negative in an older child. Also, the progression to renal damage from VUR is extremely rare in the older child.

- Over 5 years of age, only an ultrasound examination is required. No further imaging should be done if this is normal.
- Under 5 years of age, the initial investigation is an ultrasound examination with a DMSA (see Table 3.2) 3–6 months after the UTI. The rationale is that a normal DMSA excludes significant reflux. If the DMSA is abnormal some form of cystography is required and this will depend on the child's age and sex.
- In children who are not yet potty-trained, males require a conventional contrast micturating cystourethrogram (MCU) in order to demonstrate the urethra. Females can have a direct radioisotope cystogram (DIC) as there is no pathology of the urethra and the radiation burden is less.
- In older potty-trained children a MAG3 and IRC (see Table 3.2) are sufficient to show differential function of the kidneys, drainage and VUR.[22-24]

The use of ultrasound contrast cystography and urosonography has been reported, mainly in Germany. The only advantage it really offers over other means of cystography is that there is no radiation burden, as ultrasound is used. Children still need to be catheterized in order to instill the contrast and the urethra is not shown. Ultrasound contrast media is expensive and not universally licensed for use in children.

Children should not be overinvestigated, and excessive investigation in the search for the single 'scar' should be resisted. The evidence is that hypertension occurs in severely damaged kidneys, which ultrasound should be able to detect.

Recurrent urinary tract infections

Recurrent urinary tract infections require a full ultrasound and DMSA scan after 3–6 months. Depending on the findings, cystography may be indicated.

THE URINARY TRACT

Unusual infections

Xanthogranulomatous pyelonephritis (XPN)

This is an unusual form of chronic infection of the kidney. These children present with an abdominal mass, failure to thrive, anemia and weight loss. Urine cultures may be positive, particularly for *Proteus* and *E. coli*.[25] The pathogenesis is controversial and is thought to be related to an abnormal response to obstruction and infection, with infiltration of the kidney by lipid-laden macrophages or xanthoma cells.

XPN may involve whole or part of a kidney and there is usually calcification present (Fig. 3.29). It is sometimes mistaken for a neoplasm as it appears solid on ultrasound, but there are two features that should alert the sonographer: one is the presence of dense calcification, and the second is rupture and extrarenal extension as the infected mass ruptures through the renal capsule. There may be cystic areas of breakdown and necrosis. These children will go on to further cross-sectional imaging, and the treatment is removal of the non-functioning kidney.

Renal candidiasis

This may occur most typically in pre-term infants who have had long term antibiotic treatment or in immunocompromised children. Infants with obstructive uropathies, such as posterior urethral valves, are also highly susceptible.

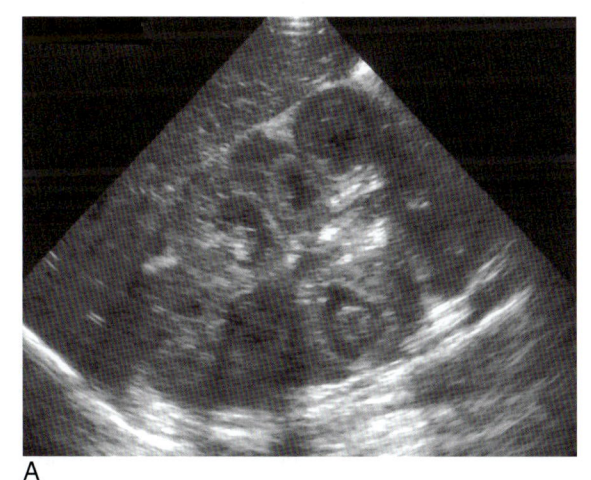

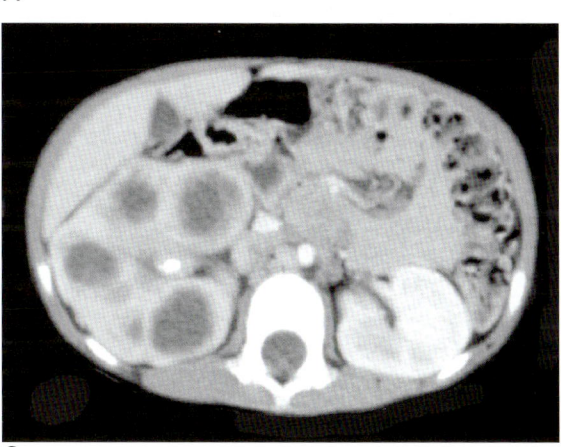

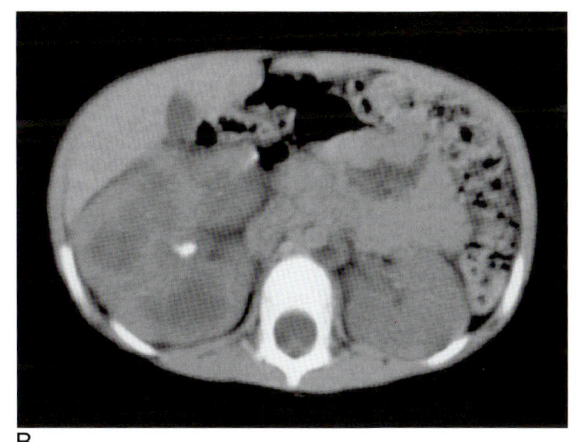

Figure 3.29 Xanthogranulomatous pyelonephritis (XPN). (A) Longitudinal sonogram of the right kidney. There are markedly echogenic calcific foci. The kidneys are usually non-functioning on nuclear medicine studies and may be mistaken for a solid renal tumor.
(B) Unenhanced CT examination showing the large right kidney and the calculus in the renal pelvis. (C) Enhanced CT on the same child showing the calculus in the renal pelvis and the dilated calices.

Sonographic appearances The kidney may be globally hyperechoic with loss of the corticomedullary differentiation. There may be dilation of the calices with clumping of the fungal balls, or mycetoma, in the collecting system, causing obstruction (Fig. 3.30). Simple bacterial infection usually produces a diffuse increase in particulate matter in the collecting system, such as in a pyonephrosis. There may be small parenchymal hypoechoic abscesses within the kidney.

Tuberculosis

Tuberculous involvement of the kidney is uncommon. The appearances are typically described as infundibular stenosis and localized cavitation of the parenchyma. The other typical appearance is the so-called autonephrectomy where the kidney is completely destroyed by the caseating mass.

CYSTIC KIDNEYS

Cystic disease of the kidneys in childhood is a confusing and complicated subject. Also the complex and often contradictory nomenclature used to describe cystic kidneys is not an aid to understanding the subject. This section aims to provide the sonographer with a simple approach to cystic kidneys in children.[26]

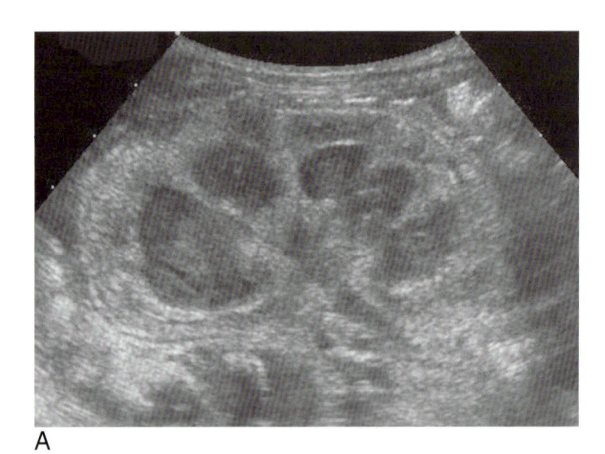

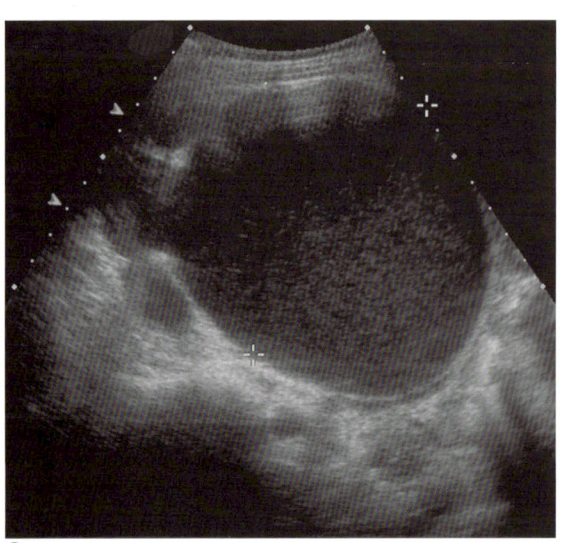

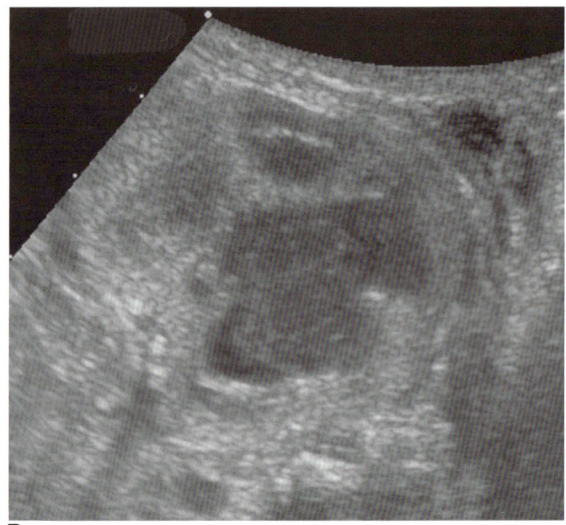

Figure 3.30 Renal candidiasis. (A) & (B) Longitudinal and transverse sonogram of the left kidney. The renal parenchyma has an increased echogenicity. The collecting system is dilated, and there are solid clumps of fungal balls obstructing the system. These appearances are almost exclusively seen in candidal fungal balls. Premature infants on long-term antibiotics are particularly vulnerable. (C) Transverse sonogram of the left kidney in a large bacterially infected pelviureteric junction obstruction (between calipers). There are diffuse echoes throughout the dilated collecting system without clumping. This reflects the cellular debris seen within the system. Clumping does not usually occur in infected systems, but layering of particulate debris may occur as in this kidney. These appearances may also be seen in infected urine in the bladder.

Terminology

- Multicystic kidney or multicystic dysplastic kidney—this refers to many cysts in one kidney often containing some dysplastic elements. Not all multicystic kidneys are dysplastic. The condition is still considered to be non-hereditary. If the multicystic kidney is unilateral, the other kidney may be normal, hydronephrotic or dysplastic. If bilateral, it is incompatible with life, and infants die soon after birth with hypoplastic lungs and/or renal failure.
- Cystic dysplasia—dysplastic kidneys can be unilateral or bilateral, usually contain cysts and are disorganized, containing ectopic tissue such as cartilage and muscle. They may function. Ultrasonically they usually appear small and echogenic with small peripheral cortical cysts. While dysplastic kidneys are often hypoplastic, not all small kidneys are dysplastic. The clinical features are very variable from a normal appearing neonate to a very dysmorphic infant. Dysplastic kidneys are associated with urinary tract obstruction, and many syndromes are associated with cystic dysplastic kidneys. Bilateral renal dysplasia will result in progressive renal failure.
- Polycystic kidney disease refers to two conditions: autosomal recessive polycystic kidney disease and autosomal dominant renal disease.
  —Autosomal recessive polycystic kidneys were previously known as infantile polycystic kidneys. Confusingly these kidneys appear highly echogenic on ultrasound. There is generalized dilation of the collecting tubules.
  —Autosomal dominant renal disease was previously known as adult polycystic kidney disease. Cysts develop anywhere along the nephron.

The ultimate diagnosis of the cystic renal disorder is not dependent on any one imaging modality and will depend on many factors. Sources of information when trying to come to the diagnosis should be collated from many areas, such as:

- obstetric history of the mother
- prenatal history and fetal ultrasonography
- family history information
- clinical examination of the child
- radiology of patient and parents
- laboratory data, for example DNA
- pathology if a biopsy is taken or from any other family members that may have had a biopsy or nephrectomy in the past.

Ultrasound is still the imaging modality of choice in children, and the findings on ultrasound will direct further imaging as required. The ultrasound approach to any cystic renal disease in children must include observations about the following, which should be carefully stated in the ultrasound report.

- unilateral or bilateral renal cysts (bilateral involvement is more common in the genetically inherited conditions)
- size of the kidneys—are they large or small?
- localization to one part of the kidney or diffuse involvement of the whole kidney. Is there a capsule around the cysts?
- extrarenal cysts, in particular in the liver or pancreas
- liver size and hepatic parenchyma appearance
- presence of a large spleen and portal hypertension.

Renal cysts are common and may be hereditary, developmental or acquired. The classification of cystic renal disease varies according to the perspective from which it is written, and despite a vast amount of literature on the subject, there is still no generally accepted classification in existence. The early Potter classification is of limited value for clinical practice because not all types represent clinical entities.

The following classification is by no means all inclusive but aims to emphasize the important clinical cystic disorders likely to be encountered by the sonographer. Broadly speaking, cystic disease of the kidneys can be divided into two groups—genetic disease and non-genetic disease:

- Genetic disease
  —autosomal recessive polycystic kidney disease (ARPKD)
  —autosomal dominant polycystic kidney disease (ADPKD)
  —juvenile nephronophthisis and medullary cystic disease complex
  —glomerulocystic kidney disease
  —cysts with multiple malformation syndromes;

- Non-genetic disease
    - —simple cysts
    - —multicystic dysplastic kidney
    - —multilocular cysts
    - —acquired renal cystic disease (chronic renal failure)
    - —caliceal diverticulum
    - —medullary sponge kidney.

Genetic disease

Autosomal recessive polycystic kidney disease (ARPKD)

This is a generalized cystic dilation of the renal collecting tubules so that the kidneys are packed to a greater or lesser degree with tiny little cysts (Fig. 3.31). It is much rarer than the autosomal dominant form and occurs in 1 in 50 000 people. Prenatal diagnosis can be made but there are false positive and false negative diagnoses.[27] Congenital

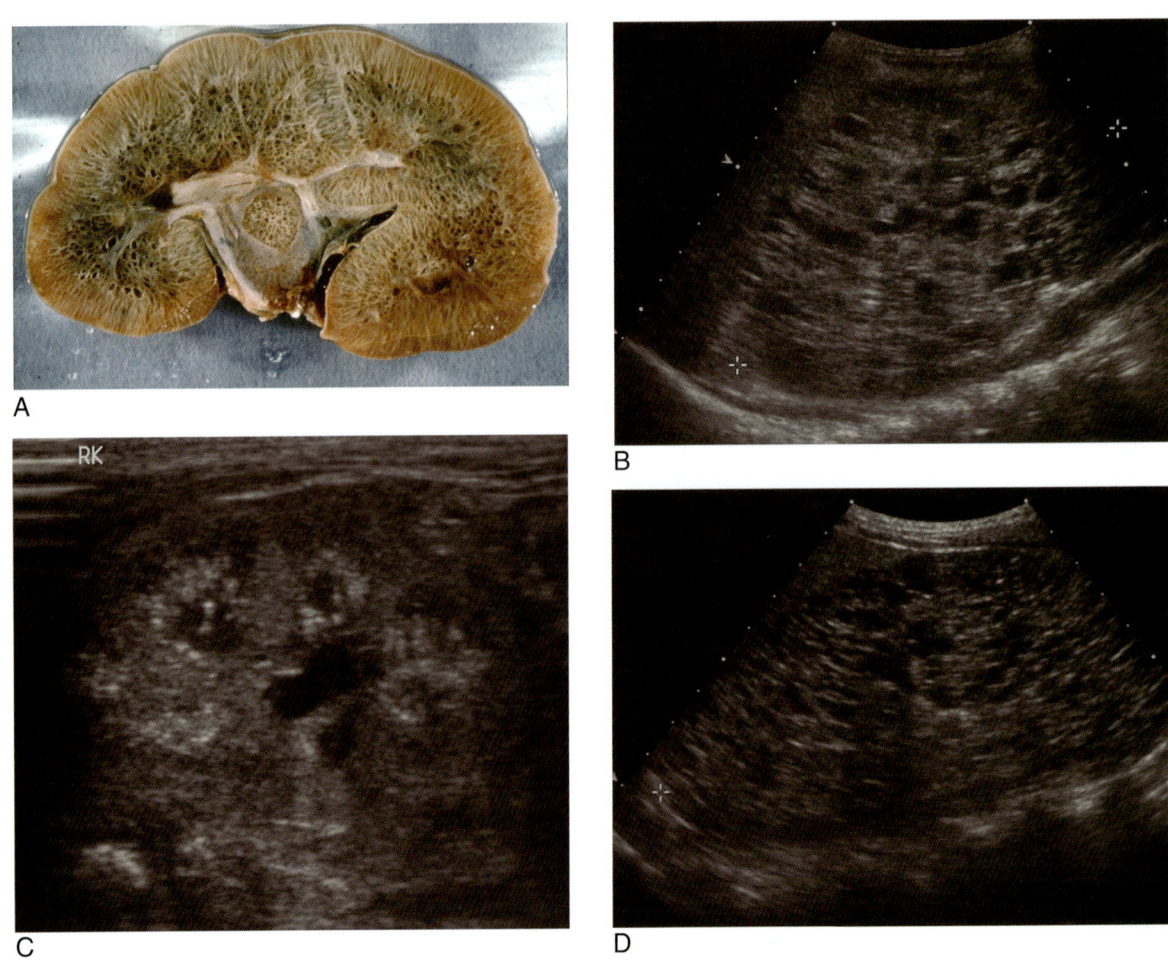

Figure 3.31 Autosomal recessive polycystic kidney disease (ARPKD). (A) Cut section of a postmortem specimen in a patient with ARPKD. There are multiple small cysts throughout the whole of the renal substance. It is these multiple cysts with their posterior acoustic enhancement which give the hyperechogenic appearances on ultrasound. (B–D) Sonograms of the kidney in three patients with ARPKD to demonstrate the wide variation in appearance. The kidneys are all large, over the 95th centile, and are globally hyperechoic. The visible cysts are generally small, rarely exceeding 2 cm. Sometimes the increase in echogenicity is primarily medullary.

hepatic fibrosis is a prerequisite for the diagnosis of ARPKD.

There are two types of presentation of ARPKD depending on the age of the patient and the dominance of the renal or the hepatic disease. In those children who present at birth or during the neonatal period the renal disease dominates, while in those who present later in childhood or adolescence the liver disease dominates, with much milder renal manifestations. The hepatic disease in these children is called congenital hepatic fibrosis with renal tubular ectasia and comes to medical attention because of the problems associated with hepatic fibrosis, such as splenomegaly, portal hypertension, varices and bleeding.

Gross cystic dilation of the intrahepatic biliary tree is usually called Caroli syndrome. The original description was purely of the hepatic disease, but dilation of the bile ducts is seen in early presenting ARPKD and in the milder end of the renal spectrum of renal tubular ectasia.

The risk for a sibling of having this condition is 25%, and the parents' kidneys should be normal.

Sonographic Appearances

- There is a wide spectrum of appearances from birth and with increasing age throughout childhood.
- There is bilateral equal involvement of the kidneys, and the reniform shape is usually maintained.
- The kidneys must be big and are generally over the 90th centile for age in the young. With increasing age and progression of the renal disease, fibrosis may result in stabilization and comparative decrease in the renal size.
- The inhomogeneous global increase in echo texture is due to the myriad of microcysts presenting multiple acoustic interfaces.
- In some a subcapsular rim of normal hypoechoic cortex is diagnostic.
- Medullary pyramids may be hypoechoic at birth in some less severely affected but over time become hyperechoic. In older children the corticomedullary differentiation is usually lost.
- Visible macrocysts are uncommon but can be seen, and they are generally no more than 1–2 cm in diameter. They become more common with age.

- Hepatic fibrosis is always present. The hepatic echo texture may be normal but, with increasing fibrosis, will become coarse and increased particularly in the periportal region.
- The liver must be carefully examined for lesions which are cystic dilations of the biliary tree. The hepatic cystic lesions are not true cysts but rather 'out-pouchings' of the bile ducts (Fig. 3.32).
- In older children, because of the hepatic fibrosis and liver disease, portal hypertension may be present. Evidence of portal hypertension with an enlarged spleen and varices must be sought.
- Doppler examination of the liver, spleen and portal system is an essential part of the examination in these children.

Further imaging When the child is older and over the neonatal period, an IVU is performed. This will demonstrate the streaky radiating pattern of contrast which is almost pathognomonic of ARPKD (Fig. 3.33). The importance of doing this examination is that in showing the caliceal pattern it will help exclude other causes of large echogenic kidneys in the neonatal period, such as dysplasia.

A hepatic iminodiacetic acid (HIDA) scan should be performed at about 1 year of age. If performed too early the HIDA scan will be normal

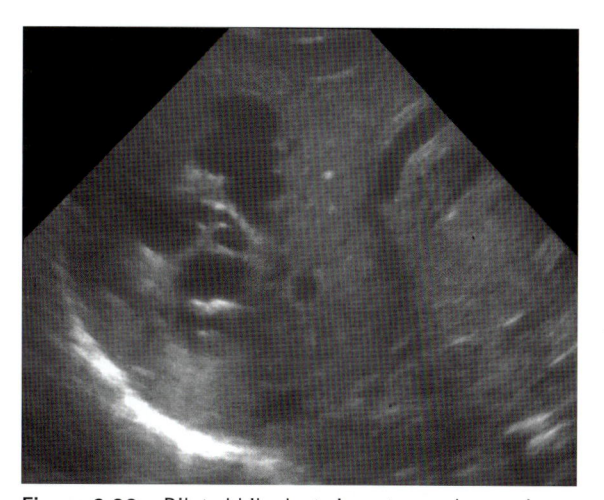

Figure 3.32 Dilated bile ducts in autosomal recessive polycystic kidney disease (ARPKD). Longitudinal sonogram of the liver showing the dilated cystic spaces. These are not cysts but dilations of the bile ducts. The liver should always be carefully examined in all children suspected of having ARPKD.

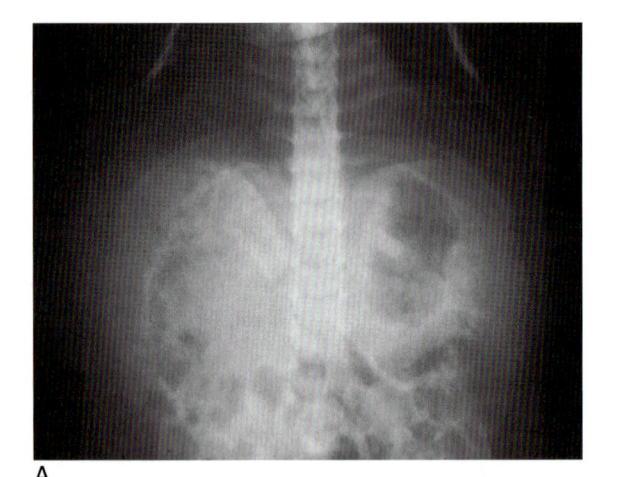

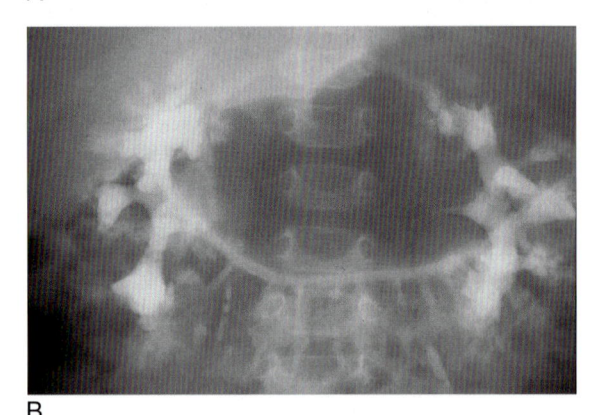

Figure 3.33 Intravenous urogram (IVU) in autosomal recessive polycystic kidney disease (ARPKD). (A) & (B) Two examples of the IVU appearances of ARPKD. The urogram should always be performed to demonstrate the caliceal pattern. This will demonstrate the typical radiating appearance of the contrast as it passes through the collecting system and help differentiate the dysplastic 'bright' kidneys.

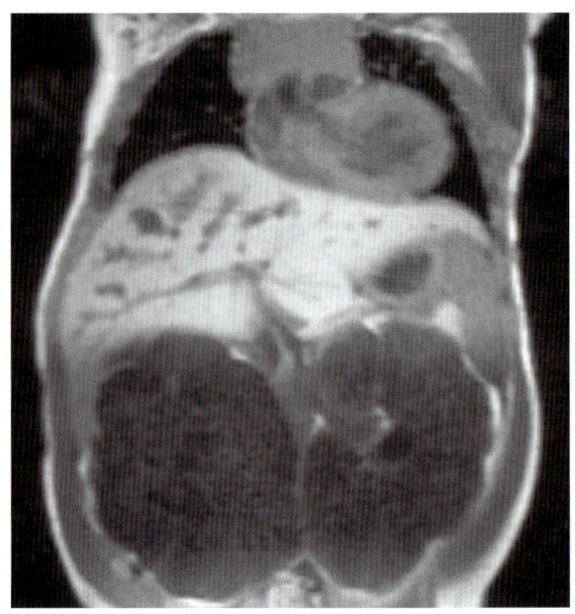

Figure 3.34 MRI examination in autosomal recessive polycystic kidney disease (ARPKD). This infant with ARPKD had an MRI because of apnoeic attacks. The examination was done to exclude a pulmonary artery sling, which was not present. The kidneys are huge, filling the abdomen and compressing the lungs. Note also the cystic areas in the liver, which are areas of bile duct dilation as seen in Figure 3.32.

but, if delayed, the effects of the hepatic fibrosis will have had time to manifest. This involves a radioisotope tracer excreted in the bile and will demonstrate accumulation and stasis of isotope in the cystic areas and delayed clearance from the abnormal liver. A large left lobe of liver may also be seen.

CT and MRI are rarely needed except in uncertain cases (Fig. 3.34). DMSA scan is not always performed but may show focal defects in the kidney.

Autosomal dominant polycystic kidney disease (ADPKD)

ADPKD is a cystic renal disorder which usually becomes manifest after the third decade of life. It is common with an estimated prevalence of approximately 1 in 1000. Two, possibly three genetic loci have been identified. There is considerable variability in the severity of the disease, and some affected individuals may present in childhood and are even detected prenatally. Cysts are found in the kidneys of 64% of children with *PKD1* under 10 and in 90% under 19 years of age.[28]

ADPKD is a systemic disease with renal and extrarenal manifestations. The extrarenal manifestations, such as liver, pancreatic and splenic cysts, are much more likely to present in adulthood. The risk of a sibling having the condition is 50%, but in the extremely rare case of a spontaneous mutation there will be no risk. There should be one affected parent (unless they are too young to demonstrate cysts or also in the rare case of a spontaneous mutation). A positive family history or the demonstration of one affected parent is one of the major criteria for the diagnosis of ADPKD in a child.

Intravenous urogram IVU is generally not indicated in suspected ADPKD as it does not provide any more information than obtained with an ultrasound. The IVU will show displaced calices around the intrarenal cystic masses, and the appearances are indistinguishable from other intrarenal masses such as lymphoma.[29]

Sonographic features Well-defined cysts can be identified in otherwise normal-looking kidneys. It is very rare to have unilateral cysts. If cysts are only found in one kidney another diagnosis should be considered. The kidneys are generally affected unequally and vary from a kidney with just a few isolated cysts to one packed full of cysts (Fig. 3.35). The more cysts in the kidneys the larger the renal size with a lobulated outline. In an infant with an early neonatal presentation, the kidneys may be very large and echogenic and the appearances indistinguishable from those of ARPKD. When bilateral cystic kidneys are found in a young child with no family history, the differential diagnosis of tuberous sclerosis must be actively excluded.

Tuberous sclerosis

This is an autosomal dominant multisystem disease with a reported prevalence of 1 in 10 000. Increasing awareness and recognition of the condition probably accounts for the increased prevalence in the reported literature. Tuberous sclerosis complex is the preferred term as it emphasizes the multiple organs involved. The condition is characterized by multiple hamartomas in the brain, skin, heart, kidneys, liver, lungs and bone. The lesions become clinically detectable at different ages, and the following are more frequently seen in children.

The most common clinical manifestations are those of the nervous system and skin. Fibrous forehead plaques may be present at birth whereas facial angiofibromas appear after 3 years with a peak at about 10 years. Subependymal giant cell astrocytomas develop between 5 and 15 years and stop growing at 20 years. The other lesions in the central nervous system include cortical tubers and subependymal glial nodules. Children who have seizures at an early age are at particular risk of mental retardation. Other manifestations in children include symptoms related to the cardiac

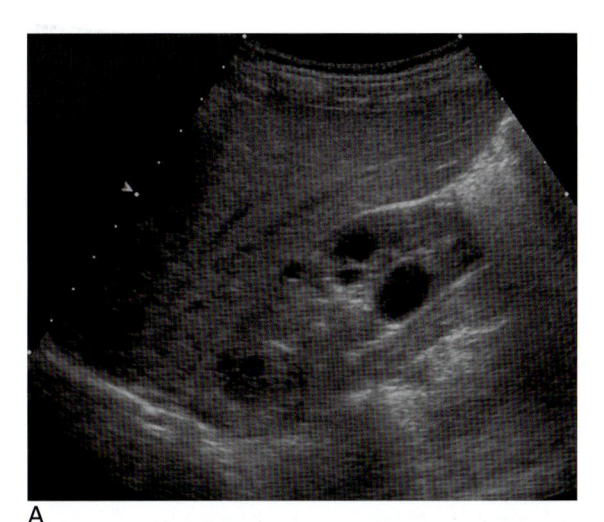

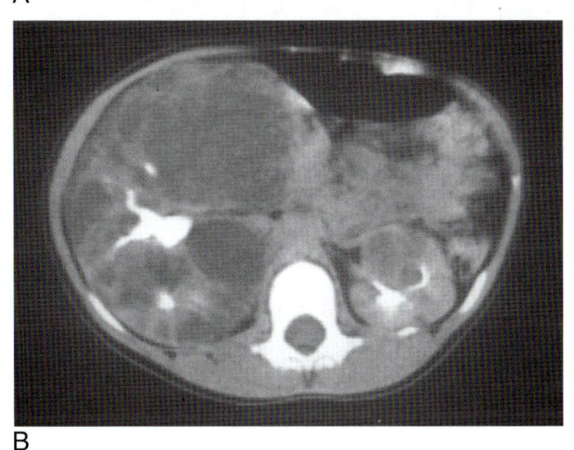

Figure 3.35 Autosomal dominant polycystic kidney disease (ADPKD). (A) Longitudinal sonogram of the kidney in a child with familial *PKD1*-type ADPKD. The kidney has a basically normal sonographic appearance but contains varying numbers and sizes of cysts. The kidneys may be involved asymmetrically, and eventually the cysts will come to occupy the whole kidney, squashing any normal renal parenchyma and ultimately leading to renal failure. This is rare in children and usually occurs later in adult life. (B) CT examination in another girl with ADPKD. The kidneys are asymmetrically involved, with multiple cysts replacing most of the right kidney and a few cysts on the left.

rhabdomyomas which are present at birth and diminish in size and even disappear in later years. They are often multiple and are most frequently located in the ventricular septum. They occur in up to 50% of affected children, with a higher frequency in the first 2 years.

The frequency of renal involvement is second only to that of the nervous system. Cysts are seen in the kidneys which are indistinguishable from those in ADPKD, but the children are usually young and generally within the first year of life.

Characteristic small echogenic angiomyolipomas are found in older children since they develop and grow in childhood and adolescence. They are benign tumors composed of abnormal thickened wall vessels and varying amounts of smooth muscle-like cells and adipose tissue. They are not noted to be locally invasive in children. Later the coexistence of cysts and angiomyolipomas is pathognomonic for tuberous sclerosis.

The main complications of renal angiomyolipomas relates to their potential to hemorrhage and, very rarely in children, tumor formation.[30]

Sonographic appearances These may be threefold:

- multiple well-defined cystic areas indistinguishable from those of autosomal dominant ADPKD (Fig. 3.36)
- small echogenic foci scattered throughout the otherwise normal-looking renal parenchyma (Fig. 3.37)
- a mixture of small cysts and angiomyolipomas (Fig. 3.38).

In a young child presenting with cystic kidneys indistinguishable from ADPKD and no family history, further imaging should include a cranial MRI and cardiac echo to exclude the intracranial tumors and cardiac rhabdomyomas (see Fig. 3.36B,C).

Juvenile nephronophthisis / medullary cystic disease complex

This is a heterogeneous group of disorders originally described as two different conditions. At least two forms are recognized on the basis of inheritance and clinical presentation: a juvenile recessive form and an adult dominant form.

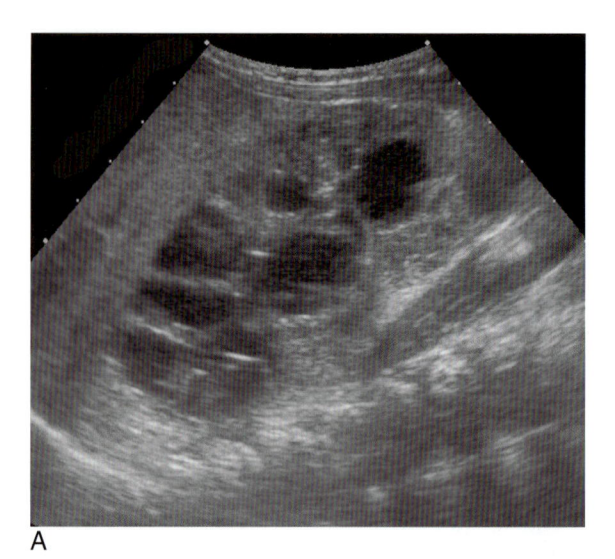

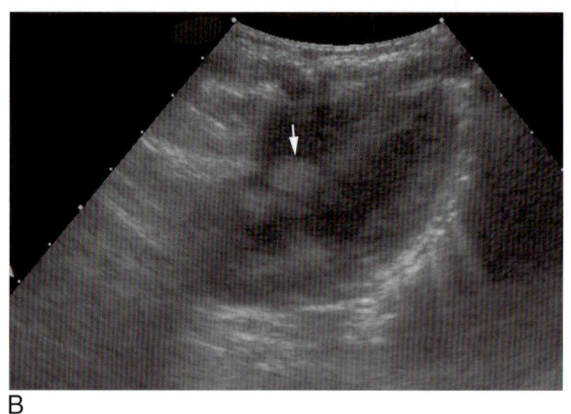

Figure 3.36 Cystic kidneys in tuberous sclerosis. (A) Longitudinal sonogram of the right kidney in a young child diagnosed as having tuberous sclerosis. Both kidneys appeared similar and contained multiple cysts of varying sizes. The appearances are indistinguishable from those of ADPKD. (B) Longitudinal sonogram of the heart in the same infant showing the echogenic rhabdomyoma (arrow).

Medullary cystic disease is an important cause of end stage renal disease in children, and the finding on ultrasound of normal size echogenic kidneys is the clue to the diagnosis. There is no other condition that will present clinically as chronic renal failure and have normal size kidneys on ultrasound. All other conditions resulting in end stage kidneys will ultimately lead to small, usually echogenic kidneys. Cysts are only seen late in the disease process and they are most likely to be small and at the

THE URINARY TRACT 77

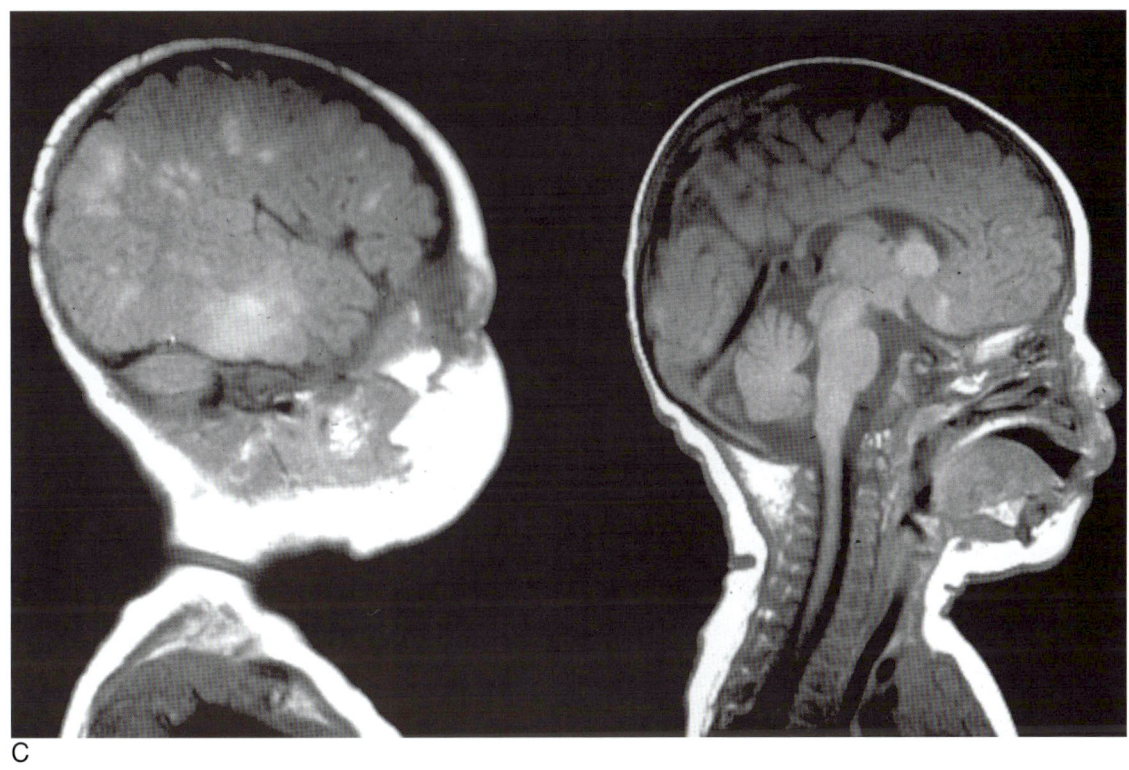

C
Figure 3.36, cont'd (C) Sagittal cranial MRI on the same infant at 6 weeks of age. Patients with tuberous sclerosis may have giant cell astrocytomas at the foramen of Monro and parenchymal lesions as seen in this child.

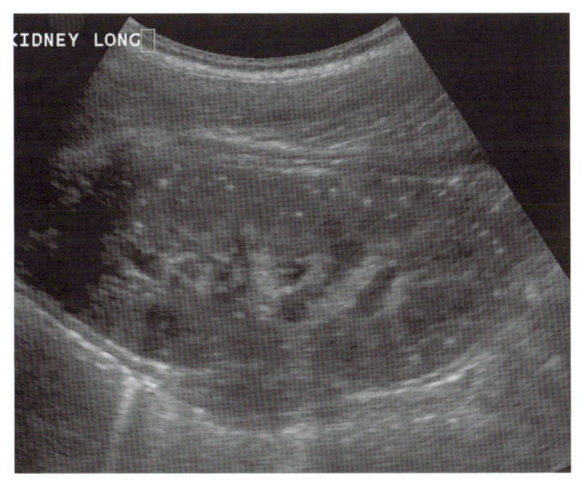

Figure 3.37 Angiomyolipomas in tuberous sclerosis. Longitudinal sonogram of the left kidney in an older child with tuberous sclerosis. There are multiple tiny echogenic foci scattered throughout the renal parenchyma which are the typical appearances of angiomyolipomas in this condition.

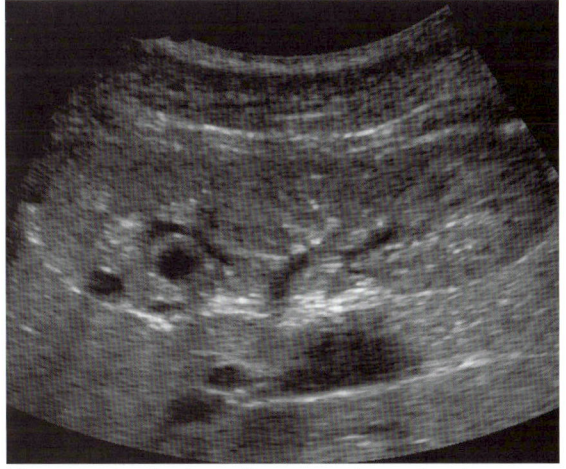

Figure 3.38 Angiomyolipomas and cysts in tuberous sclerosis. Longitudinal prone sonogram of the right kidney showing the combination of small echogenic angiomyolipomas and cysts.

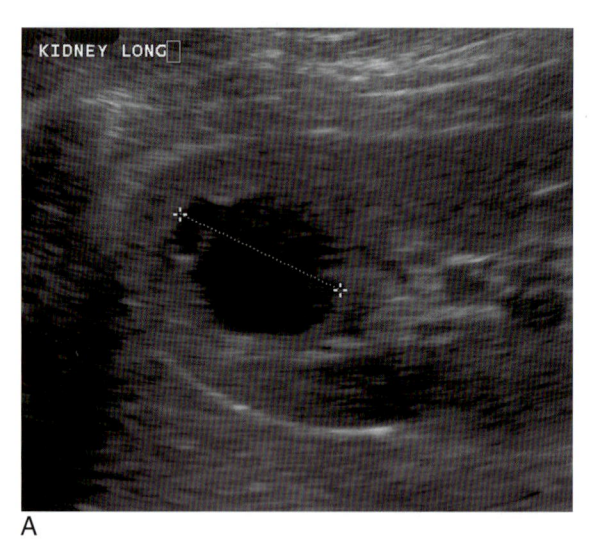

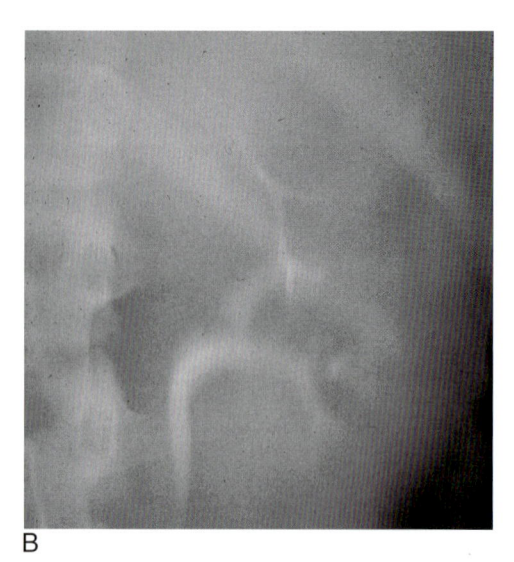

Figure 3.39 Simple cyst. (A) Incidental finding of a single simple cyst in the upper pole of the kidney in a child. (B) Intravenous urogram demonstrating that the 'cyst' does not connect with the collecting system.

corticomedullary junction or in the cortex. The childhood form is recessively inherited and is associated with other extrarenal abnormalities such as retinitis pigmentosa, congenital hepatic fibrosis and skeletal malformations.

Glomerulocystic kidneys

The indiscriminate use of this term has caused much confusion in the literature. Glomerulocystic kidneys are found in several syndromes, most notably tuberous sclerosis, orofaciodigital syndrome and Zellweger syndrome. A rare familial form with hypoplastic kidneys and with an autosomal dominant inheritance has also been described. The diagnosis is not made on sonography alone but usually in conjunction with clinical presentation, history and biopsy.

Non-genetic disease

Simple cysts

Simple cysts in children are extremely rare and usually detected incidentally. The largest reported series of 16 102 pediatric sonograms reported an overall frequency of 0.22%. The incidence of cysts was not related to age in this population, but it is well recognized that with increasing age in adulthood the incidence of simple cysts also increases. Simple cysts commonly occur in the upper poles (Fig. 3.39). Simple renal cysts may be seen in oncology patients who have had previous chemotherapy or abdominal radiotherapy.

The diagnosis of a simple renal cyst in children should, however, be one of exclusion. The differential diagnosis includes a duplex kidney with an obstructed upper moiety, a caliceal cyst/diverticulum or part of another cystic condition such as ADPKD.[31]

Children with a 'simple' cyst seen on ultrasound should have:

- a careful family history taken regarding renal disease
- an intravenous urogram to exclude a caliceal diverticulum
- follow-up examinations until late adolescence to determine whether other cysts develop.

Ultrasound exams every 5 years to monitor any development of new cysts (and therefore potentially the diagnosis of ADPKD) should be sufficient.

Caliceal cysts

Sonographic identification of a 'cyst' should be further investigated to determine whether a caliceal cyst or diverticulum is present. Its importance lies in the possibility of a calculus, with infection developing within it, or the possibility that TB has caused infundibular stenosis. An IVU is required with full pelvicaliceal distension in order to opacify the diverticulum (Fig. 3.40).

Multilocular cystic nephroma

The multilocular cystic nephroma is an uncommon, generally benign cystic tumor. It occurs in boys less than 4 years of age. The tumor is distinguished by the well-defined capsule surrounding the mass and absence of renal tissue in the septae.

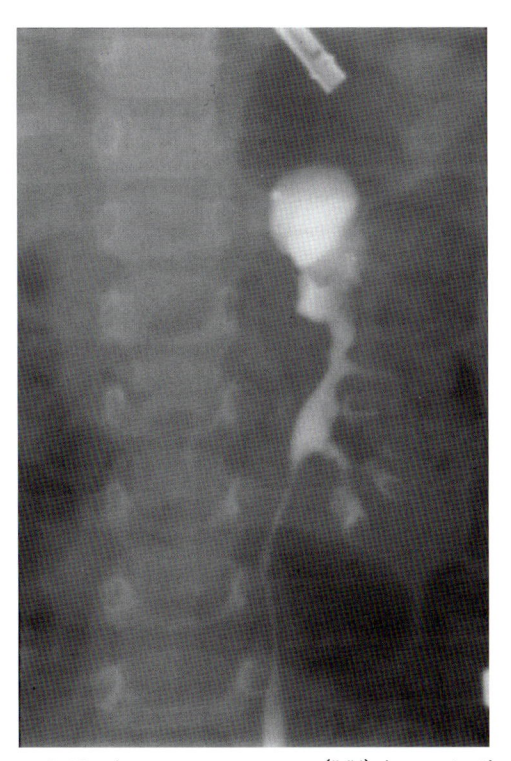

Figure 3.40 Intravenous urogram (IVU) demonstrating a caliceal cyst. This child presented with what appeared to be a simple renal cyst on ultrasound. This demonstrates the importance of doing an IVU in children with a 'simple' renal cyst. The appearances may be identical on ultrasound. It is important to differentiate between simple cysts and caliceal cysts as the latter may become infected and develop stones.

CT and MRI are generally required for better delineation. All such tumors are removed because of their malignant potential.

Medullary sponge kidney

Medullary sponge kidney is a term used to describe changes found on intravenous urography which shows brush-like linear striations in the renal papillae, frequently in association with renal calculi. It may be focal or involve the whole of the kidney and usually is associated with some enlargement of the kidney. It is not usually a disease of childhood although isolated cases are sometimes seen with hematuria, nephrolithiasis and infections. Medullary sponge kidney is probably a developmental abnormality.

On IVU the blush in the medulla related to the calices has a very similar appearance to that seen in ARPKD and at times may be indistinguishable if the entire kidney is involved. The term renal tubular ectasia is more widely accepted as the correct term to describe these renal changes in children. The ultrasound appearance of renal tubular ectasia without calculi is simply an increased echogenicity of the medullae in normal kidneys of normal size.

Acquired cystic renal disease

This term usually refers to the cysts which develop in the native kidneys of patients in chronic renal failure. There is no underlying cystic renal disorder and no other organ involvement. Acquired cysts can be found in up to 22% of patients in chronic renal failure, but their frequency increases with time on dialysis to up to 90% for those on dialysis for over 10 years. The incidence is similar for those on hemo- and chronic peritoneal dialysis. After successful transplantation, the cysts tend to regress in size. The importance of maintaining surveillance of these kidneys is because of a potential for malignant change, namely renal cell carcinoma. The cysts may also be complicated by hemorrhage or infection. Diagnosis is easily achieved with ultrasound (Table 3.3).

THE 'BRIGHT' KIDNEY

The kidney is termed 'bright', or echogenic, when the parenchymal and renal cortical echogenicity is greater than that of the parenchyma of the liver or

Table 3.3 Cystic kidneys

Diagnosis	Inheritance	Unilateral or bilateral	Extrarenal manifestations	Clinical features
ARPKD	Recessive; chromosome 6p	Bilateral and symmetrical Dilated collecting ducts Enlarged size	Liver CHF Portal hypertension	Neonatal period Respiratory distress Hypertension Renal insufficiency and portal hypertension in older children
ADPKD	Dominant: (*PKD1*)16p, 85% (*PKD2*)4q, 15%	Bilateral Unequal Cysts in all parts of nephron Enlarged size	Cystic liver, pancreas, spleen are rare in children Berry aneurysm and SAH Cardiac valvular abnormalities Thoracic aortic aneurysm	Usual onset 3rd–5th decade Childhood onset probably only *PKD1*
Tuberous sclerosis	Dominant	Bilateral Cysts in young Angiomyolipomas &/or cysts in older children	Hamartomas in brain, heart, skin, lung	Fits and mental retardation Renal failure late
Cystic dysplasia	None	Unilateral or bilateral	Only when syndromic	Associated with urinary obstructive lesions
Simple cyst	None	Uni- or bilateral (rare)	None	
Multicystic dysplastic	None	Unilateral Bilateral incompatible with life		30% abnormal contralateral kidney such as dysplasia, PUJ and ureteral stenosis Bladder ureterocele VUR
Multilocular cystic (Wilms)	None	Unilateral	None	

CHF, congenital hepatic fibrosis; PUJ, pelviureteric junction; SAH, subarachnoid hemorrhage.

the spleen. It is essential to know something about the

- size of the kidney
- what the corticomedullary differentiation looks like
- whether cysts are present or not
- age of the child
- clinical presentation.

It is important to recognize that ultrasound, while sensitive, is not specific. The causes of increased echogenicity are extensive and multiple and reflect the pathologies seen in the neonate and the older child.[32] Rarely can imaging with ultrasound alone make the diagnosis.

The neonate

The conditions causing bright kidneys in the neonate are different to those seen in the older child. Table 3.4 lists the commonest causes of bright kidneys seen in the neonate. The ultimate diagnosis

Table 3.4 Differential diagnosis of enlarged hyperechoic kidneys in the neonate

Diagnosis	Pathological and imaging features	Clinical features
Acute tubular necrosis (ATN)	Bilateral symmetrical hyperechoic kidneys	Perinatal event Cardiac patients Anuria or polyuria Normal prenatal scan
Renal vein thrombosis (RVT)	Unequal renal involvement Hyperechoic interlobular vessels Renal vein and IVC thrombosis and clot Associated with adrenal hemorrhage	Hematuria Renal failure Normal prenatal scan
ARPKD	Bilateral symmetrical renal involvement Hepatic fibrosis and biliary dilation Later portal hypertension	Detected prenatally Large palpable kidneys Hypertension
ADPKD	Big hyperechoic kidneys identical to ARPKD IVU showing 'puddling' may differentiate from ARPKD	Detected prenatally
Autosomal dominant glomerulocystic kidneys	Large echogenic kidneys	Rare condition Familial renal biopsy for diagnosis
Dysplastic kidneys	Large echogenic kidneys Renal compromise	May be associated with VUR
Dysplastic kidneys associated with a syndrome	Clinical evidence of a syndrome, e.g. polydactyly	Edwards syndrome Lawrence–Moon–Biedl syndrome Meckel syndrome Beckwith–Wiedemann syndrome Opitz–Lemi syndrome Oto-brachial-digital syndrome

ADPKD, autosomal dominant polycystic kidney disease; ARPKD, autosomal recessive polycystic kidney disease; VUR, vesicoureteric reflux.

will depend on the prenatal and perinatal history. It must also be recognized that in the neonate, normal kidneys may appear echogenic but are not enlarged.

Renal vein thrombosis

The following is a typical clinical scenario. A neonate presents with hematuria having had a difficult birth. The pregnancy had been uneventful with a normal prenatal scan. Varying degrees of renal failure may be present.

The ultrasound examination may demonstrate a large echogenic kidney and it may be impossible to differentiate between renal vein thrombosis, acute tubular necrosis and medullary necrosis. However, a number of features should be noted:

- whether the kidneys are affected equally and bilaterally
- whether there is asymmetric involvement
- what the spectral Doppler trace looks like in the renal artery, vein and IVC
- whether there is intraluminal thrombus in the IVC.

Renal vein thrombosis starts as an intrarenal event, and the severity really depends on whether it extends into the renal veins and IVC. There is typically increased echogenicity of the interlobular

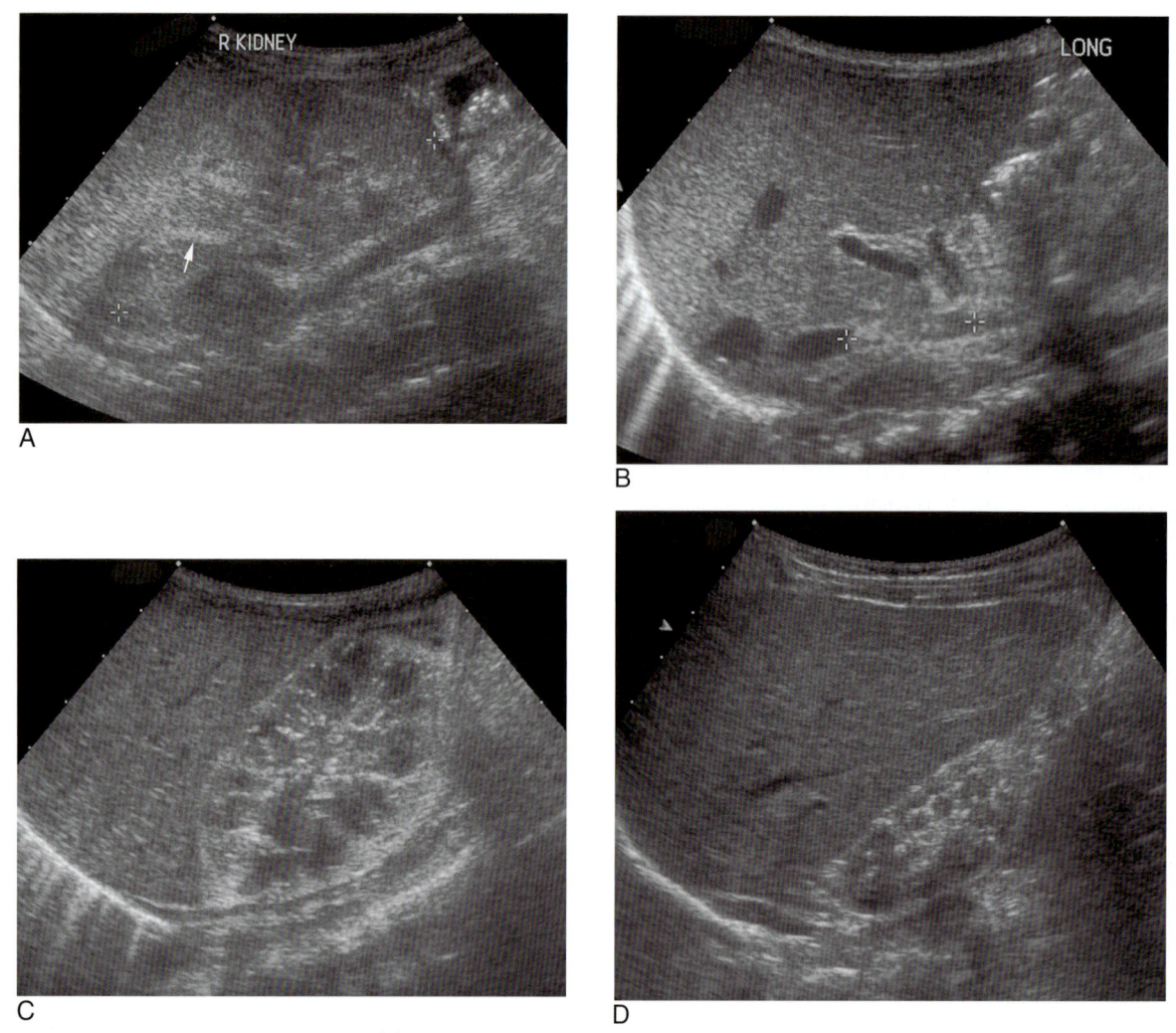

Figure 3.41 Renal vein thrombosis. (A) Longitudinal sonogram of the right kidney (between calipers). The kidney appears enlarged and swollen with a patchily bright echonephrogram. There is poor corticomedullary differentiation. Bright interlobular vessels are just visible (arrow). (B) Longitudinal sonogram of the IVC showing thrombus within the IVC (between the calipers). (C) Sonogram of the right kidney 2 weeks later. The kidney is smaller and not so swollen, with a grossly abnormal echo texture. The interlobular vessels are very echogenic. (D) Longitudinal sonogram of the right kidney 6 months later. The kidney is small and shrunken and there was no function on DMSA scanning.

vessels with a patchy echo nephrogram and some preservation of the corticomedullary differentiation (Fig. 3.41). Often the kidneys are unequally involved, and measurement of size is very important in this diagnosis.

Acute tubular necrosis and medullary necrosis may simply demonstrate enlarged echogenic kidneys. They are usually equally and symmetrically involved. No further imaging is undertaken at this stage, and infants will generally recover with renal support.

Cystic disease of the kidney

Polycystic kidney disease (ARPKD and ADPKD) together with renal dysplasia and glomerulocystic kidneys can all produce kidneys that are equally and symmetrically enlarged and echogenic. The medullae are usually involved too. Some forms of dysplastic kidneys associated with different syndromes, especially the Beckwith–Wiedemann syndrome, may look identical and will only be differentiated on further imaging.

Dysplastic kidneys

Cystic dysplasia can usually be diagnosed without difficulty on ultrasound. The overall disorder represents a nonspecific reaction of the kidney to disturbances in early development.

Generally the globally echogenic, small, poorly functioning kidney is considered to be dysplastic, but the size may range from the enlarged hyperplastic form to the hypoplastic form. All these kidneys function, but very poorly. There is usually complete loss of the normal architecture. The condition may be unilateral or bilateral and when bilateral the child will go into end stage renal failure. Dysplasia is seen in association with other renal abnormalities and in obstructing conditions such as duplex systems and posterior urethral valves.

The ultrasound appearances are classically those of small, highly echogenic kidneys with a variable number of small, typically subcortical cysts around the edge of the renal cortex (Fig. 3.42). The collecting system may or may not be dilated, depending on the underlying pathology. There is an increased incidence of reflux in these dysplastic kidneys and so generally a cystogram is performed.[33]

There are numerous well-defined syndromes where renal dysplasia is a feature, and the following are some of the important ones seen in children.

VACTERL syndrome Renal anomalies are found in over 50% of infants with VACTERL syndrome and range from uni- or bilateral dysplasia to single kidneys and crossed-fused ectopia. All infants with this diagnosis should have a renal ultrasound examination.

Renal-hepatic-pancreatic dysplasia This combination of renal-hepatic-pancreatic dysplasia was first described by Ivemark. The renal lesions consist of cystic dysplasia.

Branchio-oto-renal dysplasia This is a syndrome of branchial arch anomalies, hearing loss

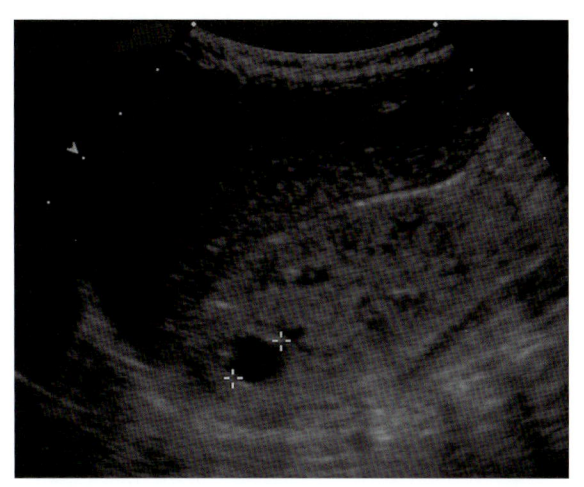

Figure 3.42 Dysplastic kidney. Longitudinal sonogram of the right kidney. The kidney is globally hyperechoic with loss of the corticomedullary differentiation. Typically there may be subcortical cysts and sometimes parenchymal cysts to aid diagnosis (between calipers). See also Figure 3.22c.

and renal hypoplasia. About two thirds have cystic dysplasia of the kidneys.

Chromosomal disorders Chromosomal disorders where renal dysplasia is a feature include, in particular, Down syndrome (trisomy 21), Patau syndrome (trisomy 13), Edward syndrome (trisomy 18) and Turner syndrome.

The older child

Ultrasound is usually the first imaging method used to evaluate the kidneys in a child presenting with proteinuria, hematuria or renal failure. The detection of echogenic kidneys is a common occurrence in pediatric practice, and, while sensitive in the detection of parenchymal abnormalities, it is not specific (Fig. 3.43). By far the commonest causes of bright kidneys seen in children are:

- glomerular disease such as acute nephrotic/nephritic syndrome
- tubular interstitial conditions such as acute tubular necrosis (ATN), toxic drugs or sepsis
- storage disorders such as glycogen storage disease
- renal dysplasia
- end stage renal disease

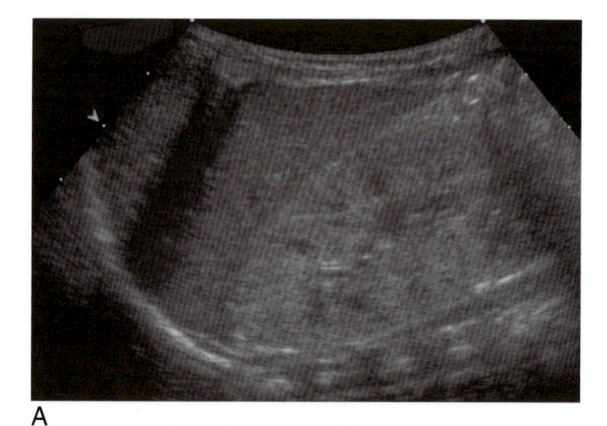

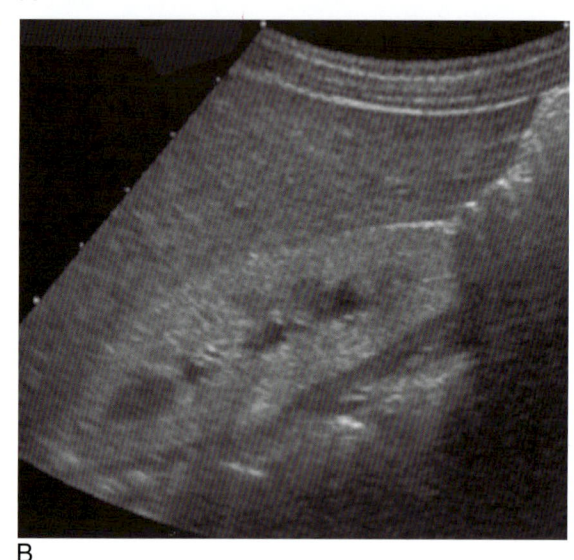

Figure 3.43 Bright kidneys. (A) & (B) Longitudinal sonogram of the right kidney in two children. The renal cortex and medullae are more echogenic than the liver parenchyma. While ultrasound is sensitive there are a number of causes of this appearance in children. Age and clinical presentation are important considerations when coming to a diagnosis.

- hypertensive nephrosclerosis
- tumor such as leukemia or lymphoma
- congenital nephrotic syndrome
- glomerulonephritis, tubular interstitial nephritis and the vasculitides
- bilateral nephroblastomatosis.

The typical ultrasound appearances are of a global increase in echogenicity with poor cortico-medullary differentiation. The kidneys may be enlarged. In conditions such as IgA nephropathy and minimal change glomerulonephritis (GN), cortical echogenicity is usually normal.

A good clinical history together with the ultrasound findings will go some way towards making the diagnosis, but in clinical practice the ultimate diagnosis is usually made with a renal biopsy.

RENAL CALCULI AND NEPHROCALCINOSIS

Renal calculi or urolithiasis refers to the macroscopic calcification that occurs in the renal collecting system. Nephrocalcinosis (NC) refers to the microscopic calcification that occurs in the tubules or interstitial tissue of the kidney. It is classified according to the anatomical area involved. Medullary calcification is differentiated from cortical and diffuse NC. Urolithiasis and NC can occur together.

Renal calculi

Renal stones are uncommon in childhood and when they occur predisposing causes must be sought, for example:

- urinary tract infection
- structural abnormalities of the urinary tract
- metabolic abnormalities.

The stones most commonly associated with infection are phosphate stones, and these are particularly associated with *Proteus* infections. The infective stones tend to occur in infants and young children. Calcium-containing stones occur in idiopathic hypercalciuria, the most common metabolic abnormality, and with increased urinary and oxalate excretion. Cysteine and xanthine stones are rare.

Renal calculi in children have a wide geographic variation, being more common in hotter climates such as the Far and Middle East.

Types of calculi

A few specific types of calculi that the sonographer should be aware of are mentioned below.

Hyperoxaluria Primary hyperoxaluria is a rare autosomal recessive inherited disease (Fig. 3.44). Infants may present with highly echogenic kidneys and it may be fatal.

Secondary (enteric hyperoxaluria) is a complication in patients with diseases involving fat malabsorption, for example, cystic fibrosis and inflammatory bowel disease. Normally oxalate is bound to calcium, which is not absorbed. In patients with enteric hyperoxaluria, calcium instead binds to fatty acids, so the water soluble oxalate is absorbed. It has been reported that nearly 15% of patients with cystic fibrosis develop renal calculi. Oxalate stones are extremely dense on plain abdominal radiography.

Cysteine stones These may develop as small stones or also assume a staghorn configuration. They are less opaque than calcium stones and are sometimes difficult to see on plain abdominal radiography (Fig. 3.45).

Uric acid stones These stones are rarely found in children. Most commonly they occur after treatment of myeloproliferative disorders has caused tumor lysis and release and deposition of the tumor tissue products into the urinary tract. They may also be seen in the Lesch–Nyhan syndrome, a metabolic disorder affecting the uric acid pathway.

Infectious stones Infectious stones are mainly composed of struvite. Urease-producing bacteria are responsible for the formation of these calculi. They are mainly seen in boys under the age of 5 years, and there is commonly an associated anomaly in the urinary tract such as a megaureter. Patients with a neurogenic bladder and extrophy are particularly prone.

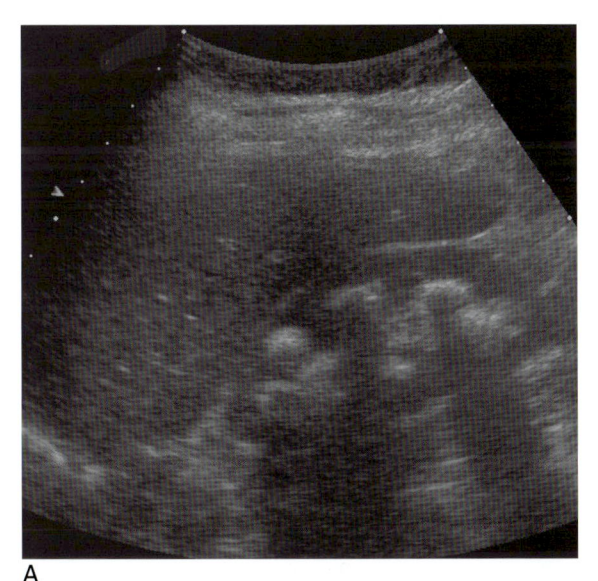

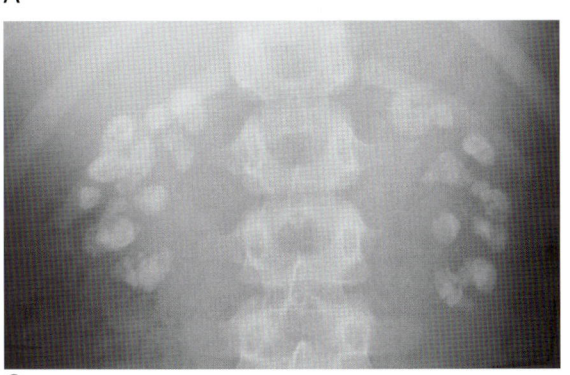

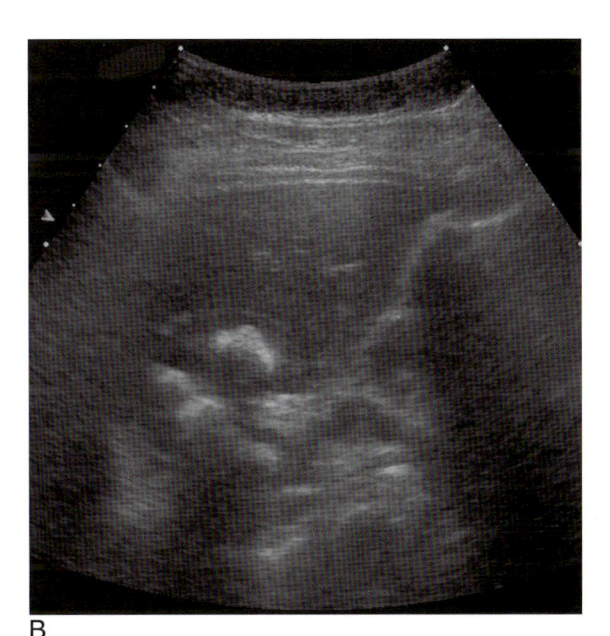

Figure 3.44 Hyperoxaluria. (A) & (B) Longitudinal and transverse sonogram of the right kidney in a child with hyperoxaluria. The stones are very dense and echogenic, casting acoustic shadows typical of this condition.
(C) Plain abdominal radiograph showing the very dense calcification in the kidneys in this child with oxalate stones.

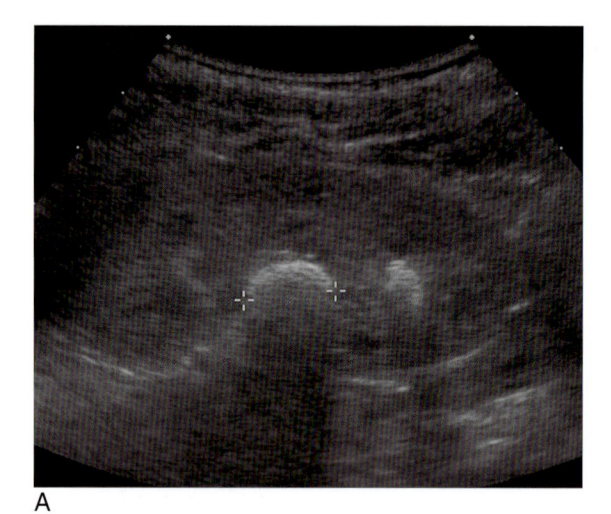

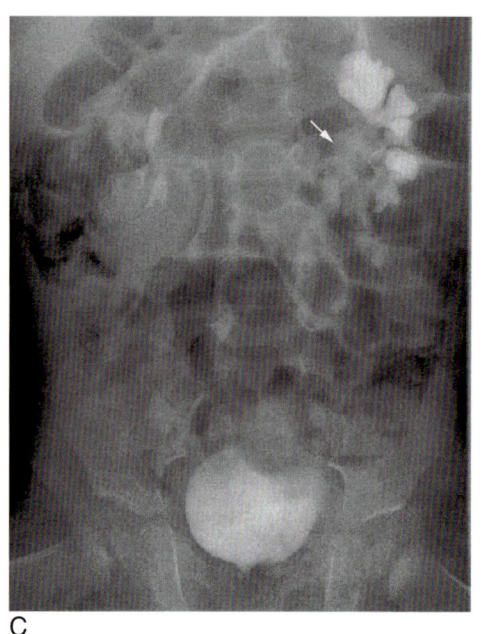

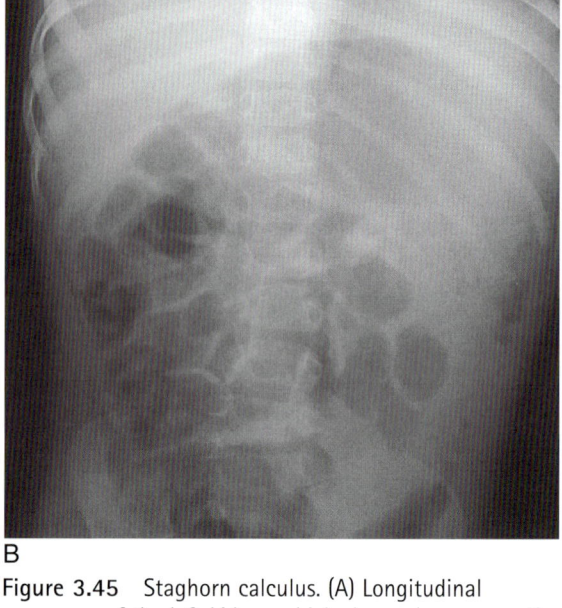

Figure 3.45 Staghorn calculus. (A) Longitudinal sonogram of the left kidney which shows dense acoustic shadowing in the central collecting system (between calipers). A staghorn calculus should be suspected when this coalition of echoes is seen within the renal pelvis. (B) Plain abdominal radiograph showing the staghorn calculus on the left. (C) Intravenous urogram on the same child showing the filling defect of the staghorn calculus in the renal pelvis (arrow) with dilation of the calices.

Imaging and treatment

High resolution ultrasound is an excellent modality for detecting and monitoring renal calculi. There are some advocates for using careful ultrasound alone in children, but when combined with plain abdominal radiography the detection and diagnosis is definitely more secure.

Ureteric stones may notoriously be missed with ultrasound but, when the stones are associated with a dilated ureter, ultrasound combined with plain abdominal radiography is usually sufficient (Fig. 3.46).

Intervention is required if there is persisting or severe obstruction or infection of the urinary tract. Cysteine stones and uric acid stones can be dissolved chemically. Extracorporeal shockwave lithotripsy (ESWL) is possible in children, and percutaneous nephrolithotomy can also be performed (Fig. 3.47).

Nephrocalcinosis

The clinical presentation of nephrocalcinosis may be asymptomatic, especially in infancy.

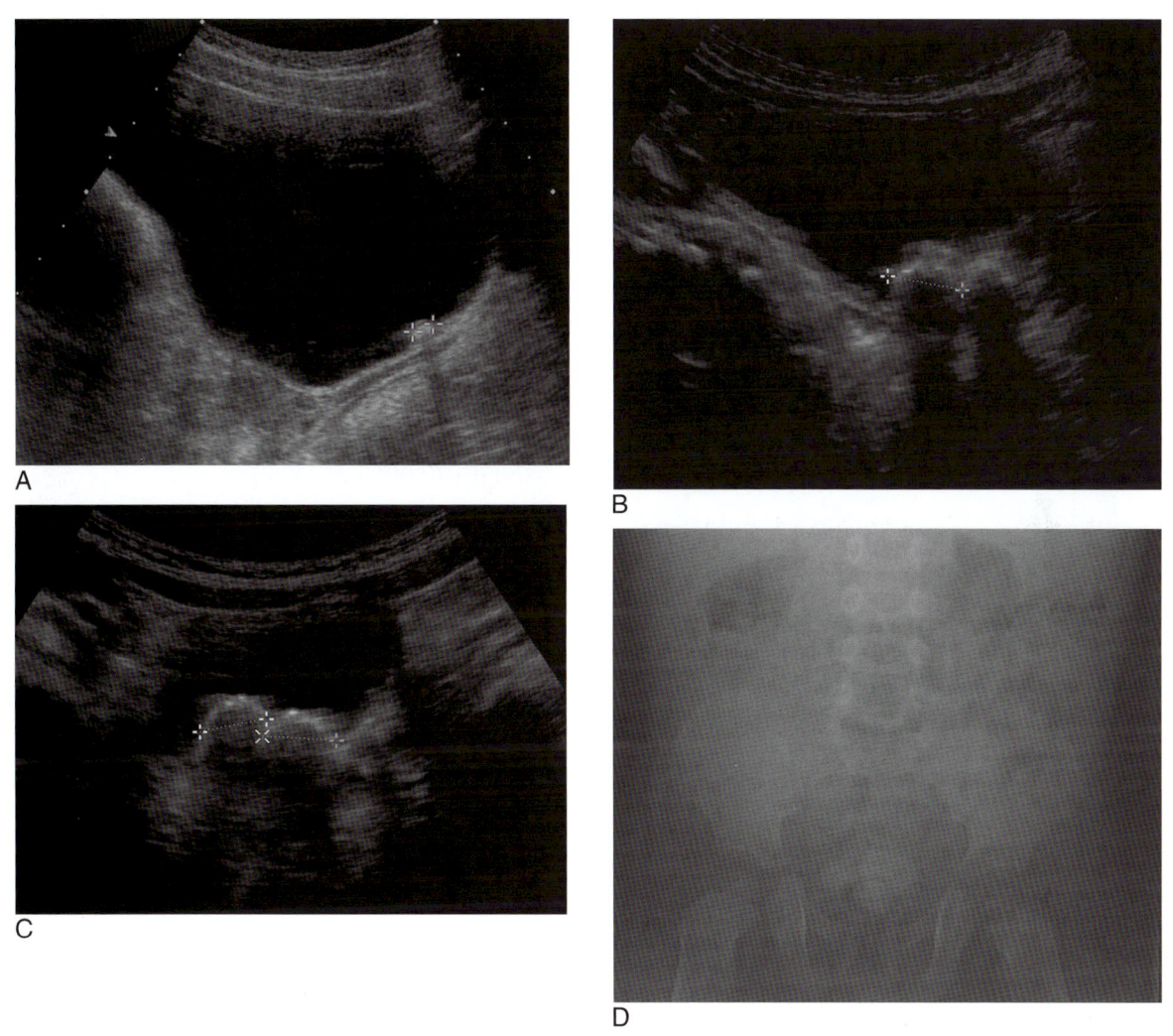

Figure 3.46 Stones in the ureter and bladder. (A) Longitudinal sonogram of the right lower ureter. There is a well-defined stone at the vesicoureteric junction, casting an acoustic shadow, and a proximally dilated ureter. Ureteric stones in the middle third of the ureter are often missed with ultrasound because of overlying bowel gas. (B) & (C) Longitudinal and transverse views of the full bladder showing multiple echogenic calculi in the bladder, casting acoustic shadows. (D) Abdominal radiograph on the same child showing multiple calculi in the bladder.

Nephrocalcinosis is described as being medullary, cortical or parenchymal.[34]

Increased medullary echogenicity of the kidneys in children, while sonographically non-specific, may be an unexpected finding and should not be ignored, as it may be indicative of severe underlying metabolic disease. In every patient it requires a clinical explanation. Iatrogenic nephrocalcinosis is the single most common cause, in infants, of increased echogenicity of the medullary pyramids. If this diagnosis can be excluded a large differential diagnosis remains.[35]

Imaging

Ultrasonography is much more sensitive in the early stages of calcium deposition in the kidneys than plain abdominal radiography, which only becomes positive when the calcium starts casting acoustic shadows on ultrasound. Initially there is a mild

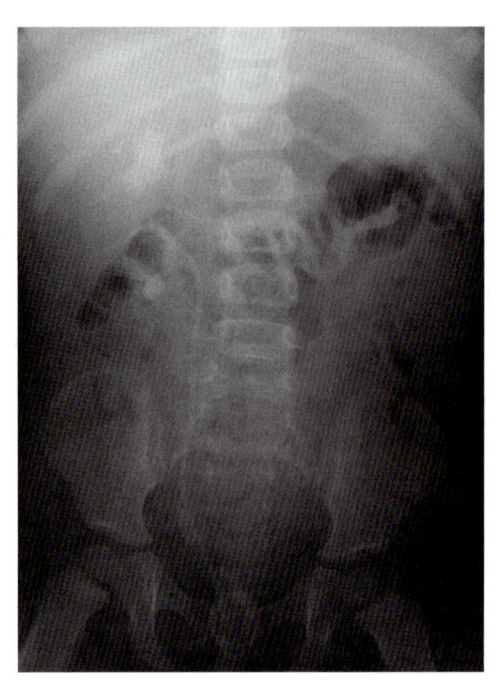

Figure 3.47 Treatment of renal calculi. Abdominal radiograph on a child after lithotripsy treatment for renal calculi. There is a JJ-stent in the right flank and residual calculi in the kidney. The ends of the JJ-stent should lie within the renal pelvis and within the bladder.

increase in echogenicity and ringing of the pyramids which, in more severely affected patients, eventually fills in the medullae and then casts acoustic shadows (Fig. 3.48). A normal plain abdominal radiograph should therefore not deter the sonographer from making this diagnosis. The earliest changes of calcium deposition in the medullae can be very subtle on ultrasound, but should be suspected when the echogenic 'dot' of the arcuate artery is lost in the increased echogenicity at the periphery of the medullae. The severity of nephrocalcinosis has been graded using an ultrasound grading scale (Box 3.8).[36] A grading scale is valuable for long term monitoring and follow-up.

Nephrocalcinosis is always bilateral and symmetrical unless there is an underlying renal artery occlusion or an old renal vein thrombosis. Coexistent hydronephrosis can obscure the nephrocalcinosis. The most important biochemical test in nephrocalcinosis is to identify hypercalcemia and hypercalciuria.

Cortical nephrocalcinosis

This is most commonly due to acute or chronic cortical necrosis and is occasionally seen in cardiac patients or in drug intoxication. It may also be seen in chronic hypercalcemia and primary hyperoxaluria.[37]

Causes of cortical nephrocalcinosis in children are:

- chronic hypercalcemia
- acute cortical necrosis
- primary hyperoxaluria
- sickle cell disease.

Medullary nephrocalcinosis

Common causes of increased medullary echogenicity in children are:

- nephrocalcinosis
  —iatrogenic, e.g. treatment for hypophosphatemic rickets, or frusemide for bronchopulmonary dysplasia or cardiac failure in a premature infant[38]
  —non-iatrogenic, e.g. idiopathic hypercalcemia in William syndrome, or absorptive hypercalciuria
- tubulopathies, e.g. renal tubular acidosis
- protein deposits giving transient increased medullary echogenicity in newborns (so-called Tamm–Horsfall proteinuria)
- vascular congestion, e.g. sickle cell anemia and renovascular hypertension
- infection, e.g. candidiasis or cytomegalovirus infection
- metabolic disease, e.g. urate deposits as in Lesch–Nyhan syndrome; also seen in tyrosinemia, glycogen storage disease and Wilson disease (dRTA)
- oxalosis
- cystic medullary renal disease, e.g. ARPKD, congenital hepatic fibrosis with renal tubular ectasia.

Uncommon causes are:

- Bartter syndrome
- Cushing syndrome
- hyper- and hypothyroidism
- lipoid necrosis
- Lesch–Nyhan syndrome

THE URINARY TRACT 89

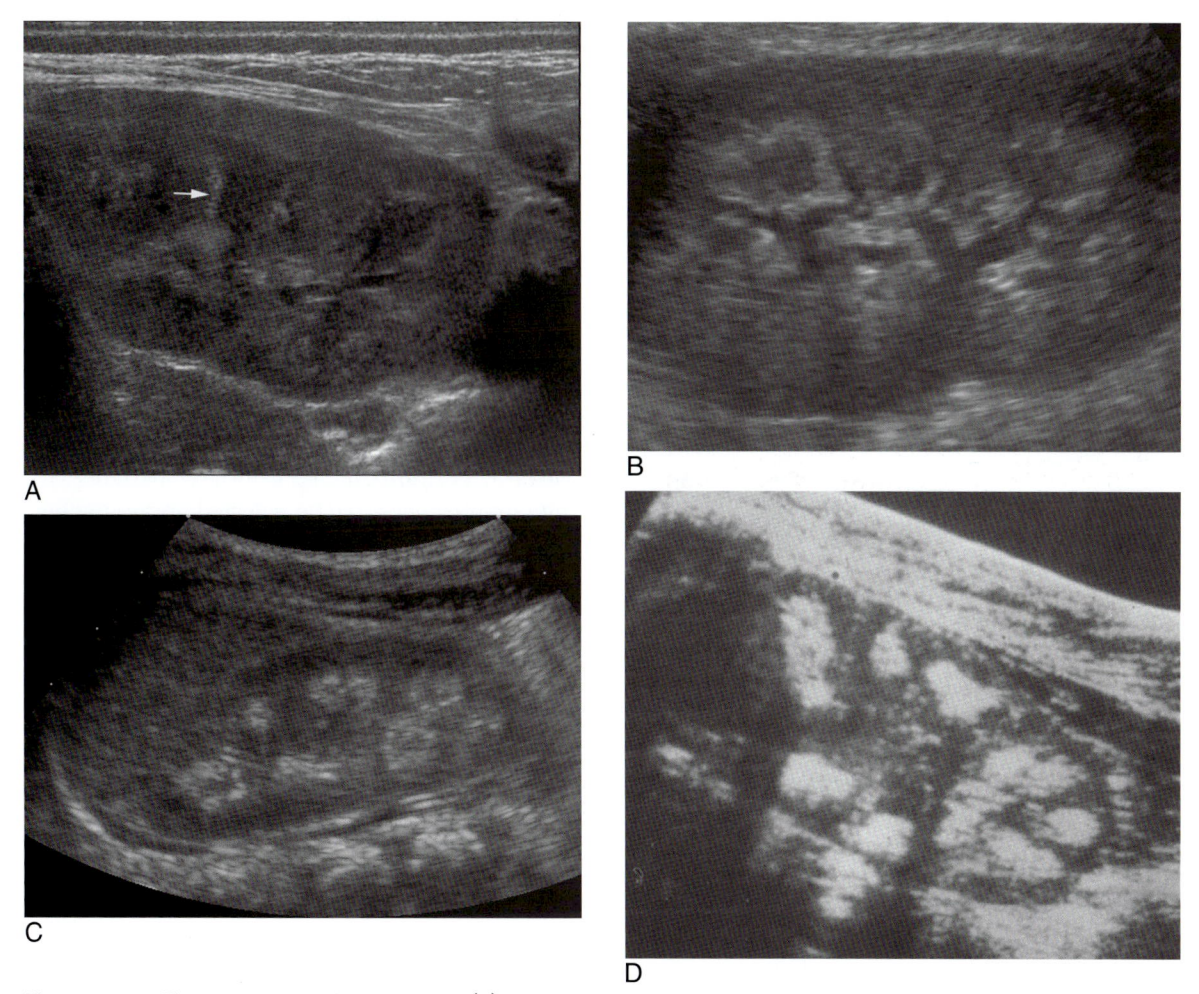

Figure 3.48 The stages of nephrocalcinosis. (A) The earliest sonographic appearance of nephrocalcinosis, with just an increased echogenicity of the lateral walls of the medullae (arrow). (B) Longitudinal sonogram showing the early appearances with ringing of the medullae. (C) Longitudinal sonogram of the right kidney showing the medullae filled in, with an increased echogenicity throughout. (D) Longitudinal sonogram showing the echogenic medullae casting acoustic shadows. It is only at this stage that nephrocalcinosis will become evident on plain abdominal radiograph.

Box 3.8 Nephrocalcinosis grading scale[36]

- Grade I: mild increase in echogenicity around the border of the medullary pyramids
- Grade II: mild diffuse increase in echogenicity of the entire medullary pyramids
- Grade III: greater, more homogeneous increase in the echogenicity of the entire medullary pyramid

- Lowe syndrome
- sickle cell disease
- vitamin D and A intoxication.

HYPERTENSION IN CHILDREN

Symptomatic hypertension in children is usually secondary and of renal origin. Most commonly this is due to parenchymal disease from renal damage and scarring following reflux nephropathy. In over 90% of children with hypertension after 1 year of age, renal disease is the cause. Coarctation of the aorta is another important cause.[39] Other causes in children are rare.

Early detection of the hypertension is important so any child with known renal damage and scarring should have their blood pressure checked twice a year.

Clinical presentation includes vomiting, headaches, facial palsy, hypertensive retinopathy, convulsions or proteinuria. Failure to thrive and cardiac failure are the most common features in infants.

Causes of hypertension include the following.

- Renin dependent
  —Renal parenchymal disease. Any kidney abnormality, such as renal scarring or glomerular disease, may produce renin and so generate hypertension
  —Tumors such as Wilms tumors
  —Renovascular disease, accounting for approximately 10% of cases. Fibromuscular dysplasia is the commonest cause of renal arterial disease in childhood, but other associations are neurofibromatosis, idiopathic hypercalcemia of infancy, an arteritic illness or middle aortic syndrome
- Coarctation of the aorta
- Catecholamine excess as in neuroblastoma or pheochromocytoma
- Endocrine causes such as congenital adrenal hyperplasia (CAH), Cushing disease and steroid treatment
- Essential hypertension is also encountered, usually in borderline, milder cases, often with a positive family history of hypertension.

Imaging

Generally speaking, the younger the child and the greater the degree of hypertension, the more chance of finding an abnormality on imaging. The role of imaging investigations in children with hypertension depends largely on the results of a thorough history, clinical examination and laboratory tests. There is no set imaging protocol applicable to all children. How aggressively one pursues the underlying renal parenchymal or renovascular disorder is dependent on a number of factors such as.

- severity of hypertension
- clinical symptoms and signs of hypertension
- effectiveness of medical treatment
- compliance of the patient in taking the medication.

Much has been written and the expectations are high regarding the role of ultrasound in hypertension. For pediatric sonographers, often with restless, crying young children, performing a prolonged complex Doppler examination has often proved to be difficult and very unrewarding. However, children with hypertension do need some form of reliable non-invasive screening examination because the appropriate patients for angiography need to be selected. Sonographers must concentrate their efforts in children on performing an excellent standard examination and learning to recognize the abnormalities that are important to detect with ultrasound. The commonest finding is a scarred kidney, in which case much time, effort and goodwill will have been wasted trying to obtain Doppler traces of little or no value, not to mention the sonographer's feeling of performing an inadequate examination. So, if the diagnosis is clearly one of bilateral scarred kidneys from reflux nephropathy, don't waste time performing a Doppler examination. Ultrasound can be easily repeated, so rather keep the Doppler examinations for those children really suspected of having renovascular disease, where it may be of some value.

The small numbers of patients that will need angiography are those with suspected renovascular disease. The aim of imaging, then, is to exclude all other causes of hypertension so that the child does not have to undergo invasive angiography unnecessarily. Ultrasound, nuclear medicine, cystography and intravenous urography are all used but the investigations are tailored to the child rather than following a set regime. Ultrasound and nuclear medicine are the commonest modalities used in the investigative work-up. Renal scintigraphy is generally good in experienced hands but is limited particularly in the setting of bilateral renal artery stenosis and renal failure.

Ultrasound is therefore the first investigation, and the findings will direct further imaging. A meticulous ultrasound examination should be performed, with the sonographer knowing exactly what to look for.

Ultrasound examination

The examination should achieve the following.
- Document the size and echogenicity of the kidneys (Fig. 3.49). A 10% difference in size warrants further investigation, such as a DMSA scan.
- Detect any renal parenchymal thinning and 'scars'.
- Note any dilation of the collecting systems or ureters.
- Carefully evaluate the abdominal aorta for coarctation. Check the caliber of the aorta above and below the renal vessels. The middle aortic arch syndrome will have narrowing of the aorta below the level of the kidneys.
- Evaluate the main renal vasculature for aneurysms or narrowing both on conventional

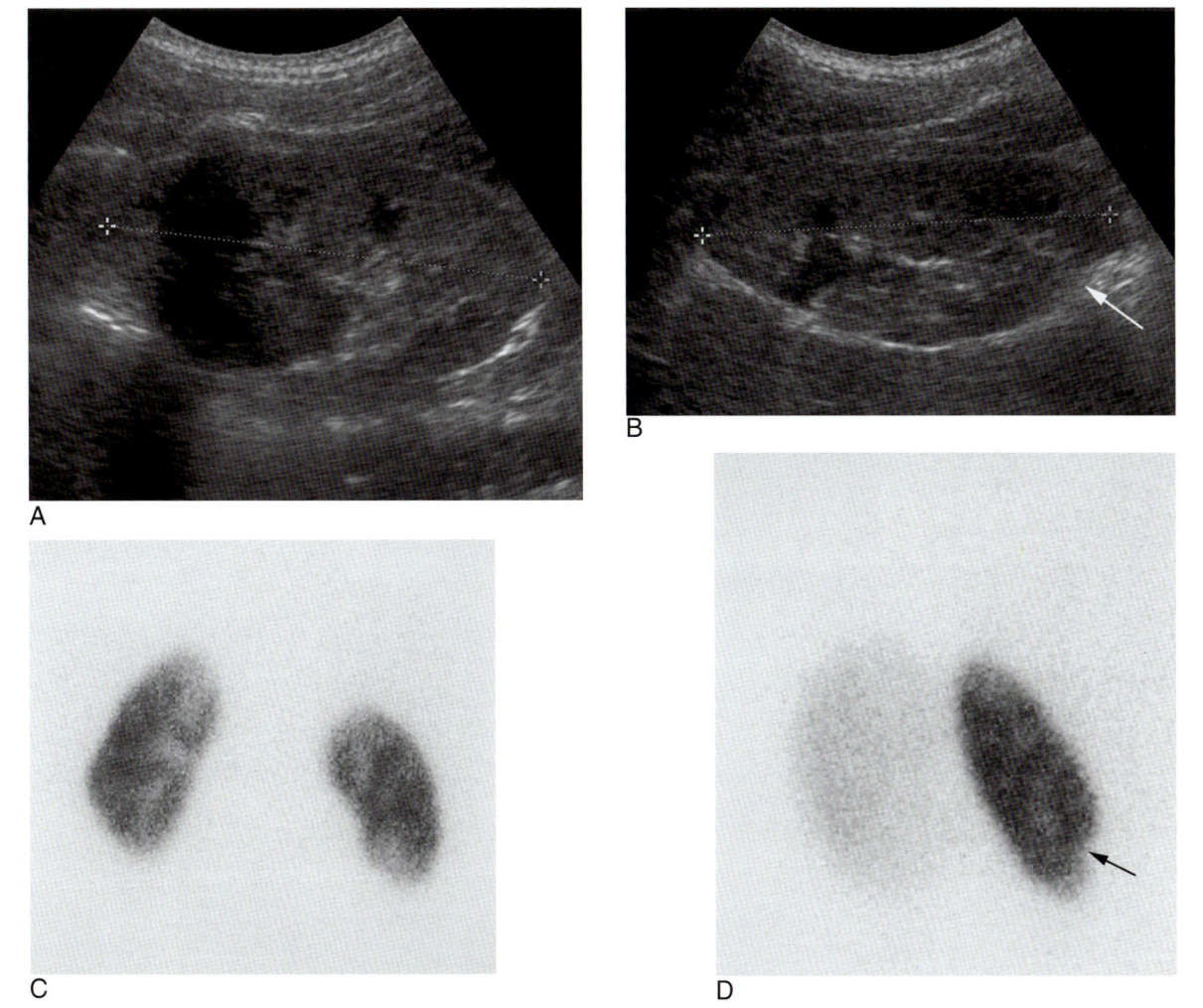

Figure 3.49 Size of kidneys in hypertension. (A) & (B) Longitudinal sonograms of both left and right kidneys in a boy presenting with hypertension. There was a 10% difference in the size of the kidneys. On very careful evaluation there is a small localized area of cortical thinning in the lower pole on the right (arrow). (C) & (D) DMSA examination on the same patient showing the very subtle difference in the size of the kidneys and the small defect in the lower pole on the right (arrow).

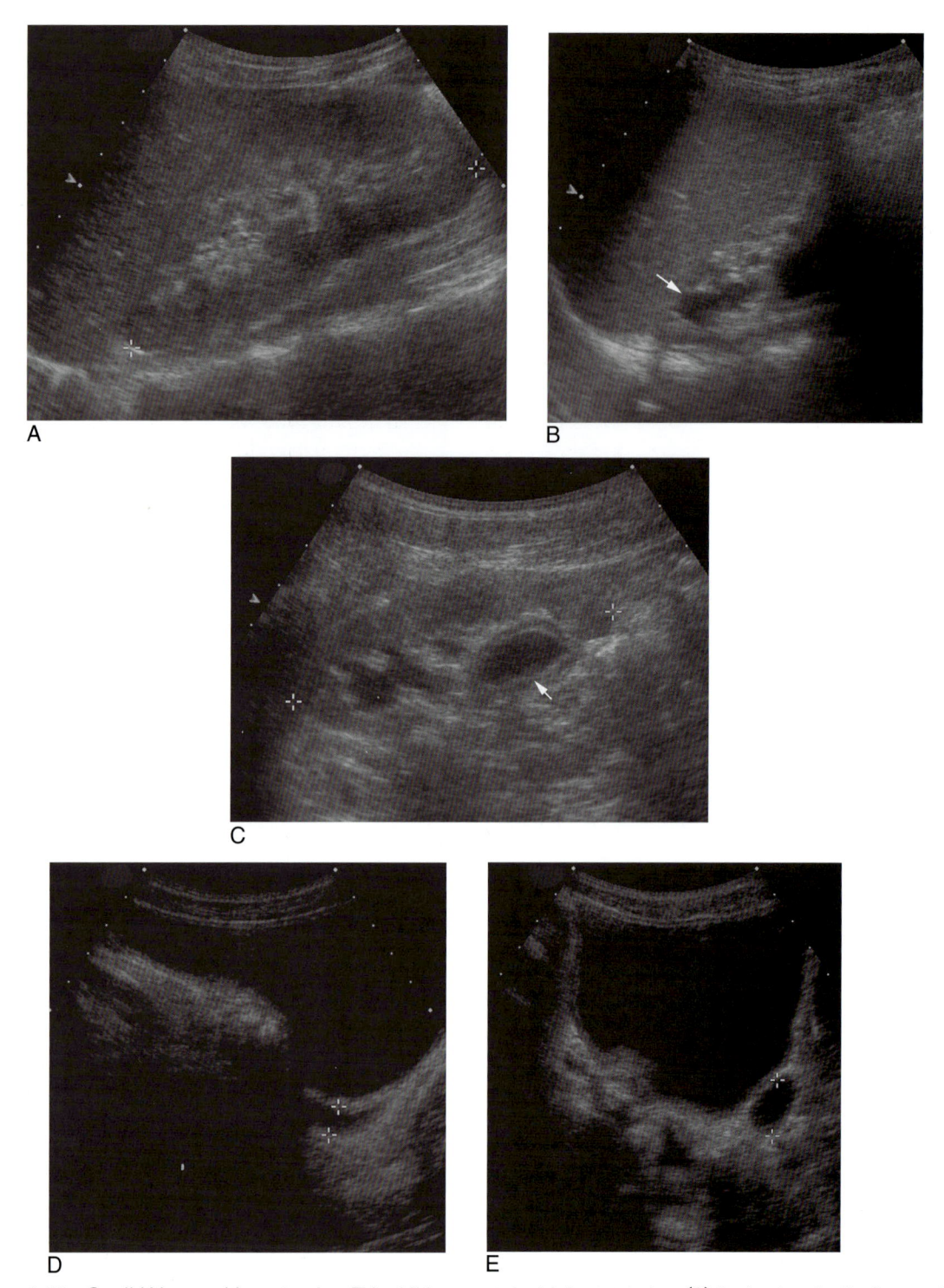

Figure 3.50 Small kidney and hypertension. This child presented with hypertension. (A) Supine longitudinal scan of the normal right kidney. (B) Supine longitudinal scan of the small left kidney. The calices extend up to the edge of the cortex (arrow). (C) Prone longitudinal scan of the same small left kidney. There is irregular cortical thinning and uroepithelial thickening (arrow). (D) & (E) Longitudinal and transverse scans of the bladder showing the dilated left ureters (between calipers). This boy had a scarred left kidney associated with VUR.

gray scale and then Doppler. Examine with the patient both supine and prone, evaluating the renal artery origins if possible. A clinical history of a renal bruit is closely associated with renal artery abnormalities.

- Obtain spectral Doppler traces in the interlobular vessels in particular, looking for the parvus tardus appearance which occurs downstream of a renal artery stenosis. The appearance is one of flattening or dampening of the intrarenal spectral trace. (Remember to compare the intrarenal spectral trace in both kidneys using the same parameters.) This is probably the easiest test to perform and most reliable finding in children.
- There should be raised catecholamine levels in suspected pheochromocytomas, so the clinical findings are important in this situation. Check for intra-abdominal tumors, in particular both the adrenal glands for a pheochromocytoma. Remember that in children pheochromocytomas are often extra-adrenal and multiple, so look around the abdomen and the pelvis for any intra-abdominal or pelvic mass.

Ultrasound is best at detecting the small kidney, the severely scarred kidney, significant hydronephrosis and most adrenal tumors. A normal ultrasound does not exclude a single renal scar, renovascular pathology or a small extrarenal pheochromocytoma.

The doppler examination Doppler ultrasound evaluation in children, particularly of the main renal arteries, is highly related to operator experience. The examination needs to be quick, especially in the younger child who has only a relatively short period of goodwill.

There are two methods of interrogating the renal vasculature:

- The direct method, in which the entire length of the renal artery must be visualized with color flow and spectral Doppler from the aortic origin to the renal hilum. This is extremely difficult in an uncooperative child and is often unsuccessful. However, it is worth the attempt.
- The indirect method—this technique is confined to intrarenal vessels which are first identified with color flow or power Doppler. Once these are identified, spectral traces are obtained. Technically this is easier and shorter to perform and is better suited to children. Identification of a significant renal artery stenosis (RAS) depends upon the demonstration of the parvus–tardus effect within the intrarenal vasculature downstream from a proximal stenosis. This results in a spectral trace of low amplitude with a slowly rising curve. If the downstream vessels are compliant then the parvus–tardus effect is preserved. However, if they are non-compliant then this effect may be masked. Many pitfalls remain, and diagnostic angiography generally remains the gold standard. In the future, contrast agents may be of value, but they are not currently in general use in children.

If the ultrasound is abnormal, then further investigation dependent upon the ultrasound findings is warranted. The primary role of ultrasound in pediatric practice still remains a careful baseline examination as outlined above.

Small kidney The discovery of a small kidney on ultrasound (Fig. 3.50) necessitates further imaging such as a ^{99m}Tc DMSA study and cystograms, to assess the degree of function of the kidney and to look for VUR. In the older child a ^{99m}Tc MAG3 plus IRC may obviate the need for both ^{99m}Tc DMSA and MCU (see Table 3.2). In the absence of VUR an IVU may be indicated to outline the calices in an attempt to establish the cause of a small kidney. The differential diagnosis lies between an old renal vein thrombosis, renal dysplasia, reflux nephropathy, postobstructive atrophy and arterial pathology. The presence of normal calices on IVU would suggest renovascular disease is likely and that arteriography is indicated. Some, however, would argue that arteriography is needed in all children with suspected renovascular hypertension and would have a low threshold for an arteriogram, as many of the stenotic lesions are potentially treatable with angioplasty.

Normal kidney With a normal ultrasound examination, a ^{99m}Tc DMSA scan is the next recommended investigation. This can detect a focal parenchymal abnormality such as renal scarring.

The major limitation of the combination of a normal ultrasound and normal ^{99m}Tc DMSA scan is in the possible failure to detect renovascular disease.

The exclusion of renovascular disease ultimately requires angiography. Fibromuscular hyperplasia, middle aortic syndrome, and osteal stenosis in neurofibromatosis are the commonest vascular pathologies encountered.

With modern angiographic catheters and advances in balloon technology, it is possible to undertake angioplasty in children with disease of the main or major intrarenal arteries. These examinations should ideally be performed by those with expertise in pediatric angiography as well as in angioplasty, so as to cause the least complications possible.

Suspected pheochromocytoma If a pheochromocytoma is proven biochemically, then a careful ultrasound examination of the abdomen should be carried out as outlined above. After the ultrasound study, an iodine–123 metaiodobenzylguanidine (^{123}I MIBG) scan is performed in order to detect particularly the extra adrenal sites which will help direct further imaging. It is important to undertake this examination before cross-sectional imaging so that further imaging can be targeted. A CT examination with specific attention focused on the areas of abnormality as seen on the ^{123}I MIBG scan should then be done, which reduces the need to examine the entire chest, abdomen and pelvis with CT. MRI although still not widely available appears to be an adequate substitute for CT when feasible in these children. With MRI there is also at least the theoretically reduced risk of a hypertensive crisis, as no iodinated contrast medium is used.

RENAL TRAUMA

Renal trauma is not uncommon in children, because of the lack of surrounding tissues, and may be blunt trauma that occurs in sporting injuries or falls. The other less common types of renal injury in childhood are penetrating injuries that occur in stab wounds or gunshot wounds and, lastly, deceleration or acceleration injuries that occur in motor vehicle accidents or airplane accidents.

The main imaging modality of choice in abdominal injury is a CT examination, and ultrasound is used either as an alternative if CT is not available or as a first line investigation. There is a definite role for ultrasound in the follow-up of renal trauma.[40]

Renal trauma is classified according to the type of injury sustained:

- parenchymal laceration
- a shattered kidney (a deeper laceration which communicates with the caliceal system)
- a shattered kidney which has shattered into numerous small bits
- an avulsion from the vascular and pelvic pedicle.

If the renal injury is classified as minor then the patient can be treated conservatively. If the patient has any vascular compromise then surgery is indicated. It is vitally important to demonstrate a functioning contralateral kidney, which can be done using CT or, if necessary, an intravenous urogram.

Color flow Doppler imaging must be used in order to evaluate the renal hilum and perfusion of the kidney. In a restless child, color Doppler energy should be the first line of Doppler examination which will immediately detect if there is any flow at all in the kidney. Ultrasound can also evaluate the collecting system for clots.

Complications that may occur with renal trauma include a perirenal or intrarenal hematoma, a urinary leak and a perinephric collection of urine.

RENAL TRANSPLANTATION IN CHILDREN

There are many causes of inadequate function of native kidneys, and when the number of functioning nephrons falls sufficiently, a state of chronic renal failure (CRF) exists. CRF implies a relentless progression with further deterioration resulting in clinical signs and symptoms and leading to end stage renal failure (ESRF) without the potential for a medical cure. Renal transplantation is the optimal renal replacement therapy for infants and young children with ESRF. It is usually followed by growth and improved psychomotor development giving a significantly improved quality of life for the child and family.[41]

The incidence of ESRF in Europe and North America appears to be similar, although the databases and reporting of the underlying cause differs, thus accounting for the apparent difference in causation. The commonest causes of ESRF leading to transplantation are: obstructive uropathy, renal dysplasia, aplasia and hypoplasia, glomerular disease (glomerulosclerosis), reflux nephropathy and ARPKD. The French reportedly have a high incidence of transplantation in children with juvenile nephronopthisis. Congenital urinary tract anomalies dominate in children under 2 years of age, whereas glomerulosclerosis is more common in older children.

In children with malignancy such as bilateral Wilms tumors, at least 5 years post-nephrectomy and treatment is observed before transplantation. This is in case of recurrence of the primary tumor.

Transplant anatomy

An understanding of the normal transplant anatomy is crucial to the performance of ultrasound examination. The surgical notes of the transplant should always be read prior to the examination being performed.

There are two ways of obtaining a renal transplant, either by having a living relation donate the kidney (LRD) or receiving a transplant from someone who has died (CAD). Generally live-related transplants do better overall than cadaveric transplants as the match may be better and there is no long cold ischemia time as the transplant is a planned procedure.

The left kidney is usually used as the left renal vein is longer and therefore easier to manipulate. When the left kidney is anastomosed onto the right vessels the kidney is rotated so that the renal pelvis comes to lie more anteriorly. This rotation of the kidney has the advantage that if access to the renal pelvis is needed post-transplant, it is more superficial and accessible. The transplanted kidney is generally placed extraperitoneally, and in the older child it may be anastomosed to the iliac vessels. In the very young child the kidney may be anastomosed to the aorta and IVC. If the kidney is cadaveric, it is harvested with the main renal artery and a piece of aorta. In live related donors the kidneys are harvested only with the main renal artery, hence renal artery stenosis is higher in this group. Venous anastomosis is usually end-to-side to the recipient's external iliac vein.

The ureter is particularly prone to ischemia because the arteries supplying the ureter are not separately harvested and the principal blood supply is from the main renal artery (Fig. 3.51). The ureter is sometimes shortened at surgery to avoid the lower ureter becoming compromised by ischemia with resulting stricture and fibrosis. To avoid reflux the ureter is usually tunneled through the bladder wall.[42]

Pre-transplantation

Some children being considered for transplantation may have had multiple lines for venous access during hemodialysis and potentially may have had a venous thrombosis. In addition children with multiple anomalies such as the VACTERL association may have underlying congenital anomalies of the major vessels, such as a high bifurcation of the aorta, which the transplant surgeon needs to know about. It is important to be aware of any congenital anomalies of the aorta and IVC as well as any thromboses of the leg vessels after catheters, as this

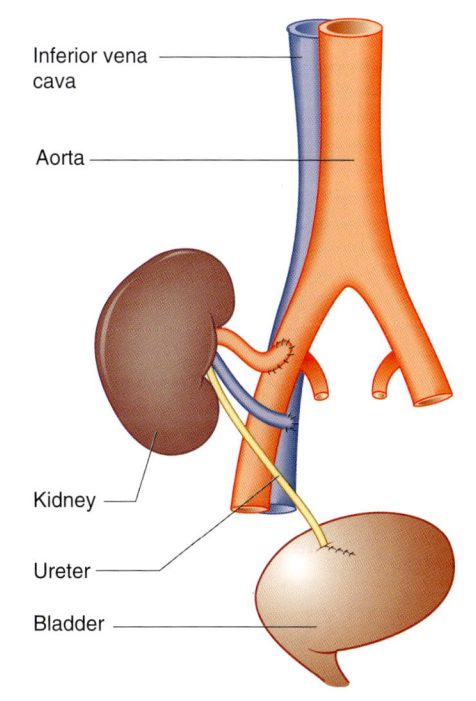

Figure 3.51 Transplant anatomy. The method in which the renal artery and vein and ureter are anastomosed during transplantation.

may influence the surgical approach. Ultrasound is generally sufficient, but more detailed anatomy of the vasculature may occasionally be required if ultrasound is inconclusive. Contrast venography or preferably MR angiography/venography should also be used.

Assessment of bladder function is an important part of the work-up, in particular in boys with obstructive uropathies. Often gastrostomies are placed so as to improve the overall nutrition of the child both for the transplant and post-surgery.

Post-transplantation

The major post-transplant complication in young children is thrombosis, primarily of the renal vein but also of the artery (Table 3.5). It has been shown that thrombosis can be reduced by avoiding young CAD donors and by heparinizing patients for 10 days post-transplant. Ensuring graft survival with prompt detection and diagnosis of complications is essential.

There are considerable variations in positioning of the artery and vein depending on the patient's size and access, and it is best to consult the surgical notes when assessing the vasculature of the pediatric renal transplant.[43,44]

The ureter is prone to developing stenoses and strictures anywhere along its course but particularly in the lower ureter, and any degree of new dilation in the transplanted kidney should be actively investigated.[45]

The major imaging techniques used are ultrasound and nuclear medicine studies, with the occasional need for cross sectional imaging or interventional techniques.

The ultrasound examination

The ultrasound examination of the renal transplant is generally easier than that of a native kidney because the transplant is more superficial. In addition the position of the transplant makes Doppler more accessible both for the intrarenal vessels and transplant artery.

Generally a curvilinear probe is the best for a good overall view of the transplant, but the choice of probe will depend on the patient's size and depth of transplant. The parenchyma is well defined peripherally and the medullae are also easier to see. The transplant vessels at hila level should not be confused with the renal pelvis, and power Doppler or color should be used. Spectral Doppler is needed for quantification.

Table 3.5 Type, incidence and timing of complications following renal transplantation

Complication	Incidence	Time after transplantation
Vascular		
Arterial stenosis	10%	Any time, usually within 3 years
Arteriovenous fistulae/pseudoaneurysms	1–18%	Any time, usually after renal biopsy
Graft thrombosis		
Renal vein thrombosis	0.3–3%	
Renal arterial thrombosis	0.2–3.5%	Early postoperative course, usually within 10 days
Non-vascular		
Rejection (hyperacute, acute, chronic)		
Ureteral obstruction	2–10%	Usually within 3 months
Urinary leak	1–5%	Usually within 2 weeks
Perirenal collections	14%	Early postoperative course, usually 2–6 weeks
–urinoma		
–hematoma		
–abscess		
–lymphocele		

Stents are often used in pediatric transplantations, and the position of the stent should be commented on. Any dilation of the collecting system should be further investigated as a matter of urgency because ureteral stenoses are common in children.

The bladder should be visualized. It is normally echo free, and any echoes will be from particulate matter which may be infection or hemorrhage.

The Doppler examination The Doppler examination is done to give a global assessment of the renal vasculature and the renal artery and vein. In children who are not cooperative after a transplant, start off by using color Doppler energy for the overview. Once an interlobular vessel has been identified then the gate is placed and a trace obtained. The trace is similar to that of the native kidney and reflects a low resistance bed with a ski slope appearance. The resistive index (RI) and pulsatility index (PI) are the most commonly used indices although the importance of their role in clinical management is very much dependent on the center.

It is essential to identify the iliac artery and vein so as not to confuse them with the transplant vessels. The transplant artery can be quite difficult to interrogate, as it is tortuous. Flow in the renal vein must be seen.[46]

In children who are hypertensive after transplantation it has been reported that the most sensitive indicator of renal artery stenosis is an increase in peak systolic velocity, generally over 2.5 m/s.

The complications arising from transplantation can be either early or late and related to the surgical procedure, ischemia, rejection, urinary tract infection, drug toxicity, obstruction or the recurrence of pre-existing disease.

Primary non-function

Primary non-function refers to a transplanted kidney that never starts working and producing urine. It is usual once the artery and vein and ureter have been successfully anastomosed that the transplant starts producing urine on the table. The immediate causes of primary non-function are acute tubular necrosis (Fig. 3.52), renal artery thrombosis or renal vein thrombosis. Other less common causes are obstruction from blood clot or ureteric anastomoses problems, acute rejection, urinary leak and collections. A good Doppler examination will help differentiate the first three primary diagnoses. In ATN there will be excellent arterial and venous traces. In renal artery thrombosis there will be no arterial or venous trace as there will be no blood entering the kidney. In renal vein thrombosis there will be no venous trace, but a systolic rise most times without any diastolic flow or reversal of flow in diastole will be seen, i.e. the blood can get into the kidney but not out. The treatment is different in the three conditions, and if a vascular problem is suspected the patient will be taken back to theater as an emergency to try to salvage the kidney. Accurate diagnosis is essential.

In children, especially the younger child with smaller vessels, there is a higher incidence of vascular complications in the immediate post-transplant period than seen in adults.

Ultrasound monitoring

Imaging children post-transplantation is broadly similar to that in adults, with a few exceptions. A young child may have a large adult kidney transplanted, usually from a parent, into the abdomen. This adult kidney may make it difficult to close the abdominal wall once anastomosed, although delayed closure of the abdomen has not been problematic in our group of patients.

Realistically ultrasound has a large and clearly defined role in monitoring the transplant, detecting vascular thrombosis, detecting dilation of the pelvicaliceal system and hence detecting ureteric obstruction, and finally in documenting any postoperative collections of blood, urine or lymph. The expectation that ultrasound can differentiate acute rejection from toxicity of the immunosuppressant cyclosporin remains a dream.

Once the immediate post-transplantation period has passed, Doppler energy to look at the general 'perfusion' of the transplant kidney as a quick assessment is very useful in an uncooperative child (Figs 3.53 and 3.54). If there is a clinical history of persisting hypertension, every effort must be made to evaluate the main renal artery with color flow Doppler and spectral flow traces. The Doppler indices, however, have been disappointing in their ability to differentiate causes of graft dysfunction,

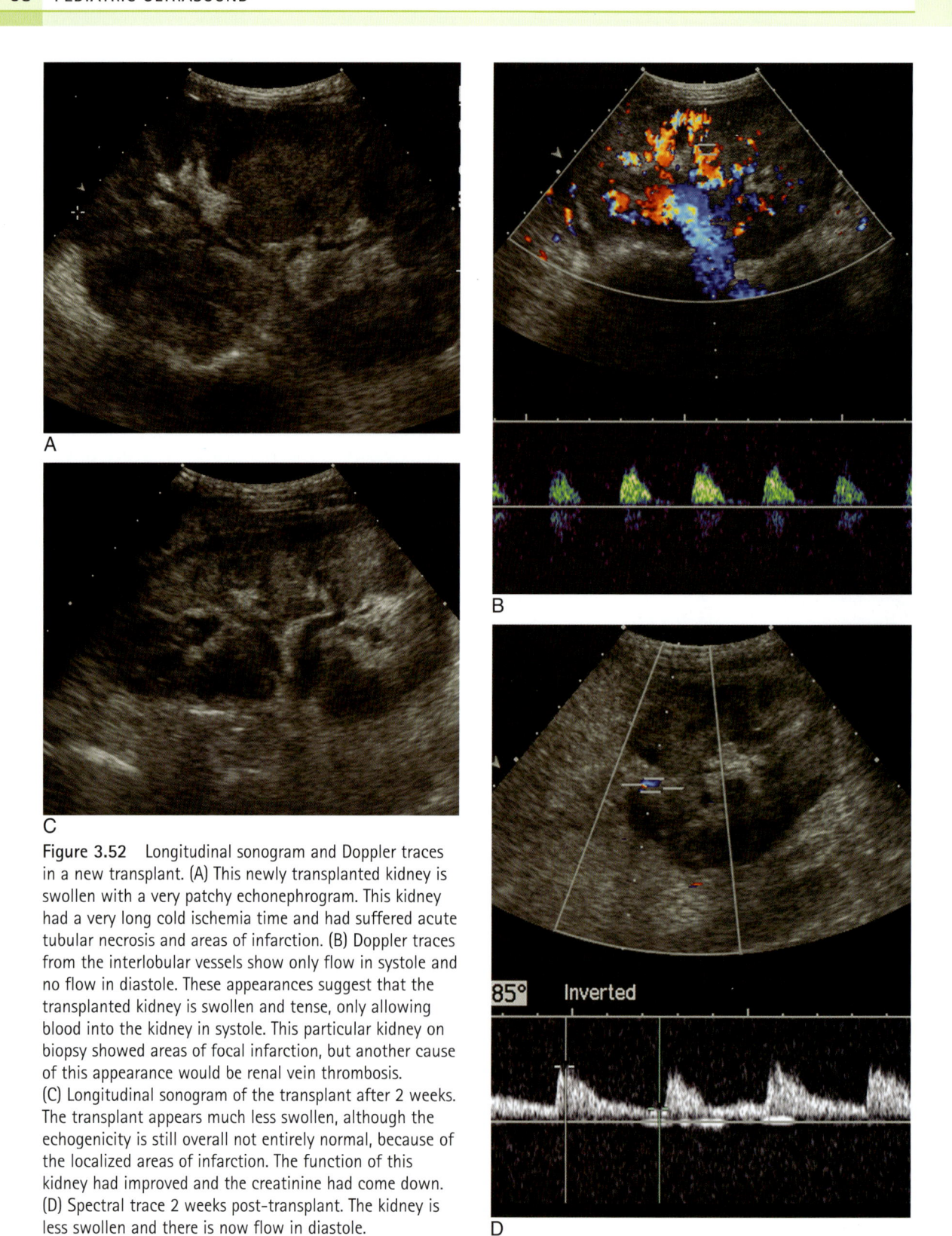

Figure 3.52 Longitudinal sonogram and Doppler traces in a new transplant. (A) This newly transplanted kidney is swollen with a very patchy echonephrogram. This kidney had a very long cold ischemia time and had suffered acute tubular necrosis and areas of infarction. (B) Doppler traces from the interlobular vessels show only flow in systole and no flow in diastole. These appearances suggest that the transplanted kidney is swollen and tense, only allowing blood into the kidney in systole. This particular kidney on biopsy showed areas of focal infarction, but another cause of this appearance would be renal vein thrombosis.
(C) Longitudinal sonogram of the transplant after 2 weeks. The transplant appears much less swollen, although the echogenicity is still overall not entirely normal, because of the localized areas of infarction. The function of this kidney had improved and the creatinine had come down.
(D) Spectral trace 2 weeks post-transplant. The kidney is less swollen and there is now flow in diastole.

THE URINARY TRACT 99

in particular ATN, rejection and cyclosporin toxicity. Some institutions use serial PI or RI together with biochemical and clinical findings to guide biopsy, but we find them non-specific and not particularly useful.

Ultrasound will help to differentiate surgical from non-surgical complications in children who present later with a non-specific rise in creatinine. Caliceal, pelvic or ureteric dilation should be sought, as well as imaging the bladder. The position and size of any perirenal or pelvic collections should be monitored and, if causing obstruction to the collecting system, should be drained.

Although ultrasound is the prime imaging modality in use, results should be compared with those of the ^{99m}Tc DTPA when performed. The importance of this integration is that often a specific diagnosis can be more accurately achieved by combining these results, which may obviate the need for a biopsy. MRI will allow visualization of the transplant artery, particularly with gadolinium-enhanced techniques. The value of MRI in distin-

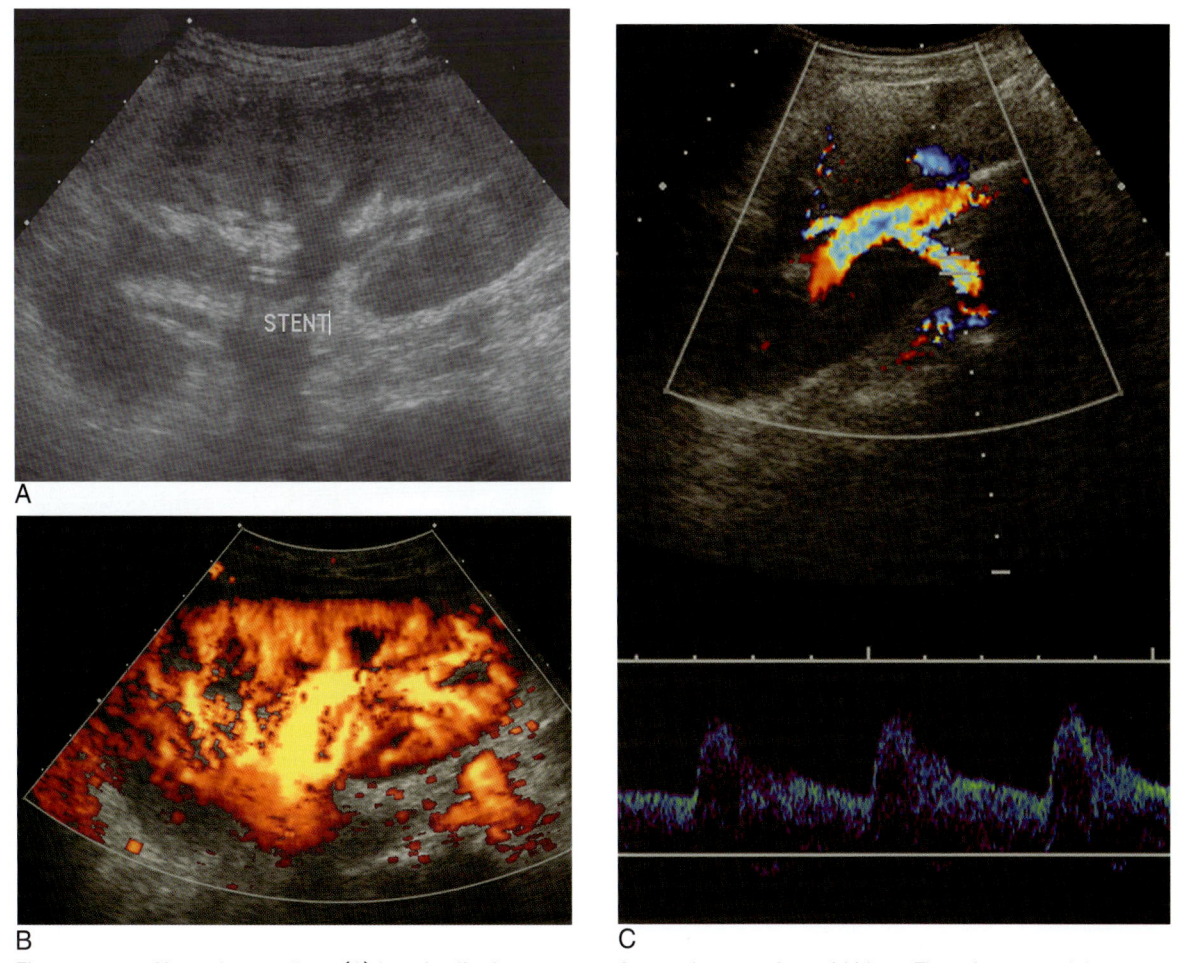

Figure 3.53 Normal transplant. (A) Longitudinal sonogram of a newly transplanted kidney. There is a stent lying within the central collecting system, and there is no dilation of the collecting system. (B) Longitudinal sonogram of the same kidney in power Doppler mode. Power gives a good overall view of the transplanted kidney and is very useful in a fractious child. (C) Demonstration of the spectral trace after renal transplantation. There is forward flow in systole and diastole. The arterial and venous trace should be easily identifiable within the kidney and renal hilum.

guishing the different causes of graft dysfunction has yet to be evaluated.

Obstruction

Early obstruction is generally caused by a blood clot, whereas late obstruction is generally caused by ureteric narrowing or compression from a lymphocele. A collection of fluid can be drained, whereas a ureteric stenosis may require a nephrostomy.[47]

Ureteral obstruction occurs in up to 10% and may result from ischemia, kinking, unrecognized PUJ stenosis, position of lower ureteric anastomosis in the bladder, extrinsic compression such as a collection, or intrinsic obstruction such as a clot. The commonest cause in children is ischemia, which is usually in the lower ureter. The diagnosis of obstruction may be difficult because hydronephrosis may or may not be present, especially in early obstruction. Also, mild collecting system distension is occasionally seen with a full bladder. It is important to repeat the ultrasound with an empty bladder. If dilation is new or persistent then either an IVU or antegrade study is warranted. Antegrade ureteric stenting is also used, with definitive treatment being delayed.

Interference with the blood supply to the ureter will result in a narrowed, stenotic ureter and a hydronephrosis/hydroureter detectable by ultrasound. The late development of a PUJ stenosis in the transplanted kidney is a well-recognized complication. Any new dilation of the pelvicaliceal system requires further imaging, e.g. IVU or ante-

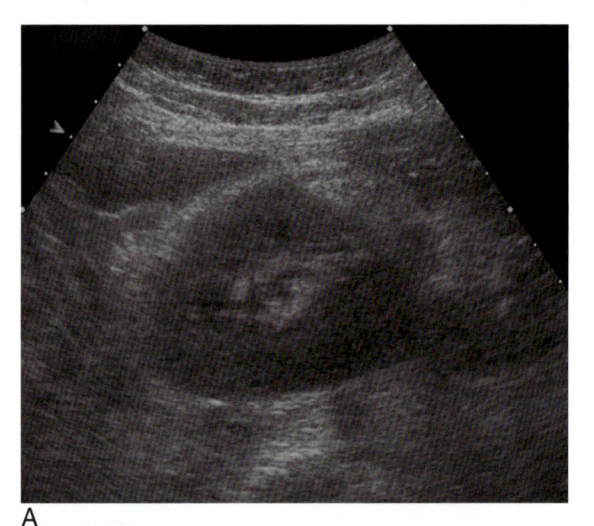

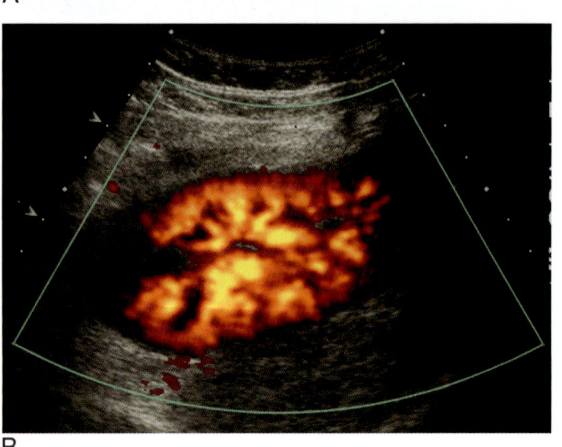

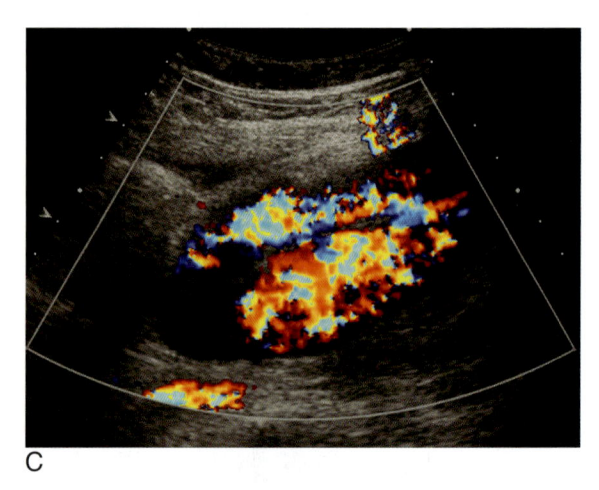

Figure 3.54 Infarcted transplant. (A) Gray scale ultrasound on a newly transplanted kidney. (B) Power mode in this newly transplanted kidney. There is a triangular wedge defect in the upper pole. (C) Color Doppler confirming there is a wedge defect in the upper pole. This kidney had an accessory artery, which was lost at surgery, supplying the upper pole. This is the area of infarction.

grade studies (Fig. 3.55), to show the level of obstruction.

The IVU has an important but limited role. When ultrasound detects a change with dilation of the collecting system despite an empty bladder, then an IVU is indicated to assess the exact level of the partial hold-up, provided the renal function will allow adequate opacification of the system. Progress to an antegrade study and then either a double J stent or a balloon dilation may be needed, depending on what is found, to relieve a stenosis of the ureter.

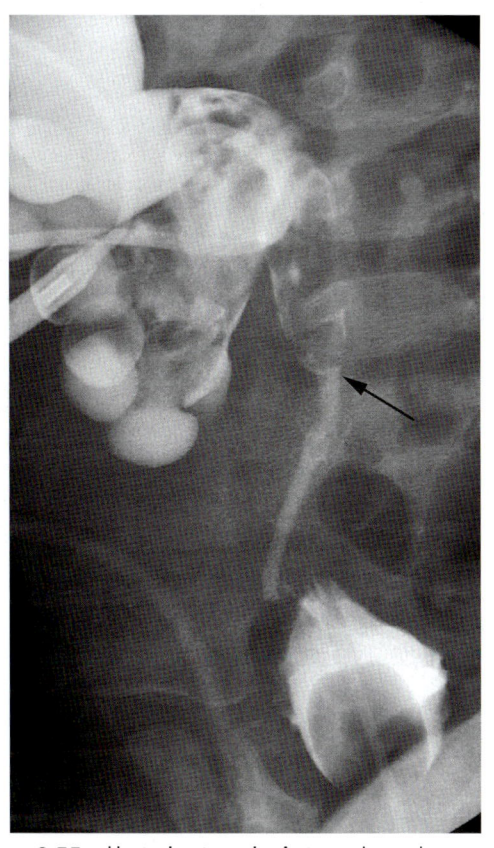

Figure 3.55 Ureteric stenosis. Antegrade pyelogram on a transplanted kidney demonstrating clot within the collecting system and a tight tubular narrowing of the upper ureter. The ureter had strictured around the stent (arrow). Ureteric stenosis post-transplant is not an unusual occurrence, as the blood supply to the ureter is compromised at transplantation. Any new dilation of the collecting system of a transplanted kidney on ultrasound should be actively investigated.

Late dysfunction

A late decrease in renal function may be due to rejection. This is a constant problem after transplantation and must be distinguished from drug toxicity, recurrence of the original disease, or late development of obstruction. All modalities of imaging have been generally disappointing in differentiating between rejection and drug toxicity, so that ultimately all patients have renal biopsies in order for the definitive diagnosis of rejection to be made.

Urinary leaks, usually from the ureter, have decreased in incidence with the routine placement of ureteric stents and are now more commonly seen after removal of the stent. Ultrasound will demonstrate the collection and, if necessary, drainage and/or nuclear medicine studies will confirm it is urine.

Lymphoceles are readily detected by ultrasound as large cystic septated collections, but cannot be reliably differentiated from urinomas or large hematomas. A ^{99m}Tc MAG3 scan will show whether these is urine going into the collection, i.e. a urinoma, or if this is a photon deficient area and therefore more likely a lymphocele. Lymphoceles will require treatment if the patient is symptomatic or if compression of the ureter occurs. Simple percutaneous drainage is ineffective, as they recur, and a sclerosing agent may be needed to permanently collapse the lymphocele.

When children develop hypertension then arterial stenosis at the site of surgery must be considered. This is uncommon with cadaveric donor kidneys since the renal artery usually comes on a patch of aorta but is more likely with live living donor transplant. In the context of hypertension, arteriography is required. The role of magnetic resonance angiography (MRA) is being evaluated, and the results are promising, but formal catheter angiography remains the reference technique currently used, particularly in children. The preferred method of treatment is angioplasty, so that formal angiography in this clinical setting is readily undertaken.

Arteriovenous fistula (AVF) and pseudoaneurysms

AVFs and pseudoaneurysms can complicate up to 20% of transplants and are generally the result of percutaneous renal biopsies (Fig. 3.56). They may present acutely with a large bleed, but more commonly the majority of AVFs and pseudoaneurysms resolve. These fistulas can be readily detected with duplex ultrasound as the findings are highly specific. If potentially life threatening the fistula can be treated by selective arterial catheterization and embolization, which will be curative.

Malignancy

Lymphoproliferative disorder is a well-recognized complication of all transplantation with concomitant immunosuppression. The children may present with local or generalized lymphadenopathy, and simply curtailing the immunotherapy may resolve the enlarged lymph nodes. There is a well-recognized association with Epstein–Barr virus. Occasionally children may present with an aggressive lymphoma requiring full chemotherapy.

TUMORS OF THE KIDNEY

The commonest solid renal tumor of childhood is a Wilms tumor (nephroblastoma). It accounts for 90% of the renal tumors of childhood. Wilms tumors usually occur in children aged about 3–5 years, and outside this age range they are rare. The other histological types of renal tumors are much less common, such as a rhabdoid tumor, which occurs in younger children and is highly malignant, and the clear cell sarcoma which metastasizes to bone. Renal carcinoma occurs in older children

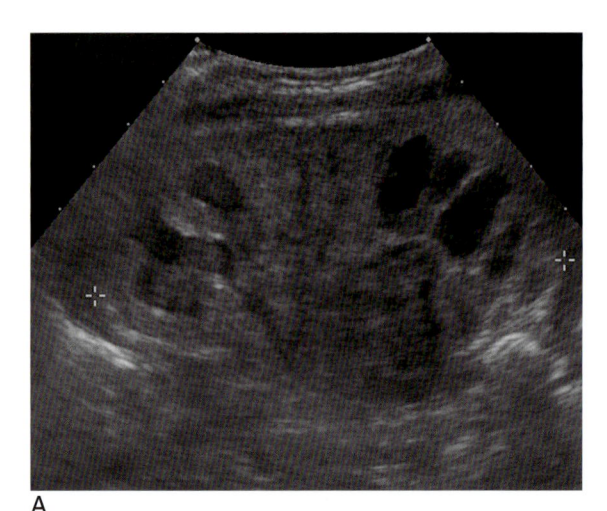

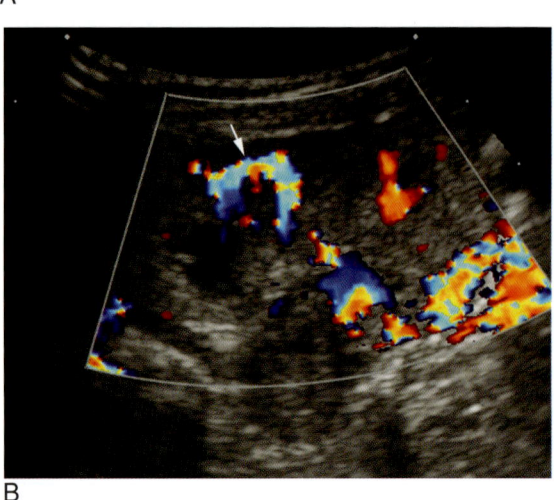

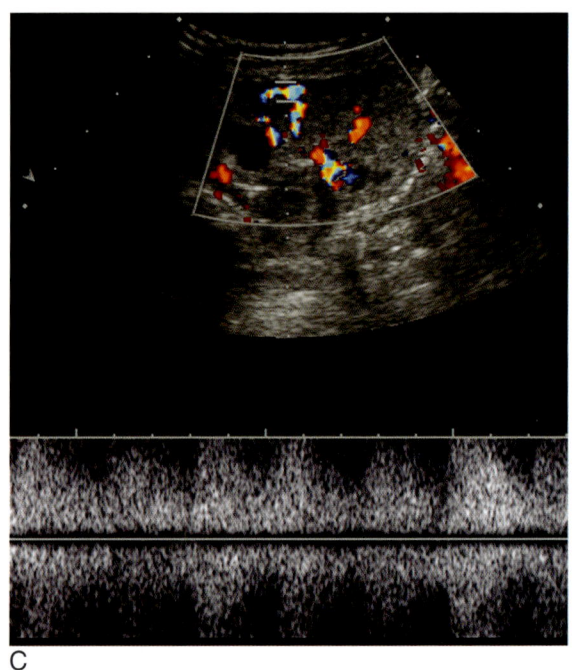

Figure 3.56 Arteriovenous malformation after post-transplant renal biopsy. (A) Longitudinal sonogram on a kidney after renal biopsy. The collecting system is dilated and there is blood clot within the calices and pelvis. (B) On color flow there is a localized area where the vessels connect (arrow). (C) Spectral Doppler taken at this localized area shows spectral broadening with no proper arterial or venous trace. This is a typical appearance of an AV shunt. It is very useful to try and identify the shunt first on color flow and then confirm on careful examination with spectral Doppler that it is an AV shunt.

> **Box 3.9 Sonographic features of Wilms tumor**
>
> *Typical*
> - Well-defined, solid renal mass
> - Small sliver of remaining normal kidney
> - Mass usually shows 'venous lakes'. Unusual to be completely solid
> - If IVC not seen, it may be compressed by right sided tumor
> - Tumor thrombus usually expands IVC
> - Aorta displaced rather than undermined
> - Lymphadenopathy not a feature
> - Liver metastases rare at presentation. Usually hypoechoic
> - Carefully examine contralateral kidney for size and focal areas of nephroblastomatosis
>
> *Atypical*
> - Rarely presents with tumor rupture
> - If extends beyond renal capsule, consider another diagnosis
> - If dense calcification consider XPN
> - If visible lymph node masses consider NBL
> - If vascular encasement consider NBL
>
> NBL, neuroblastoma; XPN, xanthogranulomatous pyelonephritis.

whereas the mesoblastic nephroma is the primary solid malignancy in the neonate. Secondary deposits from lymphomas and leukemia do occur.[48]

Wilms tumor

Clinical presentation

These children usually present with an abdominal mass. There may be associated hematuria, fever and hypertension. Wilms tumors usually present in the under 5 age group and are unilateral in 95%. These tumors are extremely rapidly growing, and the clinical presentation may be related to tumor hemorrhage or rupture. Rarely are they found during screening.[49]

Ultrasound is the first examination on any child presenting with an abdominal mass.[50]

Sonographic appearances

Typical sonographic features of Wilms tumor are listed in Box 3.9. The appearances are very much dependent on the stage and size of the renal tumor at presentation. The tumor is usually well defined with no definite normal renal parenchyma seen. Sometimes a sliver of compressed kidney may be visible on the edge of the tumor mass. Very occasionally the Wilms tumor may be completely exophytic, i.e. arising from the kidney but completely extrarenal (Fig. 3.57).

The mass is predominantly solid, but hypoechoic areas or venous lakes are a common feature. The renal vein and IVC must be carefully examined as invasion may occur with tumor thrombus (Fig. 3.58). The contralateral kidney must be carefully examined both for nephroblastomatosis and a distinct renal tumor. A small number of Wilms tumors calcify (as opposed to a neuroblastoma) and the calcification is generally coarse and linear. Lymphadenopathy is not usually a feature of Wilms tumors but rather that of neuroblastoma. The role of ultrasound is to make the diagnosis and thus direct further imaging.

It is important for the sonographer not to misdiagnose solid renal lesions and in particular xanthogranulomatous pyelonephritis, which will show dense calculi with or without extrarenal rupture.[51] Occasionally the intrarenal mass may be cystic throughout (Fig. 3.59). The liver must

- hemihypertrophy (3%)
- Beckwith–Wiedemann syndrome
- Perlman syndrome
- sporadic aniridia (33%)
- Wagr syndrome
- Drash syndrome—pseudohermaphrodite
- renal anomalies—horseshoe kidney
- neurofibromatosis.

Screening for Wilms in high risk conditions

If patients with high risk conditions are to be screened it must be remembered that Wilms tumors are very rapidly growing and tend to occur usually within the first 3–5 years. It is therefore suggested that ultrasound examinations should take place with a minimal interval of 3 months. However, this does cause a great deal of parental anxiety, and some have suggested abdominal examination by the parent as an alternative.[52–54]

Wilms tumor staging

Wilms tumors are staged as follows:[55]

- Stage I: tumor confined to the kidney without capsular or vascular invasion
- Stage II: tumor beyond renal capsule; vessel infiltration
- Stage III: positive lymph nodes in the abdomen or pelvis, peritoneal invasion or residual tumor at surgical margins; tumor spillage
- Stage IV: metastatic disease outside the abdomen or pelvis
- Stage V: bilateral tumors at presentation.

Figure 3.60 shows a series of scans on a girl with bilateral Wilms tumor with recurrence.

Other renal tumors of childhood

Mesoblastic nephroma

Mesoblastic nephroma is the commonest solid renal tumor seen in the neonatal period. It generally has a good prognosis, and surgical excision is curative. Some have been diagnosed prenatally. Ultrasound appearances are slightly different to those seen in a Wilms tumor. The renal mass is generally more solid in appearance, without

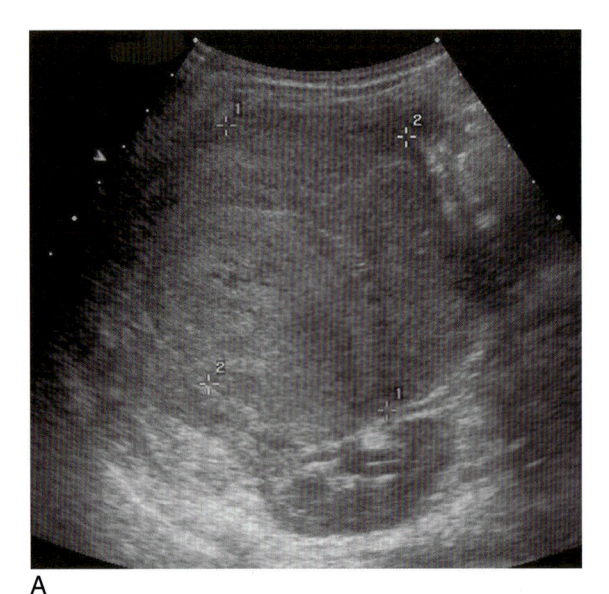

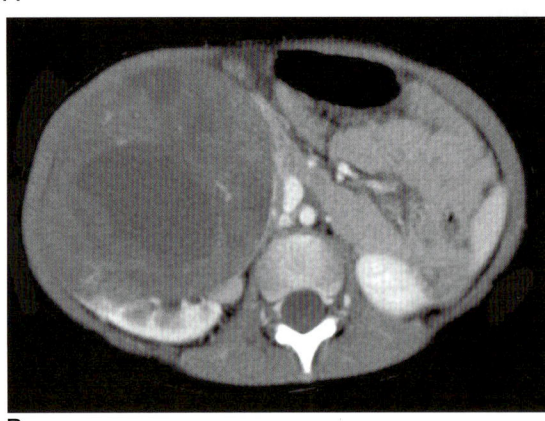

Figure 3.57 Exophytic Wilms tumor. (A) Transverse sonogram in a child presenting with an abdominal mass (between calipers). The normal kidney is squashed posteriorly by the large extrarenal mass. This was a Wilms tumor which was predominantly extrarenal. This can sometimes confuse the unsuspecting sonographer. (B) CT examination on the same child, showing this largely extrarenal mass pushing the IVC across the midline.

be carefully examined for hypoechoic metastases (see Ch. 4 for ultrasound differences with neuroblastoma).

Occasionally the children present with trauma, and the use of Doppler will help differentiate between a hematoma and tumor.

A number of conditions are associated with Wilms tumors:

THE URINARY TRACT 105

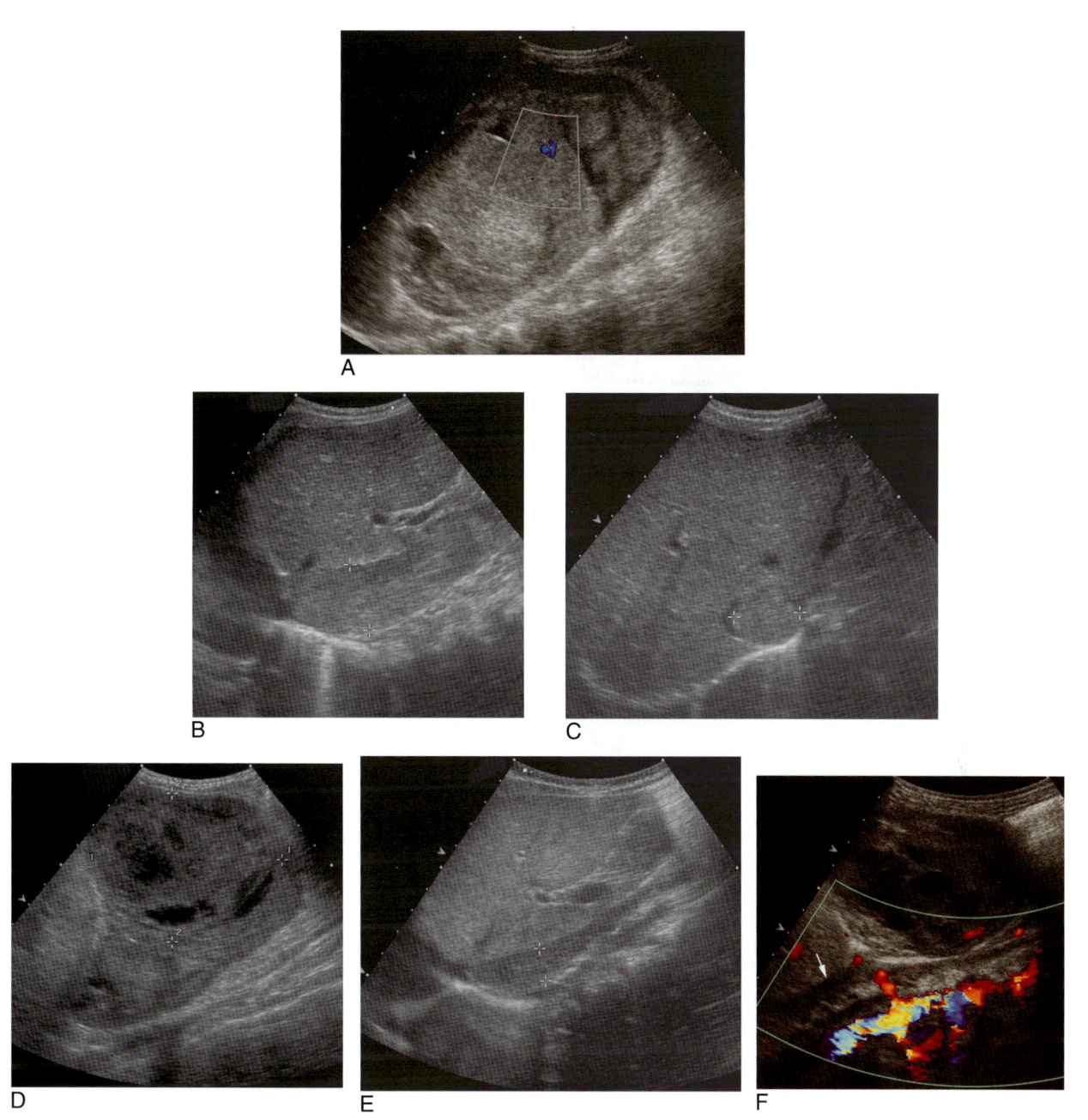

Figure 3.58 Wilms tumor with tumor in the IVC. (A) Longitudinal sonogram of a right-sided abdominal mass. The mass is heterogeneous with a small amount of compressed normal renal tissue superiorly. On Doppler this mass was not particularly vascular. (B) Longitudinal sonogram of the IVC. The IVC (between the calipers) is dilated and filled with tumor thrombus. The tumor thrombus is extending up to the right atrium. (C) Transverse sonogram of the IVC. There is a thin hypoechoic rim around the edge of the dilated tumor thrombus filling the IVC (between calipers). (D) Longitudinal sonogram of the right renal mass 6 weeks later and after chemotherapy. The mass is significantly smaller in size with areas of breakdown centrally. The mass is lying within the calipers. Also, normal renal tissue can be seen superiorly and posteriorly. (E) Longitudinal sonogram at the same time of the IVC (between calipers). The tumor thrombus is still within the IVC but is less distended. (F) Doppler examination. There is no flow in the IVC because of the tumor thrombus (arrow). The aorta is located posteriorly because of the oblique projection on ultrasound, and the origins of the two renal arteries can be seen.

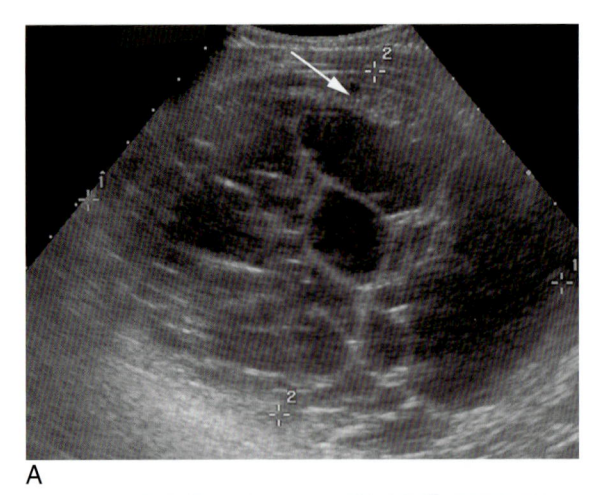

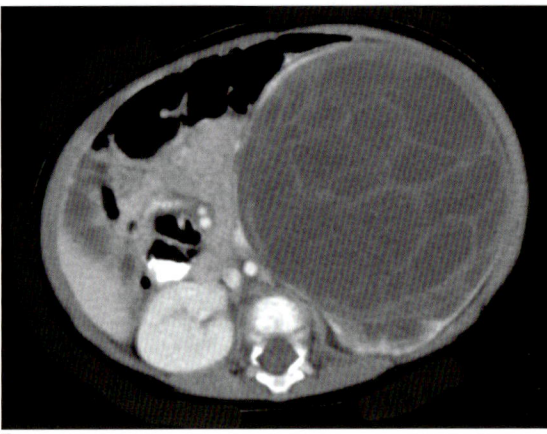

Figure 3.59 Cystic Wilms tumor. (A) Prone longitudinal sonogram of a large predominantly cystic Wilms tumor (between calipers). There is some compressed renal tissue seen posteriorly (arrow). (B) CT examination of the abdomen on the same child showing the large cystic mass arising from the left kidney. The aorta and IVC are pushed to the right.

the lakes, and it may have a whorled appearance (Fig. 3.61).

Rhabdoid tumor

This is a highly aggressive renal malignancy that occurs in younger children and it is not unusual at presentation for them to have metastases to the lungs, liver, brain and skeleton.[56]

Clear cell sarcoma

This accounts for a small percentage (4%) of childhood solid renal masses. It is almost indistinguishable from a Wilms tumor on imaging. The important differentiating feature of this type of renal tumor is that it metastasizes to bone. These children need radioisotope bone scans complemented by MRI scans. It is more common in males and does not occur bilaterally.

Renal cell carcinoma

This rare form occurs in the older child, generally over 10 years of age.

Lymphoma/Leukemia

Bilateral renal involvement is not uncommonly seen in children. The appearances are very similar to those seen in adults, usually with evidence of disease elsewhere. Ultrasound diagnosis of renal enlargement with hypoechoic areas of cellular infiltration is a typical appearance. This is associated with other sites of disease such as the liver, spleen and lymph nodes. Usually these other sites are known clinically. Renal ultrasound should be performed in all children with leukemia, particularly ALL and lymphoma, prior to the commencement of treatment. Disease should be sought elsewhere within the abdomen—in particular abnormalities of size and echogenicity of the liver and spleen, upper abdominal lymphadenopathy or a lymphomatous nodal mass.

Nephroblastomatosis

Nephroblastomatosis is residual embryonic blastema rests within the kidney. It is known to be premalignant and is found in almost all patients with bilateral Wilms tumors. It may be perilobar or intralobar. It may be difficult to diagnose on ultrasound as it has a mixed appearance and may be hypo-, hyper- or isoechoic. This is one of the reasons why CT and/or MRI plus contrast is needed in all children (Fig. 3.62).[57–59]

Rhabdomyosarcoma

The genitourinary tract is the second most common site for rhabdomyosarcoma tumors. They

THE URINARY TRACT 107

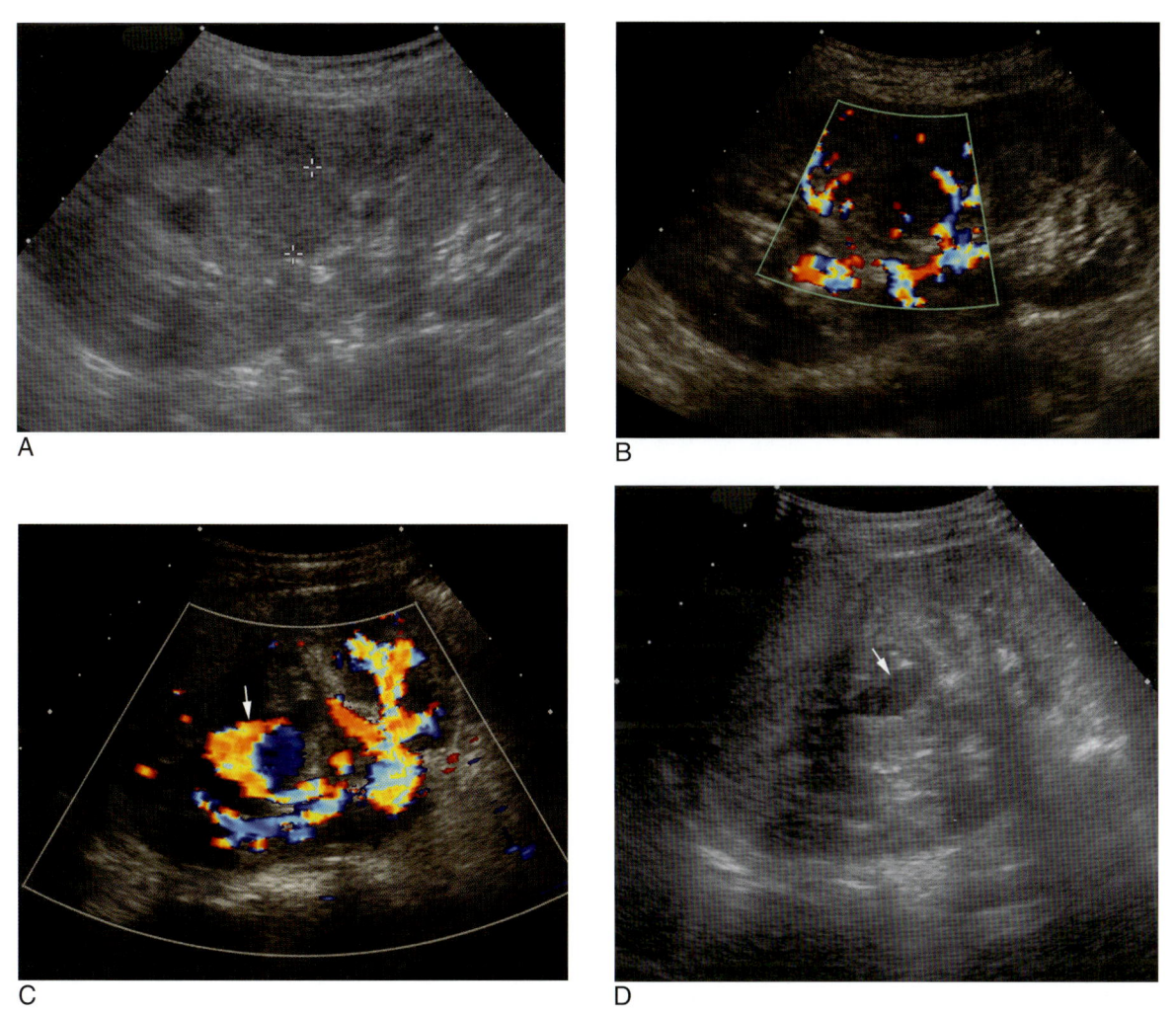

Figure 3.60 Bilateral Wilms tumor with recurrence. (A) Longitudinal sonogram of the left kidney. This girl's right kidney had been removed because of a Wilms tumor. There is a nodule (between the calipers) lying adjacent to the collecting system. On biopsy this was found to be a small nodule of Wilms tissue within her contralateral kidney. (B) Longitudinal sonogram of the left kidney with Doppler. The central nodule is hypovascular, with displacement of the vessels around it. (C) Longitudinal sonogram after resection of that centrally located Wilms tumor. There is an unusual configuration of the kidney arising from surgery. In addition this child had developed an AV shunt (arrow) as a complication of the surgery. This settled down on conservative treatment. (D) Longitudinal sonogram of the same area without Doppler. There is a hypoechoic area (arrow) centrally in the kidney which could be mistaken for a dilated calix. This demonstrates the importance of Doppler examination after resection.

Continued

may arise from the bladder wall, the prostate or the vagina in girls. The commonest presentation of a prostatic rhabdomyosarcoma is acute urinary retention. A vaginal rhabdomyosarcoma may prolapse out of the vagina on the perineum and has a botryoides or 'grape-like' appearance. If arising from the bladder wall, it will present as an abdominal mass.[60]

The ultrasound appearances are those of a solid mass, either fundal or at the bladder base, sometimes with some central areas of necrosis. It is important to carefully assess the bladder wall for invasion and thickening on the ultrasound examination. The rest of the abdomen must be evaluated for lymphadenopathy and hepatic spread (Fig. 3.63).

108 PEDIATRIC ULTRASOUND

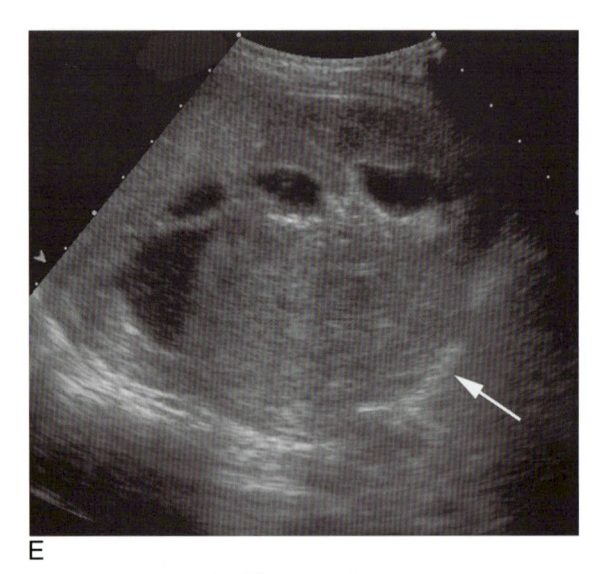

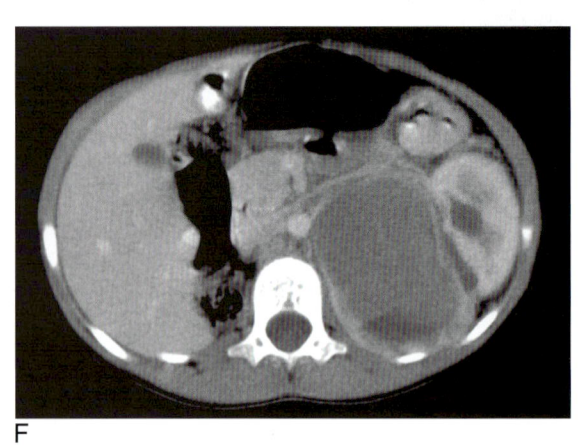

Figure 3.60, cont'd (E) Longitudinal sonogram on the same kidney 8 months later. This was a routine follow-up. Note the unusual configuration of the kidney with dilated calices and a large mass arising anteriorly from the kidney (arrow). (F) Contrast-enhanced CT examination on the same child on the same day as (e). There is a mass arising from the single remaining kidney.

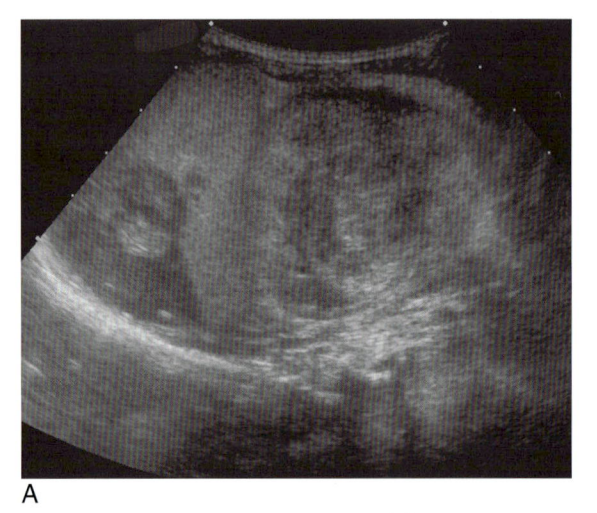

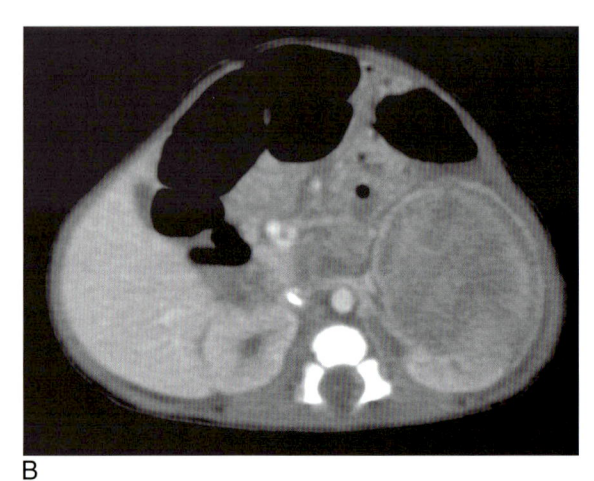

Figure 3.61 Mesoblastic nephroma. (A) Longitudinal sonogram of the left kidney in an infant. This shows the solid renal mass. The appearances are different to a 'typical' Wilms tumor in that the mass is predominantly solid and has a 'whorled' appearance. A small sliver of kidney is just about visible in the upper pole. (B) CT examination on the same child. There is a small amount of enhancing normal kidney posteriorly.

THE URINARY TRACT 109

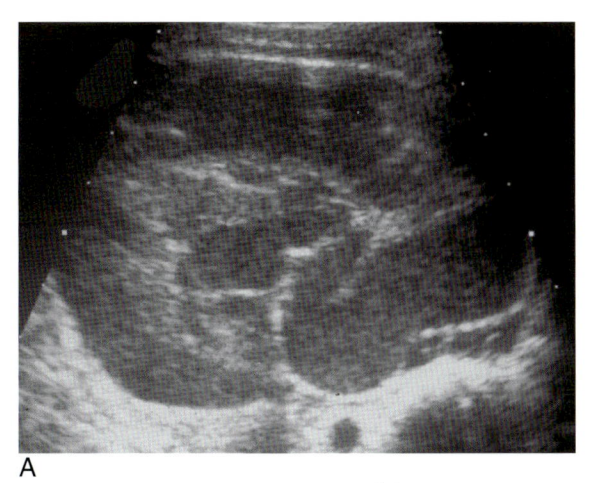

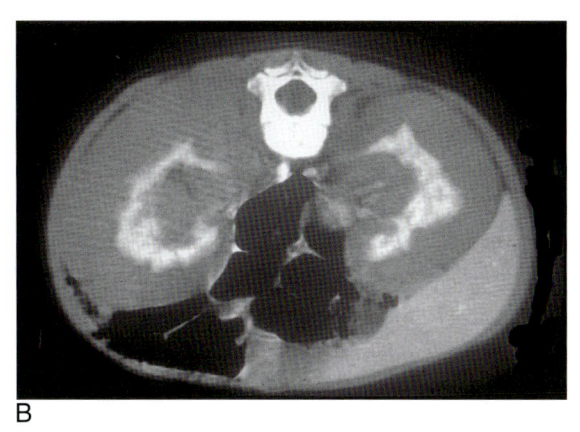

A B

Figure 3.62 Nephroblastomatosis. (A) Longitudinal sonogram on a child with hemihypertrophy. The kidneys were large with a subcortical hypoechoic layer of tissue which is the nephroblastomatosis. (B) Contrast-enhanced CT examination on the same child clearly demonstrating the nephroblastomatosis with the normal renal tissue squashed centrally. This child was examined prone as she was about to have a renal biopsy.

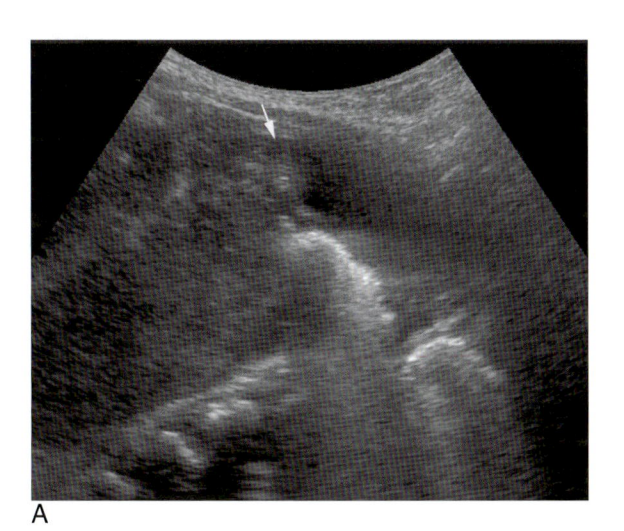

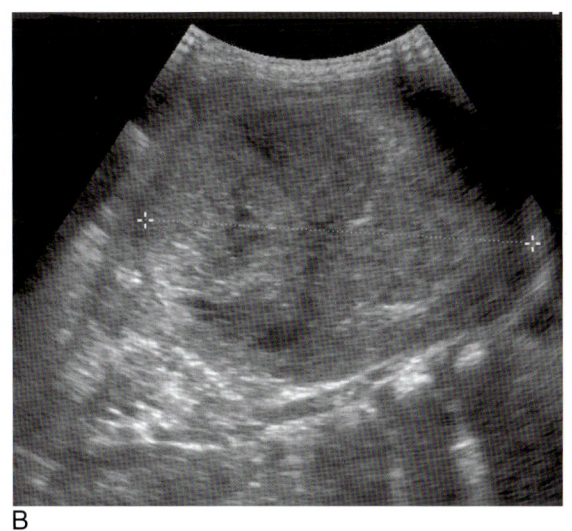

A B

Figure 3.63 Rhabdomyosarcoma of the bladder. (A) & (B) Longitudinal and transverse sonogram of the abdomen in a 2 year old presenting with an abdominal mass. There is a well-defined solid mass abutting and arising from the fundus of the bladder (arrow) which on biopsy was a rhabdomyosarcoma. Other typical sites are the prostate in boys. If they arise from the vagina in girls, this is rarely diagnosed on ultrasound as they present clinically with a protruding mass or bleeding.

Continued

Figure 3.63, *cont'd* (C) Contrast-enhanced CT examination on the same child, demonstrating the large solid mass filling the abdomen.

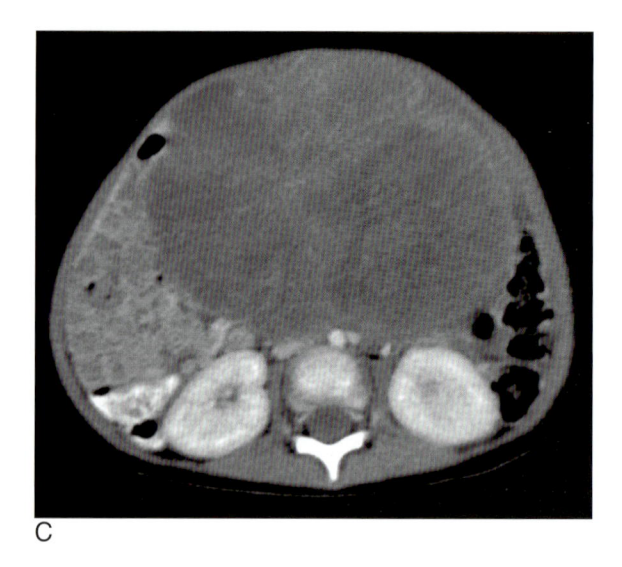

SUMMARY

Ultrasound is the major imaging modality in the pediatric renal tract, which provides the bulk of the workload in most departments. It is used both for the initial diagnosis and the follow-up of renal conditions. The sonographer must learn to perform a meticulous examination and have a standard examination protocol.

References

1. Hellstrom M, Hjalmas K, Jacobsson B, et al. Normal ureteral diameter in infancy and childhood. Acta Radiol 1985; 26:433–439.
2. Fernbach SK, Maizels M, Conway JJ. Ultrasound grading of hydronephrosis: introduction to the system used by the Society for Fetal Urology. Pediatr Radiol 1993; 23:478–480.
3. Dinkel E, Ertel M, Dittrich M, et al. Kidney size in childhood. Sonographical growth charts for kidney length and volume. Pediatr Radiol 1985; 15:38.
4. Holloway H, Jones TB, Robinson AE, et al. Sonographic determination of renal volumes in normal neonates. Pediatr Radiol 1983; 13:212.
5. Rosenbaum DM, Korngold E, Littlewood-Teele R. Sonographic assessment of renal length in normal children. AJR Am J Roentgenol 1984; 142:467.
6. Rottenberg GT, de Bruyn R, Gordon I. Sonographic standards for single functioning kidney in children. AJR Am J Roentgenol 1996; 167:1255–1259.
7. Jequier S, Rousseau O. Sonographic measurements of the normal bladder wall in children. AJR Am J Roentgenol 1987; 149:563.
8. Anderson PJ, Rangarjan V, Gordon I. Assessment of drainage in PUJ dilatation: pelvic excretion efficiency as an index of renal function. Nucl Med Comm 1997; 18:823–826.
9. Crabbe DCG, Thomas DFM, Gordon AC, et al. Use of Tc99m DMSA to show patterns of renal damage associated with prenatally detected vesicoureteral reflux. J Urol 1992; 148:1239–1241.
10. Elder JS. Importance of antenatal diagnosis of vesicoureteral reflux. J Urol 1992; 148:1750–1754.
11. Sheridan M, Jewkes F, Gough DCS. Reflux nephropathy in the first year of life – The role of infection. Ped Surg Int 1991; 6:214–217.
12. Tibballs JM, de Bruyn R. Primary vesicoureteric reflux – how useful is postnatal ultrasound? Arch Dis Child 1996; 75:444–447.
13. Zerin JM, Ritchey ML, Chang ACH. Incidental vesicoureteral reflux in neonates with antenatally detected hydronephrosis and other renal abnormalities. Radiology 1993; 187:157–160.
14. Avni EF, Aradi K, Rypans F, et al. Can careful ultrasound examination of the urinary tract exclude vesicoureteric reflux in the neonate. Br J Radiol 1997; 70:977–982.
15. Koff SA. Neonatal management of unilateral hydronephrosis. Role of delayed intervention. Urol Clinics North Am 1998; 25:181–186.
16. Ransley PG, Dhillon HK, Gordon I, et al. The postnatal management of hydronephrosis diagnosed by prenatal ultrasound. J Urol 1990; 144:584–587.

17. Tsai TC, Lee HC, Huang FY. The size of the renal pelvis on ultrasonography in children. J Clin Ultrasound 1989; 17(9):647–651.
18. Jaswon MS, Dibble L, Puri S, et al. Prospective study of outcome in antenatally diagnosed renal pelvis dilatation. Arch Dis Child Fetal Neonatal Ed 1999; 80:F135–138.
19. Jodal U, Winberg J. Management of children with unobstructed urinary tract infection. Paed Nephrol 1987; 1:647–656.
20. Fettich JJ, Kenda RB. Cyclic direct radionuclide voiding cystography: increasing reliability in detecting vesicoureteral reflux in children. Pediatr Radiol 1992; 22(5):337–338.
21. Lebowitz RL, Olbing H, Parkkulainen KV, et al. International system of radiographic grading in vesicoureteric reflux. Pediatr Radiol 1985; 15:105–109.
22. Peters AM, Morony S, Gordon I. Indirect radionuclide cystography demonstrates reflux under physiological conditions. Clin Radiol 1990; 41(1):44–47.
23. van der Vis Melsen MJE, Baert RJM, Rajnherc JR. Scintigraphic assessment of lower urinary tract function in children with and without outflow obstruction. Br J Urol 1989; 64:263–269.
24. Lonergan GJ, Pennington DJ, Morrison JC, et al. Childhood pyelonephritis: comparison of gadolinium-enhanced MR imaging and renal cortical scintigraphy for diagnosis. Radiology 1998; 207:377–384.
25. Cousins C, Somers J, Broderick N, et al. Xanthogranulomatous pyelonephritis in childhood: ultrasound and CT diagnosis. Pediatr Radiol 1994; 24:210–212.
26. Fick GM, Gabow PA. Hereditary and acquired cystic disease of the kidney. Kidney Int 1994; 46:951–964.
27. Kaplan BS, Fay FM, Shah VM, et al. Autosomal recessive polycystic kidney disease. Pediatr Nephrol 1989; 3:43–49.
28. Bear JC, Parfrey PS, Morgan JM, et al. Autosomal dominant polycystic kidney disease: new information for genetic counselling. Am J Med Genet 1992; 43:548–553.
29. Hayden CK, Swischuk LE, Davis M, et al. Puddling: a distinguishing feature of adult polycystic kidney disease in the neonate. AJR Am J Roentgenol 1984; 142:811–812.
30. Webb DW, Super M, Normand ICS, et al. Tuberous sclerosis and polycystic kidney disease. Br Med J 1993; 306:1258–1259.
31. McHugh K, Stringer DA, Hebert D, et al. Simple renal cysts in children: diagnosis and follow-up with ultrasound. Radiology 1991; 178:383–385.
32. Bernstein J. Developmental abnormalities of the renal parenchyma: renal hypoplasia and dysplasia. Path Ann 1968; 3:213.
33. Garber SJ, de Bruyn R. Laurence Moon Biedl syndrome: renal ultrasound appearances in the neonate. Br J Radiol 1991; 64:631–633.
34. Alon US. Nephrocalcinosis. Pediatrics 1997; 9:160–165.
35. Dyer RB, Chen MYM, Zagoria RJ. Abnormal calcifications in the urinary tract. Radiographics 1998; 18:1405–1424.
36. Dick PT, Shuckett BM, Tang B, et al. Observer reliability in grading nephrocalcinosis on ultrasound examinations in children. Pediatr Radiol 1999; 29:68–72.
37. Haller JO, Berdon WE, Friedman AP. Increased renal cortical echogenicity: a normal finding in neonates and infants. Radiology 1982; 142:173–174.
38. Downing GJ, Egelhoff JC, Daily DK, et al. Furosemide-related renal calcifications in the premature infant. Pediatr Radiol 1991; 21:563–565.
39. Deal JE, Snell MF, Barratt TM, et al. Renovascular disease in childhood. J Pediatr 1992; 121:378–384.
40. Ruess L, Sivit CJ, Eichelberger MR, et al. Blunt abdominal trauma in children: impact of CT on operative and non-operative management. AJR Am J Roentgenol 1997; 169:1011–1014.
41. Kari JA, Romagnoli J, Duffy P, et al. Renal transplantation in children under 5 years of age. Pediatr Nephrol 1999; 13(9):730–736.
42. Baxter GM. Ultrasound of renal transplantation. Clin Radiol 2001; 56:802–818.
43. Maia CR, Bittar AE, Goldani JC. Doppler ultrasonography for the detection of renal artery stenosis in transplanted kidneys. Hypertension 1992; 19:207–209.
44. Snider JF, Hunter DW, Muradian GP, et al. Transplant renal artery stenosis: evaluation with duplex sonography. Radiology 1989; 172:1027–1030.
45. Kashi SK, Lodge JPA, Giles GR, et al. Ultrasonography of renal allografts: collecting system dilatation and its clinical significance. Nephrol Dial Transplant 1991; 6:358–362.
46. Bakir N, Sluiter WJ, Ploeg RJ, et al. Primary renal graft thrombosis. Nephrol Dial Transplant 1996; 11:140–147.
47. Berger PM, Diamond JR. Ureteral obstruction as a complication of renal transplantation: a review. J Nephrol 1998; 11:20–23.
48. Strouse PJ. Pediatric renal neoplasms. Radiol Clin North Am 1996; 34:1081–1100.

49. Applegate KE, Ghei M, Perez-Atayde AR. Prenatal detection of a Wilms' tumor. Pediatr Radiol 1998; 29:64–67.
50. Scott DJ, Wallace WHB, Hendry GMA. With advances in medical imaging can the radiologist reliably diagnose Wilms' tumors? Clin Radiol 1999; 54:321–327.
51. Groenveld D, Robben SG, Meradji M, et al. Intrapelvic Wilms' tumor simulating xanthogranulomatous pyelonephritis. Pediatr Radiol 1995; 25:568–569.
52. Goske MJ, Mitchell C, Reslan WA. Imaging of patients with Wilms' tumor. Semin Urol Oncol 1999; 17:11–20.
53. Geller E, Smergel EM, Lowry PA. Renal neoplasms of childhood. Radiol Clinics North Am 1997; 35(6):1391–1413.
54. Choyke PL, Siegel MJ, Craft AW, et al. Screening for Wilms' tumor in children with Beckwith–Wiedemann syndrome or idiopathic hemihypertrophy. Med Pediatr Oncol 1999; 32:196–200.
55. Cohen MD. Commentary: imaging and staging of Wilms' tumors: problems and controversies. Pediatr Radiol 1996; 26:307–311.
56. Agrons GA, Kingsman KD, Wagner BJ, et al. Rhabdoid tumor of the kidney in children: a comparative study of 21 cases. AJR Am J Roentgenol 1997; 168:447–451.
57. Lonergan GJ, Martinez-Leon MI, Agrons GA, et al. Nephrogenic rests, nephroblastomatosis and associated lesions of the kidney. Radiographics 1998; 18:947–968.
58. Gylys-Morin V, Hoffer FA, Kozakewich H, et al. Wilms' tumor and nephroblastomatosis: imaging characteristics at gadolinium-enhanced MR imaging. Radiology 1993; 188:517–521.
59. Beckwith JB, Kiviat NB, Bonadio JF. Nephrogenic rests, nephroblastomatosis, and the pathogenesis of Wilms' tumor. Pediatr Pathol 1990; 10:1–36.
60. McHugh K, Boothroyd AE. The role of radiology in childhood rhabdomyosarcoma. Clin Radiol 1999; 54:2–10.

Chapter 4

The adrenal glands

CHAPTER CONTENTS

Normal appearances and ultrasound
 technique 113
Abnormalities of the adrenal glands 115
 Congenital adrenal hyperplasia 115
 Adrenal hemorrhage 115
 Adrenal abscess 116
 Adrenal cystic lesions 116
Tumors of the adrenal glands 117
 Neuroblastoma 117
 Ganglioneuroblastoma/neuroma 123
 Other childhood adrenal tumors 124

Embryology

The cortex and medulla of the adrenal glands have different origins. The medulla originates from neural crest cells of the adjacent sympathetic ganglion, whereas the cortex develops from mesoderm of the posterior abdominal wall. The cortex eventually comes to encircle the medulla. The adrenal glands of the fetus are nearly 20 times larger than the adult gland relative to body weight.

An adrenal gland may be absent, hyperplastic or fused, but sonography plays little role in these conditions.

NORMAL APPEARANCES AND ULTRASOUND TECHNIQUE

Normal appearances

The adrenal glands lie above the kidneys in an anteromedial position. They have a typical wishbone appearance and form a cap or an inverted V over the kidneys. They are most easily seen at birth and in the neonate until about 1 month, when they are large and have a typical hypoechoic cortex and hyperechoic medulla (Fig. 4.1). They lose about a third of their weight during the first 4 weeks of life, because of the regression of the primitive fetal cortex. They continue to regress and do not regain their original weight till about the end of the second year of life. After the early neonatal period the gland appears essentially very similar to that seen in the adult.[1]

If there is an absent kidney, it is interesting that the adrenal stays in the normal position but spreads out in the renal bed.

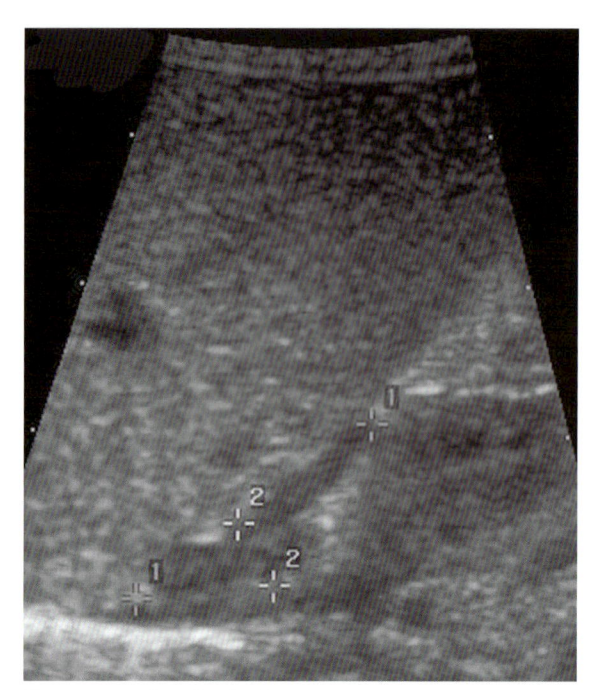

Figure 4.1 Longitudinal sonogram of a normal neonatal adrenal gland. The adrenal cortex is hypoechoic with a hyperechoic medulla. The gland is wishbone-shaped and very prominent in a neonate. This appearance disappears within the first few months of life.

Size

Normal measurements are quoted in the literature for the pediatric adrenal gland and are included here for completeness (Table 4.1). In reality these measurements are of little use clinically and are not routinely used in clinical practice.

Ultrasound technique

A 5 MHz curved array is generally best for the abdomen of most young children, although a higher frequency vector probe can also be used in a young baby. Always start at the highest frequency and move down in MHz if there is insufficient penetration. The adrenal glands in neonates are large and easily visualized, and the sonographer should expect to see them in the majority of neonates.

The adrenal glands in adults and in children are more consistently seen on the right side, because of the acoustic window provided by the liver. To adequately visualize the left adrenal requires more perseverance and time.

The right adrenal There are two ways to visualize the right adrenal in a child:

Table 4.1 Normal range of ultrasonographically determined adrenal diameters in the normal neonate

Age (days)	Transverse	Anteroposterior	Length
1	10.4–22.0	4.1–12.3	9.1–19.9
2	10.0–21.2	4.1–11.9	8.7–19.0
3	9.7–20.6	4.1–11.5	8.5–18.3
4	9.5–20.1	4.0–11.2	8.2–17.7
5	9.3–19.6	4.0–10.9	8.0–17.2
6	9.1–19.2	4.0–10.7	7.8–16.7
7	8.9–18.9	4.0–10.5	7.6–16.3
14	8.0–16.8	3.9–9.2	6.7–13.8
21	7.2–15.2	3.8–8.2	5.9–12.0
28	6.6–13.8	3.8–7.4	5.3–10.4
35	6.0–12.6	3.7–6.7	4.7–9.1
42	5.6–11.5	3.7–6.1	4.2–7.8

After Scott EM, Thomas A, McGarrigle HHG, Lachelin GCL. Serial adrenal ultrasonography in normal neonates. J Ultrasound 1990; 9:279.

THE ADRENAL GLANDS

- Start off conventionally in the right flank using the liver as an acoustic window. Identify the right kidney and then angle medially to locate the area between the right crus of the diaphragm and IVC.
- Alternatively, start scanning longitudinally over the IVC. Gradually rotate the transducer 45° to the right so that an image of the upper IVC and right upper pole of the kidney is obtained. The adrenal lies in the angle between these two structures (Fig. 4.2).

The left adrenal The left adrenal is much more difficult to demonstrate, largely because of food and air in the stomach which lies directly in front of the adrenal. One can give a drink of clear fluid which will enable the stomach to be used as an acoustic window. Gradually compress the gas out of the way with the transducer. The more conventional method is to use the extreme left flank approach or intercostal approach and, by using deep inspiration or expiration, to bring the adrenal gland into view. Turning the patient into the right oblique position is sometimes also helpful.

ABNORMALITIES OF THE ADRENAL GLANDS

Congenital adrenal hyperplasia (CAH)

This is a recessively inherited condition caused by an enzyme deficiency in the adrenal cortex. In the majority of patients the deficient enzyme is 21-hydroxylase. Clinically there is an accumulation of steroidal precursors proximal to the enzyme deficiency, with a resulting diversion into the androgen (therefore male) biosynthesis pathways. This results in virilization of females and early masculinization in males. In the majority, aldosterone cannot be synthesized, and some infants may present with severe salt wasting in the neonatal period which may be fatal. While the adrenal glands may be detectably enlarged in some, ultrasound plays little role in assessing the glands.[2] However, CAH is the most common cause of female pseudohermaphroditism, with female infants presenting with ambiguous genitalia. The role of ultrasound in these infants with ambiguous genitalia is to demonstrate the presence of internal female structures (uterus and ovaries). The uterus is occasionally associated with a small hydrometrocolpos, as the insertion of a vagina may be anomalous and narrowed, sometimes inserting into the urethra with a persistent urogenital sinus[3–5] (see Fig. 7.11).

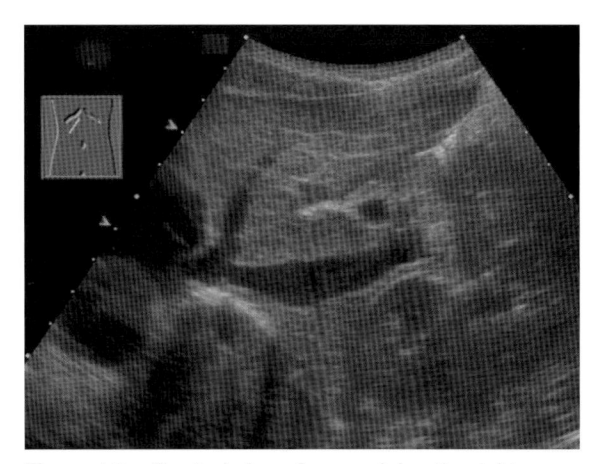

Figure 4.2 The technique for examining the right adrenal. The upper IVC and upper pole of the right kidney are on the image. The triangle between the two is where an adrenal mass will be found.

Adrenal hemorrhage

Adrenal hemorrhage is a common cause of an abdominal mass in a neonate. This has been reported in the literature as sometimes occurring as an antenatal event, and the sonographic appearances postnatally often confirm this. Conditions which are associated with adrenal hemorrhage are hemoconcentration caused by shock, hypoxia, septicemia, birth trauma or stress, and this occurs particularly in infants of diabetic mothers.[6,7]

Clinically the neonates present with a palpable abdominal mass, anemia due to the hemorrhage, jaundice, hypertension and, if the mass is large enough, vomiting and small bowel obstruction.

There is a common association with renal vein thrombosis, which must be actively excluded, and this is more commonly left sided because of the insertion of the left adrenal vein into the left renal vein. Bilateral adrenal hemorrhages can occur. Hemorrhages may be complicated by abscess formation.[8]

In older children adrenal hemorrhage is associated with meningococcal septicemia, trauma and anticoagulants.

Ultrasound appearances The adrenal hemorrhage has differing appearances depending on when in the evolution of the hemorrhage the ultrasound examination is performed. In the early stages when there is fresh hemorrhage, the adrenal is enlarged and echogenic. As the blood starts to liquefy, the central area becomes increasingly hypoechoic with some internal echoes; this can take 1–2 weeks from the time of hemorrhage. In a short space of time the hemorrhage starts shrinking (Fig. 4.3) and may ultimately be left with a rim of calcification. On plain abdominal radiography this is typically triangular in shape.

When an adrenal hemorrhage is found, the kidneys must be carefully scanned and measured and the echogenicity evaluated for renal vein thrombosis. The features to look for are an echogenic enlarged swollen kidney with the typical increase in echogenicity of the interlobular vessels[9] (Fig. 4.4).

A much rarer condition, neuroblastoma, is the main differential diagnosis. Normally a neuroblastoma is more solid in appearance and will not change its internal echo texture with time. Serial examination is therefore recommended in the uncertain cases. However, urinary catecholamines (VMAs) will be elevated in over 90% of patients with neuroblastoma. Neuroblastoma may also undergo hemorrhage and be cystic in appearance.[10] This coexistence with neuroblastoma may require further cross sectional imaging, and it is in these instances that an MRI scan may improve diagnostic accuracy. Sonography, however, remains the prime imaging modality of choice.

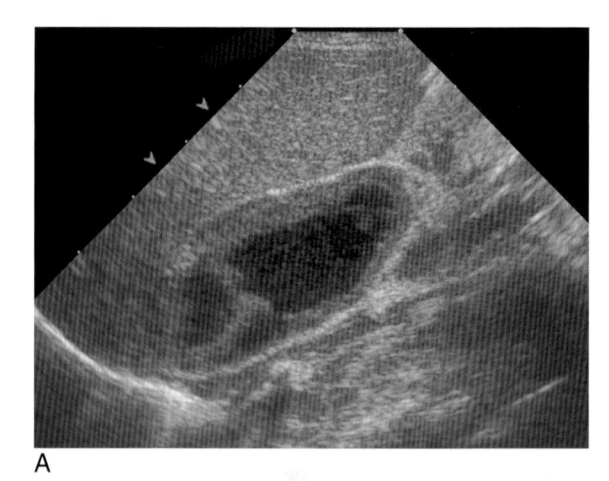

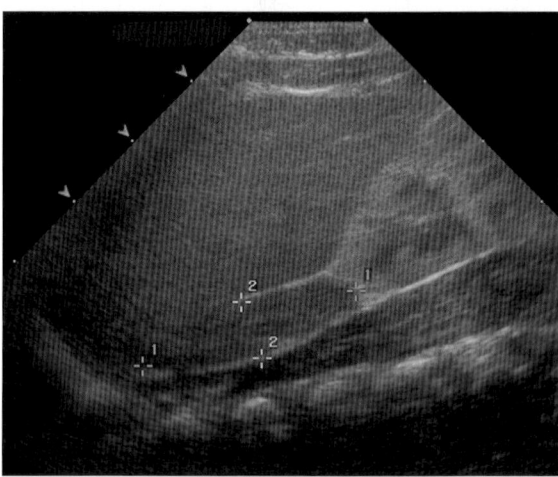

Figure 4.3 Resolution of an adrenal hemorrhage. (A) Longitudinal sonogram of an old right adrenal hemorrhage. The adrenal is predominantly cystic with some internal echoes. (B) Longitudinal sonogram of the right adrenal 1 month later (between calipers) showing that it has shrunk in size considerably. Adrenal hemorrhages change in their appearances very quickly.

Adrenal abscess

Adrenal abscess is a very rare condition and sometimes complicates the pre-existing adrenal hemorrhage. It is thought that hematogenous seeding of some common bacterial infections such as *E. coli* and *Staph. aureus* occurs.

Sonographically, one cannot differentiate an abscess from a hemorrhage, but clinically the child may have evidence of infection with a fever and a high white cell count.

Adrenal cystic lesions

Cystic adrenal masses are rare, but there are some conditions in which lesions may appear cystic:

- A resolving adrenal hemorrhage may appear complex, with internal echoes, and is usually seen after 2–3 weeks.
- Cystic neuroblastoma is very rare.
- True adrenal cysts are very rare and appear purely cystic with a thin wall and no internal

THE ADRENAL GLANDS 117

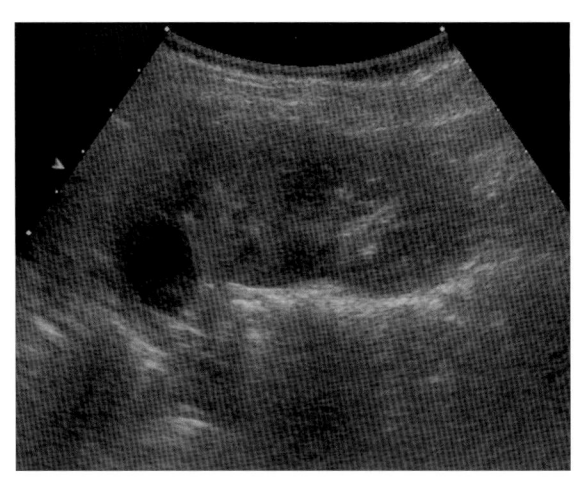

Figure 4.5 Adrenal cyst found incidentally in a well child. Prone longitudinal scan showing a well-defined cyst above the left kidney. These are very rare but are sometimes seen in Beckwith–Wiedemann syndrome. Neuroblastoma can sometimes be purely cystic. The sonographer must ensure this is not an obstructed duplex.

TUMORS OF THE ADRENAL GLANDS

Neuroblastoma, ganglioneuroblastoma and ganglioneuroma are all tumors of the sympathetic nervous system (Fig. 4.6). They may be found in the neck, mediastinum and adrenals down to the pelvis. Their main difference is in their malignant potential. Neuroblastomas are the most malignant, have the most immature cells (neuroblasts) and occur in younger children usually under two years. Ganglioneuromas are at the benign end of the spectrum with the most mature (ganglion) cells. They are often found incidentally on a chest radiograph. Ganglioneuroblastomas contain both immature and mature cells and are therefore of intermediate malignant potential.

Neuroblastoma

Neuroblastoma (NBL) is one of the commonest solid tumors of childhood. Together with Wilms tumor, it is the second commonest abdominal solid tumor of childhood. Because of its aggressive nature and late staging at presentation, it accounts for approximately 15% of childhood cancer deaths. These children are usually younger than those presenting with a Wilms tumor: the median age of

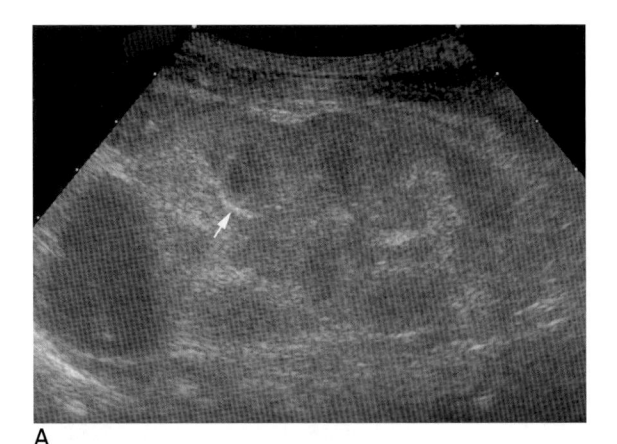

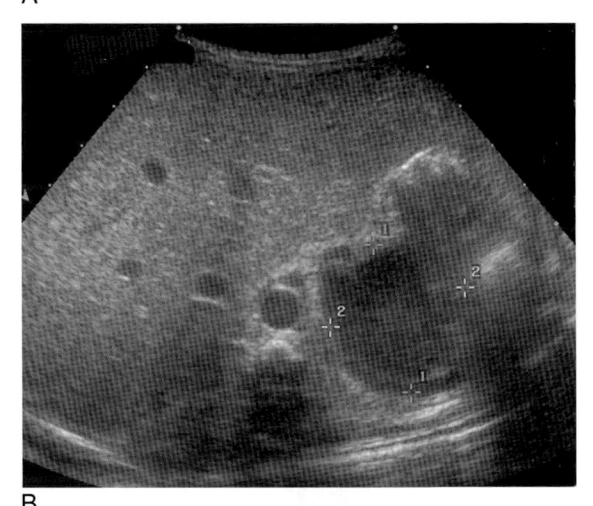

Figure 4.4 Adrenal hemorrhage and renal vein thrombosis. (A) & (B) Longitudinal and transverse sonogram on a large left cystic adrenal above the left kidney. This is the appearance of an adrenal hemorrhage which has liquefied. The kidney also appears abnormally swollen, with a patchy echo nephrogram and ill-defined bright interlobular vessels (arrow). This was an adrenal hemorrhage in association with renal venous thrombosis. This association is more common on the left, because of the drainage of the left adrenal vein into the left renal vein.

  echoes. They may be associated with Beckwith–Wiedemann syndrome (Fig. 4.5).
- Lesions that may mimic an adrenal cyst are an obstructed upper moiety of a renal duplex system or a localized upper moiety multicystic kidney. An MCU may help by showing reflux into the lower moiety and an 'incomplete' kidney.

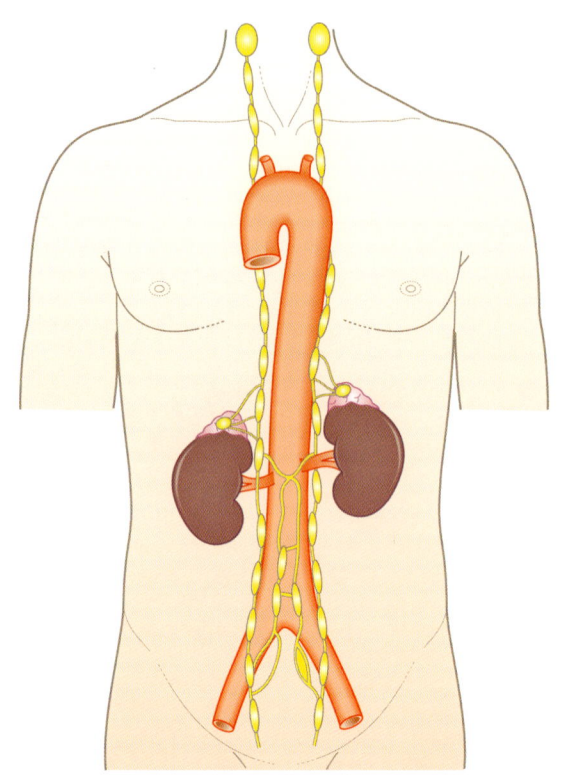

Figure 4.6 Sympathetic chain and adrenal glands. It is along this line that all the neurogenic tumors may be found.

diagnosis is 22 months, and the majority of patients present under 4 years of age. There is an equal sex incidence. There is an association of other disorders such as Beckwith–Wiedemann syndrome, Hirschsprung disease, DiGeorge syndrome and neurofibromatosis.[11]

Neuroblastomas may arise anywhere along the sympathetic chain, as they are derived from neural crest cells. The commonest sites are the adrenal gland, retroperitoneum and posterior mediastinum. They may also occur less commonly in the neck and pelvis. The ultimate prognosis depends on a number of parameters such as histology, electron microscopy, cytogenetic and molecular and biological information.

Screening for NBL has only been undertaken in the early 1970s in Japan in the hope that early detection would improve the cure rate. However, the epidemiological analysis showed that the incidence of tumors in older children did not change but that the early detection resulted in an increase in stage 1 tumors. Those discovered at screening were of low stage and favorable histology. This suggested that the tumors discovered at urinary screening are most likely those to remain occult, to regress or mature. Screening for NBL in infancy does not appear to decrease the incidence of advanced NBL in older children or improve survival.[12,13]

Clinical presentation Neuroblastoma has often metastasized at presentation, so that these children are ill with bone pain, anemia and weight loss. They usually present with an abdominal mass, and other presenting complaints are malaise and irritability. They may be short of breath because of the large abdominal mass. The 'dancing eye' syndrome (opsoclonus–myoclonus) is sometimes the presenting symptom, where these children have typical jerking of the eyes and abnormal movements of the limbs. The cause is unknown but the syndrome is associated with a better outcome.

Neuroblastomas may secrete catecholamines. Vasoactive intestinal peptide (VIP) secretion may result in the children presenting with watery diarrhea and hypokalemia.

Imaging There are two main features of NBL tumors. If they arise within the adrenal, they may appear well defined. They may also appear infiltrative, in which case they may have a lobulated outline and there may be small areas of hemorrhage. Lymphadenopathy is often a feature of the tumor mass, and sometimes it may be difficult to differentiate the two (Fig. 4.7).

Calcification is one of the features of NBL that helps differentiate it from a Wilms tumor. Approximately 30% will show calcification on plain abdominal radiographs, and this is typically a very fine stippled calcification[14] (Fig. 4.8). After treatment this may become dense and punctate.

Plain radiography is extremely helpful in NBL, as it may show a number of features. In the chest there may be erosions seen posteriorly in the ribs or pedicle erosion from the intraspinal extension. In the abdomen there may be paravertebral widening, which is a hallmark of NBL (Fig. 4.9). In the abdomen, calcification may be seen with evidence of bony metastases to the metaphyses.

On ultrasound the tumor mass is generally solid, occasionally with small punctate echogenic areas.

THE ADRENAL GLANDS 119

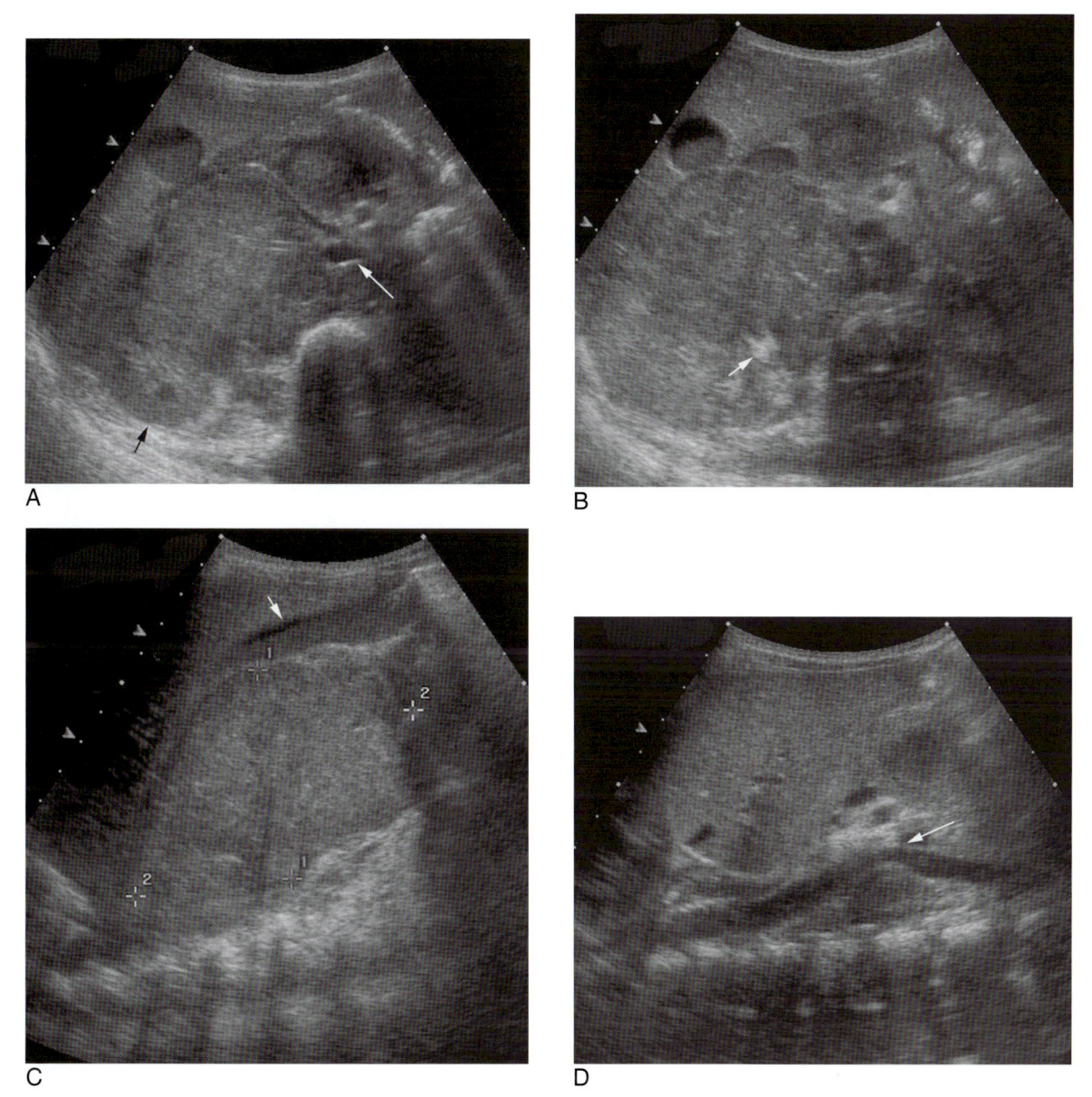

Figure 4.7 Neuroblastoma right with displacement. This young child presented with a right-sided abdominal mass. (A) Transverse scan of the right-sided mass. The right kidney (black arrow) is pushed posteriorly, and the mass is growing medial to it. There is anterior displacement of the hepatic vessels, and the aorta is undermined and pushed laterally (white arrow). The pancreas and mesenteric vessels are also pushed to the left. There is sludge in the gallbladder. (B) Transverse scan at a higher level. The mass has echogenic areas of calcification (arrow). The upper abdominal vessels must be carefully examined for encasement and displacement. (C) Longitudinal scan on the same patient showing the large solid mass with calcification (between calipers). The gallbladder is full of sludge lying anteriorly from stasis of bile (arrow). (D) Longitudinal ultrasound at the level of the IVC. There is elevation of the IVC (arrow) by tumor mass and lymph nodes. This appearance is one of the features to look for in NBL.

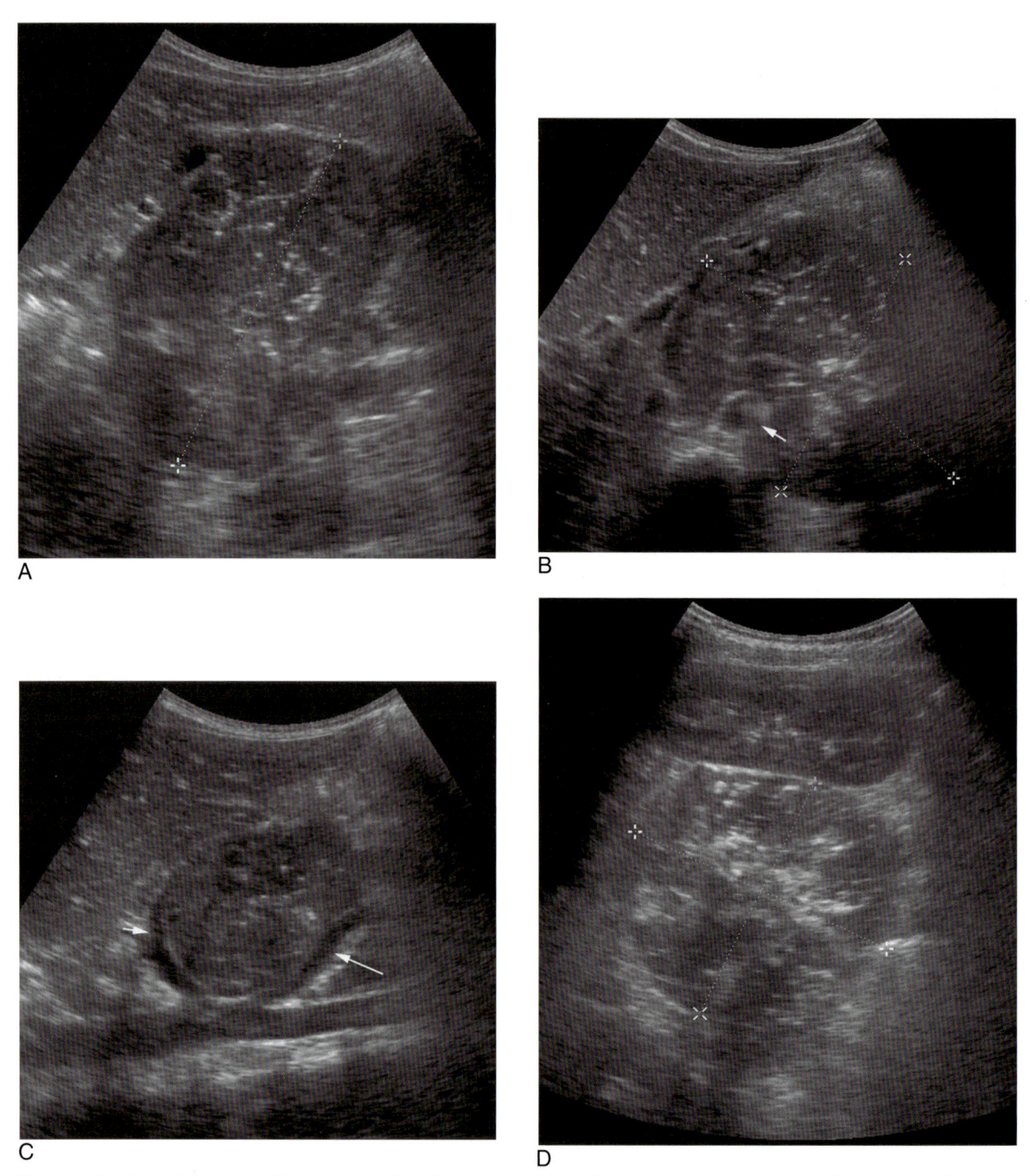

Figure 4.8 Neuroblastoma with echogenic foci. This young, pale child was very irritable, presenting with a left adrenal mass. (A) & (B) Longitudinal and transverse sonogram of the left adrenal mass. The mass has typical small echogenic foci of fine calcification and is crossing the midline passing anteriorly to the aorta (arrow). The aorta is not encased. (C) Longitudinal sonogram just at the level of the aorta, showing displacement of the celiac axis (short arrow) and superior mesenteric artery (long arrow) around this mass which is lying centrally in the abdomen. (D) Prone sonogram of the left showing how the mass is lying anterior to the left kidney, which is squashed posteriorly. The mass is lying between the crosses and contains echogenic calcific areas.

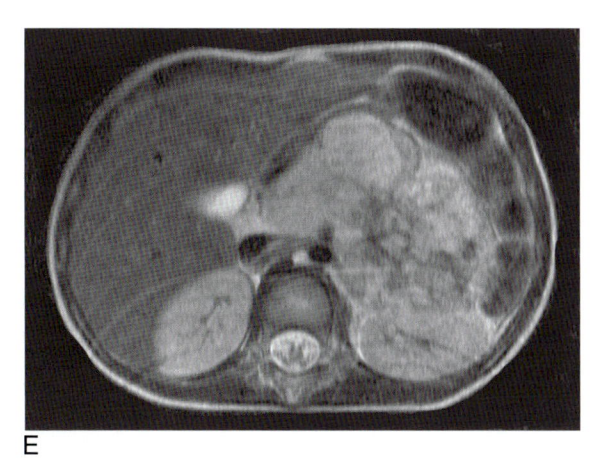

Figure 4.8, cont'd (E) MRI scan on the same child, showing the large left mass crossing the midline anterior to the left kidney, which is compressed posteriorly by the mass.

Acoustic shadowing behind the areas of calcification may or may not be present (Fig. 4.10). Neuroblastoma rarely invades the kidney, and when it does this makes differentiation from a Wilms tumor difficult. Ultrasound evaluation of the liver for metastatic disease should be always included in the examination. Metastatic disease in the liver appears either as diffuse infiltration as in 4S neuroblastoma (see below and Box 4.1)—the so-called 'pepper pot' appearance—and focal hypoechoic areas which are not enhancing at CT (Fig. 4.11). Doppler is essential to evaluate encased and displaced IVC, aorta and mesenteric vessels.[15]

The role of ultrasound is to make the initial diagnosis, which will thus direct further imaging and investigation. The main features to look for are:

- extent of tumor
- organ of origin
- region of invasion
- vascular encasement
- adenopathy
- calcification
- metastatic liver disease.

Neuroblastoma and Wilms tumors are the two common childhood malignancies which need to be differentiated. Table 4.2 provides some differentiating sonographic features.

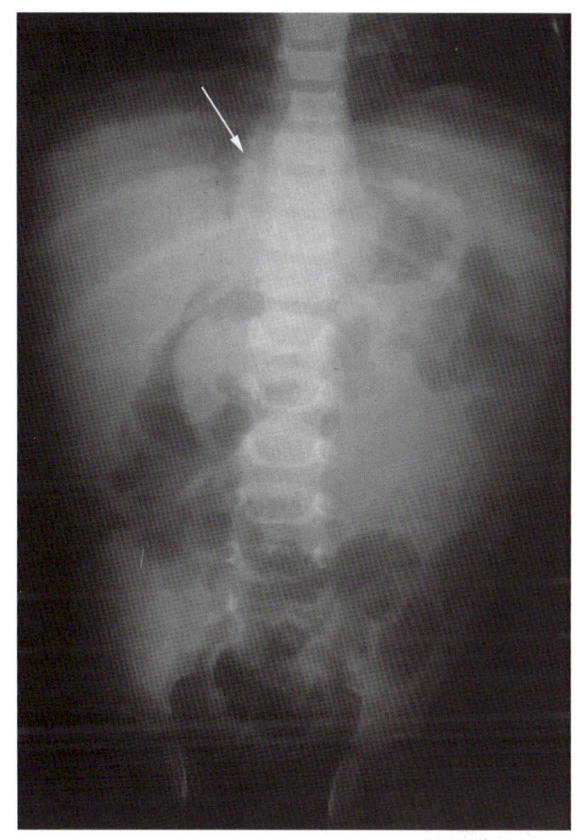

Figure 4.9 Abdominal radiograph in neuroblastoma. Plain AXR on a child with an abdominal mass. There is upper abdominal paravertebral widening on either side of the spine (arrow). This is one of the features to look for on the abdominal radiograph in neuroblastoma.

If intraspinal extension is present it is best demonstrated on MR imaging, which should be performed on any patient with tumors close to the spine. In addition, MR will demonstrate marrow disease.[16]

Nuclear medicine studies are generally required to show the bony involvement. MIBG (metaiodobenzylguanidine) labeled with iodine-123 shows uptake in the primary tumor and metastases. MIBG is taken up by all catecholamine-producing tumors, such as pheochromocytoma, carcinoid and medullary thyroid cancer in addition to the neuroblastoma spectrum. The evaluation of bone disease is most routinely done by technetium-99m MDP (methylene diphosphonate), and this is more sensitive than plain radiography in the detection of bone disease.

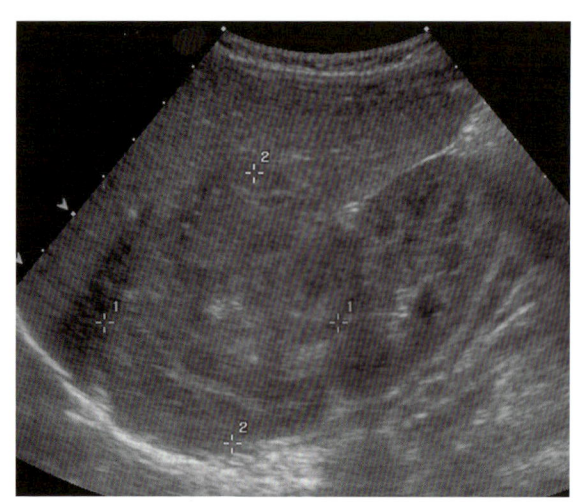

Figure 4.10 Neuroblastoma well defined in a young child presenting with a right abdominal mass. Longitudinal sonogram of the right flank showing a well-defined mass (between calipers) containing very echogenic specks that are typical of neuroblastoma. Notice how the right kidney can still be seen but is just displaced inferiorly. It is unusual for NBL to invade the kidney.

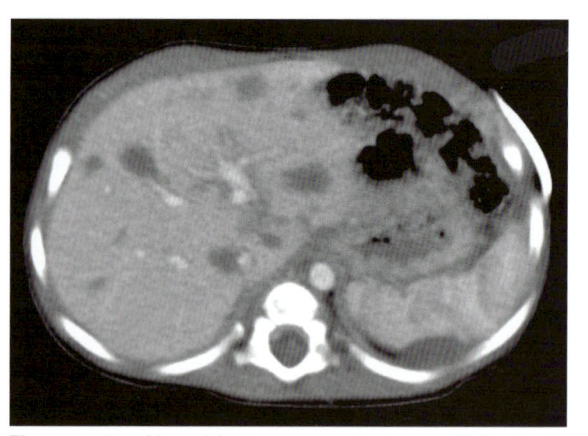

Figure 4.11 Neuroblastoma secondaries on CT. Contrast-enhanced CT examination on a child with neuroblastoma and extensive secondary deposits in the liver. The secondary deposits in the liver do not enhance with contrast. There is also a deposit posteriorly in the spleen.

Once the child has had a full pre-treatment evaluation then ultrasound will be used for follow-up examination and to monitor treatment.[17]

Box 4.1 gives the staging classification for NBL. Stage 1 tumors are completely resected with no other disease, regardless of whether they cross the midline. Tumors invading one side of the canal are Stage 2. Stage 3 are those extending across the midline. In bilateral tumors the mass with the higher tumor staging is given.

4S Neuroblastoma

This is a special form of neuroblastoma occurring in the neonatal period and has a much more benign course. It accounts for nearly 50% of malignant tumors in neonates.

Clinical presentation Infants usually present with a hugely enlarged and enlarging liver, sometimes causing respiratory embarrassment. They may also have skin lesions described as 'blueberry

Table 4.2 Differences between Neuroblastoma and Wilms tumor

Neuroblastoma	Wilms tumor
Separate to kidney—rarely invades kidney	Arises from kidney
Kidney displaced, compressed and rotated	Depends on stage, but generally difficult to identify normal kidney
	Venous lakes
Solid with fine pinpoint calcification	10% calcify
May be ill-defined and infiltrating retroperitoneum	Usually well defined unless ruptured
Undermines and encases aorta SMA/SMV and IVC	Pushes and displaces aorta and IVC
No invasion of renal veins and IVC	Invades and grows into renal vein and IVC
May have abdominal lymphadenopathy	Unusual to have prominent lymphadenopathy
Contralateral kidney normal	10% bilateral

IVC, inferior vena cava; SMA/V, superior mesenteric artery/vein.

> **Box 4.1 International Neuroblastoma staging system**
>
> Stage 1: Localized tumor confined to the area of origin; complete gross excision, with or without microscopic residual disease; identifiable ipsilateral and contralateral lymph nodes negative microscopically
>
> Stage 2A: Unilateral tumor with incomplete gross excision; identifiable ipsilateral non-adherent lymph nodes negative microscopically
>
> Stage 2B: Unilateral tumor with complete or incomplete gross excision; positive ipsilateral non-adherent lymph nodes; identifiable contralateral lymph nodes negative microscopically
>
> Stage 3: Tumor infiltrating across the midline (vertebral column) with or without regional lymph node involvement; or unilateral tumor with contralateral regional lymph node involvement; or midline tumor with bilateral regional lymph node involvement or extension by infiltration
>
> Stage 4: Dissemination of tumor to distant lymph nodes, bone, bone marrow, liver, or other organs (except as defined in stage 4S)
>
> Stage 4S: Localized primary tumor as defined for stage 1 or 2 with dissemination limited to liver, skin and/or bone marrow (<10% tumor) in infants younger than 1 year
>
> Adapted from Brodeur GM, Pritchard J, Berthold F, et al. Revisions of the international criteria for neuroblastoma diagnosis, staging and response to treatment. J Clin Oncol 1993; 11:1466–1477.

muffin' appearance. They may appear as dark purple or blue masses.

The adrenal primary is not always found and occurs in approximately 45% of patients. It is usually small and stage 1 or 2. The bone marrow is involved, so it will be positive on bone marrow aspiration, whereas bone scanning will be normal.

Fetal neuroblastoma has been discovered as early as 19 weeks, and is almost always adrenal in origin. 4S neuroblastoma has a favorable outcome. Regression of known neuroblastoma most often occurs in stage 4S and takes up to 1 year on average. The cause of regression is unknown.

Ultrasound The liver is very large and has a heterogeneous texture—typically described as a 'pepper pot' appearance. On CT scanning this extensive infiltration may be missed because of the patterns of tumor enhancement and uniform increase in parenchymal attenuation. Primary adrenal lesions may not be detectable or very small—usually stage 1 or 2 and well defined.

Other imaging Radioisotope bone scans will be normal, but bone marrow aspirates will be abnormal (Fig. 4.12).

Ganglioneuroblastoma/neuroma

Characteristics of this tumor are:

- usually an incidental finding or found on chest radiograph
- wide spectrum from malignant to completely benign
- usually a well-defined solid mass.

It occurs in older patients, with a median age of diagnosis of 7 years, and it is much less common than neuroblastoma. The tumor is found in the posterior mediastinum, retroperitoneum and adrenal gland. It manifests as an asymptomatic mass discovered on a routine examination. Sometimes it may cause a local mass effect, particularly on the adjacent bones. Rarely it may secrete catecholamines which will cause flushing.

Ultrasound examination will show a generally well-defined mass which is homogeneous. Up to 60% will show calcification and are typically fine and speckled. Plain radiography may show rib changes or foraminal erosion.

Treatment is complete surgical resection with follow-up surveillance.

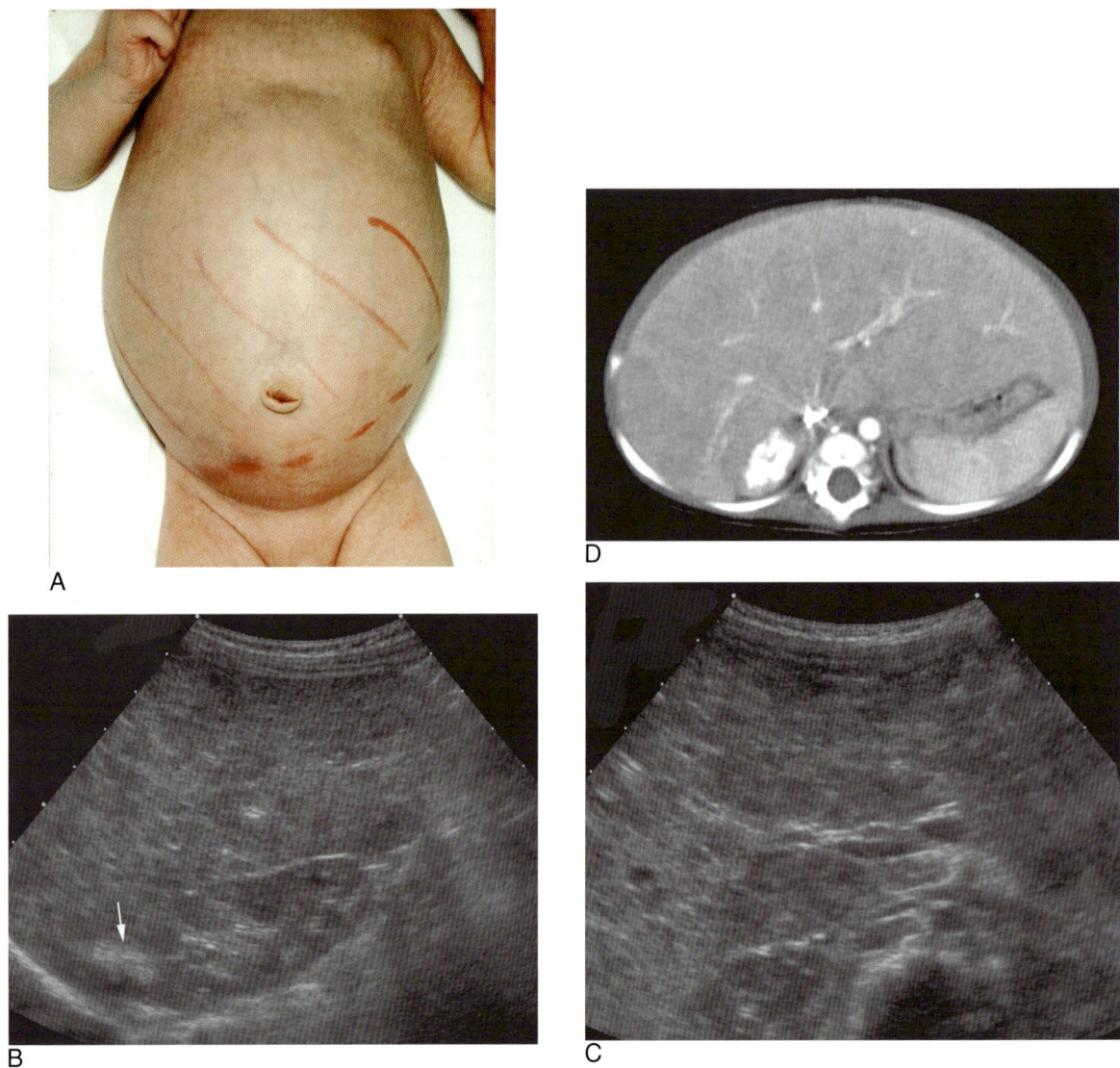

Figure 4.12 4S Neuroblastoma. (A) This young infant presented with a rapidly enlarging liver. The liver edge has been marked, and it occupies almost the whole of the abdomen. (B) Longitudinal sonogram on the same child demonstrating a small echogenic adrenal mass (arrow) and a very heterogeneous appearance to the liver. (C) Transverse sonogram of the liver showing the generalized heterogeneous appearance which is typical of 4S neuroblastoma. (D) Contrast enhanced CT examination on the same child. This shows the right adrenal mass. In addition there is massive hepatomegaly with a very heterogeneous appearance with contrast enhancement.

Other childhood adrenal tumors

Other childhood adrenal tumors are difficult to differentiate on ultrasound criteria alone, as all are usually solid and well defined. Table 4.3 outlines some of the differing clinical presentations and associations to consider when arriving at a diagnosis.[18]

Adrenocortical tumors

These tumors arise from the adrenal cortex and are collectively known as adrenocortical neoplasms. They may be adenomas or carcinomas, but the two types are difficult to distinguish histopathologically and indeed radiologically. Both adenomas and carci-

Table 4.3 Other childhood adrenal tumors

	Adrenal carcinoma	Pheochromocytoma
Clinical presentation	Hormonal effects Precocious puberty Cushing syndrome	Hypertension Urinary catecholamines raised
Associated anomalies	Hemihypertrophy Beckwith–Wiedemann Li–Fraumeni	Tuberous sclerosis Neurofibromatosis Von Hippel–Lindau Sturge–Weber Multiple endocrine neoplasia types IIA and IIB
Ultrasound appearances	Solid, well defined Adenoma < 4 cm or < 50 g Carcinoma > 4 cm or > 100 g	Solid, well defined May be multiple extra adrenal masses in abdomen
Other imaging	CT or MRI	Radioisotope MIBG scan CT or MRI to show other lesions in chest or abdomen Adrenal vein sampling

MIBG, metaiodobenzylguanidine.

nomas are rare in children younger than 5 years, and girls are affected more than boys. There are known associated syndromes such as hemihypertrophy, Beckwith–Wiedemann and Li–Fraumeni syndromes. Rarely, the tumors have been reported in association with congenital urinary tract abnormalities, congenital adrenal hyperplasia (CAH) or ganglioneuroma/blastoma. Clinically they present with endocrine disturbances such as precocious puberty, virilization or Cushing syndrome (Fig. 4.13).

Adenomas are smaller, usually solid and well defined, whereas carcinomas are larger and may have areas of hemorrhage with central necrosis and cystic areas. Generally it is not possible to differentiate adenomas and carcinomas on imaging, but diagnostic differentiation is based on metastatic spread, which is more common in the larger carcinomas. Overall, these tumors rarely present as large abdominal masses but may at presentation have tumor extension into the IVC and right atrium, which must always be sought on ultrasound. A small percentage may calcify.

Ultrasound is a very good screening tool for any child suspected of having an adrenal tumor.

The diagnosis is not difficult to make, as the majority present clinically with hormonal disturbances such as virilization, acne, hypertension, weight gain and fatigue and have biochemical changes and a mass on imaging (Fig. 4.14).

Other pediatric adrenal masses have a different clinical presentation. Neuroblastoma may present

A

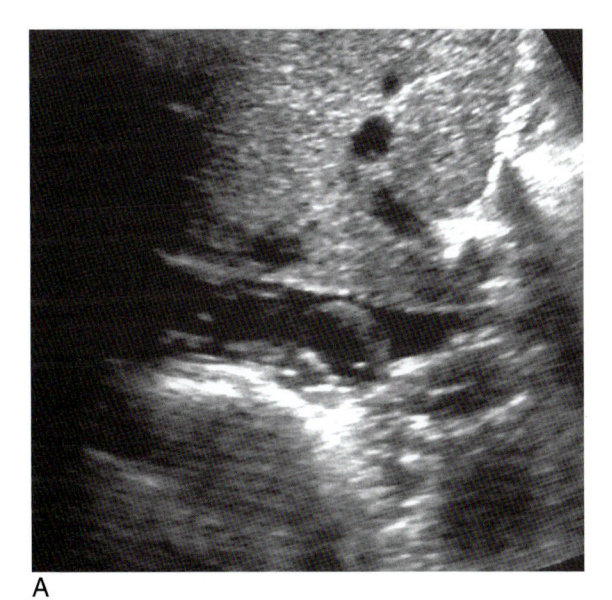

Figure 4.13 Cushing syndrome. A 2-year-old boy presenting with Cushing syndrome.

Continued

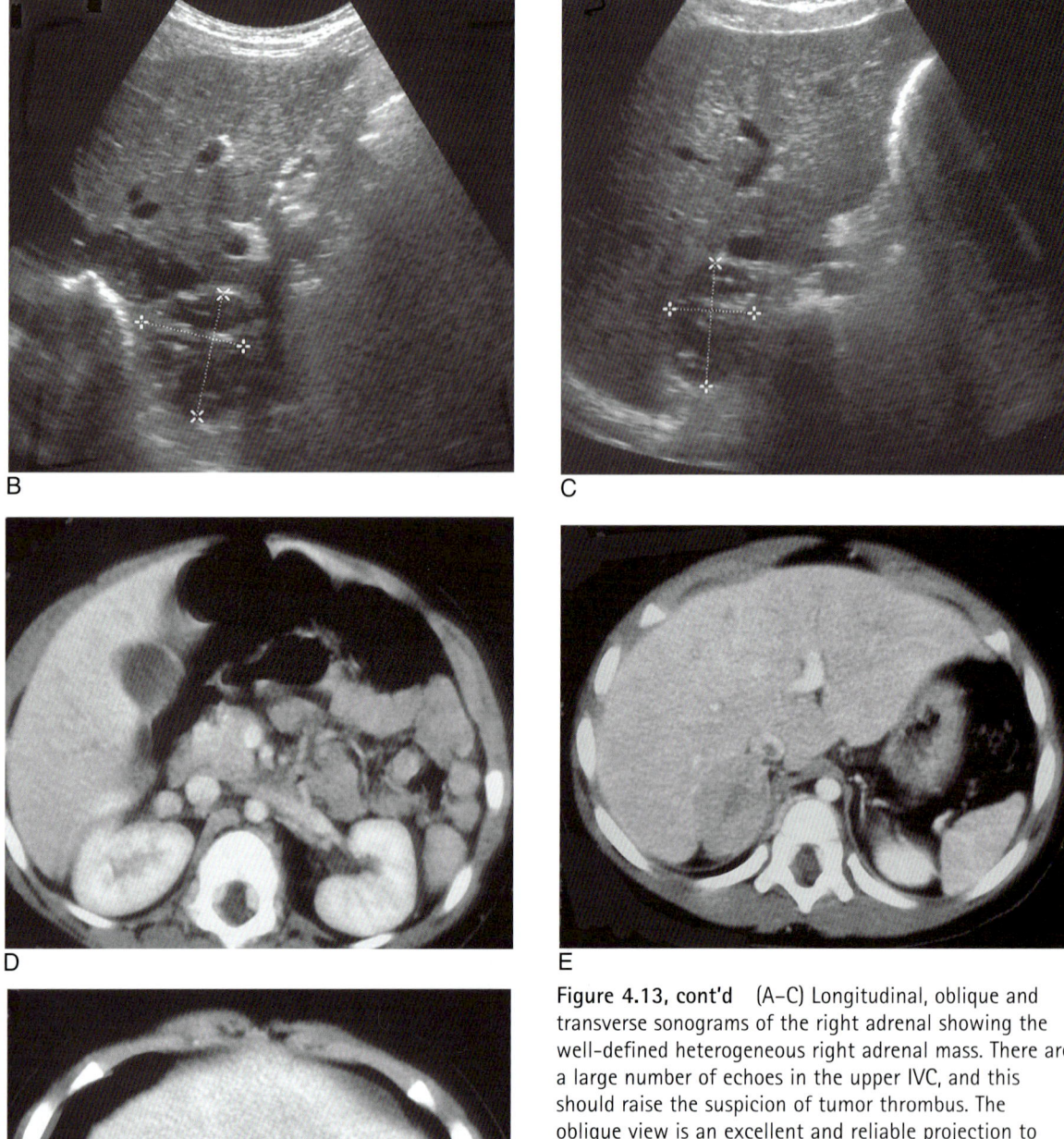

Figure 4.13, cont'd (A–C) Longitudinal, oblique and transverse sonograms of the right adrenal showing the well-defined heterogeneous right adrenal mass. There are a large number of echoes in the upper IVC, and this should raise the suspicion of tumor thrombus. The oblique view is an excellent and reliable projection to demonstrate the right adrenal. (D–F) Three slices from the CT scan on the same child at the level of the kidneys, at the level of the right adrenal mass and at the entry of the IVC into the right atrium. There is a right adrenal mass and tumor thrombus on the higher scan, extending into the right atrium (arrow).

THE ADRENAL GLANDS 127

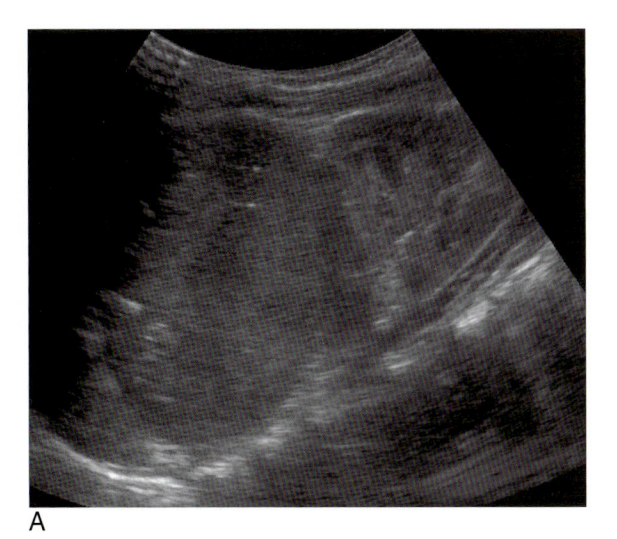

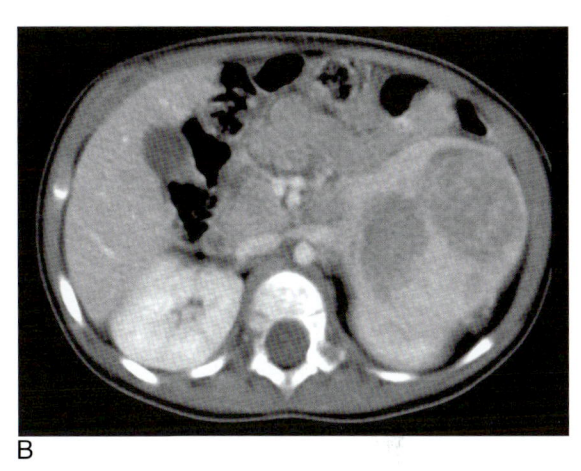

Figure 4.14 This child presented with virilization and hypertension. (A) Longitudinal scan of the left kidney and adrenal mass. Notice how there is a whole left kidney but it has just been compressed inferiorly. Always assess how much of the kidney is seen when trying to differentiate adrenal from renal masses. (B) Contrast-enhanced CT scan on the same child at the level of the renal vein. The left kidney was compressed posteriorly but was separate from the mass. This was an adrenal tumor secreting hormones which resulted in the virilization of the child.

with elevated VMAs, 'dancing eye syndrome' and with evidence of VIP secretion (diarrhea and hypokalemia). Pheochromocytomas arising from the adrenal gland secrete catecholamines and present with hypertension but may have very similar appearances on imaging.

Pheochromocytomas

These children typically present with paroxysmal headaches caused by hypertension. In children pheochromocytomas may be multiple and extra-adrenal in origin. Less than 10% are malignant.

Imaging with radionuclide MIBG is essential before cross sectional imaging is performed, in order to locate the mass so that a targeted examination can be performed. On ultrasound the pheochromocytoma will appear very similar to other adrenocortical tumors (Fig. 4.15), but the clinical presentation will be different. It is essential to examine the whole abdomen for extra-adrenal masses.[19]

Wolman disease

This is an extremely rare lipidosis, and the features in the adrenal are markedly enlarged, densely calcified glands. Infants die early, and the adrenal changes may be accompanied by hepatosplenomegaly.[20]

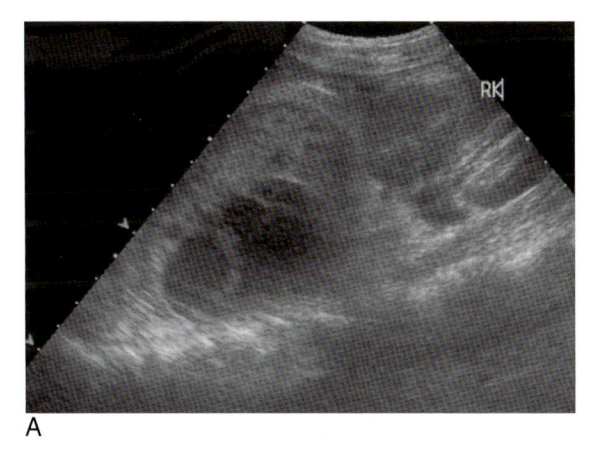

Figure 4.15 Pheochromocytoma. This boy presented with a 2-year history of headaches and had massively raised catecholamines in the blood. (A) Longitudinal ultrasound of the right adrenal showing a large cystic adrenal mass above the right kidney (RK). Notice the echogenic rim around the mass from fresh hemorrhage.

Continued

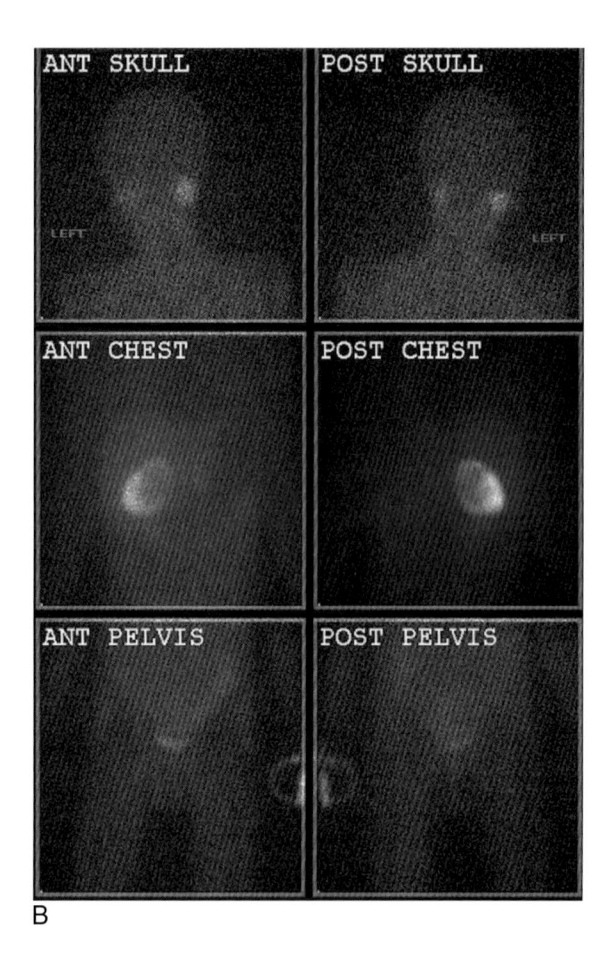

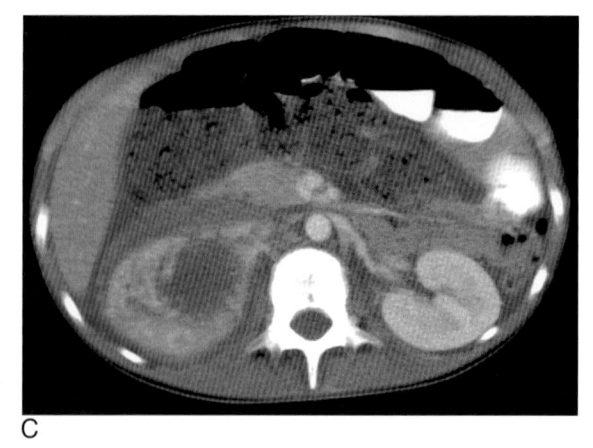

Figure 4.15, cont'd (B) MIBG scan shows avid uptake of isotope in the pheochromocytoma. The central photon-deficient area was the cystic area on ultrasound. No other tumors are showing up. There is normal uptake in the salivary glands. (C) CT scan at the level of the cystic right adrenal pheochromocytoma. The tumor had ruptured and bled.

References

1. Oppenheimer D, Carroll B, Vousem S. Sonography of the normal neonatal adrenal gland. Radiol 1983; 146:157–160.
2. Wright NB, Smith C, Rickwood AMK, et al. Review imaging children with ambiguous genitalia and intersex states. Clin Radiol 1995; 50:823–829.
3. Avni EF, Rypens F, Smet MH, et al. Sonographic demonstration of congenital adrenal hyperplasia in the neonate: the cerebriform pattern. Pediatr Radiol 1993; 23:88–90.
4. Bryan PJ, Caldamone AA, Morrison SC, et al. Ultrasound findings in the adreno-genital syndrome (congenital adrenal hyperplasia). J Ultrasound Med 1988; 7:675–679.
5. Sivit CJ, Hung W, Taylor GA, et al. Sonography in neonatal congenital adrenal hyperplasia. AJR Am J Roentgenol 1991; 156:141–143.
6. Lee W, Cornstock CH, Jurcak-Zaleski S. Prenatal diagnosis of adrenal haemorrhage by ultrasonography. J Ultrasound Med 1992; 11:369–371.
7. Levin TL, Morton E. Adrenal haemorrhage complicating ACTH therapy in Crohn's disease. Pediatr Radiol 1993; 23:457–458.
8. Carty A, Stanley P. Bilateral adrenal abscesses in a neonate. Pediatr Radiol 1973; 1:63–64.
9. Black J, Williams DI. Natural history of adrenal haemorrhage in the newborn. Arch Dis Child 1973; 48:183–190.
10. Croitoru DP, Sinsky AB, Laberge JM. Cystic neuroblastoma. J Pediatr Surg 1992; 27: 1320–1321.
11. Lonergan GJ, Schwab CM, Suarez ES, et al. Neuroblastoma, ganglioneuroblastoma and ganglioneuroma: radiologic-pathologic correlation. RadioGraphics 2002; 22:911–934.
12. Lukens JN. Neuroblastoma in the neonate. Semin Perinatol 1999; 23:263–273.

13. Acharya S, Jayabose S, Kogan SJ, et al. Prenatally diagnosed neuroblastoma. Cancer 1997; 80:304–310.
14. White SJ, Stuck KJ, Blane CE, et al. Sonography of neuroblastoma. AJR Am J Roentgenol 1983; 141:465–468.
15. Amundsen GM, Treven CL, Mueller DL, et al. Neuroblastoma: a specific sonographic tissue pattern. AJR Am J Roentgenol 1987; 148:943–945.
16. Berdon WE, Ruzal-Shapiro C, Abramson SJ, et al. The diagnosis of abdominal neuroblastoma: relative roles of ultrasonography, CT and MRI. Urol Radiol 1992; 14:252–262.
17. Bousvaros A, Kirks DR, Grossman H. Imaging of neuroblastoma: an overview. Pediatr Radiol 1986; 16:89–106.
18. Abramson SJ. Adrenal neoplasms in children. Radiol Clin North Am 1997; 35:1415–1453.
19. Daneman A. Adrenal neoplasms in children. Semin Roentgenol 1988; 23:205–215.
20. Ozmen MN, Aygun N, Kilic I, et al. Wolman's disease: ultrasonographic and computed tomographic findings. Pediatr Radiol 1992; 22:541–542.

Chapter 5

The liver, spleen and pancreas

CHAPTER CONTENTS

Liver   131
The normal pediatric hepatobiliary system   133
   Ultrasound technique   133
   Normal appearances of the liver   134
   Normal appearances of the gallbladder and biliary tree   135
Abnormalities of the neonatal liver   136
   Hepatomegaly   136
   Hemangioma and hemangioendothelioma   136
   Liver tumors in the neonate   140
Abnormalities of the neonatal biliary system   140
   Neonatal jaundice   140
Cystic dilation of the biliary system   144
   Congenital hepatic fibrosis   144
   Caroli disease   145
   Choledochal cysts   145
Diffuse abnormalities of the pediatric liver   148
   The bright liver   148
   Cirrhosis   149
   Portal hypertension   150
   Hepatitis   152
   Veno-occlusive disease   153
   Cystic fibrosis   154
Focal lesions of the pediatric liver   154
   Benign focal liver lesions   154
   Liver tumors   157
Abnormalities of the gallbladder and bile ducts in childhood   160

Liver transplantation   162
Spleen   163
The normal spleen   163
Congenital variants   164
Splenomegaly   167
The small spleen   167
Focal splenic lesions   167
Splenic trauma   169
Pancreas   170
Congenital anomalies   171
Normal anatomy   172
   Ultrasound technique   173
The abnormal pancreas   174
   Cystic fibrosis   174
   Other diffuse pancreatic conditions   175
   Focal lesions   177

LIVER

Embryology

Early in development of the caudal foregut the liver, gallbladder and bile duct arise as a ventral outgrowth. The developing liver bud grows into the septum transversum, which is a mass of mesoderm between the developing heart and midgut. The septum transversum ultimately goes on to form the ventral mesentery and central part of the diaphragm. The liver bud grows rapidly, filling a large part of the abdominal cavity in the first 10 weeks. The right and left lobes are about the same size but the right lobe soon becomes larger as a result of the supply of oxygenated blood from the umbilical vein. The liver starts producing blood cells at about 6 weeks, and bile formation starts by the 12th week. A small caudal outpouching of the hepatic diverticulum becomes the gallbladder, and the stalk of the diverticulum forms the cystic duct. The stalk connecting the hepatic and cystic ducts to the duodenum becomes the common bile duct (see Fig. 5.25).

Fetal vascular anatomy

In the fetal circulation the umbilical vein enters the left branch of the portal vein at the umbilical recess, lying in the free border of the falciform ligament from the umbilicus to the liver (Fig. 5.1). The left portal vein connects with the hepatic vein via the ductus venosus, and the blood then flows into the right atrium of the heart. The ductus venosus effectively forms a large venous shunt and bypasses the liver, allowing most of the blood from the placenta to pass directly to the heart. This fetal anatomy is important, as umbilical venous catheters should follow this route. If they enter the right portal vein then there is the potential for portal vein thrombosis to occur. After birth the umbilical vein obliterates and goes on to form the ligamentum teres in the falciform ligament. The ductus venosus also obliterates and goes on to form the ligamentum venosum. Within a few hours of birth and in very early neonatal life these structures can be readily identified with careful sonography. In the older child the ligamentum teres can be seen as an echogenic structure arising from the left branch of the portal vein (Fig. 5.2). When the pressure in the liver rises, as in cirrhosis, this channel re-canalizes and opens so that portal venous blood can flow away from the liver towards the umbilicus. This is how umbilical varices develop.

The inferior vena cava has a complex developmental anatomy, but anomalies are surprisingly infrequent. The most common anomaly is a persistent left sided IVC which drains into the right atrium through the enlarged orifice of the coronary sinus.

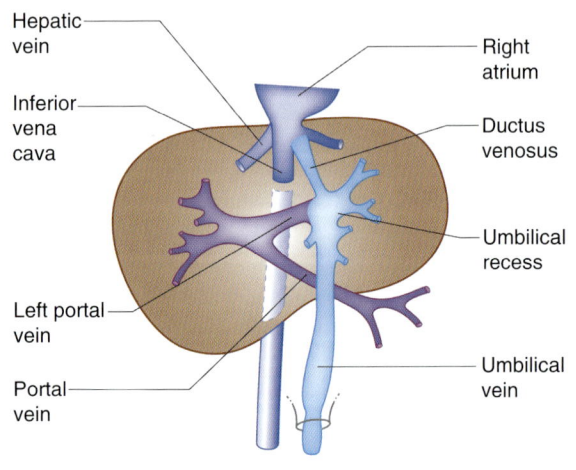

Figure 5.1 Fetal hepatic blood system. The diagram shows the relationship of the umbilical vein to the portal and hepatic venous systems in the fetus. The ductus venosus connects the left portal vein to the hepatic vein/right atrial region. The ductus venosus goes on to become the ligamentum venosum. The umbilical vein goes on to form the ligamentum teres of the liver, which is found on the lower margin of the falciform ligament. It is easy to understand how, if a catheter from the umbilical vein is misplaced, the portal vein can occlude with thrombus.

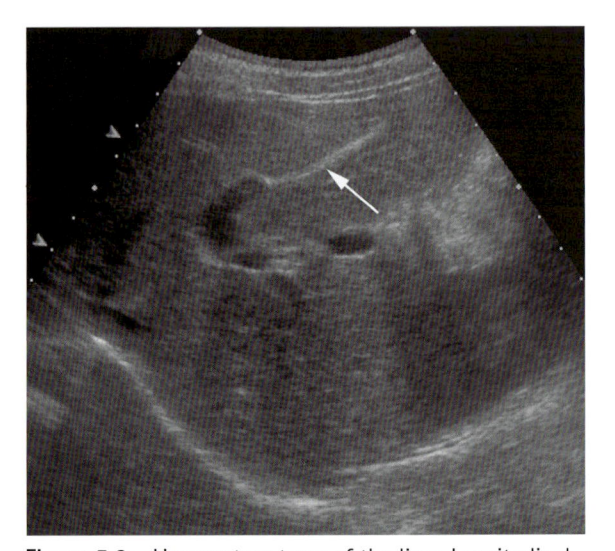

Figure 5.2 Ligamentum teres of the liver. Longitudinal sonogram in an older child showing the echogenic line of the obliterated ligamentum teres. This is occasionally seen in children, most commonly in a newborn, where it sometimes takes hours or days to close. It can be identified arising from the left portal vein.

In the abdomen the commonest anomaly is an interrupted IVC with failure of development of the hepatic segment. As a result the blood from the lower body drains via the azygous and hemi-azygous system of veins. The hepatic veins drain separately into the right atrium. There may also be a double IVC, which usually occurs below the renal veins, with the left IVC being smaller than the right.

THE NORMAL PEDIATRIC HEPATOBILIARY SYSTEM

Ultrasound is the first line investigation in any suspected abdominal pathology in children. Liver disease may be suspected clinically, in which case the findings of ultrasound will guide further imaging. However, lesions in the liver are often detected incidentally. Hence, abdominal examinations, regardless of the clinical history, should include a full examination of the major abdominal organs and their vasculature. This is particularly true in children, where many conditions are congenital. The liver has a very large functional reserve and may need to suffer extensive disease before dysfunction becomes clinically apparent. Also, there are many conditions, for example, renal, which are associated with liver disease, which will not be detected unless they are specifically sought.

A thorough basic knowledge of the normal anatomy of the liver is essential but, in addition in children, knowledge of the congenital anomalies that may simulate disease is also required. Perhaps nowhere else in the abdomen is the use of Doppler so important both to characterize focal lesions and evaluate the portal and hepatic vasculature.

Ultrasound technique

Curved linear array transducers are undoubtedly the best probes to use for the liver and spleen and upper abdomen. They give a good overview with little degradation of the near field. Changing to a linear transducer is essential if there is any suspicion of disease causing subtle small foci, such as candida (see Fig. 5.16B), as these can be easily overlooked. High quality Doppler is essential, as vascular abnormalities such as hemangiomas are common. Also, normal hepatic vascular anatomy and flow patterns should be confirmed.

Guidelines on technique are as follows.

- In children read the request carefully and check any previous reports or examinations. Always know what you are potentially looking for before you start, as the window of opportunity and period of goodwill for a quiet child is limited. Sedation, while rarely used for abdominal ultrasound, may be the only alternative when trying to clarify complex pathology, particularly when a good Doppler examination is needed.
- Children are best scanned supine at first, and visualization of organs is best enhanced by deep inspiration or expiration depending on which is better in any individual child. This exaggerated respiration brings the organs into better view. In inspiration the lungs inflate and the liver, spleen and kidneys descend below the ribs. This technique is also useful when trying to displace bowel. Sometimes in older children, organs will be better seen in the oblique and even decubitus position. The unwary sonographer must, however, accommodate the unusual views and appearances of the other organs such as kidney, IVC and aorta. An intercostal approach is very useful for a liver tucked high underneath the ribcage.
- Unless there is a suspicion clinically and a specific request to examine the biliary tree, children are not starved for routine abdominal examinations. If gallbladder or biliary disease is suspected during the examination, it is best to bring them back fully prepared and repeat the examination. One of the major advantages of ultrasound is that it can be repeated often and frequently.
- Ensure that the equipment is set optimally and a wide range of transducers is available for every eventuality.
- Have a systematic plan for examining the abdomen so that all the intra-abdominal structures are evaluated routinely. Leave any pathological process until last so that an important organ is not forgotten in the excitement of trying to come to a diagnosis.
- Remember to examine the intra-abdominal organs, both in longitudinal and transverse sections, in their entirety.

- The major abdominal vessels are important in children because organs, and in particular the liver, may have anomalous arterial supply and venous drainage. The IVC is particularly important and may be interrupted or may contain tumor or thrombus or a congenital web. The portal vein and porta hepatis should also be carefully examined for collateral vessels such as cavernous transformation.
- Don't forget to look in areas often overlooked such as the subphrenic spaces, i.e. above the liver and spleen, the retroperitoneum and pelvis.
- Pay meticulous attention to the ultrasound examination first. Remember it is a dynamic examination and it is not always easy to produce images of what you are seeing.

Normal appearances of the liver

It is assumed that the sonographer undertaking pediatric examinations should have a thorough knowledge of liver anatomy, and the following serves only to highlight the differences seen in children.

The pediatric liver has a homogeneous echo texture and is normally more echogenic than the parenchyma of the renal cortex. The medullae of the kidneys are darker still. The margins of the liver are sharp, and there is a thin, echogenic capsule surrounding the liver. When the liver enlarges, the edges become rounded. The portal vasculature is readily distinguished and, if doubt exists about dilated bile ducts, use Doppler to differentiate bile ducts and vessels. Dilated bile ducts typically produce the 'too many tubes' appearance or 'double barrel shotgun' appearance in the porta hepatis. If the parenchyma is involved in a process that increases the echogenicity, the portal walls may merge with this increased echogenicity and the portal vein walls appear less prominent. This is a good way to assess increased echogenicity of the liver.

Size of lobes and segments

Requests for sonography in children with clinically suspected hepatosplenomegaly are common. Volumetric measurements are available in the literature, although they are not used in routine clinical practice.[1]

The size and shape of the liver varies from child to child, and so in routine scanning the size is best assessed subjectively. The right lobe of the liver usually extends to just below the right kidney but, if a Riedel's lobe (a normal anatomical variant) exists, this may extend further. The left lobe of the liver on transverse scanning usually extends just to the left of the aorta, and in hepatomegaly this may extend well to the left and come to lie above the spleen and displace it inferiorly. This is sometimes erroneously thought to be splenomegaly on clinical examination. In young babies the left lobe is normally relatively large and may extend well over the midline.

Situs inversus is when the liver is on the left and the stomach and spleen on the right. In polysplenia or asplenia the liver has a transverse lie across the abdomen.

Broadly speaking, the liver is divided into the right and left lobes. The right lobe has two segments—the anterior and posterior segments—the division being by the right hepatic vein. The left lobe has a medial and lateral segment, the division being the left hepatic vein. In addition, there is a caudate lobe. It is important to distinguish the latter as it has a different blood supply and in certain conditions, such as Budd–Chiari syndrome (obstruction to the hepatic veins), it may enlarge and have a different echogenic appearance. However, when a mass is present in the liver, it is far more accurate, both for surgery and staging, to carefully locate the position of the mass in relation to the segment of the liver. This system of segmenting the liver was described by Couinaud and is used in CT and MRI and by surgeons when surgery is planned. It is essential to be familiar with this system.

Hepatic vasculature

Figure 5.3 shows Doppler waveforms of the hepatic vessels.

Hepatic veins The hepatic veins drain blood from the liver into the IVC and right atrium of the heart. The normal waveform is triphasic, toward the liver in diastole and a brief reversal in systole.

The hepatic vein waveform is affected by:

THE LIVER, SPLEEN AND PANCREAS 135

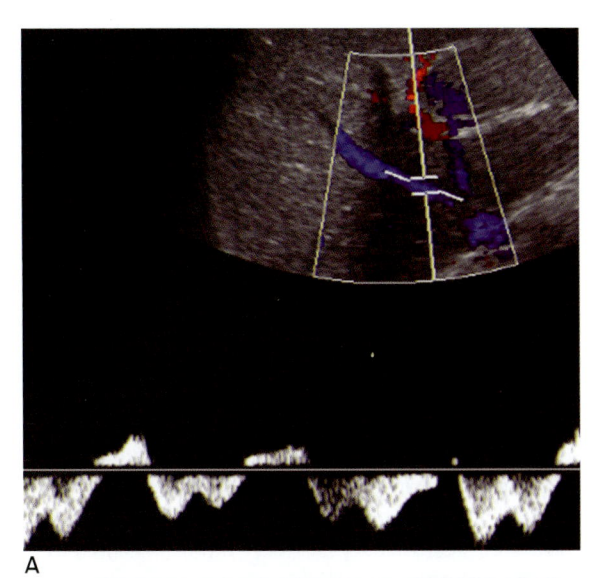

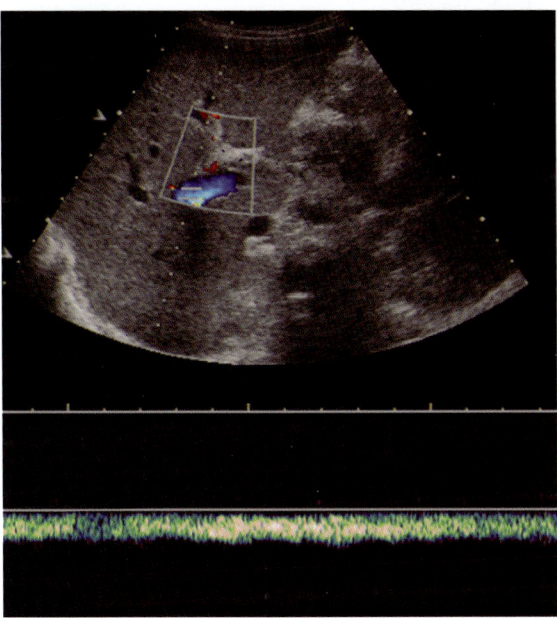

Figure 5.3 Doppler waveforms of hepatic vessels. (A) Hepatic vein waveform. This is triphasic. (B) Portal vein. The waveform is undulating and continuous. It is very important that sonographers learn to carry out Doppler examination of this vessel in the pediatric abdomen.

- compliance, that is the flexibility of the liver, so that conditions affecting the liver parenchyma and 'stiffening' the liver will dampen the waveform
- cardiac status—there is normally reversal of flow in atrial systole but, if the heart is failing, the

veins may massively dilate. In addition the IVC also dilates. There is loss of the normal fluctuation in the size of the lumen of the IVC and hepatic veins with respiration

- extra-hepatic conditions such as ascites, which may compress the veins and change the normal waveform.

Portal vein The portal vein brings blood to the liver from the spleen and bowel. The portal vein enters the liver in the porta hepatis and divides into the right and left branch. In the liver its branches have echogenic walls and are the most prominent vessels.

Normal diameter under 10 years of age should be in the region of 8 mm; over 10 years, it is 10 mm. Diameter is highly variable and varies with deep inspiration, food and posture. Normal waveform is monophasic with modulations due to respiration and cardiac activity.[2,3]

Congenital variations of the portal vein include a pre-duodenal portal vein which is frequently associated with situs inversus, duodenal stenosis, annular pancreas, malrotation of the bowel and other congenital malformations. Double portal vein and agenesis of the portal vein also occur.

Hepatic artery The hepatic artery carries oxygenated blood to the liver from the aorta. It is pulsatile with forward flow throughout the cardiac cycle.

Inferior vena cava The IVC drains the venous blood from the lower body. It should always be carefully examined, in particular for its normal course and anatomy, size and any intraluminal obstruction or pathology.

Normal appearances of the gallbladder and biliary tree

The gallbladder and biliary tree in a child are best examined after a fast. In infants, time the examination for the next feed if they are fed 4-hourly; in older children, a minimum of 6 hours' fast is needed. Alternatively, give older children appointments for the first examination of the morning so that they can have an overnight fast. After an adequate fast, the normal gallbladder will be well distended with bile. The shape and size of the gallbladder are very variable (Table 5.1). In children, as in adults, folding of the gallbladder may be mistaken for a septum and, when this occurs, patients should be examined in the decubitus position, or even erect.

Congenital anomalies of the gallbladder are also quite rare, and intrahepatic gallbladder and duplication are probably the anomalies one is likeliest to see. Provided the infant or child is adequately prepared the sonographer should always expect to see the gallbladder in pediatric practice.[4,5]

Gallbladder wall thickness and common hepatic duct diameter show no significant change with age:[6,7]

- gallbladder wall thickness 1–3 mm
- common hepatic duct diameter 1–4 mm.

ABNORMALITIES OF THE NEONATAL LIVER

Pathological conditions encountered in the neonate and in childhood differ, so this and subsequent sections divide liver abnormalities into neonatal and childhood conditions. There will be some overlap, but the intention is to provide a better understanding and help narrow the diagnosis for the sonographer.

Hepatomegaly

One of the commonest clinical indications for examining the neonatal abdomen is hepatomegaly. Box 5.1 lists the differential diagnoses.

Congestive cardiac failure

The liver may appear enlarged and echogenic. The most striking feature is dilation of the hepatic veins and the inferior vena cava. The infant will usually have a clinical history of heart failure. Ascites may also be present.

Hemangioma and hemangioendothelioma

A hemangioma is a primary, benign, frequently symptomatic, vascular neoplasm. Infantile vascular hemangioendothelioma is the most common hepatic

Table 5.1 Normal ranges (−2 SD to +2 SD) for the anteroposterior and coronal diameter as well as length of the gallbladder and diameter of the right portal vein

Age (years)	AP diameter (mm)	Coronal diameter (mm)	Length (mm)	Right portal vein diameter (mm)
0	5.7–9.7	5.1–18.1	11.4–25.2	2.1–4.0
1	7.8–15.5	7.6–22.9	19.8–40.0	3.0–5.6
2	8.7–17.9	8.6–24.9	23.2–46.1	3.4–6.3
3	9.3–19.8	9.3–26.5	25.8–50.8	3.7–6.8
4	9.9–21.3	10.0–27.7	28.1–54.7	4.0–7.3
5	10.4–22.7	10.5–28.9	30.0–58.2	4.2–7.7
6	10.8–23.9	11.1–29.9	31.8–61.3	4.4–8.0
7	11.3–25.1	11.5–30.9	33.4–64.2	4.6–8.4
8	11.6–26.1	12.0–31.7	35.0–66.9	4.8–8.7
9	12.0–27.1	12.4–32.6	36.4–69.5	5.0–9.0
10	12.4–28.1	12.8–33.3	37.7–71.9	5.1–9.2
11	12.7–29.0	13.2–34.1	39.0–74.1	5.3–9.5
12	13.0–29.8	13.5–34.8	40.3–76.3	5.4–9.7
13	13.3–30.6	13.9–35.5	41.4–78.4	5.5–10.0
14	13.6–31.4	14.2–36.1	42.6–80.4	5.7–10.2
15	13.9–32.2	14.5–36.8	43.7–82.3	5.8–10.4

After McGahan et al.[6]

> **Box 5.1 Causes of hepatomegaly in the neonate**
>
> *Diffuse*
> - 4S Neuroblastoma
> - Cardiac failure
> - Fatty infiltration, metabolic liver disorders
> - Hepatitis
> - Leukemia
>
> *Focal*
> - Angiomatous lesions
> - Metastases from Stage IV neuroblastoma
> - Hepatoblastoma

mass in the neonate, and over 80% present within the first 6 months of life.

Infants typically present with hepatomegaly or are thought to have an abdominal mass. Other clinical presentations include high output heart failure (25%) caused by intratumoral, high flow, arteriovenous shunts. Disseminated intravascular coagulation occurs as the platelets are damaged and trapped as they pass through the AV shunt, and so thrombocytopenia results and the potential to bleed is high (Kasabach–Meritt syndrome). If rupture of the hemangioma has occurred during delivery, they may even present with a hemoperitoneum. Occasionally these infants may be asymptomatic and are referred, from dermatologists, with skin hemangiomas. The reported incidence of associated hepatic hemangiomas varies in the literature, because of selection of patients, but generally about half of those with multiple skin hemangiomas will have them in the liver as well. There is also an association with hemangiomas in the lung, trachea, thymus, spleen, lymph nodes and meninges.

Diagnosis may be made in utero, and fetal hydrops may occur as a result of the AV shunting of blood.

Ultrasound appearance

There are two different types of hemangiomas: Type I has proliferation of small vascular channels and cavernous areas, and Type 2 has an irregular structure and tendency to fibrosis. Hemangioendotheliomas may be solitary, multiple or diffuse, ranging in diameter from a few millimeters to several centimeters, and reflect the capillary nature of the hemangioma. Asymptomatic and sometimes even symptomatic tumors can undergo complete involution by 2 years.

There is a wide spectrum of ultrasound appearances, from a single small hyper- or hypoechoic nodule to multiple similar nodules throughout the liver parenchyma (Fig. 5.4). Lesions may be present in the spleen as well. Calcification occurs in approximately 15%. They are highly vascular on Doppler examination but settings must be optimal for slow flow. Spectral traces should always be obtained from the hemangioma, which will demonstrate the AV shunting. Ultrasound is particularly useful to look at vessels both feeding and draining the hemangiomatous mass, so the aorta, celiac, superior mesenteric feeding vessels, and hepatic veins draining the mass need to be examined carefully. In addition this will also help in the differential diagnosis—if a mass is found in the liver in a neonate, with large feeding arteries and large draining veins, the diagnosis is most likely to be a hemangioma. In massive intratumoral AV shunting the patient may be in severe congestive heart failure. Ultrasonically the multiple small hemangiomas appear hypoechoic. The single hemangiomas may appear hyperechoic, as seen in adult hemangioma. An enhanced CT examination will show early peripheral enhancement with delayed progression to the center of the lesion. Occasionally the central portion of large masses will remain hypodense, and this corresponds to central fibrosis.

Angiography will show the associated abnormalities of the hepatic artery and large tortuous draining veins with shunting.

Cavernous hemangiomas contain large cystic spaces (Fig. 5.5). The sonographer must carefully evaluate the mass and examine the aorta and major blood vessels, as shunting of blood to the liver may be large and the diversion of blood may increase the size of the hepatic artery and superior mesenteric artery. Ultrasound is an excellent modality for demonstrating this in the neonate, as other cross sectional imaging does not generally produce

138   PEDIATRIC ULTRASOUND

images of such exquisite detail due to the small size of the infant. Blood flow in the cavernous hemangioma may be slow and difficult to detect on Doppler but with newer equipment and optimal settings for slow flow this can be overcome. Very rarely these hemangioendotheliomas may fill the whole of the liver, producing a very specific and extraordinary appearance (Fig. 5.6). These infants may be in severe heart failure and have major problems with a bleeding diathesis. Sometimes extreme measures have to be taken in order for the infant to survive, and embolization of the hepatic artery has been attempted in order to prevent the shunting of blood.

Interferon and steroids have been used with variable success to decrease the size of the mass. The natural history of hemangiomas is to decrease in size with time.

Carefully performed dynamic enhanced CT scanning and MRI will help show the vascular nature of the mass. Calcification is occasionally seen in the vessels.

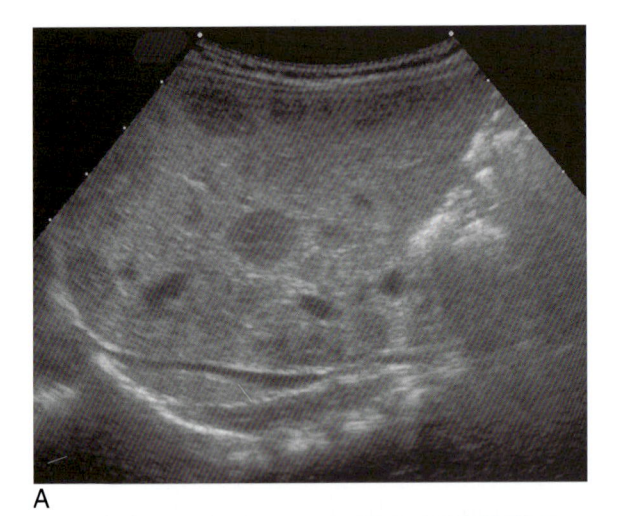

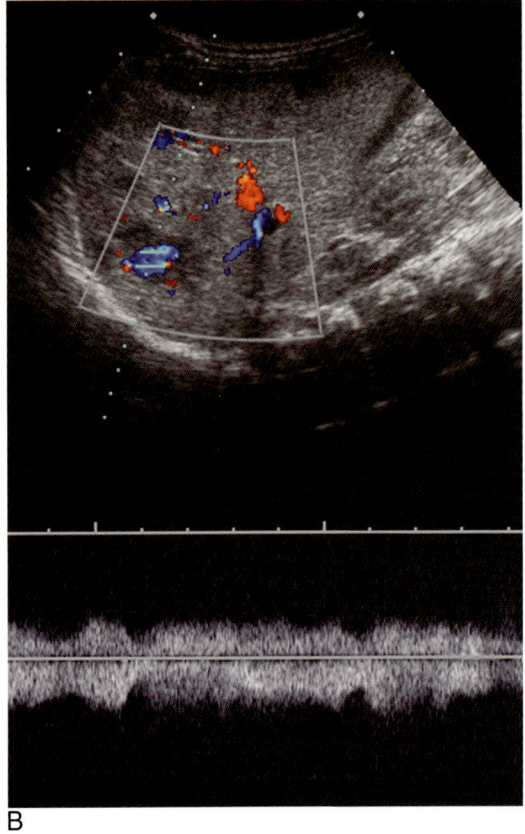

Figure 5.4 Hepatic hemangiomas. (A) Longitudinal sonogram of the liver showing multiple hypoechoic areas within the liver parenchyma. (B) Doppler examination of these multiple small hemangiomas demonstrating the AV shunting of blood within the hemangioma. The spectral waveform is abnormal, with spectral widening and no obvious arterial and separate venous waveform. When severe shunting occurs the patient will go into heart failure.

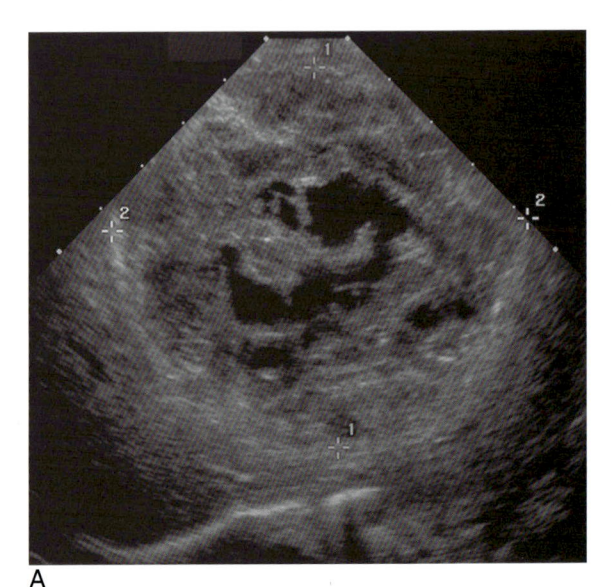

Figure 5.5 Cavernous hemangioma. (A) This newborn presented with a large palpable mass in the liver. Ultrasound examination revealed a well-defined mass containing serpiginous channels (between calipers).

THE LIVER, SPLEEN AND PANCREAS 139

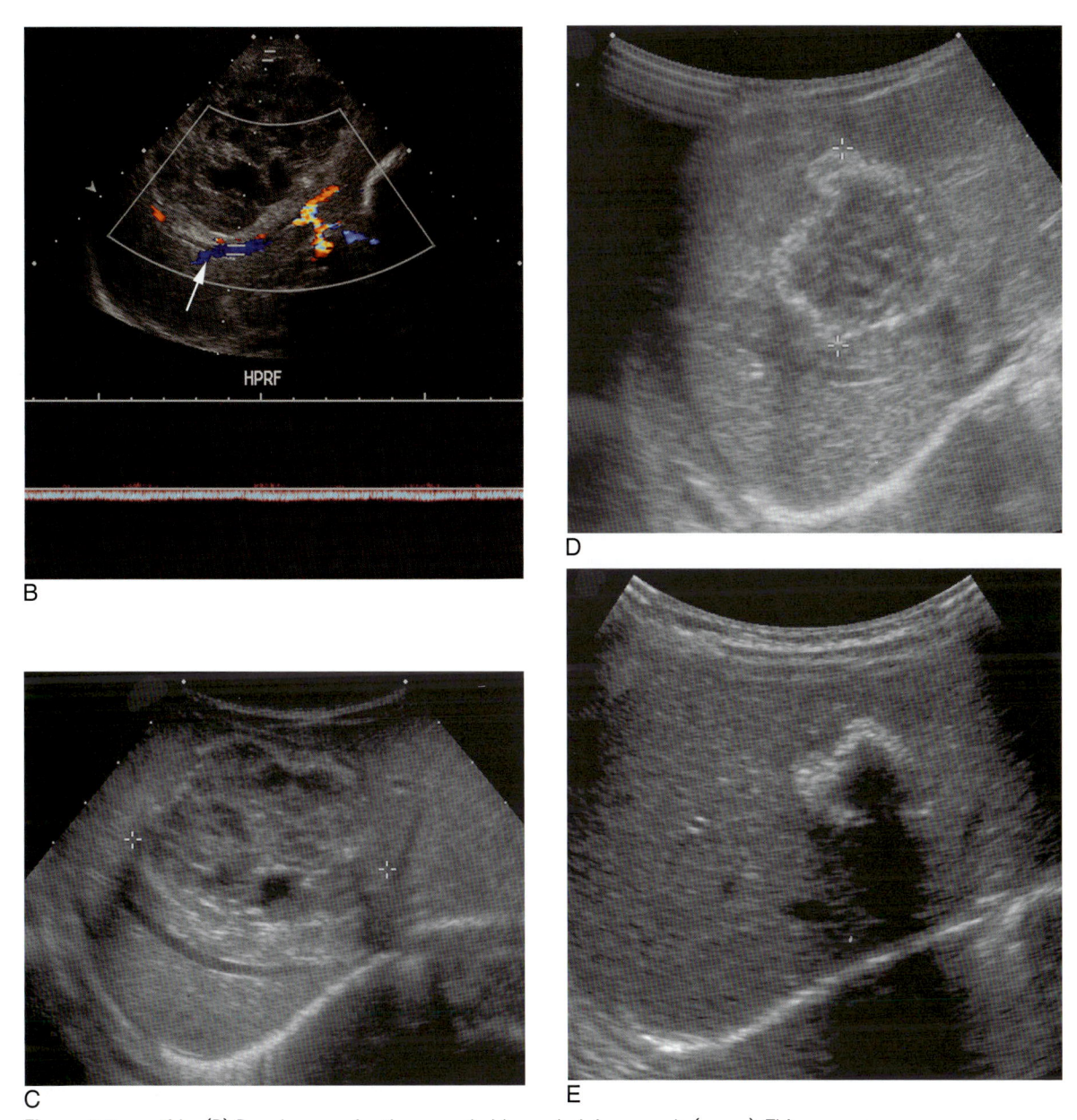

Figure 5.5, cont'd (B) Doppler examination revealed large draining vessels (arrow). This was a cavernous hemangioma of the liver. On Doppler very little flow or no flow is seen within these large dilated channels, because of the slow flow of blood. (C) Ultrasound examination of the mass 1 month later shows that the channels are still evident but the mass is better defined and smaller in size. (D) Longitudinal sonogram of the mass 1 month later revealed increased peripheral echogenicity, suggesting calcification, and once again the mass has regressed in size. (E) Follow-up 6 months after birth shows that the cavernous hemangioma has become much smaller, thrombosed its blood supply and become highly calcified.

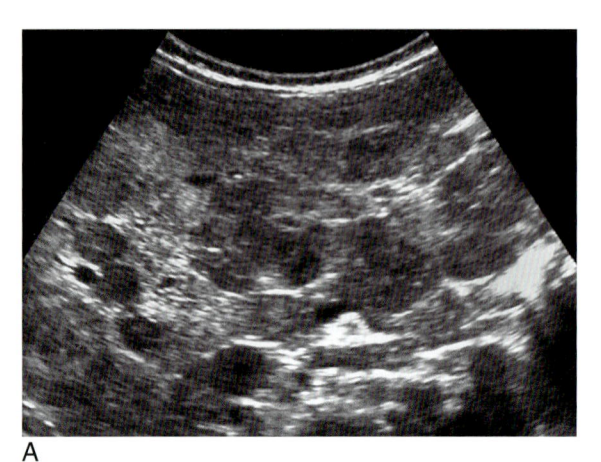

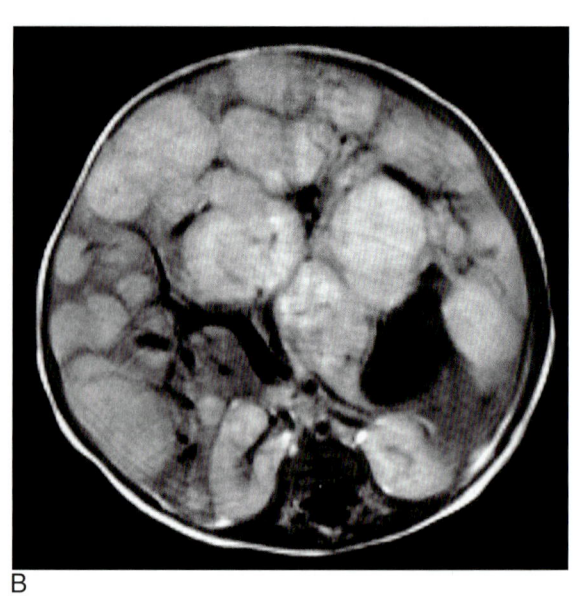

Figure 5.6 Hemangioendothelioma. (A) Transverse sonogram of the liver at the level of the superior mesenteric artery. The liver is markedly enlarged and filled with multiple hypoechoic hemangiomas. This baby was extremely ill and eventually died from an uncontrollable disseminated intravascular coagulation. (B) MRI examination on the same infant showing these extensive lesions throughout the whole liver.

These lesions are the most commonly seen hepatic masses in neonates and, provided the alfa-fetoprotein is normal, should be the first diagnosis excluded. It is for this reason that every effort must be made to perform a careful Doppler examination on all these patients (Fig. 5.7).

Liver tumors in the neonate

Hepatoblastoma

Hepatoblastoma may occasionally be seen in the neonate. It is for this reason that the alfa-fetoprotein levels should be measured in any suspicious cases, as they will be elevated in the vast majority. Alfa-fetoprotein is a glycoprotein that is made by the liver, yolk sac and gut. In the fetus it may escape into the amniotic fluid via an open neural tube defect or from open ventral wall defects. This is why it is used so successfully prenatally to help detect these defects.

Ultrasound appearances Hepatoblastomas are usually solitary, reasonably well-defined lesions. They are most common in the right lobe and may contain areas of calcification.

Hepatic tumors are very vascular and must not be mistaken for hemangiomas. One of the differentiating features to look for is the Doppler shift, which is greater in hepatoblastoma, as is vascular invasion with amputation of portal vessels (Fig. 5.8).

4S Neuroblastoma

4S NBL presents in the early neonatal period with a generalized enlargement of the liver and, on ultrasound, has a heterogeneous appearance typically described as a 'pepper pot' appearance. This should be the first differential diagnosis considered when a massively enlarged heterogeneous liver is found in the neonate and an active search for an adrenal primary tumor made. This is fully described in Chapter 4.

ABNORMALITIES OF THE NEONATAL BILIARY SYSTEM

Neonatal jaundice

Jaundice is a result of elevation of bilirubin in the blood. Bilirubin may be unconjugated, when it has been released from red cells which have been broken

THE LIVER, SPLEEN AND PANCREAS   141

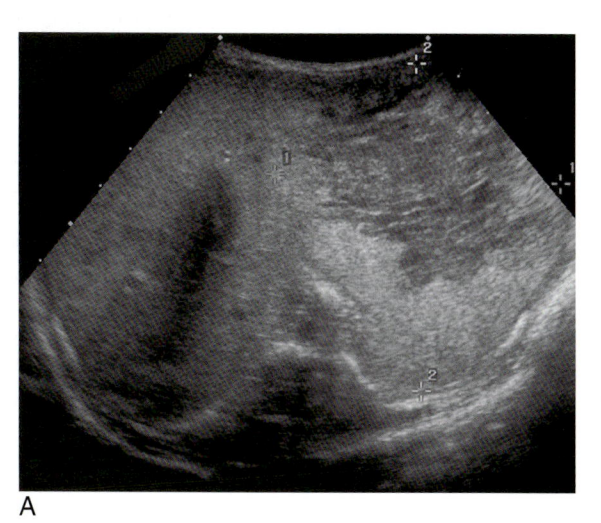

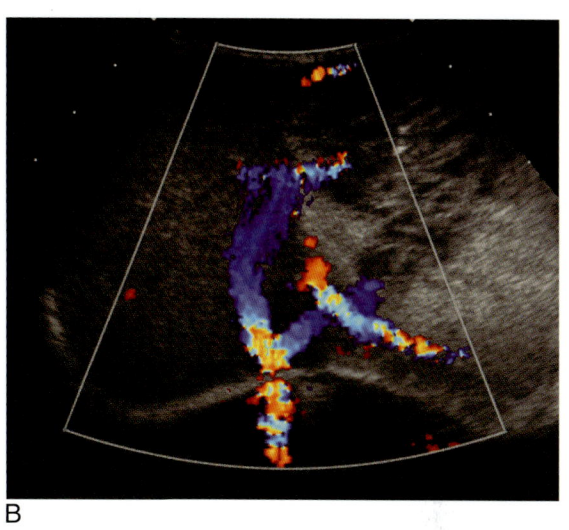

A B

Figure 5.7 Hepatic hemangioma. (A) This female neonate was discovered prenatally to have a liver mass. This is the first scan at 1 week of age. Transverse sonogram of the liver shows a large mass occupying most of the left lobe of the liver (between calipers). It has a heterogeneous appearance and centrally some tubular structures which look like blood vessels. (B) Transverse sonogram of the mass with color flow Doppler. There are huge draining hepatic veins which indicate that this mass is highly vascular with some shunting of blood. This was diagnosed at biopsy as an infantile hemangioendothelioma.

down normally or pathologically, or conjugated, when the released bilirubin is converted by liver cells to a water soluble form excreted in the bile ducts. The conjugated form normally aids fat digestion and turns stools dark.

Most newborn infants become clinically jaundiced. If the jaundice persists for more than 2 weeks it is called persistent or prolonged. This is usually an unconjugated hyperbilirubinemia which resolves.

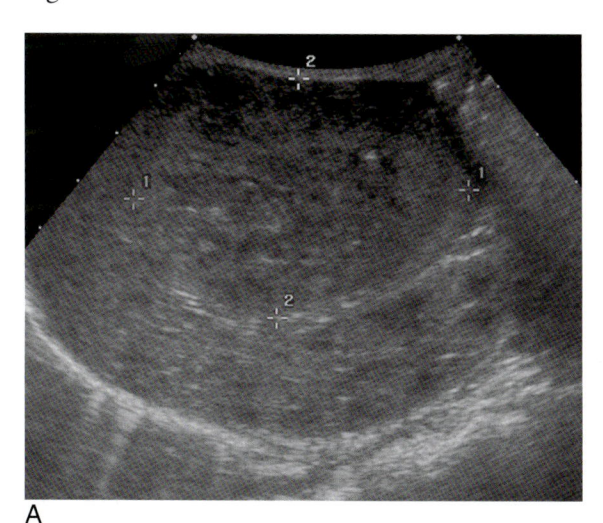

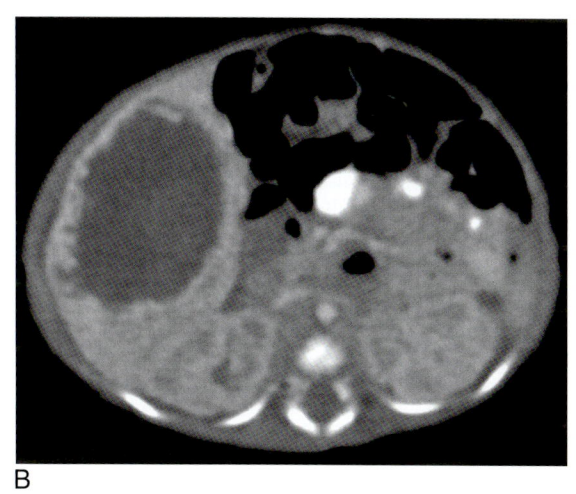

A B

Figure 5.8 Neonate hepatoblastoma. (A) Longitudinal sonogram of the right lobe of the liver and right kidney in a young infant presenting with an abdominal mass. There is a well-defined solid mass within the liver (between calipers) which on biopsy was a hepatoblastoma. (B) Contrast-enhanced CT examination of the liver in this infant. This shows what appears to be predominantly a cystic mass with rim enhancement. This is an unusual enhancing lesion. The alfa-fetoprotein level was raised.

Continued

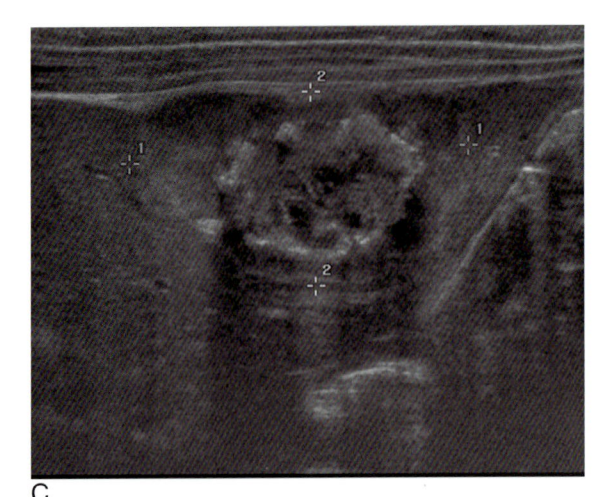

Figure 5.8, cont'd (C) Longitudinal sonogram of the mass 2 months later after treatment. The mass is much smaller in size (between calipers) but now shows some dense calcification around the edge.

Persistent jaundice caused by liver disease is conjugated hyperbilirubinemia. Clinical evaluation gives very few clues to the etiology, but typically the infants have pale stools, dark urine, hepatomegaly, bleeding disorders (as the liver is unable to synthesize prothrombin) and failure to thrive. Diagnosis of the cause of the jaundice is urgently required, as early intervention improves the ultimate prognosis.

Clinically the infants present in the first month of life with jaundice. The initial steps are:

- Confirm elevated bilirubin, of which more than 20% will be conjugated.
- Identify a potentially treatable cause such as sepsis or hypothyroidism or a metabolic condition (Box 5.2).
- Differentiate neonatal hepatitis from biliary atresia or a potentially surgically treatable condition such as a choledochal cyst. Ultrasound is an excellent modality to screen neonates with jaundice.

Biliary atresia

This occurs in 1 in 10–14 000 live births. It is a progressive disease in which there is destruction of the extrahepatic biliary tree and intrahepatic bile ducts.

> **Box 5.2 Causes of persistent neonatal jaundice**
>
> *Unconjugated*
> - Breast milk jaundice
> - Infection, particularly urinary tract
> - Hemolytic anemia, e.g. G6PD deficiency
> - Hypothyroidism
> - High gastrointestinal obstruction
>
> *Conjugated > 20% total bilirubin*
> - Bile duct obstruction, such as:
>   Biliary atresia, choledochal cysts
> - Neonatal hepatitis, such as:
>   Congenital infection
> - Inborn errors of metabolism, such as:
>   Alfa-1 antitrypsin deficiency
>   Tyrosinemia, galactosemia
> - Cholestasis, such as:
>   Intrahepatic biliary hypoplasia
>   Alagilles syndrome
>   Inspissated bile syndrome
>   Choledocholithiasis
>   Cystic fibrosis
>   Total parenteral nutrition (TPN)

Current thinking is that it is an acquired inflammatory disease of the bile ducts with resulting damage to segments of the biliary tree, giving abnormal intrahepatic ducts and an interruption of the extrahepatic bile duct. There are many types and they vary according to the extent of the sclerotic and fibrotic process in the biliary tree. All or part of the extrahepatic biliary tree may become atretic and absent. The gallbladder may be preserved, isolated or associated with a choledochocele or patent common bile duct. A choledochocele is an isolated segment of bile duct which fills with fluid. Those who have a patent extrahepatic bile duct and gallbladder have a better prognosis.

These babies have a normal birth weight but rapidly fail to thrive. They have cholestatic jaundice, with pale stools and dark urine. Hepatomegaly is present, and splenomegaly will develop secondary to portal hypertension.

Ultrasound findings Ultrasound examinations must be carefully performed with the highest resolution transducers available. Generally the findings in neonatal jaundice are non-specific, but there are a few features that need to be specifically commented on.

- *Common bile duct.* It is important to try to identify the common bile duct, which will be non-dilated in neonatal hepatitis and biliary atresia. In infants the normal common bile duct may be difficult to detect, and Doppler should always be used to confirm the position of the hepatic artery. The major differential is a choledochal cyst, so identification of a dilated common bile duct is crucial.
- *Gallbladder.* The infant must be adequately fasted. In biliary atresia the gallbladder is not always absent as previously thought but may be small and abnormal. Failure to find the gallbladder after an adequate fast is highly suggestive of biliary atresia.
- *Intrahepatic bile ducts.* These are not dilated in neonatal hepatitis or biliary atresia. They may be dilated in a choledochal cyst and in cholelithiasis or where sludge fills the biliary tree. Bile plug syndrome is a condition where pigment stones fill the biliary tree; some of the causes are total parenteral nutrition (TPN), frusemide treatment, dehydration, infection and prematurity. Sludge may be seen in the gallbladder.
- *Portal cyst.* A separate cyst may be seen in the porta hepatis in approximately 10% of patients. This is a remnant of the extrahepatic bile duct. It must not be confused with a choledochal cyst; if any suspicion exists, further imaging should be undertaken to determine the nature of the cystic structure. 'Cysts' may also be intrahepatic in location.

Other abnormalities to look for include polysplenia, pre-duodenal portal vein and an interrupted inferior vena cava which does not join the inferior aspect of the right atrium. Situs inversus is also associated.

The ultimate diagnosis of biliary atresia is made by a combination of tests. Radioisotope studies show failure of excretion of the IDA compounds by the liver with no filling of the bowel on delayed images. Percutaneous liver biopsy makes the diagnosis by demonstrating portal fibrosis.

Biliary atresia leads to chronic liver failure and death within 2 years unless surgical intervention is performed. Surgery consists of bypassing the fibrotic ducts by performing a portoenterostomy (Kasai procedure) in which the jejunum is anastomosed to the patent ducts on the cut surface of the porta hepatis. If surgery is performed before the infant is 60 days old, 80% achieve bile drainage. The success decreases with age—hence the urgency for diagnosis. If this surgery is not successful then liver transplantation is the only alternative.

Possible future complications include cholangitis and a 2% risk of malignancy in the biliary tree. Follow-up after portoenterostomy is to monitor for the development of cirrhosis.

Neonatal hepatitis

In neonatal hepatitis there is hepatic inflammation. The causes are mainly congenital neonatal infections such as cytomegalovirus, toxoplasmosis rubella and congenital syphilis but some are idiopathic in origin. In contrast to biliary atresia these infants may have intrauterine growth retardation and hepatosplenomegaly at birth.

Intrahepatic biliary hypoplasia (Alagille syndrome)

This is an autosomal dominant condition. Infants have characteristic triangular facies, skeletal abnormalities, peripheral pulmonary stenosis, renal tubular disorders, defects in the eye and intrahepatic biliary hypoplasia with severe itching and failure to thrive. Half survive into adult life without transplantation.

Inspissated bile plug syndrome

This is a rare condition where thick, inspissated bile obstructs the biliary tree usually in the lower common bile duct. It is associated with conditions which cause the bile to become thick and viscid, such as cystic fibrosis, which also causes meconium ileus in the neonate, or total parenteral nutrition in the older infant. Excessive hemolysis is also associated. Ultrasound will demonstrate a dilated common bile duct often with sludge in the gallbladder.

Spontaneous perforation of the bile duct

This is a very rare condition presenting in the early neonatal period. Infants present with jaundice and ascites resulting from the leakage of bile around the liver from the perforated duct. The biliary tree is not dilated on ultrasound.

Role of ultrasound

The major role of ultrasound in neonatal jaundice is the following.

- Identify a cause of the obstructive jaundice that may be amenable to treatment such as dilation of the biliary tree—for example, a choledochal cyst or obstruction by inspissated bile or biliary calculi.
- Once these conditions have been excluded, the role of ultrasound is to try to differentiate biliary atresia from neonatal hepatitis. It must, however, be emphasized that there is no single biochemical test or imaging procedure that is entirely satisfactory to differentiate the two (Table 5.2).

CYSTIC DILATION OF THE BILIARY SYSTEM

Congenital hepatic fibrosis

Congenital hepatic fibrosis is a condition that is most commonly associated with autosomal recessive polycystic kidney disease (ARPKD) in the infant. Older children may present to a physician with signs and symptoms of liver disease. Hepatic fibrosis is essential to the diagnosis of autosomal recessive polycystic kidney disease.

The ultrasound diagnosis of congenital hepatic fibrosis is a spectrum of appearances. The liver may appear normal, particularly in the young infant. Later, the liver may enlarge, often predominantly the left lobe. The periportal fibrosis appears as an

Table 5.2 Differentiation of idiopathic neonatal hepatitis from biliary atresia

	Neonatal hepatitis	Biliary atresia
Familial incidence	20%	None
Size	Premature or small for gestational age	Normal
Stool		Usually persistently pale (acholic)
Nasogastric aspirate		No bile
Liver parenchyma	Normal or increased echogenicity	Normal or increased echogenicity
Bile ducts	Not dilated	Not dilated
Gallbladder	Normal	Contracted and abnormal
	Contracts after a feed	15% absent
		10% normal
Associated anomalies		Polysplenia, pre-duodenal portal vein, diaphragmatic hernia, situs inversus
HIDA scan	Poor uptake, but excretion into bowel	Good uptake, with no liver excretion into bowel
Other		Intra- or extrahepatic 'cysts'; choledochocele
Liver biopsy	Non-specific	Portal fibrosis
Diagnosis	ERCP or operative cholangiography outlines normal biliary tree	ERCP or operative cholangiography fails to outline normal biliary tree
Treatment	Treatment of the underlying cause if found	Early: Hepatoportoenterostomy (surgical bypass of fibrotic ducts); Kasai procedure Late: Liver transplantation

ERCP, Endoscopic retrograde cholangiopancreatography; HIDA, hepatic iminodiacetic acid.

increase in the echogenicity around the portal veins although the changes can often be very subtle and difficult to appreciate. The most diagnostic appearances are those of cystic dilations in the liver parenchyma, which are saccular dilations of the biliary tree. It is essential to carefully examine the liver in all infants suspected of having ARPKD.

Congenital hepatic fibrosis may also be associated with Jeune syndrome, Meckel syndrome, chondrodysplasia syndromes and Zellweger syndrome (see Ch. 3, section on cystic kidneys).

Caroli disease

In the 1950s Caroli et al described a disease characterized by non-obstructive dilation of the intrahepatic bile ducts. These cystic dilations of the bile ducts were prone to developing biliary calculi, and the patients were at risk of developing cholangitis. The disorder may be associated with congenital hepatic fibrosis and medullary cystic disease of the kidneys and a choledochal cyst (Fig. 5.9). Any infant or child with large echogenic kidneys and suspected of having ARPKD should have a careful evaluation of the liver. Polycystic disease of the liver is seen in autosomal dominant polycystic kidney disease and differs in that the cysts do not communicate with the bile ducts. It rarely occurs in children.

Choledochal cysts

These are cystic dilations of the extrahepatic biliary system.[8–12] About 25% present in the neonatal period with cholestasis (Fig. 5.10). Some are detected by prenatal scanning. Choledochal cysts appear most commonly as cystic or fusiform dilation of the common bile duct. They are thought to be related to an anomalous connection between the common bile duct and pancreatic duct which results in chronic reflux of pancreatic juices and dilation of the common bile duct. Ultrasound is the initial imaging modality of choice and will generally give an excellent demonstration of the dilation of the intra- and extrahepatic biliary tree. ERCP (endoscopic retrograde cholangiopancreatography) will further delineate the anatomy of the biliary tree (Fig. 5.11). Intraoperative (i.e. during surgery) cholangiography is also sometimes performed.

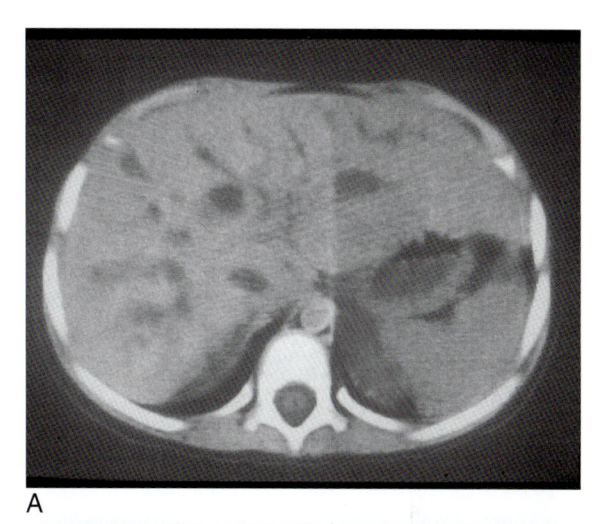

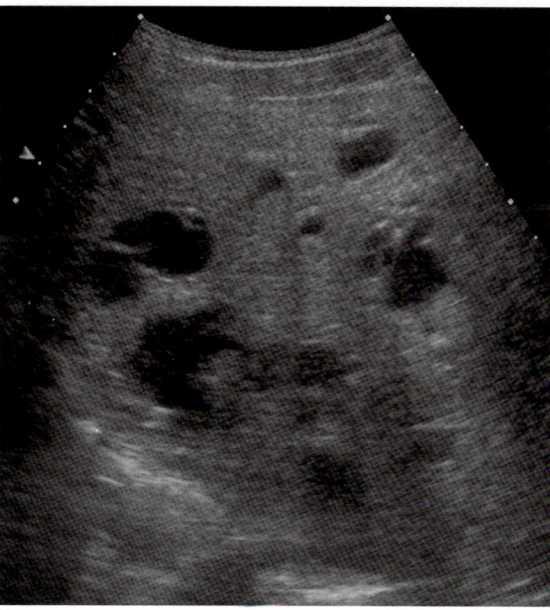

Figure 5.9 Caroli disease. (A) This boy presented with a longstanding history of liver disease. He was diagnosed as an infant with congenital hepatic fibrosis and Caroli disease. CT examination shows multiple cystic areas related to the bile ducts. (B) Ultrasound examination of the right lobe of the liver 5 years later shows the multiple cystic areas within the liver, which have enlarged. These were cystic dilations of the biliary tree and not hepatic cysts. *Continued*

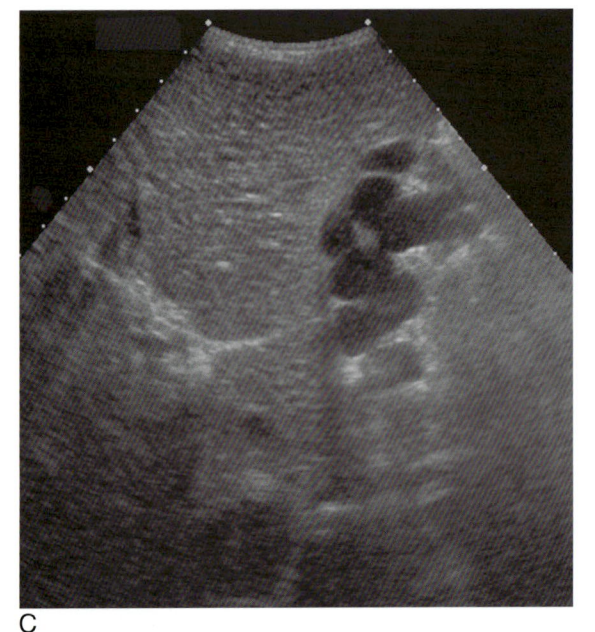

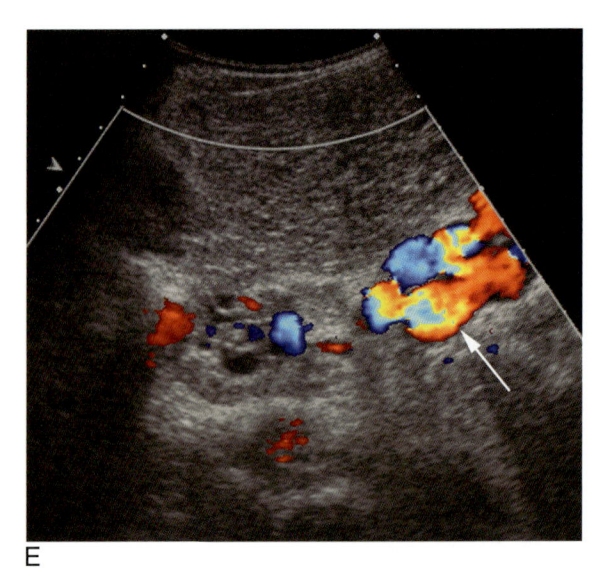

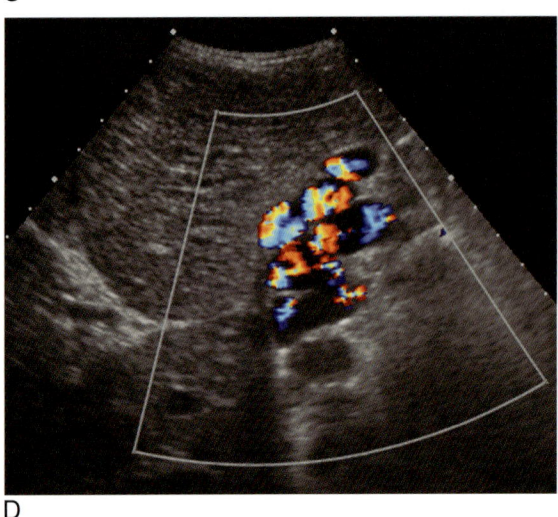

Figure 5.9, cont'd (C) He had recently had a hematemesis, and longitudinal ultrasound examination of the liver revealed a dilated tortuous vessel around the porta hepatis. (D) Doppler examination in the same projection revealed that this vessel was venous and was feeding the gastric vessels. (E) Transverse examination of the liver at the level of the pancreas revealed the multiple abnormal vessels within the porta hepatis and on the undersurface of the liver leading to the gastric fundus (arrow). In addition he had a grossly abnormal hepatic echo texture consistent with his congenital hepatic fibrosis.

Clinical presentation In infants choledochal cysts are now commonly detected prenatally. These choledochal cysts may rupture, and the infant may present with bile peritonitis.

The typical presentation in childhood is one of abdominal pain, jaundice and a palpable abdominal mass. They may also present with persistent jaundice. Choledochal cysts are more common in females. There may also be a clinical history of fever, vomiting, jaundice and abdominal pain which may be related to pancreatitis and/or cholangitis.

Pancreatitis is thought to be related to the anomalous duct anatomy. Cholangitis, an ascending infection in the bile ducts as a result of stasis of bile, may also occur. There have also been cases reported in the literature of portal hypertension developing because of compression of the portal vein by the large cyst or secondary to biliary cirrhosis.

THE LIVER, SPLEEN AND PANCREAS   147

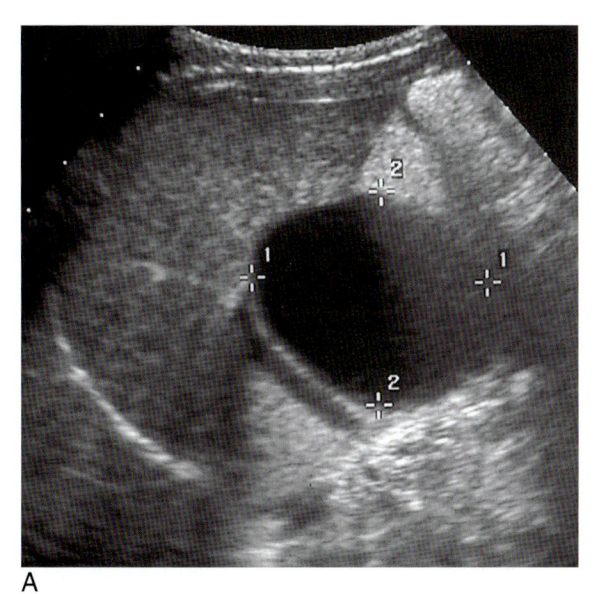

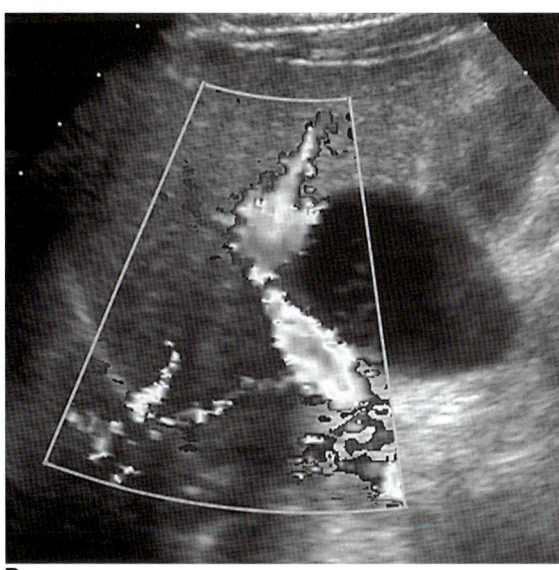

Figure 5.10 Choledochal cyst in a newborn. (A) This baby had a prenatal diagnosis of a cystic structure in the porta hepatis. Longitudinal sonogram of the porta hepatis showing the cystic structure anterior to the portal vein. The structure did not have a well-defined muscular and mucosal wall and was not associated with intrahepatic bile duct dilation. The infant was otherwise well and not jaundiced. It is important not to mistake a choledochal cyst for a choledochocele in biliary atresia. (B) Doppler examination confirms the cystic structure is anterior to the portal vein, and this was found at surgery to be a choledochal cyst.

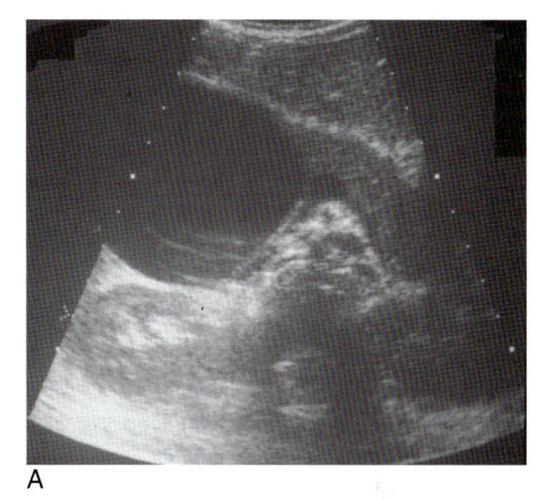

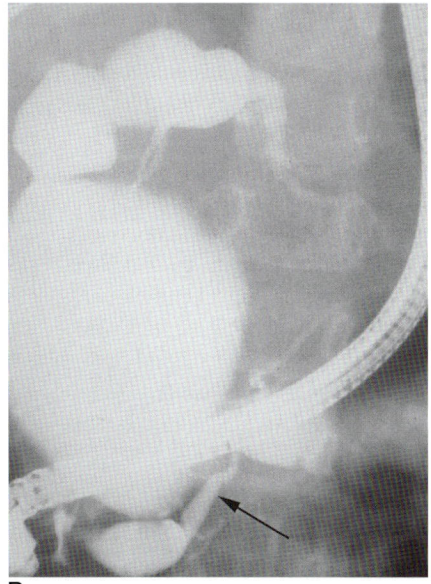

Figure 5.11 Choledochal cyst in the older child. (A) This child presented with an upper abdominal mass, jaundice and pain. Ultrasound examination demonstrated a large cystic mass in the region of the head of the pancreas. There was no appreciable wall but there was dilation of the main right and left hepatic bile ducts. The primary differential diagnosis for cystic lesions in the region of the gastric antrum is duplication cysts of the bowel. The classic triad of pain, mass and jaundice is seen in less than 30% of patients. (B) ERCP (endoscopic retrograde cholangiopancreatography) examination. A tube has been passed down the esophagus and into the duodenum. Contrast has been injected into the pancreatic and common bile duct orifice. Instead of the common bile duct there is a large dilated choledochal cyst with dilation of the intrahepatic bile ducts. Contrast has also filled the pancreatic duct (arrow).

Ultrasound examination Ultrasound is generally regarded as the imaging modality of choice in any child presenting with jaundice. The ultrasound should demonstrate the intra- and extrahepatic biliary tree together with the gallbladder. At sonography the choledochal cyst will appear as a cystic dilation of the common bile duct, separate from the gallbladder, and there may or may not be dilation of the hepatic duct or intrahepatic ducts. The main differential diagnosis of a cystic structure in the region of the porta hepatis and antrum of the stomach is a duplication cyst of the bowel. The sonographer must carefully look for the typical wall seen in a duplication cyst.

Other cysts that need to be differentiated in the older child are mesenteric or omental cysts, hepatic cysts, cystic teratomas and pancreatic pseudocysts. Choledochal cysts do not always have intrahepatic dilation, and it is in this instance that further imaging is particularly needed. Of particular use are nuclear medicine studies using a radioactive tracer which is excreted in the bile. A HIDA scan will fill the dilated ducts and choledochal cysts. Particularly important are the delayed images where there may not be any filling of the bowel.

Gallstones within the gallbladder, biliary sludge within the cyst, and dilated intrahepatic bile ducts are commonly seen. There is also the known association with malignancy. Carcinoma of the bile ducts may be found, and the risk of this seems to be related to the biliary stasis and metaplasia which occurs as the pancreatic juices reflux into the biliary tree.

The treatment is surgical resection.

DIFFUSE ABNORMALITIES OF THE PEDIATRIC LIVER

Many conditions throughout childhood may affect the liver. Some are highly specific to children but, overall, most liver pathologies have a similar appearance to that seen in the adult. The liver may be involved in a generalized or focal process, and pathology seen in childhood is best characterized into diffuse and focal conditions.

Conditions that diffusely affect the liver are generally non-specific in their ultrasound appearances. They are often associated with hepatomegaly and sometimes jaundice. The role of ultrasound is to show the extent of the liver involvement, demonstrate biliary dilation if present and then primarily to examine the upper abdomen looking for other signs of chronic liver disease such as portal hypertension and varices.

Once an abnormality is detected the liver should be examined, with a number of specific features of disease in mind:

- size of the liver, which will give an indication of whether the condition is acute or chronic—in chronic conditions the liver undergoes fibrosis and gets smaller
- reflectivity of the liver parenchyma—use the portal vein walls as a marker of increased echogenicity
- hepatic artery, vein and portal venous system—careful examination of the vessels is important in all liver pathology
- outline of the liver—smooth and angular or with a nodular outline suggesting areas of regeneration or infiltration
- evidence of disease elsewhere, in particular:
  —spleen size and presence of focal splenic lesions
  —reflectivity and size of kidneys.

The bright liver

Increase in the echogenicity of the liver parenchyma and hepatomegaly is seen in many conditions affecting the liver. Figure 5.12 shows the bright sonographic appearance of the liver in a patient with acute lymphatic leukemia.

Fatty infiltration

Fatty infiltration is the result of the accumulation of fat in the hepatocytes (liver cells) and produces an appearance of increased reflectivity of the liver parenchyma and poor ultrasound penetration. It is generally a sign of injury. In children it is related to early cirrhosis, hyperalimentation and any insult to the liver which may alter the metabolism. Fatty infiltration is also seen after chemotherapy and steroid therapy, in malnutrition, obesity, and cystic fibrosis most commonly. Metabolic conditions

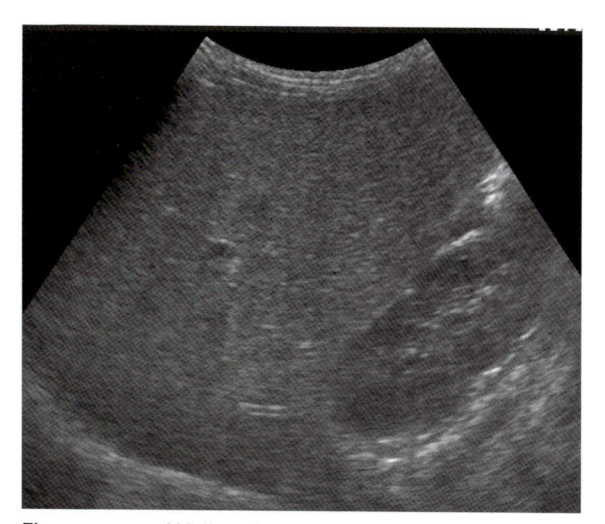

Figure 5.12 ALL liver. This patient had acute lymphatic leukemia (ALL) and presented clinically with anemia and a large liver and spleen. On ultrasound examination the liver was enlarged with a global increase in parenchymal echogenicity. This appearance is also seen in the spleen in leukemia.

such as tyrosinemia, Wilson disease and glycogen storage disease type I also cause fatty livers.

On ultrasound, fatty infiltration should be suspected when the liver appears large and hyperechoic with loss of the normally reflective walls of the portal venous system. Also normal contrast between the liver and the right kidney may be lost so that the unsuspecting sonographer may suspect the gain settings are incorrect and change to a lower frequency probe. Appearances of fatty infiltration are variable, dependent on the amount of fat. Glycogen storage disease, a condition in which glycogen is stored within the liver, is not uncommonly encountered in children. It produces a large, echogenic liver. In these patients, in particular type I, adenomas, i.e. round hypoechoic lesions of varying sizes, must be sought.

In all children the kidneys must be evaluated and in particular measured as they may appear normal but enlarged. In tyrosinemia nephrocalcinosis may occur.

Occasionally, fatty infiltration may be focal and anywhere in the liver (Fig. 5.13). It may be any size or shape and may be mistaken for a tumor.

Cirrhosis

Cirrhosis is the end stage of many forms of liver disease. It is defined pathologically as extensive fibrosis with regenerating nodules. It can occur in many conditions (Box 5.3) and is the liver's response to widespread damage of the parenchyma. It may be secondary to hepatocellular disease or to chronic bile duct obstruction (biliary cirrhosis). The main effects of cirrhosis are diminished hepatic function and portal hypertension with splenomegaly, varices and ascites. Hepatocellular carcinoma may develop. Children with compensated cirrhosis may be asymptomatic if liver function is adequate.

Ultrasound appearances In the acute process there may be fatty infiltration in which case the liver may be enlarged and echogenic. Later, fibrosis may be seen which also causes an echogenic liver but with a coarse texture (Fig. 5.14). Fibrosis occurs in bands throughout the liver and does not increase the beam attenuation as fatty infiltration does.

The liver eventually becomes small, with compensatory hypertrophy of other lobes, particularly the left and caudate lobes. The liver margins become irregular. The parenchyma becomes heterogeneous and there may be hypoechoic areas of the regenerating nodules. Because the liver becomes rigid and non-compliant the waveforms of the vessels both entering and leaving the liver undergo change.

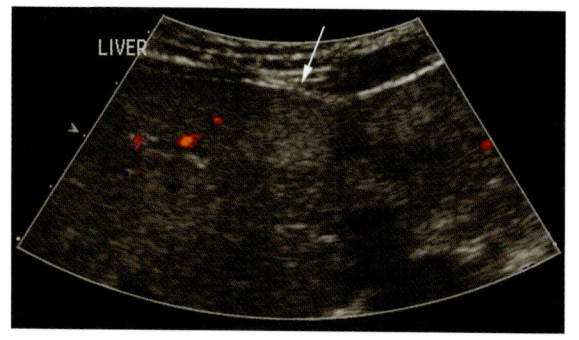

Figure 5.13 Focal fatty infiltration. Longitudinal sonogram of the right lobe of the liver showing a localized area of increased echogenicity (arrow). This was an incidental finding and considered to be a localized area of fatty infiltration in the liver.

150 PEDIATRIC ULTRASOUND

> **Box 5.3 Causes of cirrhosis and chronic liver disease in children**
>
> *Chronic hepatitis*
> Post-viral B, C
> Autoimmune hepatitis
> Drugs
> Inflammatory bowel disease
> Primary sclerosing cholangitis ± ulcerative colitis
> *Congenital forms*
> Cystic fibrosis
> Wilson disease (over 3 years): deposition of copper in the liver
> Tyrosinemia
> Alfa-1 antitrypsin deficiency
> Congenital hepatic fibrosis
> *Secondary to*
> Neonatal liver disease
> Bile duct abnormality such as Caroli syndrome

Portal hypertension

Blood from the portal system may not be able to enter or leave the liver. This may be due to prehepatic, intrahepatic or suprahepatic causes. The effect of this is for pressure to build up in the portal venous system so that there is back pressure on the spleen. In addition, because the blood cannot pass through the liver back to the heart, the back pressure results in opening up of collateral vessels. The ultimate result of this increased portal pressure is the development of varices and splenomegaly. The key to diagnosis on imaging lies in the demonstration of splenomegaly and, in particular, varices, i.e. the collateral circulation. Ascites may also be present. Ultrasound is always the first investigation and can give a large amount of information regarding the portal system.

Causes

- *Prehepatic*. Portal vein obstruction (Fig. 5.15) is one of the more common causes in children. In the neonate this may be due to umbilical vein

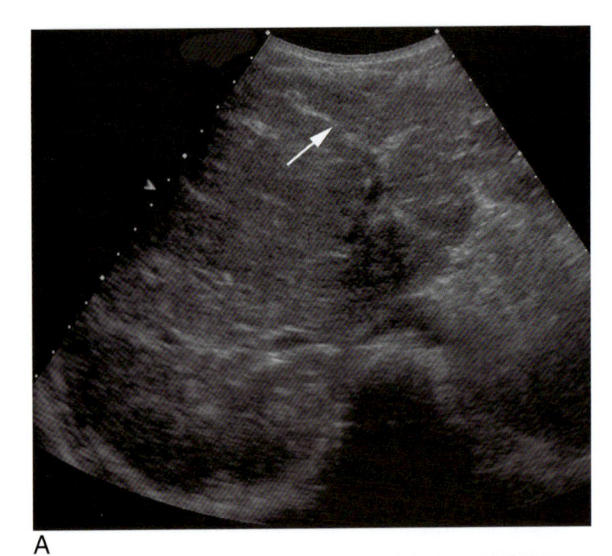

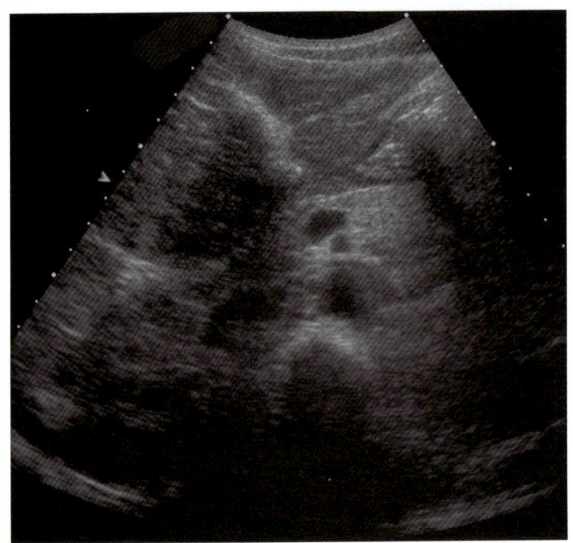

Figure 5.14 Cirrhosis. (A) Transverse sonogram of the liver in a child with longstanding cystic fibrosis. There are dense linear areas of fibrosis throughout the whole of the liver (arrow). In addition the outline of the liver margin is lobulated from regenerating nodules. (B) Transverse sonogram at the level of the pancreas. Once again the dense portal tracts are shown within the liver parenchyma from fibrosis. In addition there is a very echogenic pancreas which is a typical appearance found in cystic fibrosis.

catheterization or be idiopathic. Periumbilical infection tracking up the umbilical vein to the portal system, or appendicitis with infection tracking up the superior mesenteric vein, entering the portal vein and causing thrombosis, may all result in portal vein obstruction.
- *Intrahepatic.* Intrahepatic obstruction to the portal vein is generally caused by cirrhosis, which may be biliary, such as biliary atresia, or in inherited conditions such as tyrosinemia.
- *Suprahepatic.* This refers to conditions affecting the hepatic veins or the high IVC, such as veno-occlusive disease or Budd–Chiari syndrome.

The expected ultrasound findings will depend on the site of obstruction. There must be a careful evaluation of the portal vein (see below), which will be obstructed and difficult to visualize in prehepatic causes, and instead a portal cavernoma or cavernous transformation may be found in the porta hepatis (lots of little vessels in the porta hepatis rather than a main portal vein). The texture of the liver parenchyma must be carefully evaluated and the hepatic veins and IVC always visualized and commented on. If cirrhosis is found, many causes are associated with renal tract changes as mentioned previously.

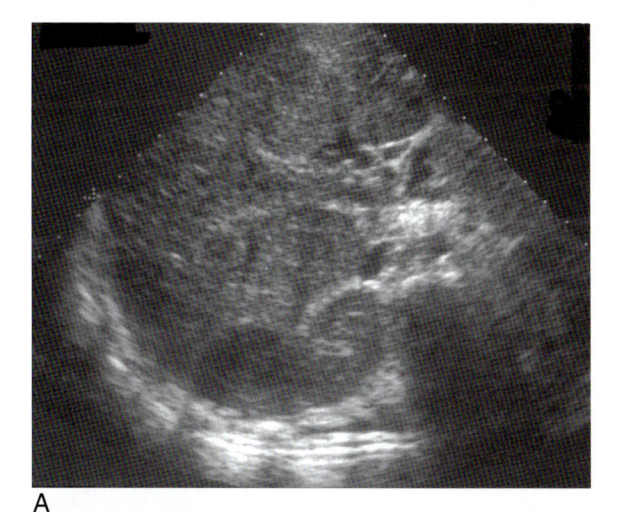

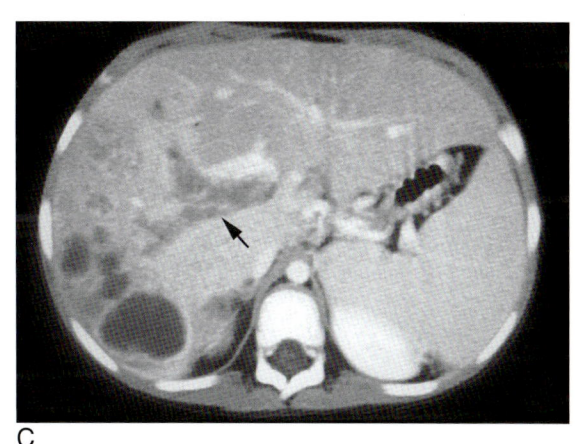

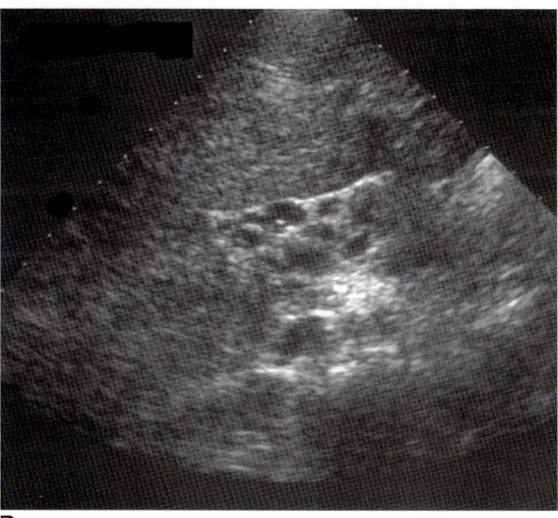

Figure 5.15 Portal vein occlusion and liver abscess. (A) Transverse sonogram of the liver in a girl presenting with a history of appendicitis. The portal vein is difficult to see and there are multiple additional vessels in the liver hilum. In addition there is a cystic area posteriorly in the right lobe of the liver next to the kidney. (B) Transverse sonogram of the liver hilum showing multiple vessels within the liver hilum and no portal flow visible. (C) Contrast-enhanced CT examination at the level of the liver hilum. The portal vein has not fully opacified with contrast, and there appear to be multiple filling defects within the portal vein (arrow). In addition there are multiple cystic lesions posteriorly in the right lobe with edge enhancement. This girl had had appendicitis with an ascending infection in the superior mesenteric vein which went on to involve the portal vein. She had further developed liver abscesses. This is a well-known complication of appendicitis.

The portal vein

Patency of the portal vein must be established with good color flow Doppler imaging. Portal flow may be damped, in which case there is lack of the normal respiratory variation. There may be reversal of flow and there may be forward and reverse flow in the portal vein. Thrombosis of the portal vein is occasionally seen. This becomes particularly obvious when no normal portal vein can be identified entering the liver but instead a number of small collateral vessels in the porta hepatis can be identified. This network of collateral vessels in the porta hepatis is called cavernous transformation.

Cavernous transformation of the portal vein consists of multiple venous channels around an occluded or stenosed portal vein. They act as periportal collaterals. Cavernous transformation can occur very soon after the portal vein thrombosis and has been reported from 1–3 weeks after the event. These veins are usually not enough to bypass the flow of blood from the spleen and gut to the liver, so other signs of portal hypertension are usually present.

When the pressure in the portal vein is consistently high, collateral channels may open up to divert the blood flow. At least twenty pathways or channels have been described, but the following are the commonest and most easily identified using ultrasound.

Paraesophageal and gastric varices These are the most frequent and easily detectable varices, and this is one of the major areas to look for abnormal vessels. Longitudinal scanning just to the left of the aorta will demonstrate the gastroesophageal junction, and color flow Doppler will show significant varices in this region on the lower surface of the liver and around the lower esophagus. Some are embedded in the esophageal wall but others are outside the wall. These are the ones that cause bleeding and are seen at endoscopy.

Splenorenal collaterals Collateral vessels developing around the spleen from the splenic hilum and draining into the left renal vein are fairly common. These are desirable shunts as they decompress the portal system without the patient bleeding. Features to look for are additional vessels between the spleen and left kidney as well as a large left renal vein from the shunting of the blood.

Paraumbilical collaterals Umbilical collaterals are not commonly seen in children and are generally found in those with hepatic causes (such as cirrhosis) of portal hypertension. They arise from the left portal vein and flow towards the umbilicus. They drain through the epigastric veins into the external iliacs. They form the caput medusae, which are varicose dilations around the umbilicus.

Other signs to look for include thickening of the lesser omentum. This should be examined longitudinally at the level of the aorta. Normally at the level of the origin of the celiac axis the extent of the lesser omentum (that is the distance from the celiac axis to the undersurface of the liver) measures one and a half times the aortic diameter. When there are collateral vessels in the omentum the measure is enlarged. A measurement in excess of 1.7 is considered to be abnormal.

Arterioportal shunts These are shunts between the hepatic artery and the portal venous system and they may be large or small. Causes include vascular malformations, trauma after liver biopsy and liver neoplasms. These fistulas may be large and cause portal hypertension and high output heart failure.

Budd–Chiari syndrome

Budd–Chiari syndrome is extremely rare in children and is caused by an obstruction in the upper IVC or hepatic veins. In most children no underlying cause is found. They may present with hepatomegaly and/or ascites. Ultrasound will show thin, attenuated hepatic veins with inverted flow. Sonography of the upper IVC may be difficult because of hepatomegaly and ascites and is less reliable for this area.

Hepatitis

Viral hepatitis

The clinical features of viral hepatitis include nausea, vomiting, abdominal pain, lethargy and jaundice. A large tender liver is common, and 30% will have splenomegaly; 30–50% of infected children do not develop jaundice.

Hepatitis, as the name implies, is the diffuse inflammation of the liver parenchyma. The most common causes are hepatitis A, B, C, D or E.

Hepatitis A This is a RNA virus which is spread by feco-oral transmission. The incidence in childhood has fallen as socioeconomic conditions have improved. The disease is mild and in some asymptomatic.

Hepatitis B Hepatitis B is a DNA virus which is an important cause of acute and chronic liver disease worldwide, with the highest incidence in subSaharan Africa and the Far East. The disease is spread by numerous routes, perinatally from the mother, horizontally in families, by blood transfusions, biting insects and by renal dialysis. The majority who contract hepatitis will recover, 2% develop fulminant hepatic failure and 10% become chronic carriers.

Chronic hepatitis B Infants infected from their mothers usually become asymptomatic carriers. About 30–50% will develop chronic liver disease which may progress to cirrhosis. There is a long-term risk of hepatocellular carcinoma.

Hepatitis C This is a RNA virus and the type associated with blood transfusions. It is also high in drug users. At least 50% develop chronic liver disease with cirrhosis and hepatocellular carcinoma in a number of years.

Other causes

Other causes of acute hepatitis are:
- cytomegalovirus
- herpes viruses
- Epstein–Barr virus
- chemotherapy or drugs ingested or inhaled
- glandular fever
- immunocompromise, e.g. in patients with AIDS. Children are particularly vulnerable.

Ultrasound appearances

In acute hepatitis the liver may be acutely enlarged with a hypoechoic appearance due to the edematous cells. Portal tracts may appear more prominent.

In chronic hepatitis the liver may become small and will have the same appearances as cirrhosis. Changes are seen in the gallbladder, with a thick edematous wall and sludge or stones.

Veno-occlusive disease

Veno-occlusive disease, as the name implies, is a partial or complete occlusion of the small hepatic veins, usually sparing the larger veins, which effectively blocks the flow of blood through the liver. It is most commonly seen in children following bone marrow transplantation but may also be seen, very rarely, after radiation or chemotherapy.

The name Budd–Chiari syndrome is often used synonymously, but in the latter syndrome the association is with hypercoagulable states or a vena cava web. Both produce similar appearances but should be differentiated for treatment purposes.

The diagnosis is not an easy one for ultrasound but features to look for are ascites, a thick-walled gallbladder, abnormal flow in the portal vein. In extensive and severe veno-occlusive disease, the portal blood flow will be towards the spleen, with reversal in the Doppler trace. The hepatic veins may be seen but will be thin and attenuated.

Causes

Causes include the following:
- congenital web in the IVC
- any condition causing polycythemia and thus thickening of the blood; coagulation disorders such as sickle cell anemia and systemic lupus erythematosus
- malignancy—liver tumor or other tumors invading the IVC or hepatic veins, e.g. Wilms
- chemotherapy for bone marrow transplantation.

The etiology may not be found in a significant number of patients.

The occlusive process usually starts in the liver and the intrahepatic venules, extending out towards the larger veins. The larger hepatic veins entering the IVC may still be patent and visualized on ultrasound, which sometimes confuses the sonographer.

Ultrasound appearances

Ultrasound features to look for are:

- a large liver and ascites with a normal size spleen in the early stages
- filling defects or thrombi in the hepatic veins
- enlargement of the caudate lobe, which has a striking appearance because of its different blood supply and venous drainage.

Pressure may build up in the liver so that collaterals are seen around the porta hepatis. As the condition progresses the liver gets smaller and the hepatic veins may be difficult or impossible to see. The spleen will progressively enlarge. The IVC must be carefully examined to look for a web. Ascites and thickening of the gallbladder may be visualized. Doppler examination of the flow in the vessels is necessary.

Hepatic veins The veins may be completely or partially occluded, and the waveform may appear flattened because of the non-compliance of the liver. However, a large liver may also compress the hepatic veins and attenuate them, making them difficult to see. Portal flow may be reversed in the acute phase but is a difficult and not entirely reliable appearance to detect on ultrasound.

Cystic fibrosis

Cystic fibrosis (CF) is the commonest cause of suppurative lung disease in Caucasians, and in the past it led to an early death by respiratory failure. It is inherited as an autosomal recessive trait with approximately 1 in 2500 affected at birth.

In CF the abnormality is an abnormal ion transport across the epithelial cells in the exocrine glands of the respiratory tract and pancreas. This results in thick, viscous secretions. Abnormal function of the sweat glands results in excessive concentrations of sodium and chloride in the sweat. This forms the basis of the diagnostic 'sweat test'.

Most children with CF initially present with malabsorption and failure to thrive from birth with recurrent chest infections. About 10% present with meconium ileus in the neonatal period, which is thick inspissated meconium causing bowel obstruction. Over 90% have malabsorption and steatorrhea due to insufficiency of pancreatic enzymes, which leads to failure to thrive.

Cystic fibrosis liver disease is seen as the child gets older and survives the respiratory complications. Clinically it may be difficult to make the diagnosis, as the overinflated lungs will push the liver and spleen down, giving an erroneous impression of hepatosplenomegaly.

Ultrasound will show the coarse multilobular cirrhosis with diffuse or patchy increase in reflectivity. The margins of the liver may appear irregular as a result of the liver nodularity. The gallbladder may contain calculi, and the diagnostic appearance of an echogenic pancreas will be seen.[13] The sensitivity of ultrasound in this condition remains to be proven in those children without biochemical evidence of liver disease.

Hepatic manifestations range from hepatomegaly and diffuse fatty infiltration, through focal biliary cirrhosis, to generalized frank cirrhosis with fibrotic change, regenerating nodules and portal hypertension.

Increased periportal echogenicity on ultrasound is thought to be related to bile duct proliferation, inflammation, edema or fibrosis. Abnormalities of the bile ducts include irregularity and tapering of the intrahepatic biliary tree. The larger bile ducts may show strictures and beading. Strictures of the distal common bile duct have been reported.

Gallbladder abnormalities and in particular gallstones are well described. Micro-gallbladders containing gelatinous material or mucus with atresia or stenosis of the cystic duct may result from the inspissated bile (see Fig. 5.14).

Liver biopsy is considered to be the gold standard but percutaneous biopsy may miss patchy early lesions.

FOCAL LESIONS OF THE PEDIATRIC LIVER

Focal liver lesions may be benign or malignant.

Benign focal liver lesions

These comprise:

- cysts
- abscesses/candida/amebic
- hydatid disease

- hematomas
- mesenchymal hamartomas
- hemangiomas.

Cysts

Pure, simple cysts in childhood are quite rare. They may be single or multiple and are well-defined and anechoic. Cysts may be at the end stage of a liver hematoma or an abscess, but these will have a thicker wall, often with internal echoes.

Liver cysts may be a feature of congenital conditions such as autosomal dominant polycystic kidney disease, but these are rarely seen in childhood. The cystic lesions seen in autosomal recessive polycystic kidney disease are in fact circular outpouchings of the bile duct. All children with apparent cystic lesions of the liver should have the kidneys carefully examined.

Abscesses

Pyogenic abscesses Pyogenic abscesses in children are occasionally encountered and generally they cannot be differentiated from any other conditions causing central necrosis and breakdown, such as a hematoma. Clinical history is of the utmost importance when trying to come to a diagnosis. Causes of pyogenic abscesses in children are different from those in adults and usually entail bloodborne bacteria from generalized sepsis or appendicitis. Local infection around the umbilicus or from umbilical vessel catheterization may also spread to the liver.

Children with depressed immunity, either from chemotherapy, transplantation, AIDS or chronic granulomatous disease, are particularly vulnerable to developing liver abscesses.

Ultrasound may demonstrate either single or multiple abscess cavities, usually with a thick wall or mixed internal echoes. There may be gas present within the abscess.

Abscesses are most commonly seen in the posterior part of the right lobe, possibly because of the portal venous flow. Fine needle aspiration and drainage is necessary to establish the diagnosis and organism.

Candida abscesses These should be particularly sought in children with known immunodeficient states. They may be multiple and small and scattered throughout the liver parenchyma. They have a number of ultrasound appearances:

- a small echo-free lesion
- a bulls-eye lesion
- a target lesion.

It must be remembered that these are different to other abscesses in that they are very small and multiple and very easy to miss on ultrasound. It is essential to perform a very careful examination of the liver parenchyma using a high frequency linear probe when this diagnosis is suspected (Fig. 5.16).

Amebic abscess This is a parasitic infection more commonly seen in the tropics. Ultrasonically the appearances are indistinguishable from other liver abscesses, with varying degrees of wall thickness and internal contents. Typically, however, on aspiration the contents are described as being 'anchovy paste'. Suspicion should be raised when there are reactive changes at the right base of the lung.

Hydatid liver disease

Hydatid liver disease is seen primarily in patients of Middle Eastern origin and also in the USA. It occurs from the larval stage of the tapeworm. They are spread to humans who eat infected cattle or sheep. Hydatid disease in the liver is bloodborne, and the hydatid abscess may be a single cyst or multiple cysts.

Ultrasound appearances The diagnosis should be suspected on the basis of the appearance of the capsule, which may be thickened and ultimately produce the 'floating lily' appearance. Daughter cysts may be evident arising from the internal capsule. Old hydatids may have a thin, calcified rim.

Chronic granulomatous disease

Chronic granulomatous disease is a recessive disorder where patients mount an inappropriate response to infection. Typically they may have small focal abscesses in the liver and spleen and also develop other signs such as thickening of the gastric antral wall and urinary bladder which produces a picture similar to that of pseudotumoral cystitis.

156 PEDIATRIC ULTRASOUND

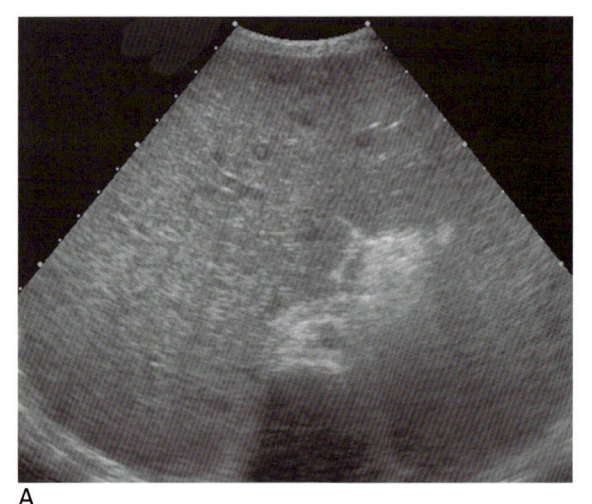

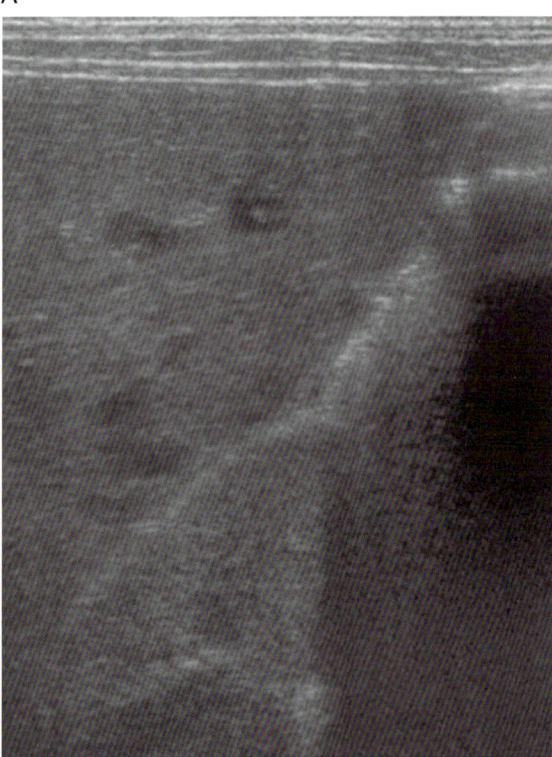

Figure 5.16 Candida of the liver. (A) Transverse sonogram of the liver using a curvilinear probe. Small hypoechoic foci can be seen within the liver but these can be easily missed if a linear probe is not used. (B) Examination of the liver using a linear probe, showing that the bullseye lesions are much easier to see and better identified using a linear probe.

These appearances basically result from an inability of the white cells to destroy bacteria. They may also have infections in the lungs, bones and lymph nodes (see Fig. 6.7).

Hematoma

Hematoma of the liver should be suspected in the correct clinical context. The ultrasound appearances depend on whether the trauma is recent or old. When the trauma is recent, the hematoma is fresh and may appear solid and echogenic. As the central area necroses, the hematoma becomes more cystic and can liquefy.

Ultrasound monitoring of the resolution of the hematoma may be all that is needed in a child that is not actively bleeding.

Angiomatous lesions

Angiomatous lesions are some of the common benign hepatic neoplasms in children, although the vast majority occur in the neonatal period and have been discussed earlier. Doppler examination is essential in all focal lesions suspected of being vascular, with particular emphasis on the vessels supplying and draining the mass lesion.

Mesenchymal hamartoma

This is usually found in children under 2 years of age and most commonly presents with a painless abdominal mass.[14–16] It is slightly more common in males. It arises from the mesenchyme of the periportal tract and accounts for 8% of hepatic tumors in childhood. The tumor is considered to be more a developmental anomaly consisting of a mixture of bile ducts, hepatocytes, vessels and mesenchyme without lymphatic vessels. Fluid accumulates in the mesenchymal tissue, and this results in cystic tumor growth.

Ultrasound appearances There are two growth patterns for these tumors: one predominantly cystic and the other predominantly stromal. The masses are usually well defined, containing multiple cystic spaces of varying sizes with more solid-looking septations. They most commonly occur in the right lobe and are generally very large.

The appearances in mesenchymal hematoma are quite variable, ranging from large cystic spaces to smaller cystic spaces. Appearances on CT are similar but in addition will show enhancement of the more solid areas with contrast. Complete surgical removal is curative.

Calcification in the liver

Calcification is relatively uncommon in the liver but when it is present it may produce some specific appearances which may be diagnostic. The following are the more common causes of hepatic calcification in children:

- infection
- granulomas particularly TB, brucellosis, histoplasmosis and coccidioidomycosis
- cytomegalovirus
- toxoplasmosis
- *Pneumocystis carinii*
- hydatid disease
- chronic granulomatous disease of childhood
- benign tumors—hemangioma or hemangioendothelioma
- malignant tumors—all malignant tumors may calcify, and 'sunburst' calcification is typically seen in hepatoblastoma
- trauma
- vascular calcification
- gallbladder and biliary calculi.

Liver tumors

After Wilms and neuroblastomas, liver tumors are the next commonest tumors seen and constitute 5% of childhood tumors. Hepatoblastomas tend to occur under the age of 3 years and hepatocellular carcinomas over that age.

Two thirds of pediatric liver tumors are malignant. Almost all liver tumors present with an abdominal mass. The role of ultrasound is primarily to establish the hepatic origin of the mass, which will then guide further cross sectional imaging.[17]

Hepatoblastoma

Hepatoblastoma is the most common primary liver tumor, accounting for up to 48% of all malignant pediatric liver tumors. The tumor arises from fetal hepatocytes. The average age at diagnosis is 18 months, ranging from birth to 3 years. They are more common in females. Presentation is with a large abdominal mass, hepatomegaly, occasionally with symptoms of an acute abdomen. Alfa-fetoprotein is elevated in 90%. There is a known association with other metabolic effects such as osteopenia and bone fractures, hypoglycemia or hypercholesterolemia. The prognosis is generally poor and dependent on the extent of liver involvement and whether the tumor is ultimately resectable.

Ultrasound appearances Ultrasonically the appearances are variable but generally they are well-defined and solid (Fig. 5.17). There may be calcification with echogenic foci or cystic areas due to necrosis. The major blood vessels, in particular the portal system, should be examined for 'cut off', and the tumor may invade the hepatic veins and IVC. On Doppler examination the tumors are generally very vascular. This appearance is also seen on angiography, which also reveals the hypervascular nature of the tumor, occasionally with a spoke-wheel pattern. Malignant neovascularization and invasion or encasement of the portal vein or hepatic artery can be seen.[18]

Hepatocellular carcinoma

Hepatocellular carcinoma (HCC) accounts for up to 20% of primary pediatric liver tumors. Histologically the appearances are similar to those of the adult type. Conditions known to be associated with and predisposing to HCC are biliary atresia, glycogen storage disease type I, hereditary tyrosinemia, hyperalimentation, hepatitis B virus infection and familial cholestasis. HCC occurs in older children, generally in the 10–12 year age range, and they present with tender hepatomegaly, jaundice, anorexia and abdominal pain due to hemoperitoneum. Serum alfa-fetoprotein levels are markedly elevated.

Ultrasound appearances The tumor shows variable patterns. It may be:

- multifocal or multinodular

158 PEDIATRIC ULTRASOUND

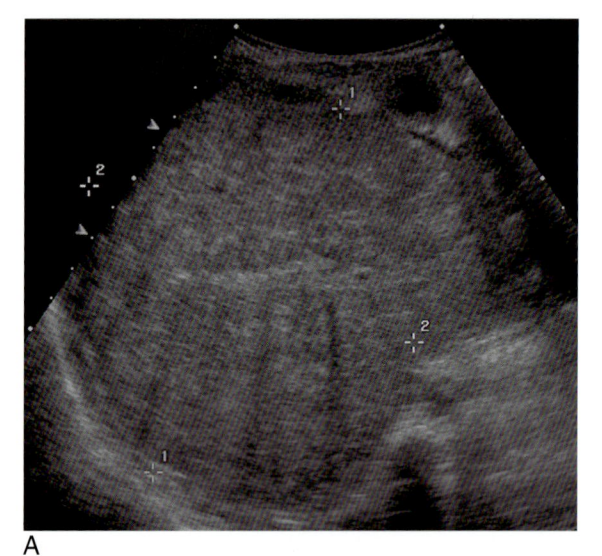

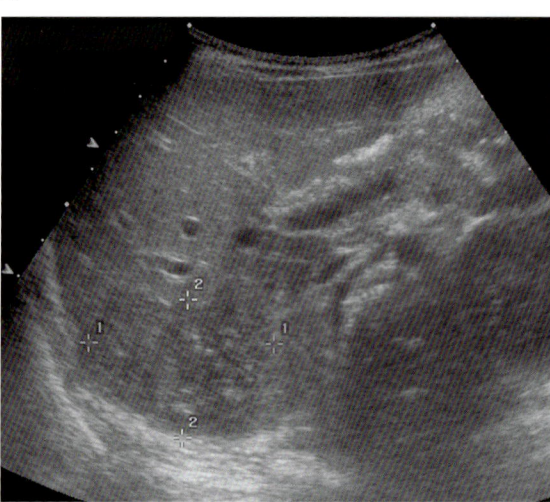

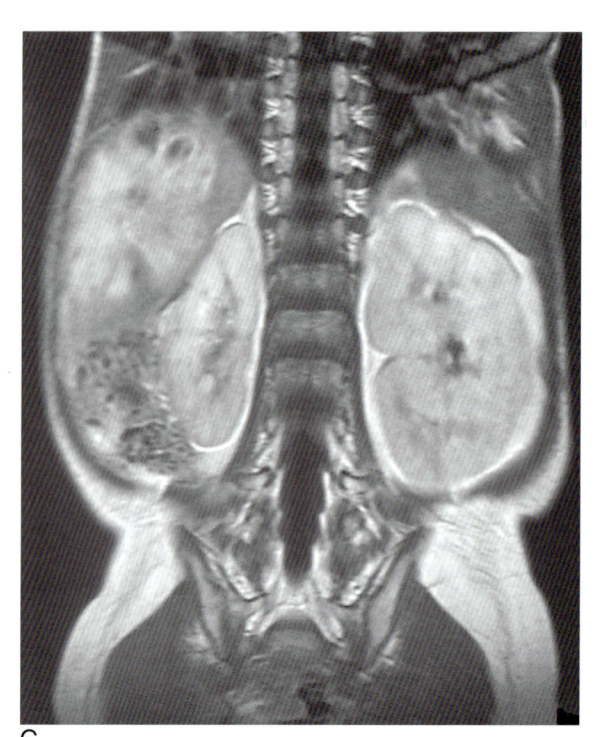

Figure 5.17 Hepatoblastoma in Beckwith–Wiedemann syndrome. (A) Transverse sonogram of the liver showing a large heterogeneous mass occupying most of the right lobe of the liver (between calipers). (B) Transverse sonogram of the liver 3 months later showing the marked reduction in size of the hepatoblastoma after treatment. It is heterogeneous and solid (between calipers). (C) MRI scan on the same child showing the abnormal area in the right lobe of the liver. There is also quite marked asymmetry in the size of the kidneys. This is due to the organomegaly in Beckwith–Wiedemann syndrome.

- solitary and extremely large
- diffuse, involving the whole liver.

The tumor cells resemble normal hepatocytes, and that is why differentiation from normal liver can be difficult. Central necrosis of the mass may result in cystic change.

On ultrasound the appearances are predominantly hypo- or isoechoic, sometimes with a thin halo representing the capsule. In diffuse HCC the appearances are subtle with just a generalized heterogeneity and disruption of the normal echo pattern.

Undifferentiated embryonal sarcoma

This is an uncommon malignant liver tumor and in the majority of cases occurs in older children and teenagers with no sex predilection. They represent 5% of pediatric liver tumors and have a number of other names such as malignant mesenchymoma or fibromyxosarcoma.

Clinical presentation, as for other liver tumors, is with an abdominal mass, with fever, jaundice and weight loss. Typically the serum alfa-fetoprotein levels are normal. The tumor consists of undifferentiated spindle cells.

The ultrasound appearances are variable from a solid mass with areas of dense calcification causing acoustic shadows to a multiseptated cystic mass. There are frequently cystic areas due to hemorrhage and necrosis. Angiographically the tumors are generally hypervascular.

Adenomas

Adenomas of the liver are rare in children. The condition with which they are most commonly associated is glycogen storage disease, particularly type I, and glucose-6-phosphatase deficiency. They may also occur in children with aplastic anemia treated with androgenic steroids. They have been reported in association with Fanconi anemia and galactosemia but are rare.

Ultrasound appearances may be a solitary, hypoechoic lesion, but may also have an isoechoic appearance.

Focal nodular hyperplasia

Focal nodular hyperplasia (FNH) is a primary liver tumor without an anatomic capsule. It comprises hyperplastic regenerating nodules divided by fibrous septae which contain hepatocytes, sinusoids and Kupffer cells. A characteristic feature of focal nodular hyperplasia is a central stellate scar from which radiate proliferating bile ducts and blood vessels (Fig. 5.18).

FNH most commonly occurs in women but has been reported in all pediatric age groups. These tumors are generally detected incidentally and on ultrasound are a single well-defined mass. Nodules may be more echogenic, less echogenic or isoechoic compared with the surrounding liver. A halo is seen in half of cases. Occasionally they may be pedunculated and hang off the edge of the liver. The mass is hypervascular.

The visibility of the mass can be improved by using harmonic imaging, and good results have been reported when using ultrasound contrast agents in adults.

The cause is unknown, but estrogen acts as a growth promoter, so that there is increased growth at puberty or when taking contraceptive drugs.

Once a diagnosis has been established, management is conservative. Regular follow-up with ultrasound is usually all that is needed.

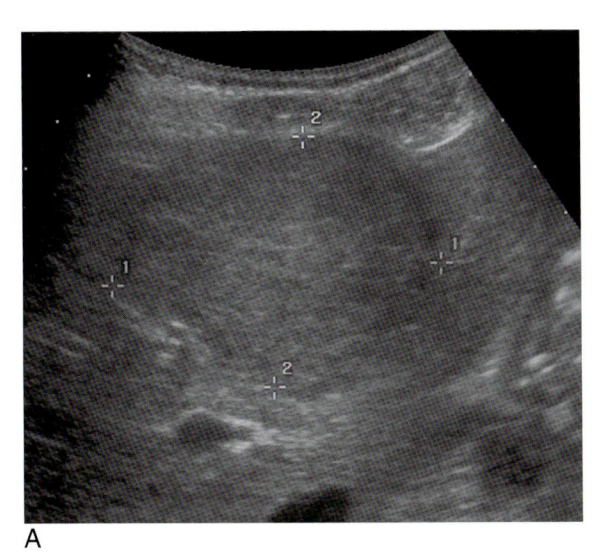

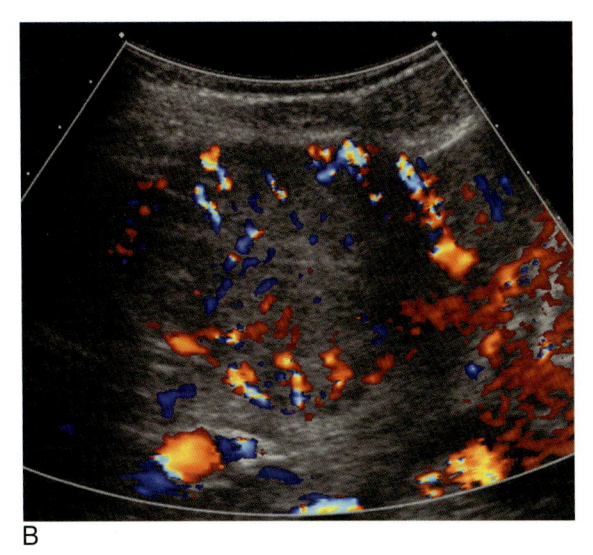

Figure 5.18 Focal nodular hyperplasia (FNH). (A) Longitudinal sonogram of the liver in an adolescent girl who was being scanned for a renal tract abnormality. This shows a well-defined solid mass with a central stellate scar typical of FNH (between calipers). FNH is thought to be related to estrogen, and this benign tumor grew as the girl went through puberty. (B) Color Doppler on the intrahepatic mass shows the stellate array of vessels around the central scar.

Secondary deposits

Metastatic disease of the liver is actually relatively rare with new treatment regimens. Tumors that typically metastasize to the liver are: Wilms Stage IV, neuroblastoma, rhabdomyosarcoma, lymphomas and teratomas.

On ultrasound, most metastases are hypoechoic. The most hypoechoic of all is hepatic lymphoma.

ABNORMALITIES OF THE GALLBLADDER AND BILE DUCTS IN CHILDHOOD

Conditions affecting the gallbladder and biliary tree are relatively rare in childhood, unlike in adults. However, there are a few conditions specific to childhood that the sonographer needs to recognize—such as the choledochal cyst and Caroli syndrome, which are described earlier in the chapter. These conditions are particularly those which dilate the biliary tree.

Cholecystitis

Inflammation of the gallbladder, or cholecystitis, may be acute or chronic. It is usually seen in association with gallstones and is a result of a superinfection of the gallbladder wall with enteric bacteria.

The sonographer must be familiar with the wide range of acute and chronic inflammatory changes seen in the gallbladder in the adult. While relatively rare in pediatrics they do occur and must be recognized.

Thickening of the gallbladder wall may be seen in a number of other conditions such as ascites due to liver, heart or kidney failure, veno-occlusive disease, localized peritonitis and sepsis, pancreatitis, hepatitis, cholangitis, leukemia and varices (Table 5.3).

Gallstones

Gallstones are more frequently recognized in children with the widespread use of abdominal ultrasound. Many are incidental findings. Cholelithiasis is not generally a problem of childhood but, when

Table 5.3 Ultrasound diagnosis of cholecystitis

Type	Ultrasound features
Acute cholecystitis (focal GB tenderness—Murphy's sign)	Presence of gallstones Symmetrical thickened GB wall > 2 mm Echo-poor halo around GB Hyperemia of GB wall on color Doppler Pericholecystic abscess Perforation and peritonitis
Chronic cholecystitis	Presence of gallstones Shrunken contracted GB Hyperechoic, irregular thick-walled GB
Gallbladder empyema (obstructed cystic duct and infected GB; acutely ill patient)	Low level echoes in bile (pus)
Gangrenous cholecystitis	Complication of acute cholecystitis Necrotic GB wall with abscesses Asymmetric GB wall thickening Sloughed mucosa with intraluminal membrane Pericholecystic collection Perforation and peritonitis
Emphysematous cholecystitis (infection with gas-forming organisms)	Gas in the GB and GB wall Hyperechoic foci with acoustic shadows and reverberations

GB, gallbladder.

found, can display all the features seen in the adult. If symptomatic, children present with right upper quadrant pain and episodes of obstructive jaundice.

Far more commonly seen in children is gallbladder 'sludge' where the gallbladder is filled with echogenic material not casting an acoustic shadow.

Ultrasound is the imaging modality of choice, and no further techniques are generally used.

Causes of gallstones in children
These include:

- hemolytic anemia, particularly sickle cell anemia, thalassemia and spherocytosis; these are pigment stones and are multiple and small (see Fig. 5.23A)
- cystic fibrosis, causing 'sticky bile'
- ileal disorders such as Crohn disease
- total parenteral nutrition
- frusemide therapy
- obstruction to the biliary tree, such as choledochal cysts, predisposing to stasis and stone formation
- Wilson disease.

Sludge in the gallbladder

Sludge in the gallbladder refers to echogenic matter within the bile which does not cast an acoustic shadow (Fig. 5.19). It may coalesce to form balls and, like biliary calculi, will be mobile. When it forms clumps it is called tumefactive biliary sludge.

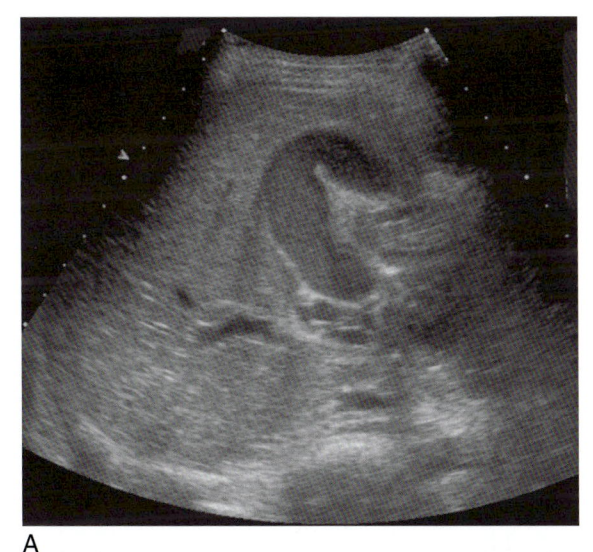

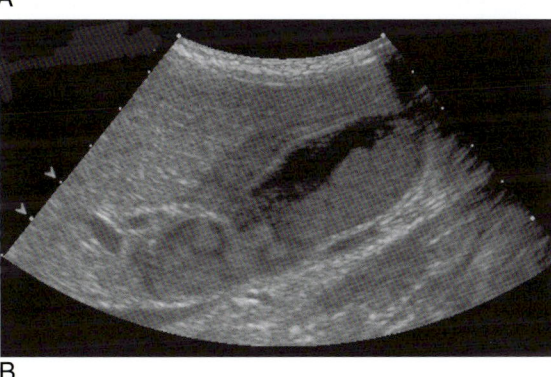

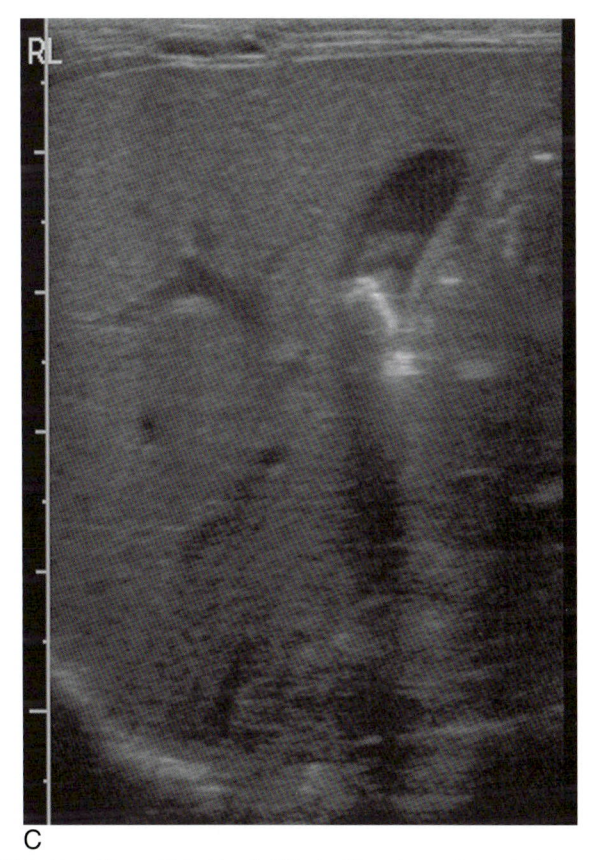

Figure 5.19 Gallstones. (A) Transverse sonogram of the gallbladder. The gallbladder is filled with echogenic material called biliary sludge. This is most commonly seen in bile stasis. This child had been extremely ill and was not eating. (B) Longitudinal sonogram of the gallbladder, which is filled with tumefactive biliary sludge (meaning that the sludge has coalesced). (C) Longitudinal sonogram of the gallbladder with a gallstone in the gallbladder neck. Gallstones are often incidental findings in children. This patient had been treated with total parenteral nutrition as a neonate.

Biliary sludge is caused by stasis of bile, most commonly seen in children who have been extremely ill and are not eating or treated with total parenteral nutrition. Other causes include an obstructed biliary tree and gallbladder.

Blood in the bile, or hemobilia, or infection such as candida, will also produce low level echoes in the bile indistinguishable from those of true biliary sludge.

Hydrops of the gallbladder

Hydrops of the gallbladder is a rare condition where there is massive dilation of the gallbladder without any obstruction to the cystic duct. It is most commonly seen in Kawasaki disease but other conditions may also cause this, such as scarlet fever, typhoid (salmonella and shigella), leptospirosis, extensive burning, sepsis and prolonged total parenteral nutrition.

Ultrasound appearances demonstrate a very large dilated gallbladder with a normal wall and no bile duct dilation. Generally the gallbladder contents are anechoic, but sometimes sludge may be present. Hydrops usually resolves with treatment of the underlying cause, generally within 1–2 weeks. Surgery is generally not indicated.

Rhabdomyosarcoma of the bile duct

This is a rare condition but is one of the malignancies seen in childhood. Children present with obstructive jaundice

Ultrasound appearances demonstrate intraluminal defects within the biliary system around the porta hepatis, with resultant intrahepatic duct dilation from the obstruction.

LIVER TRANSPLANTATION

Liver transplantation in children has had remarkable success in recent years. The indication for transplant is still primarily that of cirrhosis, and the pediatric causes include biliary atresia, alfa–1 antitripsin deficiency, both fulminant and chronic hepatitis, glycogen storage disease type I, metabolic disorders and tyrosinemia. Transplantation is carried out in specialist centers in the UK.

Liver transplantation requires a huge input of resources in the radiology department both pre- and post-transplantation.

Preoperative assessment

The role of ultrasound pre-transplant is to document the known pathology of the liver and assess the associated abnormalities such as portal hypertension. The pre-transplant ultrasound therefore includes a full evaluation of the abdomen. In addition the major vasculature related to the liver that will be involved in transplantation needs to be carefully documented. Assessment involves the following.

- The patency of the inferior vena cava needs to be demonstrated. Congenital anomalies are much higher in these children, in particular those with biliary atresia, and abnormalities such as polysplenia, situs inversus, left IVC and azygous continuation, preduodenal portal vein, and anomalies of the celiac and superior mesenteric artery supplying the liver all need to be documented.
- The portal vein needs to be identified as being patent and of a good caliber. A portal vein which is not seen or is less than 4 mm diameter needs further investigation. End stage liver disease and decompression from bleeding varices may be associated with a smaller portal vein.
- The hepatic artery should be evaluated, in particular for congenital anomalies and anomalous supply to the liver.

In essence the ultrasound examination needs to evaluate all the major vasculature which will be required for successful transplantation.

Arteriography is indicated when the portal vein is small or cannot be identified. Cavography is performed when the IVC is thrombosed or anomalous.

In addition to pre-transplant evaluation with ultrasound, patients will require evaluation of their heart and lungs and an assessment of their bone mineral density, which is often impaired in liver disease.

Postoperative assessment

Ultrasound is the examination of choice in the postoperative assessment of the liver transplant.

The major problems that can occur post-transplantation are related to the vessels and their anastomoses:

- Hepatic artery thrombosis is one of the more common complications in pediatric patients, and its exclusion relies on ultrasound and color Doppler to demonstrate flow in the artery and liver. If suspected on ultrasound the patient will need to have an arteriogram to confirm the findings. Other vascular complications of the hepatic artery include anastomotic leaks.
- Portal vein thrombosis is not as common as hepatic artery thrombosis. Stenoses can also occur at the anastomotic sites and, if present in the portal vein, portal hypertension will appear.
- Biliary complications are common and primarily related to hepatic artery blood supply. Within the liver transplant the biliary system is supplied only by the hepatic artery, and if a problem occurs with the artery then the bile ducts are vulnerable. Necrosis of the bile ducts with bile leakage can result. As in the blood vessels, anastomotic stenosis also occurs.
- Rejection can be a difficult diagnosis to make, and the diagnosis is usually reliant on a liver biopsy. An ultrasound-guided biopsy can be performed.

Other complications include infection with abscess formation and collections, pleural effusions, ascites and bile collections.

SUMMARY

Ultrasound is an excellent screening and monitoring modality for the liver and biliary tree in children. The vessels supplying and draining the liver are intimately related to the pathology, so that Doppler techniques are particularly important to perfect. Table 5.4 summarizes liver investigations in children.

SPLEEN

The spleen is an often forgotten organ that should not be overlooked when examining the intra-abdominal contents. The spleen may be involved most commonly as part of a multiorgan systemic illness or it may be part of an isolated process.

Development of the spleen

The spleen, a large, vascular and lymphatic organ, begins to develop early in fetal life. It develops from the mesenchyme of the dorsal mesogastrium. These mesenchymal cells differentiate to form the capsule, parenchyma of the spleen, and the connective tissue. As the stomach rotates, the left surface of the mesogastrium fuses with the peritoneum over the left kidney. This is why the dorsal attachment of the spleen is the splenorenal ligament and why the splenic artery follows a tortuous course anterior to the left kidney.

The lobulated appearance of the spleen can be identified by the third gestational month. The spleen consists of red and white pulp. The white pulp consists of the lymphoid follicles and the reticuloendothelial system, while the red pulp consists of the vascular sinuses. With age and increasing antigen stimulation the red pulp increases.

THE NORMAL SPLEEN

The spleen has a homogeneous echo texture similar to that of the liver and, when compared with the left kidney, is slightly more echogenic than the renal cortex. The red and white pulp cannot be differentiated on ultrasound. The normal spleen has rounded margins, and within the splenic hilum one can follow the splenic artery and the splenic vein. Normal charts are available for spleen size, and this should be measured for every abdominal examination.

A curvilinear transducer is best in most children, and the frequency will depend on the age and size of the child. The normal spleen can be satisfactorily examined in the supine position but often, if there is a large amount of bowel gas, the child will need to be examined in the right oblique position or even intercostally. A linear transducer is best for this and is essential when trying to delineate small splenic parenchymal lesions. Table 5.5 gives normal splenic size by age.[19]

Table 5.4 Liver investigations in children

Investigation	Description	Indication
Ultrasound and color Doppler ultrasound		Ideal screening modality for liver and biliary pathology
CT	Child may need sedation or general anesthesia Oral or intravenous contrast is required High radiation dose Motion artifacts degrade image	Mass lesions in the liver
MRI	No radiation dose Multiplanar image capability excellent for tissue contrast and vessels Major disadvantage is length of examination and image degradation by movement	Liver masses Parenchymal liver conditions
MR cholangiography (MRC)		Bile ducts
Radioisotope: 99mTc sulfur colloid imaging	Attaches to reticular endothelial system and produces an overall image of liver	Shows filling defects on scan but is non-specific
Radioisotope: 99mTc-labeled iminodiacetic acid (IDA)	Radionuclide which is excreted in the bile may reflect hepatic function and bile duct obstruction	Bile duct abnormalities, e.g. biliary atresia and choledochal cyst
Angiography	Vascular catheter insertion Invasive in children	Hepatic hemangiomas requiring treatment and embolization For visualization of the splenic vein in portal hypertension
Cholangiography: ERCP (endoscopic retrograde cholangiopancreatography)	Tube passed orally and pancreatic and common bile duct catheterized with retrograde injection of contrast	Suspected choledochal cysts and pancreatic duct delineation
Cholangiography: Operative cholangiogram	Contrast injected into gallbladder and biliary tree during surgery	Choledochal cyst, biliary atresia
Cholangiography: percutaneous transhepatic cholecystography	Percutaneous puncture of the biliary tree Can be done under ultrasound guidance	For delineation of the biliary tree

CONGENITAL VARIANTS

Accessory spleen

Accessory spleens are small nodules of splenic tissue which are found in addition to the main bulk of the spleen and are reportedly found in up to 30% of autopsies.[20] They arise from failure of the individual clumps of mesenchyme to fuse during the development of the spleen. They may be single and are most commonly found in the splenic hilum, or they may be multiple and located anywhere within the upper abdomen but particularly along the splenic vessels or within the omental layers. Due to the relationship of the development of the spleen, mesonephros and left gonad, splenic tissue may even be attached to the left ovary or within the scrotum. This is called splenogonadal fusion and is important as it may present as a mass related to the testis which may result in orchidectomy.[21]

Splenunculi (Fig. 5.20) vary in size from a few millimeters to a few centimeters and are similar in echogenicity to the splenic parenchyma. A blood supply can be demonstrated on Doppler. They may cause a diagnostic dilemma in that they are often mistaken for lymph nodes in the splenic hilum. If the spleen is removed, accessory splenic tissue can hypertrophy.

Table 5.5 Normal splenic size (in 230 infants and children)[19]

Age (number)	Length of spleen (cm)			
	10th percentile	Median	90th percentile	Suggested upper limit
0–3 months (n = 28)	3.3	4.5	5.8	6.0
3–6 months (n = 13)	4.9	5.3	6.4	6.5
6–12 months (n = 17)	5.2	6.2	6.8	7.0
1–2 years (n = 12)	5.4	6.9	7.5	8.0
2–4 years (n = 24)	6.4	7.4	8.6	9.0
4–6 years (n = 39)	6.9	7.8	8.8	9.5
6–8 years (n = 21)	7.0	8.2	9.6	10.0
8–10 years (n = 16)	7.9	9.2	10.5	11.0
10–12 years (n = 17)	8.6	9.9	10.9	11.5
12–15 years (n = 26)	8.7	10.1	11.4	12.0
15–20 years (n = 17)				
Female	9.0	10.0	11.7	12.0
Male	10.1	11.2	12.6	13.0

The wandering spleen

This refers to a spleen that is highly mobile and either on a long or even absent pedicle. The importance of recognizing this condition lies in the fact that the spleen may be lying abnormally low within the abdomen or may have an abnormal lie. It has been reported in children with abnormal abdominal musculature such as prune belly syndrome.[22] As a result of the abnormal pedicle, torsion or twisting of the spleen may occur with resulting compromise of the blood supply to the spleen. In the acute phase of torsion the spleen appears large and hypoechoic because of infarction and congestion, and in the chronic phase the spleen may be small and difficult to detect. Doppler will demonstrate no flow in the spleen. A radioisotope scan may be useful in determining that there is no functioning splenic tissue.

Cardiac abnormalities

Certain cardiac abnormalities may be associated with anomalies of the spleen.[23]

Polysplenia is more common in females and refers to a transverse liver, multiple aberrant nodules of spleen on the right side of the abdomen, and an interrupted infrahepatic portion of the IVC. There is azygous continuation and a tendency for bilateral distribution of left sided viscera. The associated cardiac disease is usually acyanotic left-to-right shunts. Malrotation of the bowel and an absent gallbladder have been reported.

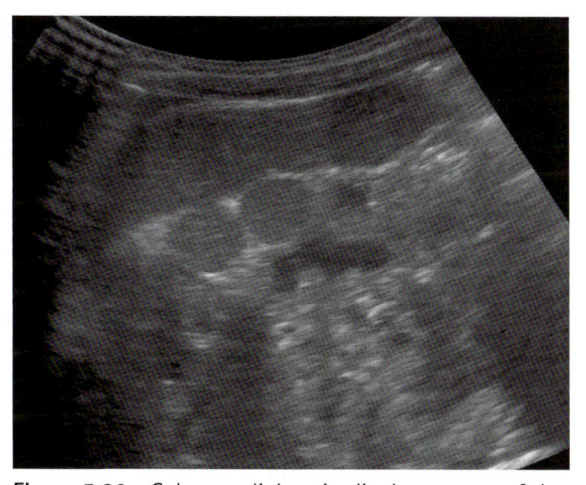

Figure 5.20 Splenunculi. Longitudinal sonogram of the hilum of the spleen. There are two well-defined splenunculi lying in the hilum. They have the same echo texture as the splenic parenchyma. Lymph nodes within the hilum must be differentiated from splenunculi. This can generally be done by ultrasound appearances and by looking for the hilum of the lymph node.

Asplenia is the absence of spleen and is more common in males. It is associated with complex cyanotic congenital heart disease with the IVC and aorta on the same side of the spine. Microgastria, midgut malrotation and duplication of the gallbladder have been described in association.

Situs inversus is where the abdominal contents appear normal but are on the opposite side from that usually expected, so that the spleen is on the right and the liver is on the left (Fig. 5.21).

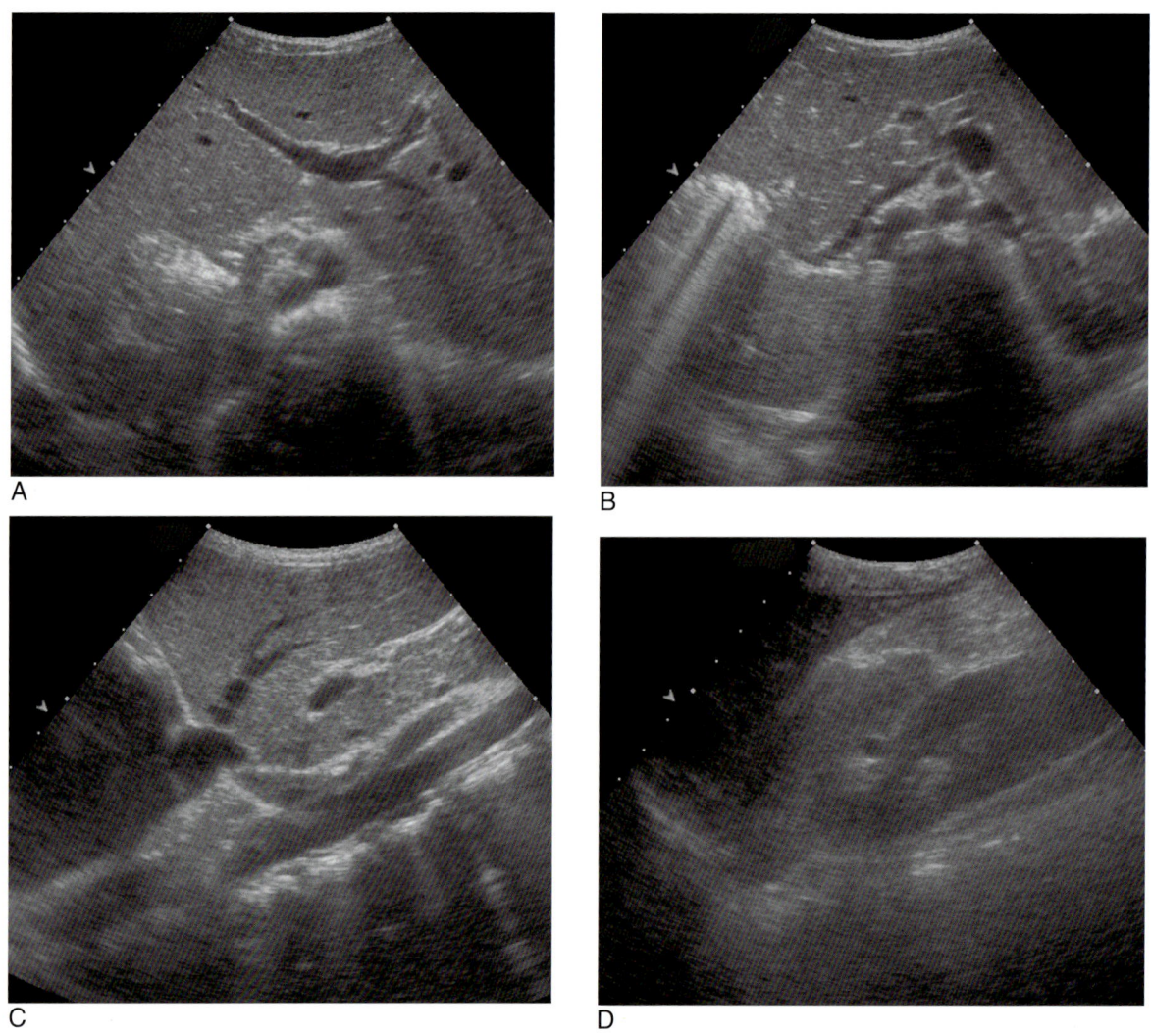

Figure 5.21 Situs inversus. (A) Transverse sonogram at the level of the liver showing that the liver is lying primarily on the left of the abdomen. The orientation of the portal system is to the left. (B) Transverse sonogram slightly lower than (A) showing the portal vein entry from the right. Notice also the bowel gas in the right flank. (C) Longitudinal sonogram at the level of the aorta. The hepatic veins are very prominent and entering the upper IVC at this level. This juxtaposition of the aorta and hepatic veins/IVC on this image could not be achieved if the liver were in the normal position. (D) Longitudinal sonogram of the right kidney showing that, instead of the liver covering the kidney, there is a small spleen above it.

SPLENOMEGALY

Causes of splenomegaly include:

- apparent splenomegaly, due to a displacement of the spleen by a large liver extending across the midline
- portal hypertension
- lymphoma and leukemia; other evidence of disease is usually present, such as hepatomegaly and lymphadenopathy
- infection—viral, bacterial, fungal, protozoal, malaria, mycobacterium and histoplasmosis
- lymphoproliferative disorders
- heart failure and splenic congestion
- infiltrative storage disorders such as Gaucher's disease, mucopolysaccharidosis and Langerhans cell histiocytosis
- hemolytic anemias with extramedullary hemopoiesis—that is, the production of blood cells outside the bone marrow when it is diseased
- focal large splenic lesion due to abscess, cyst or trauma, which may present as splenomegaly
- extracorporeal membrane oxygenation (ECMO)—this is thought to be related to damage to the red cells, with the spleen enlarging as it removes these damaged cells.[24]

THE SMALL SPLEEN

This may be caused by:

- infarction either due to a wandering spleen or conditions such as sickle cell disease
- congenital absence or hypoplasia of the spleen
- partial splenectomy
- Celiac disease
- Fanconi anemia.

FOCAL SPLENIC LESIONS

Cysts

Cysts in the spleen are occasionally detected and may be true cysts or pseudocysts. It may be difficult once the cyst is detected to determine the initial etiology, but the wall must be carefully examined to help detect whether it is a primary congenital cyst or a cyst secondary to an infective process or a hematoma; in the latter case, there will be no epithelial lining. However, it is generally not possible to differentiate between true and pseudocysts. Splenic cysts may rupture or become infected. Epidermoid cysts may also occur in the spleen and may appear as well-defined cystic lesions. There may be calcification within the cyst or within the wall and it may be multiseptated. The cyst in addition may appear complex with internal echoes resulting from hemorrhage or infection. Hydatid infections may also be seen in the spleen, and this generally results from a ruptured liver cyst or systemic infection. They are well defined, single or multiple, with wall calcification.[25]

Hemangiomas

Hemangiomas are one of the commonest benign neoplasms in the spleen. The ultrasound appearances of hemangiomas vary according to the size of the blood vessels and may be single or multiple and may have a hyperechoic appearance or may appear cystic if the blood vessels are large. Doppler examination is essential for any undiagnosed focal lesion in the spleen. They are associated with Beckwith–Wiedemann syndrome and Turner syndrome. In Kasabach–Merrit syndrome there is a large hemangioma which causes platelet trapping and damage resulting in disseminated intravascular coagulation which may be fatal. Splenic hemangiomas have a similar appearance to those found in the liver on cross sectional imaging, so that on CT examination they may demonstrate peripheral enhancement and on MRI they are hyperintense on T2-weighted images.

Lymphangiomas

Lymphangiomas in the spleen appear as they do elsewhere in the body, with multiple large cystic spaces filled with lymph. The vascular content is variable, so that some have large capillaries. Ultrasonically the lesions have multiple cystic spaces with variable thickness and vascularity of the septations.[26]

Abscesses

Abscesses in the spleen have similar ultrasound appearances to those in the liver. They are also usually spread by the blood and typically have thick walls and internal echoes. In pediatric practice, children who develop splenic abscesses are those who are immunocompromised. In this instance they are often multiple. Pyogenic abscesses are typically ill-defined hypoechoic lesions on ultrasound and may contain internal debris. These pyogenic abscesses may be hematogenously spread from a primary site of infection such as appendicitis, empyema, osteomyelitis or ear infections. They may be associated with subacute bacterial endocarditis.

Fungal abscesses, such as those particularly seen in candida, aspergillus and cryptococcus, are indistinguishable on ultrasound. They have a variable appearance and may appear similar to those seen in the liver such that they may have a well-defined hypoechoic lesion or they may have a bullseye or target appearance. They are typically very small, only a few millimeters, and a linear transducer is preferred when suspected. Usually the spleen and liver are involved together rather than in isolation. Contrast enhancement is needed to better delineate the lesions when a CT is performed.

Candida Candidal abscesses are seen particularly in children who are immunosuppressed. As in the liver, they are small and have a bullseye or hypoechoic appearance (Fig. 5.22).

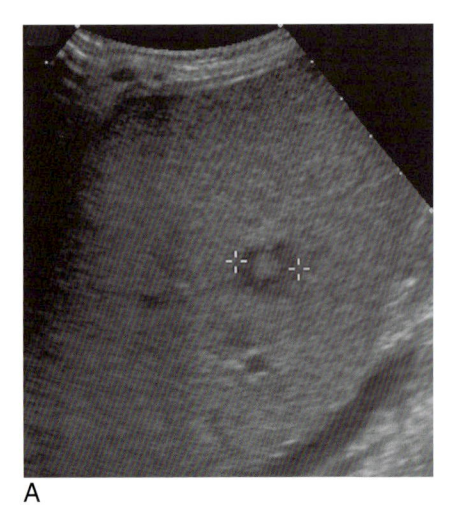

Diffuse splenic abnormalities

Neoplastic conditions Both lymphoma and leukemia may involve the spleen in a focal or diffuse manner. When the spleen is diffusely enlarged there may be no focal abnormality with an apparently normal architecture. Lymphoma (both Hodgkin and non-Hodgkin) and leukemia are the commonest neoplastic conditions involving the spleen.

Involvement of the spleen may occur in approximately a third of children with lymphoma. The spleen may be enlarged and may have focal hypoechoic nodules. In addition the spleen may

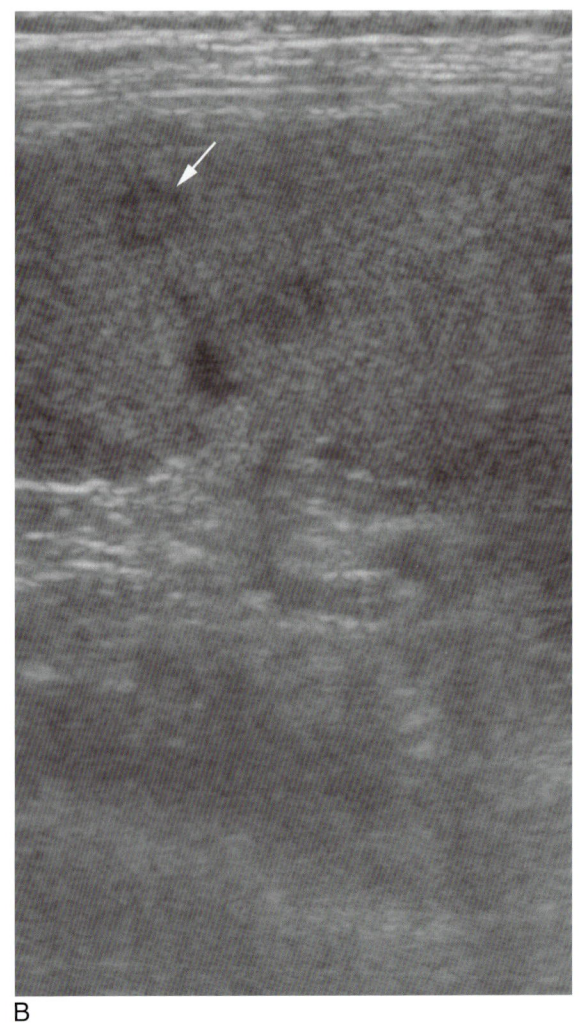

Figure 5.22 Candida of the spleen. (A) Longitudinal sonogram of the spleen showing the bullseye appearance which is one of the features of candidal infection. (B) Longitudinal sonogram of the spleen. This is another patient with a small bullseye lesion (arrow).

THE LIVER, SPLEEN AND PANCREAS

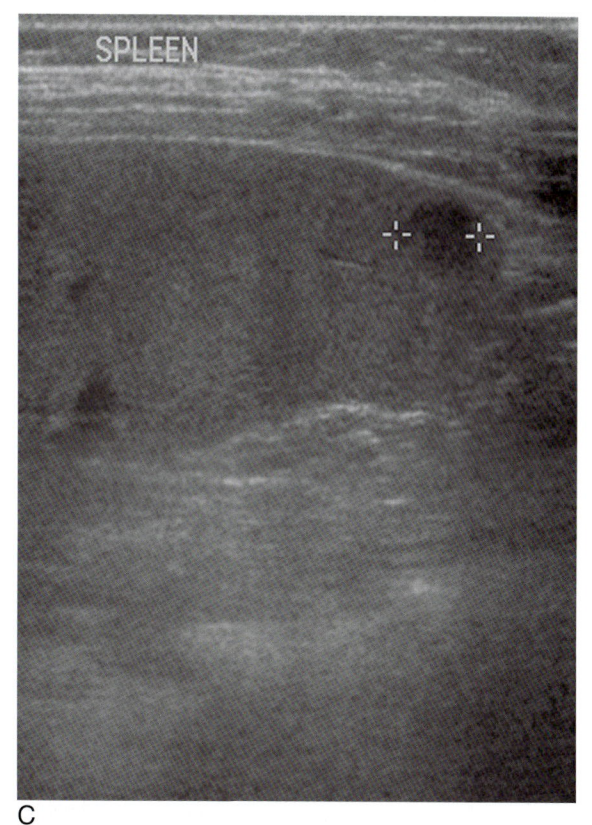

Figure 5.22, cont'd (C) Longitudinal sonogram of the spleen showing a larger focal hypoechoic lesion (between calipers) of candidal infection.

appear with a generalized hypo- or hyperechoic parenchyma.

Leukemia also involves the spleen and may also produce a generalized hyper- or hypoechoic splenic enlargement. Rarely are the lesions focal.

Langerhans cell histiocytosis is a condition primarily involving the skin, bone marrow, reticular endothelial system and lungs and is characterized by proliferation of histiocytes. The spleen may enlarge with multiple focal hypoechoic nodules.[27]

Storage disorders Hepatosplenomegaly is seen in all patients with Gaucher disease. This is a congenital disorder where there is lack of the enzyme glucocerebrosidase. Glucocerebrosidase as a result accumulates in the liver and spleen. Gaucher cells may accumulate, causing hyper- or hypoechoic nodules in the spleen. Extramedullary hemopoiesis, infarction and fibrosis may also occur.

Infarction There are a number of conditions that may cause infarction of the spleen in children, such as sickle cell disease, torsion due to an abnormal pedicle, cardiac emboli, vascular diseases and, rarely, portal hypertension. The spleen is particularly vulnerable to infarction as the splenic artery is an end artery. Once the spleen has infarcted there may be additional complications such as infection with abscess formation, pseudocyst formation and even rupture. Initially the localized areas of infarction may be wedge-shaped and eventually these organize and become fibrosed. Ultimately the spleen will appear small with echogenic areas. There may be isolated areas of infarction or the whole spleen may undergo infarction. Patients with sickle cell disease are particularly prone to developing splenic infarcts (Fig. 5.23).

Peliosis This is a rare disorder associated with disseminated tuberculosis, steroid therapy and hematologic malignancies. It is usually found incidentally and particularly affects the liver. There may be blood-filled spaces within the organs of the reticular endothelial system.

SPLENIC TRAUMA

The spleen is one of the most commonly traumatized intra-abdominal organs. In a child who has sustained abdominal trauma, CT is the prime imaging modality of choice and, in the acute abdomen, it will not only reliably detect splenic trauma but trauma elsewhere within the abdomen. In addition, ultrasound examination of an acute abdomen in a child may be difficult and should never be used in isolation. Most splenic injuries are now managed conservatively if at all possible so as to preserve splenic tissue. Children who lose their spleens are at a higher lifetime risk of sepsis, in particular from pneumococci, and are placed on long term prophylactic antibiotics.

Trauma to the spleen may involve:

- intrasplenic parenchymal lacerations
- subcapsular hematomas resulting from the parenchymal tear or laceration

- hematomas
- fractures and ruptures.

Grading systems have been used to classify splenic trauma; however, this does not always influence treatment, which is very largely dependent on the clinical status of the patient. Contrast extravasation from the site of trauma on CT is one of the prime indicators for surgery.

Ultrasound appearances As in all hematomas, the acute appearance from fresh blood may be hyperechoic and may be difficult to distinguish from that of a normal spleen. Once the hematoma starts liquefying centrally it becomes hypoechoic and easier to detect. Finally, after they have healed, they may appear as a linear echogenic line or liquefy and become cystic. Subcapsular fluid is seen just beneath the capsule of the spleen, which is usually crescent shaped. If rupture of the spleen has occurred then fluid may be seen in the flank or in the rest of the abdomen (Fig. 5.24).

When traumatized splenic tissue is scattered in the peritoneal cavity, splenosis occurs. This is the attachment of splenic tissue to the peritoneum. This splenic tissue may serve to protect the patient against infection if the spleen has been removed. However, it may be mistaken for mass lesions such as lymphoma if the sonographer is not aware of the clinical history.

CT, MRI and nuclear medicine studies with ^{99m}Tc sulfur colloid or denatured red cells can all be used to identify splenic tissue.

SUMMARY

Ultrasound is an excellent screening modality for suspected splenic pathology. The major role of ultrasound is in the detection of focal and diffuse conditions causing splenomegaly and in the diagnosis of portal hypertension.

PANCREAS

Embryology

The pancreas develops from the ventral and dorsal pancreatic buds. Most of the pancreas is derived from the dorsal pancreatic bud, which appears first

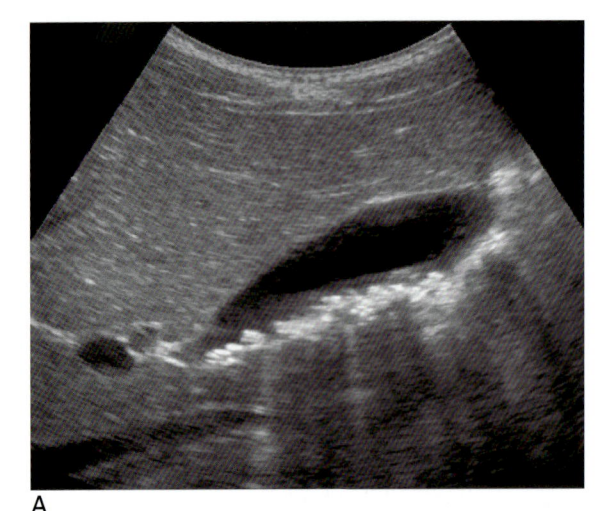

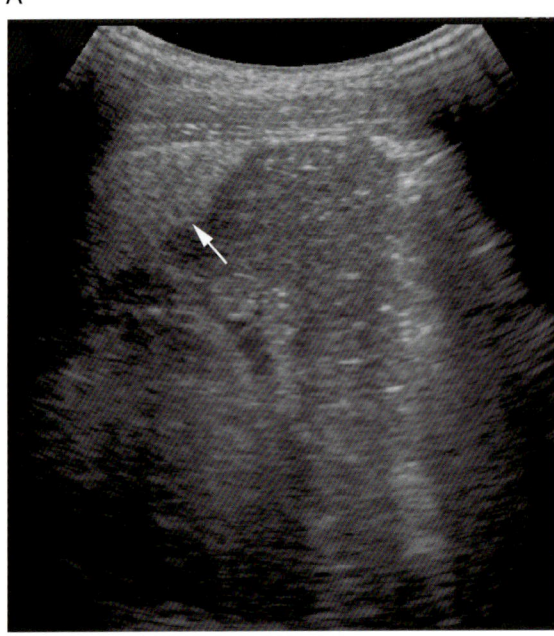

Figure 5.23 Splenic infarct in sickle cell disease. (A) Longitudinal sonogram of the gallbladder in a boy with sickle cell disease. There are multiple small echogenic calculi within the gallbladder in keeping with multiple pigment stones. (B) Longitudinal sonogram of the spleen in the same boy with sickle cell disease. The spleen is small, contracted and difficult to see from multiple infarcted areas caused by his sickle cell disease. There is a dense area of fibrosis next to the diaphragm (arrow).

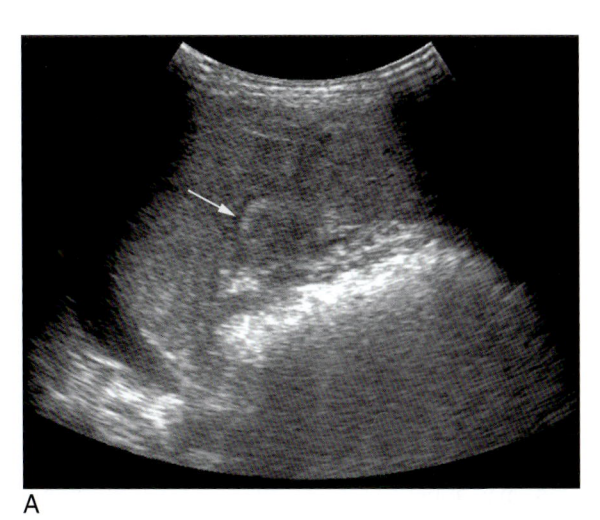

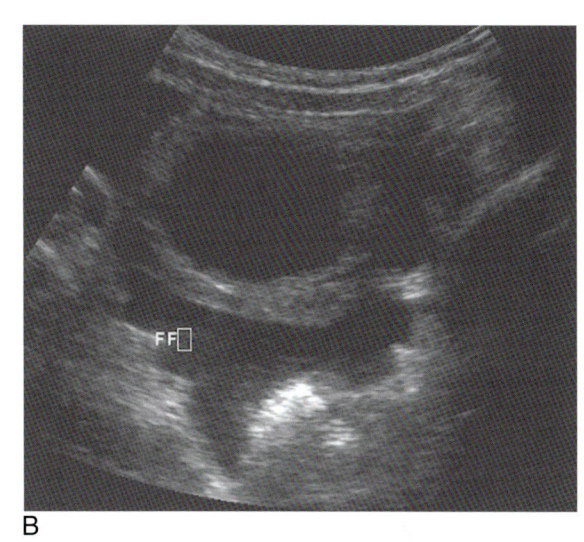

Figure 5.24 Splenic trauma. This young girl fell off a bunk-bed. (A) Longitudinal sonogram of the spleen revealed a small parenchymal tear (arrow). In addition on this view a small pleural effusion can be seen. (B) Transverse sonogram of the pelvis in the same girl revealed free fluid (FF) behind the bladder.

(Fig. 5.25). The ventral pancreatic duct develops near the entry of the bile duct to the duodenum. As the duodenum rotates, the ventral pancreatic bud is carried dorsally with the bile duct and forms the uncinate process and part of the head of the pancreas. The structures around the head of the pancreas are those related to the ventral pancreas, such as the uncinate process and head, whereas the body and the tail develop from the dorsal bud. When the two moieties of the pancreas fuse, the duct system fuses as well to form the main pancreatic duct of Wirsung. The accessory pancreatic duct, or duct of Santorini, results from persistence of the dorsal duct.

The proximal part of the dorsal bud duct sometimes persists as the accessory pancreatic duct, and the two ducts often communicate with each other. In about 10% of people the pancreatic duct system fails to fuse and the two original ducts persist.

CONGENITAL ANOMALIES

The congenital anomalies of the pancreas are related to the rotation and fusion of the two pancreatic buds. It is unusual for ultrasound to detect any of these abnormalities unless specific attention is paid to the head of the pancreas and duodenum.[28]

Congenital cysts

Congenital cysts are caused by anomalous development of the pancreatic ducts. They may be multiple. Multiple congenital cysts may be found in ADPKD and von Hippel–Lindau syndrome, although this is usually in the much older age group and not in the pediatric population.

Pancreas divisum

This is the commonest abnormality and occurs when the ventral and dorsal pancreatic buds do not fuse and each maintains a separate duct.

Annular pancreas

Annular pancreas occurs when the ventral and dorsal segments encircle the duodenum and effectively cord a ring of pancreatic tissue around the duodenum. This causes an obstruction to the gastric outlet, usually in the second part of the duodenum, and if complete the children will present early in life.

Ectopic pancreas

Ectopic pancreas usually lies in the submucosal position and most commonly occurs around the antrum or proximal small bowel. It is associated with other congenital abnormalities of the bowel, in particular the VATER association, malrotation and atresias of the duodenum (Fig. 5.26).

NORMAL ANATOMY

The anatomical landmark to look for when trying to identify the pancreas is the bullseye appearance of the superior mesenteric artery. At the level where the left renal vein passes between the superior mesenteric artery and aorta, the pancreas can be seen draped anteriorly over these structures. The head is intimately related to the duodenum, the body over the midline, and the tail drapes

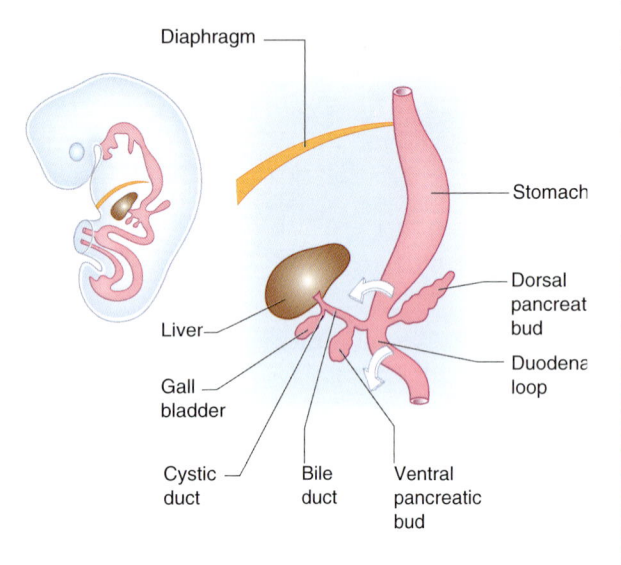

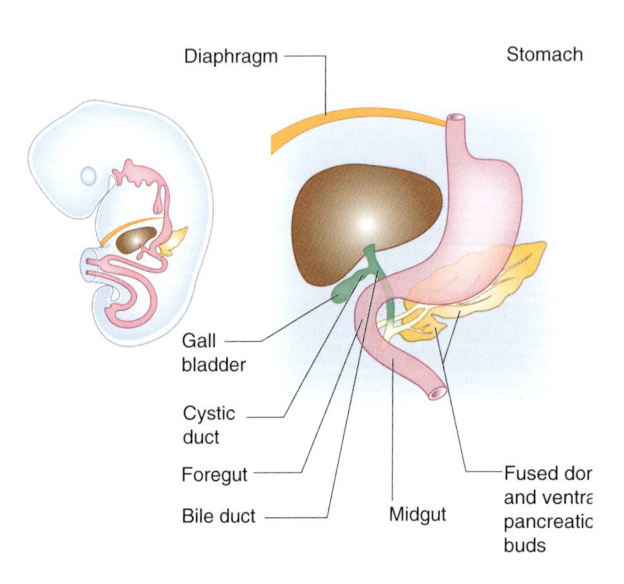

Figure 5.25 Early fetal development of the pancreas. The pancreas develops from dorsal and ventral buds that go on to fuse. The bile duct initially lies lateral to the gut but, after rotation and fusion of the pancreatic buds, it comes to lie posterior to the duodenum and head of the pancreas.

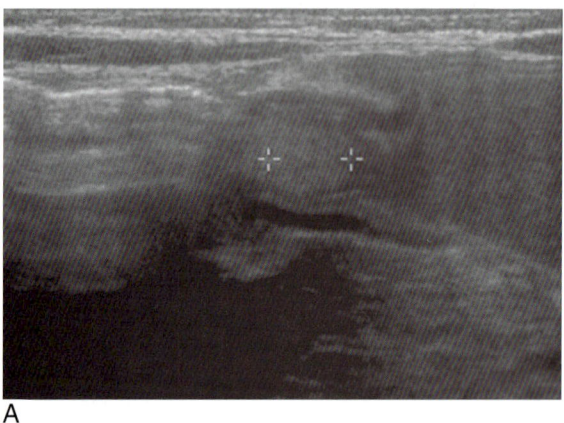

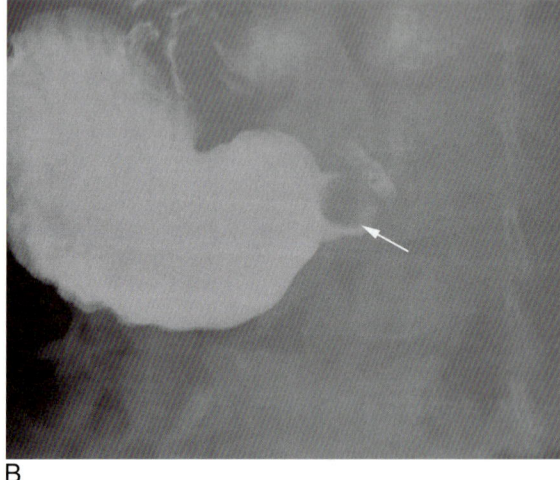

Figure 5.26 Ectopic pancreatic tissue. (A) Transverse sonogram of the gastric antrum in an 18-month-old child presenting with a longstanding history of vomiting. Ultrasound examination revealed an echogenic mass (between calipers) obstructing the gastric outlet. (B) Barium meal examination revealed a well-defined intraluminal defect (arrow) causing a delay in gastric emptying. This was found at surgery to be ectopic pancreatic tissue lying in the stomach wall.

down and comes to lie just anterior to the left kidney and splenic hilum. It is situated in the anterior pararenal space. The lesser omentum and the posterior wall of the stomach form the anterior border. The pancreas has four parts: the head and uncinate process, neck, body and tail.

Vascular landmarks are the splenic artery along the superior margin of the gland and the splenic vein along the posterior wall of the pancreas, joining the superior mesenteric vein behind the pancreatic neck to form the portal vein. The common bile duct is located just behind the head of the pancreas and ends together with the pancreatic duct at the second portion of the duodenum.[29]

The size of the pancreas varies according to the age of the child. It grows substantially in the first year of life, but the rate decreases thereafter (Table 5.6).

The echogenicity of the pancreas is similar to but sometimes less than that of the liver, particularly in the newborn (Fig. 5.27).[30,31]

Ultrasound technique

The pancreas is a relatively superficial structure, and a transducer of the highest frequency for the size of the patient should be used. Curvilinear transducers are the best although, if a localized

Table 5.6 Normal dimensions of the pancreas as a function of age in children[35]

Age (years)	Maximal anteroposterior diameter[a] (cm)		
	Head	Body	Tail
0–6	1.6 (1.0–1.9)	0.7 (0.4–1.0)	1.2 (0.8–1.6)
7–12	1.9 (1.7–2.0)	0.9 (0.6–1.0)	1.4 (1.3–1.6)
13–18	2.0 (1.8–2.2)	1.0 (0.7–1.2)	1.6 (1.3–1.8)

[a]Mean values (range in parentheses)

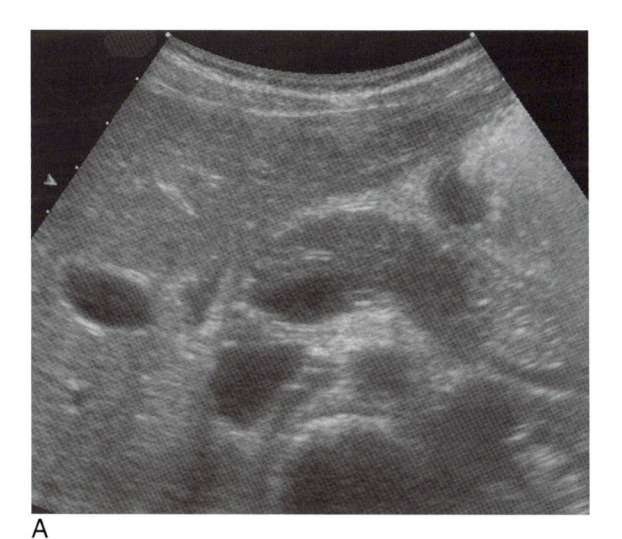

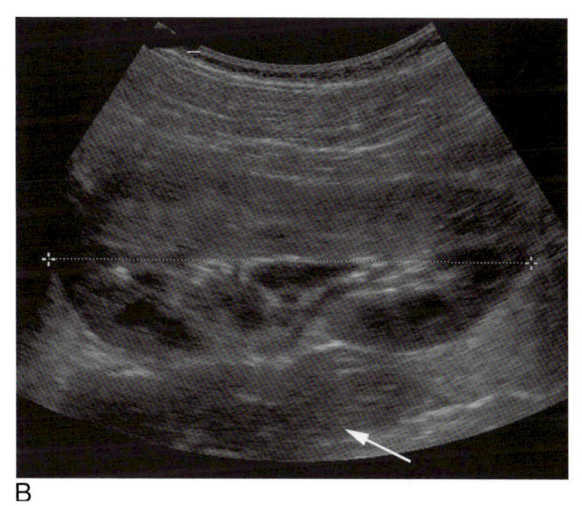

Figure 5.27 Normal pancreas. (A) Transverse sonogram showing a normal pancreas. Notice that the echogenicity of the pancreas in a child is generally slightly lower than that of the liver. Also the pancreatic duct can be easily visualized in the head of the pancreas. (B) Longitudinal sonogram of the left kidney (between calipers). The tail of the pancreas is lying anterior to the left kidney and can sometimes be mistaken for a mass (arrow).

abnormality is detected, a linear probe may produce images of better diagnostic quality, in particular when looking for duct disease. No special preparation is necessary, but a fast does help to decrease the amount of upper abdominal gas.

Transverse and longitudinal scanning of the whole pancreas is performed with the patient in the supine position. The whole of the pancreas must be evaluated for its contour and appearances. In addition the superior abdomen must be systematically and thoroughly examined. Occasionally the pancreas may be obscured by bowel gas, and it can be helpful to get the patient to drink water so that the stomach is filled and can act as an acoustic window. In addition, using graded compression, the sonographer can sometimes displace the bowel gas.

Table 5.7 lists the advantages and disadvantages of various imaging methods for investigating the pancreas.

THE ABNORMAL PANCREAS

Cystic fibrosis

Cystic fibrosis (CF) is an autosomal recessive condition which affects approximately one in every 2000 white births. It used to be called mucoviscidosis. The underlying defect is in a chloride transporter protein which lines duct epithelium. This results in inspissation of mucus in the ducts of the pancreas, bronchial and biliary trees which ultimately leads to chronic pancreatic insufficiency. The inspissated mucus in the pancreas results in dilation of the ducts and acini, which progresses to the formation of small cysts and to fibrosis of the pancreas. The obstruction and distension lead to degeneration and atrophy, and pancreatic insufficiency results with fibrosis and fatty replacement. This not only affects the exocrine tissues but also the endocrine pancreatic tissue, which may result in glucose intolerance. About 85% of children with cystic fibrosis have pancreatic insufficiency which results in steatorrhea and malabsorption.

Ultrasound appearances The pancreas is initially normal at birth but, when fibrosis and fat replacement occurs, there is an increase in the echogenicity and decrease in the size of the pancreas with atrophy.

Fatty replacement in cystic fibrosis varies with age and is most frequent in the older patient, usually in late adolescence. In addition, small punctate areas of calcification to larger granular deposits are found in up to 8%. There may be dilated pancreatic ducts as a result of obstruction by the material. Pancreatic cysts are a common finding and are typically small.

Table 5.7 Methods of investigation of the pancreas

Investigation	Advantages	Disadvantages
Ultrasound	Non-invasive Can be repeated often Good visualization of biliary tree Monitoring of fluid collections, pseudocysts, extent of pancreatic necrosis and peripancreatic inflammation	Cannot reliably detect pancreatic necrosis Pancreas obscured by bowel gas
Contrast-enhanced CT	Modality of choice for the diagnosis of acute pancreatitis	Children may require sedation or GA
Magnetic resonance cholangiopancreatography (MRCP)	Good delineation of the biliary tree	Expensive equipment Children may require sedation or GA Long examination
Endoscopic retrograde cholangiopancreatography (ERCP)	Good delineation of pancreatic duct. Collections connecting with duct also demonstrated	Pediatric expertise needed to cannulate duct

The severity of the ultrasound changes seen in the pancreas is related to increasing age. Improved treatment regimens have resulted in more patients surviving and consequently an increase in survival of patients with chronic pancreatic disease.

The major effects then on the pancreas are pancreatic insufficiency, pancreatitis and diabetes mellitus. The treatment of the intestinal complications of cystic fibrosis is with oral pancreatic supplements.

Other diffuse pancreatic conditions

Shwachman syndrome

Shwachman syndrome, after cystic fibrosis, is the next most common cause of pancreatic insufficiency in childhood. This is also an autosomal recessive condition and it is characterized by the impairment of neutrophil function. Other features seen in the syndrome include metaphyseal chondrodysplasia which manifests as shortening of the extremities, metaphyseal widening and a 'cup' deformity of the ribs, together with bone marrow hypoplasia and exocrine pancreatic insufficiency leading to malabsorption. The sweat test is normal.

The diagnosis should be considered in any child with pancreatic insufficiency with a normal sweat test and neutropenia. These children are particularly prone to recurrent infections.

The characteristic pathology in the pancreas is fatty infiltration, so that on ultrasound the pancreas is hyperechoic but normal in size.[32]

Nesidioblastosis

Nesidioblastosis is a persistence of the fetal state of the pancreas, with diffuse proliferation and persistence of nesidioblasts, which are cells that differentiate from duct epithelium. These cells secrete insulin, so that affected babies present with hypoglycemia. The treatment is subtotal pancreatectomy. Ultrasound examination is not particularly helpful in these infants, and in the few reported series in the literature the pancreas was of normal or increased echogenicity.[33,34]

Acute pancreatitis

The commonest cause of acute pancreatitis in pediatrics is blunt abdominal trauma, most commonly from road traffic accidents or non-accidental injury. Other causes include infection such as mumps, drug toxicity and biliary and pancreatic anomalies. Biliary lithiasis is a rare cause in children.

Acute pancreatitis is uncommon in childhood, and when it does occur no obvious precipitating cause can be found. Trauma as a result of child abuse is one of the commonest causes, whereas hereditary causes are most common for chronic pancreatitis.

Attacks of pancreatitis are characterized by severe epigastric or periumbilical pain which tends to be constant, radiating to the back and shoulders. The pain is made worse by eating and is not relieved by antacids. On moving, the abdomen is severely uncomfortable and when pancreatitis is prolonged, pleural effusions and pancreatic pseudocysts may occur. The diagnosis is confirmed by markedly raised amylase levels.

Clinically, patients need to be rested and all oral feeds stopped. The role of ultrasound is in the monitoring of patients with pancreatitis for the development of pseudocysts. Patients in whom the clinical diagnosis is in doubt and who do not show rapid clinical improvement or further deterioration need ERCP (endoscopic retrograde cholangiopancreatography). This is used to better delineate the duct system in suspected congenital anomalies.[35-37]

In mild pancreatitis the gland may appear normal but usually there is evidence of edema with an enlarged gland which appears hypoechoic. The ultrasound findings are diverse and may be diffuse or focal gland enlargement. The borders of the gland may be poorly defined and there may be dilation of the duct.

Severe acute pancreatitis may be complicated by complete gland necrosis, which is best demonstrated by CT. This may become infected in a significant proportion, and the presence of air either from a fistula or the infection means that this needs to be drained.

Fluid collections arise in or adjacent to the pancreas in acute pancreatitis, and the majority will resolve spontaneously. Some may persist, but others may develop into pseudocysts.

Pancreatic pseudocysts (Fig. 5.28) have fibrous capsules. Pseudocysts evolve from an acute collection and may take several weeks to develop. The majority

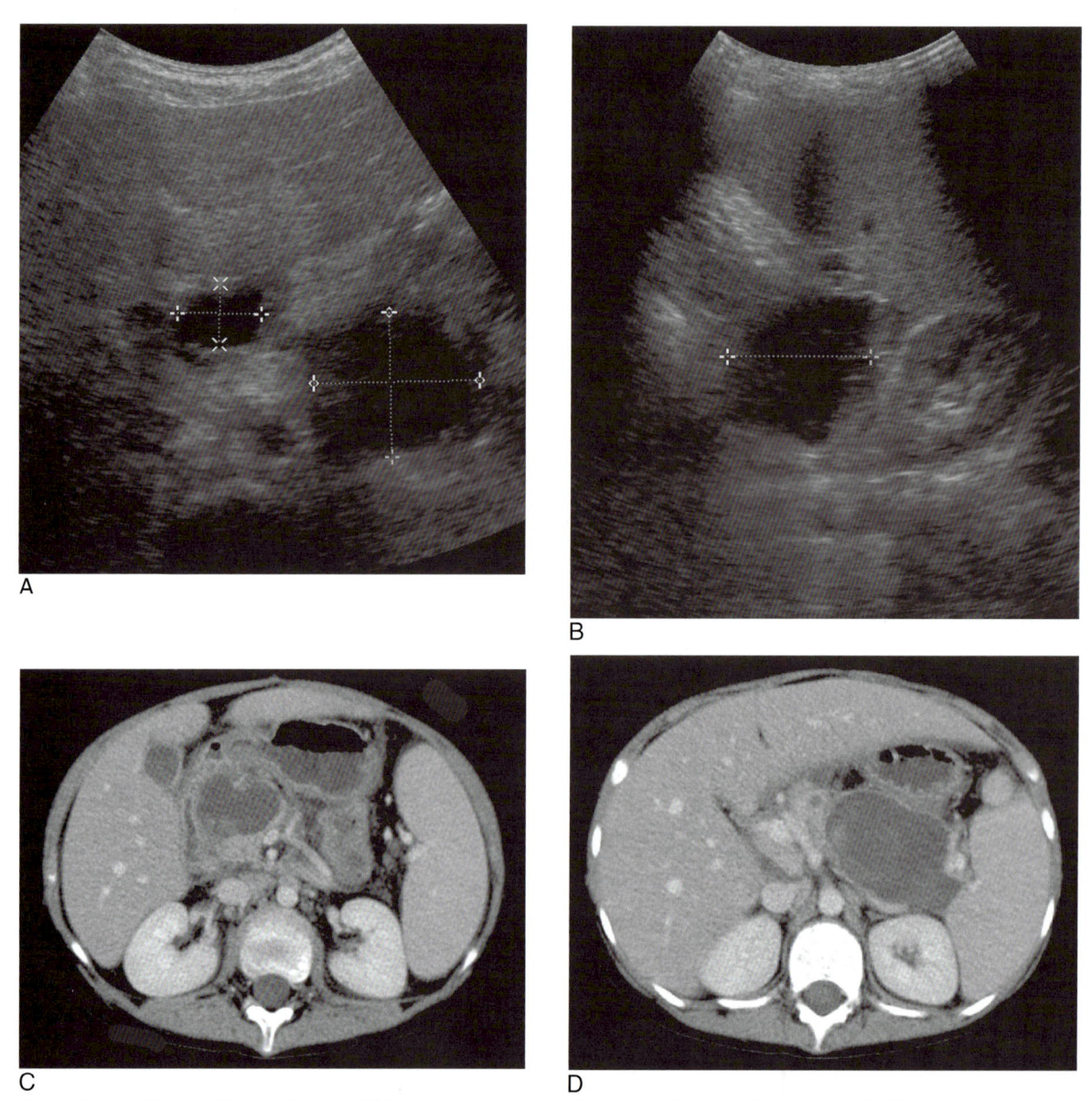

Figure 5.28 Pancreatic pseudocysts. (A) Transverse sonogram in a boy with chronic pancreatitis. There are two pancreatic pseudocysts between the markers, one in the head and one in the tail. The other visible pancreatic tissue is very echogenic. (B) Transverse sonogram from the left flank. This is a good view to demonstrate lesions in the tail of the pancreas, as the pancreatic tail lies just anterior/medial to the left kidney. (C) Contrast-enhanced CT examination on the same boy showing the pancreatic pseudocyst in the head of the pancreas. (D) Contrast-enhanced CT examination showing the pancreatic pseudocyst in the tail of the pancreas. Notice the close relationship of the splenic and portal vessels to the pseudocyst. Vascular erosion is a well-known complication in this condition.

will resolve spontaneously, but complications such as infection, hemorrhage, bile duct obstruction or even rupture may occur. Treatment is by percutaneous drainage.

Vasculature Because of the intimate relationship of the pancreas to the major superior mesenteric vessels, complications associated with these vessels may occur. This is because the pancreatic enzymes erode or cause thrombosis of these vessels. If the vessels are eroded there may be hemorrhage or there may be rupture of vessels with a pseudoaneurysm to an artery. Angiography may be required to embolize the bleeding blood vessels.

Other complications such as perforation of the bowel as a result of erosion from pancreatic enzymes, or ischemia due to the vascular complications, may occur. Bile duct dilation may be visible, resulting from edema of the pancreatic head leading to persistent stenosis or obstruction of the biliary tree.

Chronic pancreatitis

Chronic pancreatitis, longstanding inflammatory disease of the pancreas, is not reversible. This is usually the result of multiple attacks of acute pancreatitis. Patients present with abdominal pain and loss of the functions of the pancreas, so that they may be diabetic. The size of the pancreas is variable. Most commonly it is small because of the fibrosis, with a generalized heterogeneous appearance (Fig. 5.29). The gland may be calcified. There may be dilation of the pancreatic duct and of the common bile duct.

Extreme care in the examination must be taken in order to evaluate all the vessels in the region of the pancreas, looking for complications such as splenic, mesenteric or portal vein thrombosis or pseudoaneurysm formation.

Differential diagnosis

Table 5.8 relates the echogenicity and size of the pancreas to the differential diagnosis of disease with diffuse pancreatic involvement. Figure 5.30 shows the echogenic appearance of the pancreas in a child with rheumatoid arthritis.

Focal lesions

Cysts

Cysts may be found in the pancreas, the commonest being pancreatic pseudocysts found in

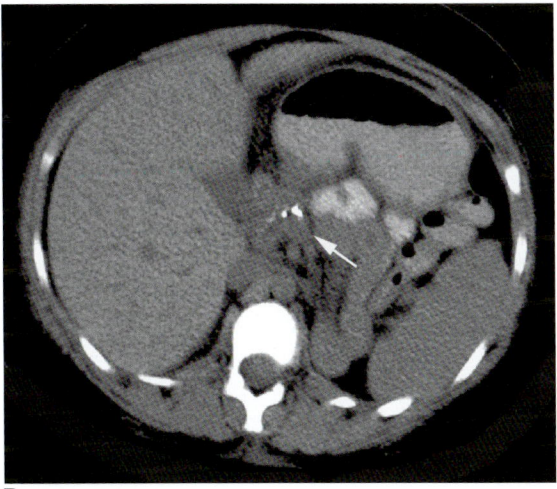

Figure 5.29 Chronic pancreatitis. (A) Transverse sonogram at the level of the pancreas. It is very difficult to see any pancreatic tissue at all, and there is just a small sliver of echogenic pancreas. This girl had longstanding pancreatitis with an atrophied pancreas and was diabetic. (B) CT examination on the same girl showing the small atrophied pancreas with areas of calcification (arrow).

Table 5.8 Differential diagnosis of disease with diffuse pancreatic involvement

Echogenicity of pancreas	Size of pancreas		
	Normal	Small	Large
Hyperechoic	• Schwachman syndrome • Cushing syndrome • Treatment with steroids • Storage disorders • Obesity • Newborn in the first month of life	• Cystic fibrosis • Chronic pancreatitis	• Nesidioblastosis • Acute pancreatitis
Hypoechoic	• Acute pancreatitis		• Acute pancreatitis • Leukemia • Lymphoma

pancreatitis. Causes of cystic lesions in the pancreas are:

- pancreatitis
- congenital
- cyst adenoma or cyst adenocarcinoma
- cystic lymphangioma
- autosomal dominant polycystic kidney disease
- hydatid disease
- cystic fibrosis
- pancreaticoblastoma.

Pancreatic neoplasms

Pancreatic neoplasms are extremely rare in childhood. They may be cystic or solid. The cystic tumors may be mucinous or serous. The mucinous are malignant (cyst adenocarcinoma) and are most commonly found in the body and tail. The serous cystic tumors are benign.[38–41]

The solid neoplasms are predominantly endocrine tumors such as insulinomas and gastronomas. Adenocarcinoma is the most common solid tumor of the pancreas, and the findings are similar to those in adults.

Pancreaticoblastomas are rare tumors of the pancreas and are associated with Beckwith–Wiedemann syndrome.

Metastatic disease is uncommon but may be lymphomatous and may have associated local lymphadenopathy.

Pancreatic trauma

Pancreatic trauma may occur in children in blunt abdominal trauma such as road traffic accidents and non-accidental injury. The pancreas may be completely transected with resulting leakage of pancreatic juices and collections of fluid in the abdomen. This release of pancreatic enzymes may

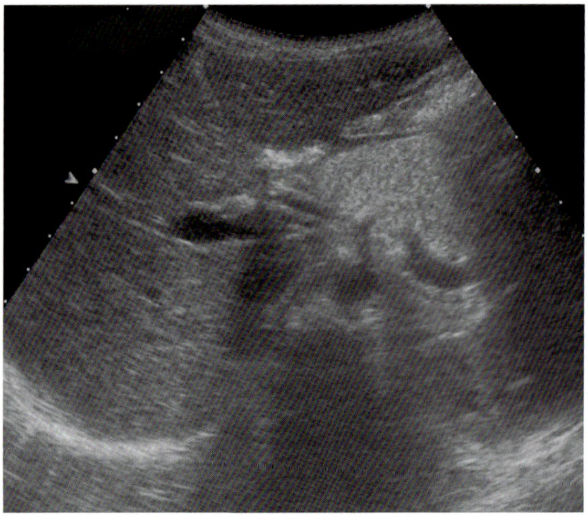

Figure 5.30 Echogenic pancreas. Transverse sonogram of the pancreas in a child with rheumatoid arthritis. She had had long term steroid therapy and fatty infiltration of the pancreas, accounting for this appearance.

initiate pancreatitis and peritonitis. As in other suspected trauma in the abdomen, CT is the examination of choice.[42]

SUMMARY

Pancreatic disease is uncommon in children. Ultrasound is excellent for monitoring the complications of pancreatitis such as pseudocysts but is often limited in its diagnostic accuracy because of overlying bowel gas and poor visualization of the pancreas. Most children will require further imaging if pathology is strongly suspected.

References

1. Dittrich M, Milde S, Dinkel E, et al. Sonographic biometry of liver and spleen size in childhood. Paed Radiol 1983; 13:206–211.
2. Patriquin H, Lafortune M, Burns PN, et al. Duplex Doppler examination in portal hypertension: technique and anatomy. AJR Am J Roentgenol 1987; 149:71–76.
3. Tessler FN, Gehring BJ, Gomes AS, et al. Diagnosis of portal vein thrombosis: value of color Doppler imaging. AJR Am J Roentgenol 1991; 157:293–296.
4. Haller JO. Sonography of the biliary tract in infants and children. AJR Am J Roentgenol 1991; 157:1051–1058.
5. Madigan S, Teele R. Ultrasonography of the liver and biliary tree in children. Semin Ultrasound 1984; 5:68–84.
6. McGahan JP, Phillips HE, Cox KL. Sonography of the normal pediatric gallbladder and biliary tract. Radiology 1982; 14:873.
7. Hernanz-Schulman M, Ambrosino MM, Freeman PC, et al. Common bile duct in children: sonographic dimensions. Radiology 1995; 195:193–195.
8. Davenport M, Stringer MD, Howard ER. Biliary amylase and congenital choledochal dilatation. J Pediatr Surg 1995; 30(3):474–477.
9. Han BK, Babcock DS, Gelfand MH. Choledochal cyst with bile duct dilatation: sonography and 99m-Tc IDA cholescintigraphy. AJR Am J Roentgenol 1981; 136:1075–1079.
10. Callahan J, Haller JO, Cacciarelli AA, et al. Cholelithiasis in infants: association with total parenteral nutrition and furosemide. Radiology 1982; 143:437–439.
11. Blickman JG, Herrin JT, Cleveland RH, et al. Coexisting nephrolithiasis and cholelithiasis in premature infants. Pediatr Radiol 1991; 21:363–364.
12. Babbitt DP, Starshak RJ, Clemett AR. Choledochal cyst: a concept of etiology. Am J Roentgenol 1973; 119:57–62.
13. McHugo JM, McKeown C, Brown MT, et al. Ultrasound findings in children with cystic fibrosis. Br J Radiol 1987; 60:137–141.
14. Donovan AT, Wolverson MK, deMello D, et al. Multicystic hepatic mesenchymal hamartoma of childhood. Pediatr Radiol 1981; 11:163–165.
15. Federici S, Galli G, Sciutti R, et al. Cystic mesenchymal hamartoma of the liver. Pediatr Radiol 1992; 22(4):307–308.
16. Wholey MH, Wojno KJ. Pediatric hepatic mesenchymal hamartoma demonstrated on plain film, ultrasound and MRI, and correlated with pathology. Pediatr Radiol 1994; 24(2):143–144.
17. Helmberger TK, Ros PR, Mergo PJ, et al. Pediatric liver neoplasms: a radiologic–pathologic correlation. Eur Radiol 1999; 9(7):1339–1347.
18. Bates SM, Keller MS, Ramos IM, et al. Hepatoblastoma: detection of tumor vascularity with duplex Doppler US. Radiology 1990; 176(2):505–507.
19. Rosenberg H, Markowitz R, Kolberg H, et al. Normal splenic size in infants and children: sonographic measurements. AJR Am J Roentgenol 1991; 157:119–121.
20. Freeman JL, Jafri SZH, Robert JL, et al. CT of congenital and acquired abnormalities of the spleen. RadioGraphics 1993; 13:597–610.
21. Cirillo RL Jr, Coley BD, Binkovitz LA, et al. Sonographic findings in splenogonadal fusion. Pediatr Radiol 1999; 29:73–75.
22. Teramoto R, Opas LM, Andrassy R. Splenic torsion wth prune belly syndrome. J Pediatr 1981; 98:91–92.
23. Chen JTT. Congenital heart disease. In: Chen JTT, ed. Essentials of cardiac imaging. 2nd edn. Philadelphia: Lippincott-Raven; 1997:301–305.
24. Klippenstein DL, Zerin JM, Hirschl RB, et al. Splenic enlargement in neonates during ECMO. Radiology 1994; 190:411–412.
25. Paterson A, Frush DP, Lane F, et al. A pattern-orientated approach to splenic imaging in infants and children. RadioGraphics 1999; 19:1465–1485.

26. Urrutia M, Mergo PJ, Ros LH, et al. Cystic masses of the spleen: radiologic–pathologic correlation. RadioGraphics 1996; 16:107–129.
27. Ferrozzi F, Bova D, Draghi F, et al. CT findings in primary vascular tumors of the spleen. AJR Am J Roentgenol 1996; 166:1097–1101.
28. Herman TE, Siegel MJ. Polysplenia syndrome with congenital short pancreas. AJR Am J Roentgenol 1991; 156:799–800.
29. Siegel MJ, Martin KW, Worthington JL. Normal and abnormal pancreas in children: US studies. Radiology 1987; 165:15–18.
30. Schneider K, Harms K, Fendel H. The increased echogenicity of pancreas in infants and children: the white pancreas. Eur J Paediatr 1987; 146:508–511.
31. Worthen NJ, Beabeau D. Normal pancreatic echogenicity: relation to age and body fat. AJR Am J Roentgenol 1982; 139:1095–1098.
32. Aggett PI, Cavanagh NPC, Matthew DI, et al. Shwachman's syndrome: a review of 21 cases. Arch Dis Child 1980; 55:331–347.
33. Schönau E, Deeg KH, Hnemmer HP, et al. Pancreatic growth and function following surgical treatment of nesidioblastosis in infancy. Eur J Paediatr 1991; 150:550–553.
34. Knight J, Garnin PJ, Danis R, et al. Nesidioblastosis in children. Arch Surg 1980; 115:880–882.
35. Coleman BG, Arger PH, Rosenberg HK, et al. Gray-scale sonographic assessment of pancreatitis in children. Radiology 1983; 146:145–150.
36. Fleischer AC, Parker P, Kirchner G, et al. Sonographic findings of pancreatitis in children. Radiology 1983; 146:151–155.
37. Jeffrey RB Jr. Sonography in acute pancreatitis. Radiol Clin North Am 1989; 27:5–17.
38. Mathieu D, Guigui B, Valette PJ, et al. Pancreatic cystic neoplasm. Radiol Clin North Am 1989; 27:163–176.
39. Ros PR, Hamrick-Turner JE, Chiechi MV, et al. Cystic masses of the pancreas. Radiographics 1992; 12:673–686.
40. Ganderer M, Stanley CA, Baker L, et al. Pancreatic adenomas in infants and children: current surgical management. J Pediatr Surg 1978; 13:591–596.
41. Gorman B, Charboneau JW, James EM, et al. Benign pancreatic insulinoma: preoperative and intraoperative sonographic localization. AJR Am J Roentgenol 1986; 147:929–934.
42. Jeffrey RB, Laing FC, Wing VW. Ultrasound in acute pancreatic trauma. Gastrointest Radiol 1986; 11:44–46.

Chapter 6

The abdomen and bowel

CHAPTER CONTENTS

Abnormalities related to embryological
 development 183
  Body wall defects 183
Ultrasound technique 184
Abnormalities of the gastrointestinal tract 184
  Gastroesophageal reflux 184
  Hypertrophic pyloric stenosis 185
  Stomach conditions 188
  Malrotation 189
  Enteric duplications 190
  Intussusception 191
  Appendicitis 194
  Bowel wall thickening/infiltrative
   disorders 197
  Anorectal anomalies 197
  Cystic abdominal masses 198
Mesentery, omentum and peritoneum 199

Embryology

Many of the gastrointestinal abnormalities seen in children and which are detectable with ultrasound arise from abnormal intrauterine development. Also, many of the anomalies are interrelated with other systems in the body. A basic understanding of the embryological development of the gastrointestinal tract will help the sonographer to perform a complete examination of all the relevant systems.

The primordial gut is divided into three parts: the foregut, midgut and hindgut.

The structures derived from the foregut are the pharynx, oral cavity, upper and lower respiratory system, the esophagus, stomach and duodenum, liver, bile ducts and pancreas. The celiac artery supplies the stomach, duodenum, liver, spleen and pancreas. During duodenal development the lumen becomes obliterated and then recanalizes. If this recanalization fails to occur then duodenal atresia or stenosis results. All atresias are distal to the second part of the duodenum (and thus entry of the common bile duct) so that infants present clinically with bile-stained vomiting. Atresias or stenoses in the jejunum and ileum are a later intrauterine event, and are thought to be related to a vascular compromise which results in a localized area of ischemia of the bowel.

The midgut forms the duodenum beyond the sphincter of Oddi (where the common bile duct enters the duodenum), the jejunum, the ileum, the cecum, the appendix and the ascending and right two thirds of the transverse colon. Due to the rapidly enlarging liver and two sets of kidneys within the abdomen there is a shortage of space within the abdominal cavity. The primitive midgut forms a loop, the midgut loop, the apex of which is continuous with the vitello-intestinal duct or yolk stalk. The midgut loop elongates rapidly on an elongated dorsal mesentery which is extruded into the extra-embryonic coelom at the umbilicus. This extrusion constitutes the physiological umbilical hernia. The major artery supplying the midgut is the superior mesenteric artery, which is central to this whole process of herniation and rotation (Fig. 6.1).

The return of the midgut to the abdomen occurs in the third month. The proximal limb (i.e. the small bowel) re-enters the abdominal cavity first. The cecum and appendix are the last structures to return to the abdomen. The cecum then descends to the right iliac fossa. The mesenteries shorten and disappear by a process of fusion, and the large bowel becomes fixed in a retroperitoneal position by a process of peritonealization. This is important because, if the bowel is malrotated, this process may result in abnormal bands from the undersurface of the liver, called Ladd bands, as the body attempts to fix the malrotated bowel in position.

Since the appendix develops during the descent of the colon, its final position frequently is posterior to the cecum or colon. These positions of the appendix are called retrocecal or retrocolic (Fig. 6.2).

The hindgut forms the left third of the transverse colon, the descending colon, the sigmoid colon, the rectum and the upper part of the anal canal. The urogenital organs are separated from the primitive rectum by the urorectal septum (Fig. 6.3). The anorectal anomalies occur when there is abnormal separation of the rectum from the urogenital system by arrested growth or deviation of the septum.

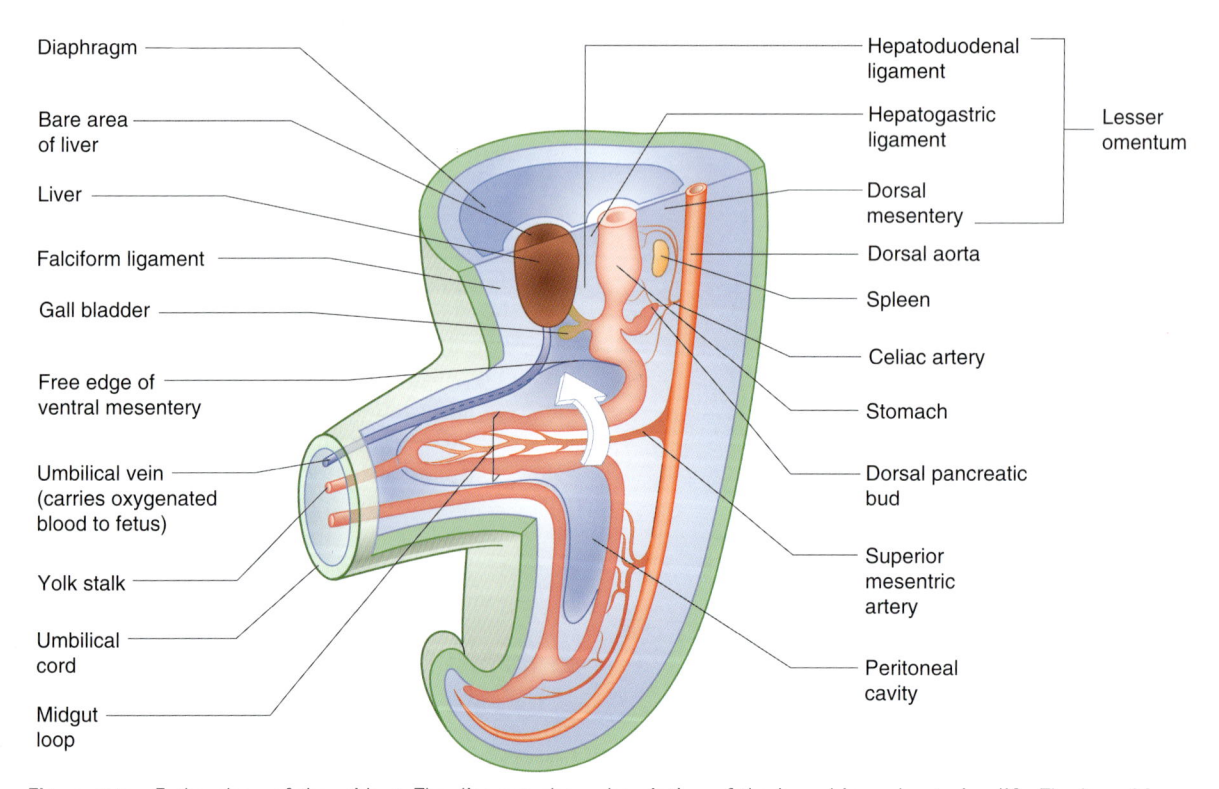

Figure 6.1 Embryology of the midgut. The diagram shows herniation of the bowel in early uterine life. The bowel is guided by the vitello-intestinal duct and rotates anticlockwise before re-entering the abdomen. The superior mesenteric artery is in the middle of the rotating bowel.

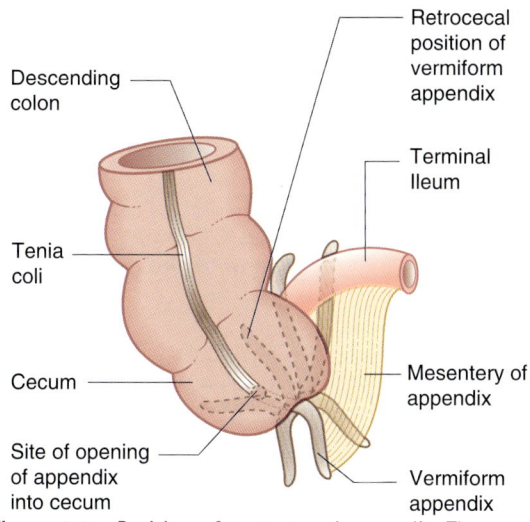

Figure 6.2 Position of a retrocecal appendix. These can be very difficult to identify on ultrasound.

This results in atresia of the rectum and fistulas to the urethra, bladder or vagina. High anorectal atresias are all associated with a fistula. In addition the development of the rectum and urogenital system takes place at the same time as that of the spine, and hence there is a high association with spinal anomalies.

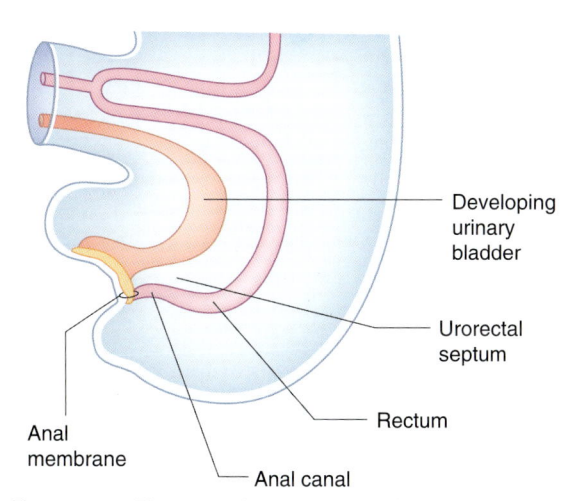

Figure 6.3 The normal separation of the rectum from the developing urethra and bladder by the urorectal septum. If the septum does not grow down, no separation occurs, resulting in a cloaca, i.e. only one orifice.

The development of the upper part of the anal canal differs from that of the lower part, and this is reflected in different epithelium, blood supply and lymphatic drainage. This is important in adults who have an anorectal malignancy, as the position of the tumor affects the lymphatic drainage and direction of metastatic spread.

The peritoneum is a membrane which surrounds the bowel and delineates the abdominal cavity. After the bowel rotates and becomes fixed, some organs come to lie behind the peritoneum, such as the kidneys and pancreas, in which case they are termed retroperitoneal. In addition, in some places the peritoneum fuses, resulting in sacs such as the lesser sac and ligaments.

ABNORMALITIES RELATED TO EMBRYOLOGICAL DEVELOPMENT

Body wall defects

Omphalocele

This involves herniation of abdominal viscera through an enlarged umbilical ring. The viscera which may be herniated include the liver, small and large intestine, stomach, spleen or gallbladder and are covered by amnion. The origin of the defect is a failure of the bowel to return to the body cavity from its physiological herniation. Omphalocele is associated with a high rate of mortality and is associated with other severe malformations.

Gastroschisis

This is a herniation of abdominal contents through the body wall directly into the amniotic cavity. It is the more common abdominal wall defect. It occurs lateral to the umbilicus, and the viscera are not covered by peritoneum. The umbilical cord is not involved. Unlike an omphalocele, gastroschisis is not associated with other abnormalities, so the survival rate is excellent. However, volvulus, that is twisting of the bowel, does occur.

Vitelline duct persistence

The vitelline duct or yolk stalk is the structure that connects the primitive gut and the yolk sac. If the vitelline duct persists it forms an outpouching of ileum which is called a Meckel's diverticulum. This occurs in roughly 2% of the population and is located about 60 cm from the ileocecal valve. It is important because, if it contains gastric mucosa, it may ulcerate and bleed or perforate. Very rarely if the vitelline duct persists and remains patent, a direct communication will exist between the umbilicus and ileum. Infants present with a 'weeping' umbilicus, even gas expulsion, and sinography reveals a connection with the ileum.

ULTRASOUND TECHNIQUE

Preparation

Ideally all children scheduled for abdominal examinations should be fasted so as to distend the gallbladder and decrease abdominal gas. In reality, this is not practical as it is far better to have a happy, drinking child with a full bladder so that the pelvis and lower abdomen can be fully examined. In addition, a hungry child is a fractious child, which makes ultrasound much more difficult. In our department we fast only those children for whom there are specific clinical queries about the gallbladder, biliary system or pancreas. No specific bowel preparation is necessary, although it is wise to ask parents to ensure the child avoids fizzy drinks.

Examination

Always start with a probe of the highest frequency and then decrease frequency if there is insufficient penetration. Generally 5–10 MHz is suitable for most children. Good near field visualization is needed. Start with a curvilinear probe and systematically examine the entire abdominal contents. Start with the intra-abdominal organs and ensure they appear normal. When looking specifically at the bowel, change and use a high frequency linear probe. Starting in the right flank, gradually move around the abdomen in a clockwise manner. Gradually compressing the abdomen and gently pushing the bowel gas away is a useful trick allowing better visualization if the abdomen is very gassy.

Observations should include bowel wall thickness, bowel motility, bowel contents, free fluid or abscess collections in the abdomen, and any masses or cysts related to the bowel. Doppler should also be used and particularly in suspected appendicitis, inflammatory bowel disease and intussusception. Ultrasound plays a major role in some conditions, in particular the cystic masses, pyloric stenosis, intussusception and appendicitis.

In most instances, contrast examinations of the bowel are still the imaging modality of choice.

ABNORMALITIES OF THE GASTROINTESTINAL TRACT

Gastroesophageal reflux

Gastroesophageal reflux (GER) is the retrograde flow of milk and solids from the stomach up the esophagus. This is particularly common in infants, where they may present with persistent vomiting and failure to thrive, but the important association in terms of the use of ultrasound is with gastric outflow obstructions such as pyloric stenosis and malrotation. It is recognized that ultrasound can detect GER (although it is not widely employed, as it is time consuming) with just a short snapshot view of the gastroesophageal junction. However, there are better, more sensitive tests available. The 'gold standard' test is a pH study where a probe is placed in the lower esophagus and monitored over a 24-hour period for acidity within the esophagus. Also a radioisotope milk scan may be used, where the baby is given milk containing tracer and then scanned for GER and even sometimes aspiration of tracer into the lungs. A conventional barium meal is probably still the examination most widely used, because of cost and availability, and it has the added advantage over all other tests of being able to demonstrate the anatomy of the gastric outlet.[1]

The ultrasound technique involves giving the baby a liquid feed prior to the examination and laying the infant supine. In the supine position the gastric fundus is filled, so this is the optimal sonographic positioning. Reflux will only be observed effectively on ultrasound if the stomach is filled with clear fluid or milk. The gastroesophageal junction lies just to the left of the aorta, in the region of the xiphi-sternum, and can be seen by scanning longitudinally over the upper abdominal aorta. By slightly angling the transducer to the left of the aorta the gastroesophageal junction and lower esophagus come into view. If GER is present, then air and gastric contents can be seen to reflux up the esophagus (Fig. 6.4). GER is common and probably physiological in most infants. It can cause major problems, however, when it is associated with hiatus hernia, severe vomiting and failure to thrive together with aspiration causing cyanotic spells and chronic lung disease.

Hypertrophic pyloric stenosis

Pyloric stenosis is an evolving condition of progressive pyloric muscle hypertrophy, which then narrows and elongates the pyloric canal. It typically occurs in male newborn infants at approximately 6 weeks and is familial. Infants present with projectile vomiting, and an epigastric mass feeling like an olive or walnut can be palpated in the majority of patients. Sometimes marked gastric peristalsis can be seen visibly on the abdominal wall. In clinically obvious cases ultrasound or barium examinations are generally not necessary. It is in the more difficult equivocal cases, where no mass can be palpated, that imaging is requested.[2-12]

Technique of ultrasound examination

The baby may have a nasogastric tube draining the stomach, or have been vomiting severely, in which case the stomach will be empty. It is useful to be able to give the baby clear fluid, and this can be done via the nasogastric tube or with a bottle. The clear fluid will fill the gastric antrum so that it can be used as an acoustic window for the pylorus. Secondly, an assessment can be made of whether any fluid is passing through the pylorus into the duodenum. Normally fluid can be seen to pass through the pylorus and into the duodenum without delay (Fig. 6.5).

Begin with the patient in the supine position, using a high frequency 15L8 MHz linear transducer.

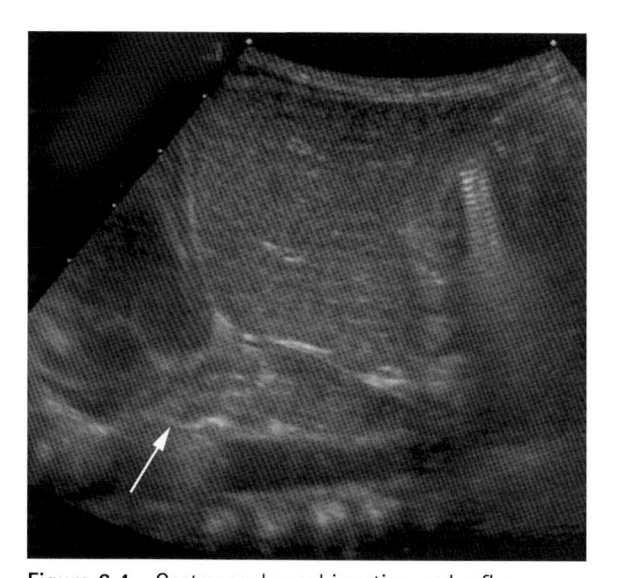

Figure 6.4 Gastroesophageal junction and reflux. Longitudinal sonogram to the left of the aorta. This shows air and food refluxing into the lower esophagus (arrow).

A

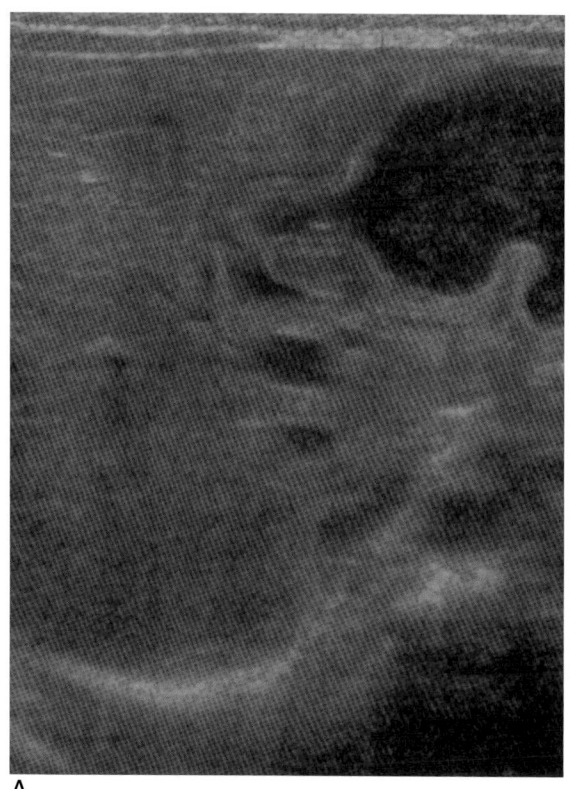

Figure 6.5 Normal pylorus. (A), (B) and (C) Transverse sonograms at the level of the pylorus. The patient has been given clear fluid in order to delineate the antrum and to observe fluid movement through the pylorus. The normal pylorus actively peristalses and fluid passes into the duodenum with ease. This is a good view to obtain when looking for pyloric stenosis.

Continued

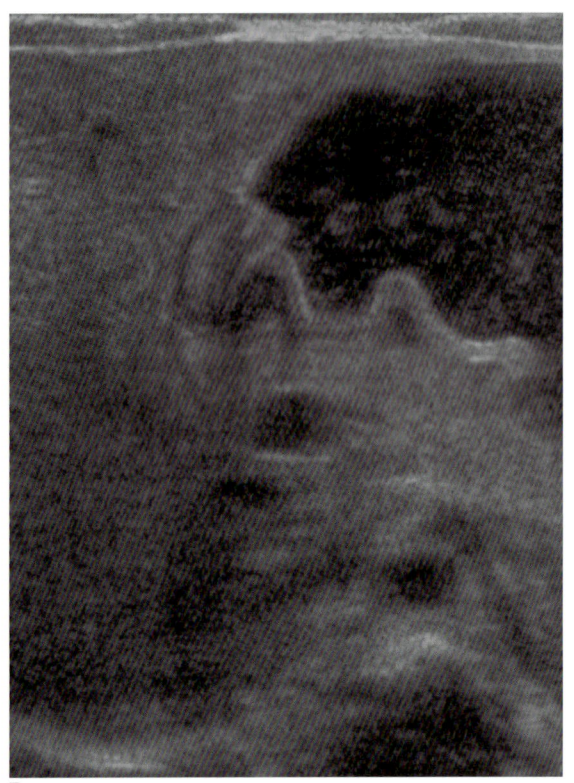

B

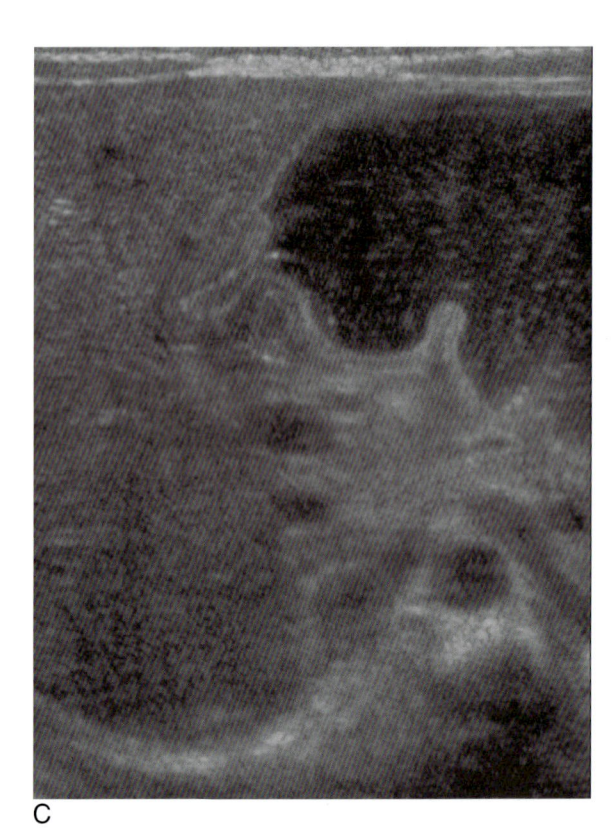

C

Figure 6.5, cont'd

If there is insufficient fluid in the stomach then fluid should be given. Be careful however not to overfill the stomach and provoke a further bout of vomiting. A very full stomach may also distort the antrum, making the pylorus difficult to see.

Start by scanning longitudinally in the right upper quadrant just medial to the gallbladder. Once the 'doughnut' of the transverse section through the hypertrophic pyloric stenosis is identified, pivot on the axis through 90° to get the longitudinal measurement. The trick in the transverse view is to identify the gastric antrum and, if the abdomen is too gassy, turn the infant right side down in order to displace gas and fill the antrum with fluid. The appearances to look for are the hypoechoic thickening of the pyloric muscle and elongation of the canal. Table 6.1 gives the published data for measurements of the canal in different series. Virtually no authors are in entire agreement, which makes remembering the measurements even more difficult! Broadly speaking, keep in mind 10 mm × 15 mm, i.e. take a pyloric length of over 15 mm and an overall width of 10 mm as abnormal in an average weight for term baby. These measurements are a slight overestimation but easily remembered. In the many series in

Table 6.1 Sonographic measurements of pyloric stenosis

Reference	Year	Measurements
3	1988	Muscle thickness 4.8 ± 0.6 mm Canal length 21 ± 3 mm
8	1994	Muscle thickness 4–4.4 mm Canal length 11–15 mm
10	1998	Muscle thickness > 3 mm Canal length > 15 mm Pyloric diameter > 11 mm Pyloric volume > 12 ml

THE ABDOMEN AND BOWEL 187

the literature there is an overlap in measurements between the normal and abnormal pylorus. To the experienced eye, if the pylorus is abnormal it is easy to identify, often without any measurements at all (Fig. 6.6).

Other important features to look for are the double mucosal channel of the pylorus, excessive antral peristalsis, delayed or absent passage of fluid into the duodenum and GER. It is important to note these additional features, as pylorospasm may mimic hypertrophic pyloric stenosis and the sonographer may make a false-positive diagnosis.

Infants who are premature, small and underweight may have pyloric stenosis in the presence of measurements that are below those quoted in the series. Pyloric volume measurements have been reported although they are not widely used or accepted.

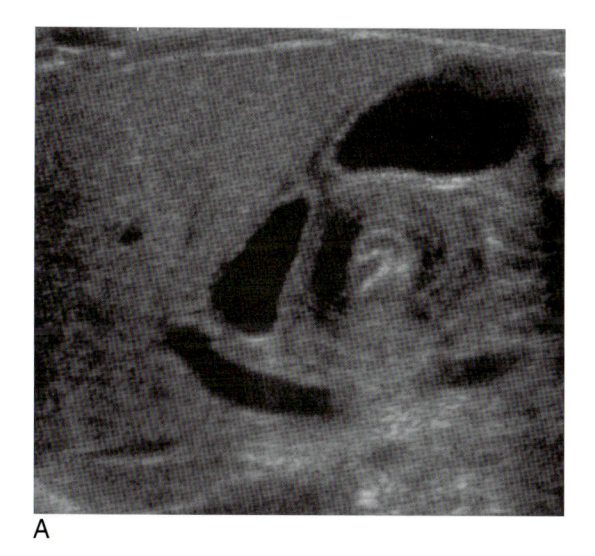

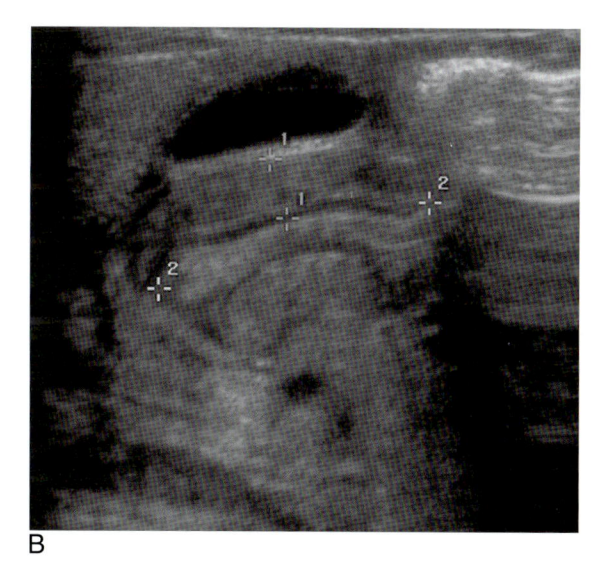

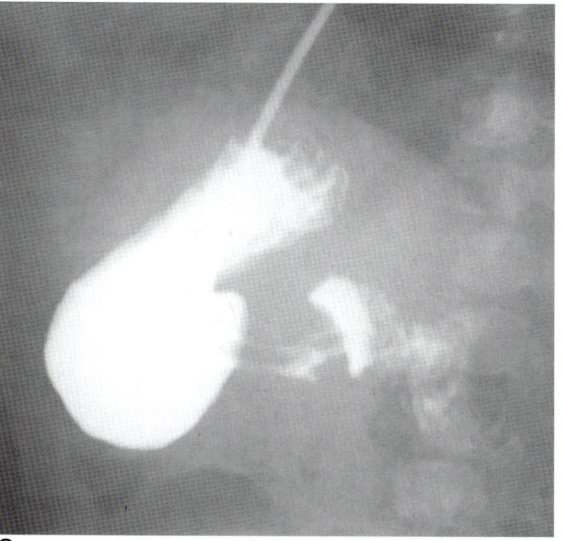

Figure 6.6 Pyloric stenosis. (A) Transverse sonogram of the pylorus in an infant with projectile vomiting and suspected of having pyloric stenosis. There is thickening of the pyloric muscle around the echogenic mucosa centrally. The gallbladder is draped over the top. (B) Longitudinal sonogram of the pyloric canal. There is marked thickening of the pyloric muscle (between calipers 1) and lengthening of the canal (between calipers 2). (C) Barium has been introduced into the stomach via a nasogastric tube. There was very active antral peristalsis and an elongated and narrowed pyloric canal. There is the typical double channel of pyloric stenosis with delay in gastric emptying because of the gastric outflow obstruction.

Stomach conditions

Pathologies involving the stomach are rare in childhood, and most are conventionally imaged using an upper gastrointestinal barium series. However, the stomach may be the site of some specific pathologies which are readily identified with ultrasound.

Thickening of the gastric mucosa or all of the stomach may be seen in a number of conditions. Lymphoma with infiltration of the bowel wall, while rare, is probably the commonest infiltrative disorder seen. Other causes such as chronic granulomatous disease (Fig. 6.7), and rarely Henoch–Schönlein purpura, and Crohn's disease may also cause thickening of the gastric wall.

Tumors of the stomach are also extremely rare, and the commonest tumor seen in the pediatric

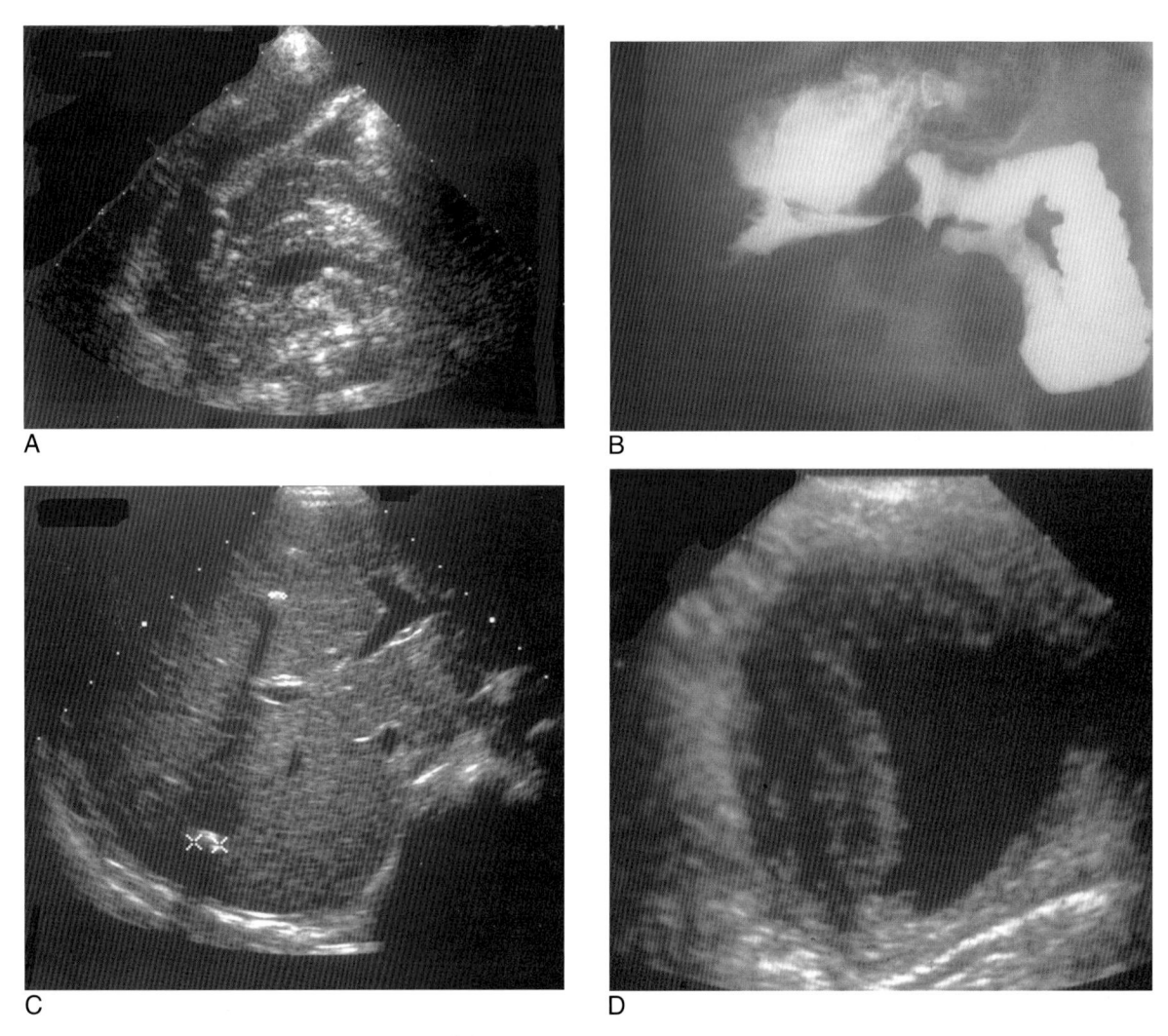

Figure 6.7 Chronic granulomatous disease. (A) Transverse sonogram of the antrum of the stomach in a child with chronic granulomatous disease. There is marked thickening of the stomach wall, particularly affecting the antrum. (B) Barium study on the same child showing the typical narrowing of the antrum of the stomach where the bowel wall has been infiltrated. (C) Longitudinal sonogram of the liver in the same child showing the multiple echogenic foci (between calipers) from chronic granulomas. (D) Longitudinal sonogram of the bladder showing the marked thickening of the bladder mucosa much like the wall of the antrum. This is pseudotumoral cystitis from the chronic granulomatous disease.

age group is the teratodermoid (Fig. 6.8). These teratodermoids appear the same as dermoids elsewhere in the abdomen and typically have a mixed echogenic appearance often containing fat, teeth and hair. Ectopic pancreatic tissue can also occur in the region of the antrum of the stomach and may be responsible for gastric outlet obstruction. Typically the pancreatic tissue lies in the wall of the stomach and produces a polypoid outpouching that may be responsible for gastric outlet obstruction (see Fig 5.26). It may also cause gastric bleeding.

Bezoars are a conglomerate mass of foreign material within the stomach. If they contain hair they are called trichobezoars, or lactobezoars if they are curds of milk in the young infant, or phytobezoars if they consist of vegetable matter. Hairs may accumulate in a girl's stomach from sucking ponytails, in a similar fashion to cats who may develop trichobezoars from grooming. Clinically these children may present with symptoms suggestive of gastric obstruction or ulceration. Ultrasonically a very echogenic mass may appear within the stomach, often casting a large acoustic shadow. Plain abdominal radiography is often diagnostic. Barium studies will show a large, generally gas-containing ball in the stomach outlined with barium.

Malrotation

Malrotation of the bowel occurs as a result of the abnormal positioning of the bowel in embryological life. The clinical history par excellence that should alert the sonographer to the diagnosis is bilious vomiting. The vomit is bilious because the obstruction is distal to the entry of the bile duct at the sphincter of Oddi. Typically this occurs in the neonatal period, and on plain film radiography the abdomen is described as being gasless with just a distended stomach and second part of the duodenum. Malrotation may occur on its own, in which case the sonographer should concentrate efforts on the orientation of the superior mesenteric artery and vein. When it is complicated by volvulus (i.e. twisting on the short mesentery around the superior mesenteric artery), ultrasound may show the so-called whirlpool sign which corresponds to the twisted ribbon on barium studies (Fig. 6.9). Malrotation complicated by volvulus is one of the pediatric surgical emergencies as the whole of the midgut may infarct as the bowel twists around and obstructs the blood flow in the superior mesenteric artery.[13–17]

In the presence of a good clinical history and no volvulus on ultrasound, the sonographer must look

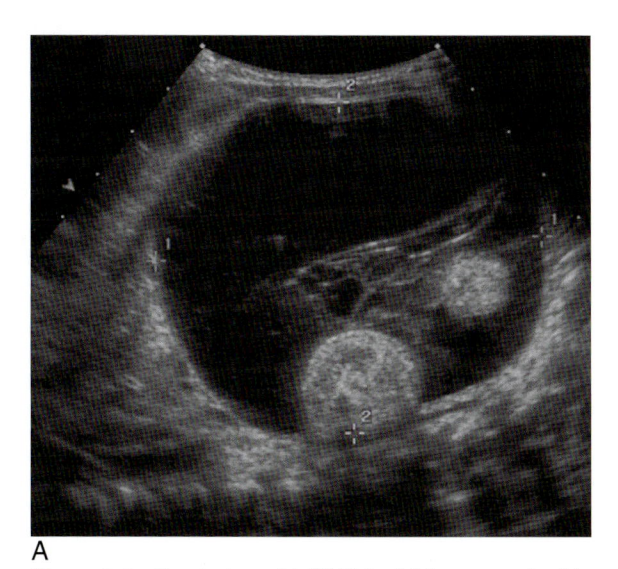

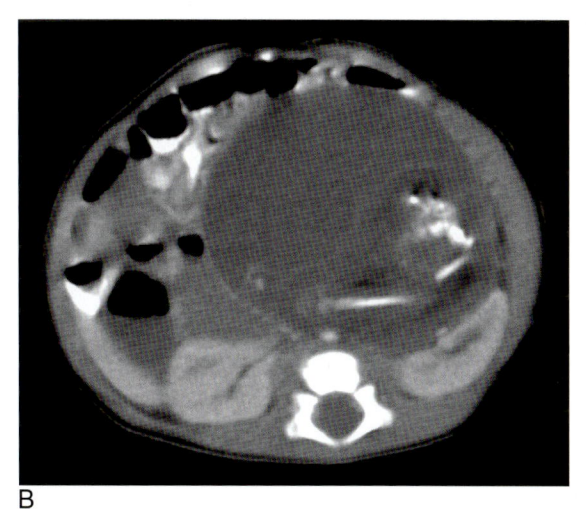

A B
Figure 6.8 Teratodermoid. (A) This child presented with an abdominal mass. Longitudinal ultrasound examination of the left flank revealed a well-defined mass with mixed cystic and highly echogenic areas of fat, hair and bone which is the typical appearance of a teratodermoid. (B) CT examination on the same child shows the mass which is also typical of a teratodermoid on CT.

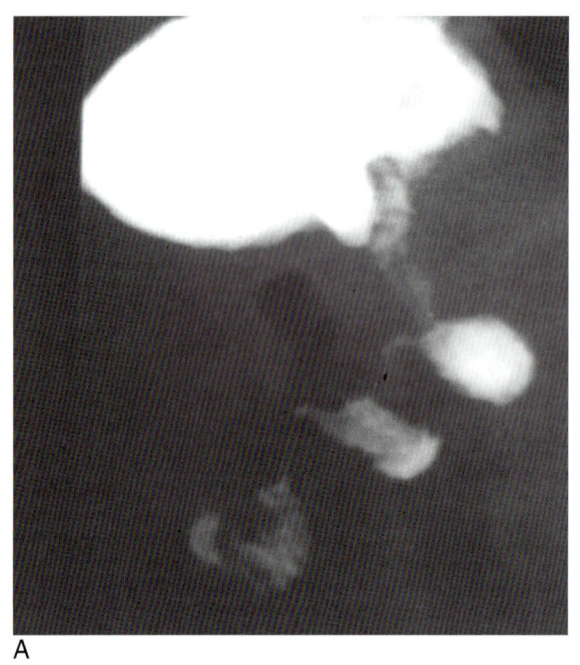

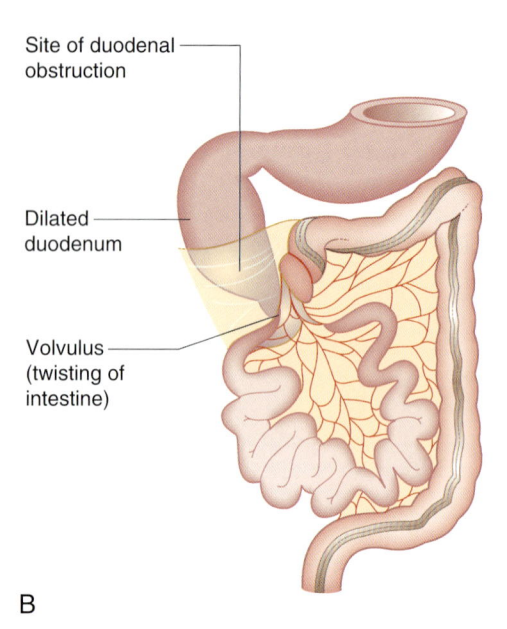

Figure 6.9 Malrotation and volvulus. (A) Barium study showing the typical twisted ribbon appearance of the proximal small bowel in malrotation and volvulus. (B) Line diagram showing the position of the bowel when malrotation and volvulus has occurred. The proximal duodenum is markedly dilated and partially obstructed. The bowel is twisted around the axis of the superior mesenteric artery. If the volvulus is severe the bowel will become ischemic and infarcted. This is a pediatric emergency.

for other abnormalities that may cause a gastric outlet obstruction, such as duodenal atresia, annular pancreas, duplication cysts or duodenal webs. Ladd bands are an abnormal process whereby the mesentery attempts to fixate the abnormally lying bowel. Opinions vary but surgeons do not generally consider that these abnormal peritoneal bands from the undersurface of the liver cause obstruction by themselves.

Technique of ultrasound examination

The patient should be lying supine. Using a linear transducer the superior mesenteric artery and vein are examined transversely. The vein normally lies immediately to the right of the artery (Fig. 6.10) but in malrotation may lie either anterior or to the left. Doppler should always be used in suspected volvulus examinations. The SMA and SMV should be followed down caudally because, if volvulus is associated, twisting will only be seen lower down to the root of these major vessels. Secondary signs such as an obstructed fluid-filled antrum and duodenum may also be seen.

While ultrasound can detect malrotation and volvulus it is not the examination of choice, and if either of these are suspected in any child, a barium study should be performed. This is one of the major pediatric surgical emergencies and if left untreated the consequences are fatal.

Enteric duplications

Duplications of the bowel may occur anywhere along the length of the gut. They are most frequently found in the ileum, although antral duplications and rectal duplications also occur.

Duplication cysts are thought to be due to the incomplete canalization of the bowel (Fig. 6.11). They may be silent and an incidental finding but may also present clinically with bowel obstruction, particularly if they occur in the antrum of the

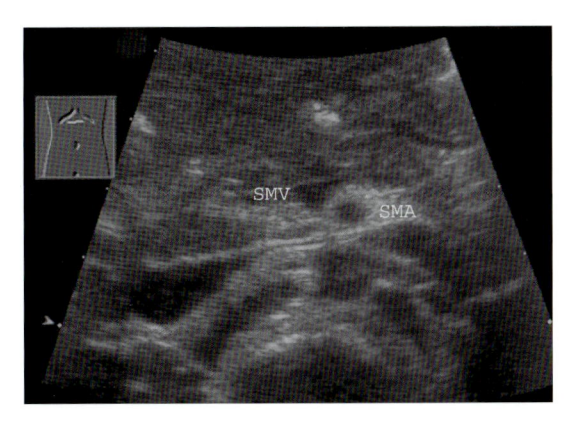

Figure 6.10 Normal SMA/SMV. The normal relationship of the superior mesenteric artery (SMA) and superior mesenteric vein (SMV) is that the vein is to the right of the artery. It is considered abnormal if the vein is in front of or to the left of the artery.

stomach. Many are now detected prenatally. A mass may be clinically palpable, and children may have symptoms related to bleeding and perforation if they contain gastric mucosa and ulcerate into the bowel lumen or peritoneal cavity. Duplication cysts are either sausage-shaped, long and tubular or rounded structures. The tubular duplications often communicate with the bowel and are more common in the lower gut and colon.

On ultrasound there are some specific features to look for such as an echogenic mucosa and a hypoechoic muscular layer which is only seen in duplication cysts (Fig. 6.12). Internal echoes are variable depending upon whether bleeding has taken place, but most are clear. Other cysts which may be confused with duplication cysts are, particularly, ovarian cysts. A choledochal cyst occurring in the region of the antrum of the stomach should also be considered, although this is sometimes associated with dilated bile ducts which will give the clue to the biliary origin. Less commonly, small mesenteric or omental cysts will appear similar, although these have no wall.[18,19]

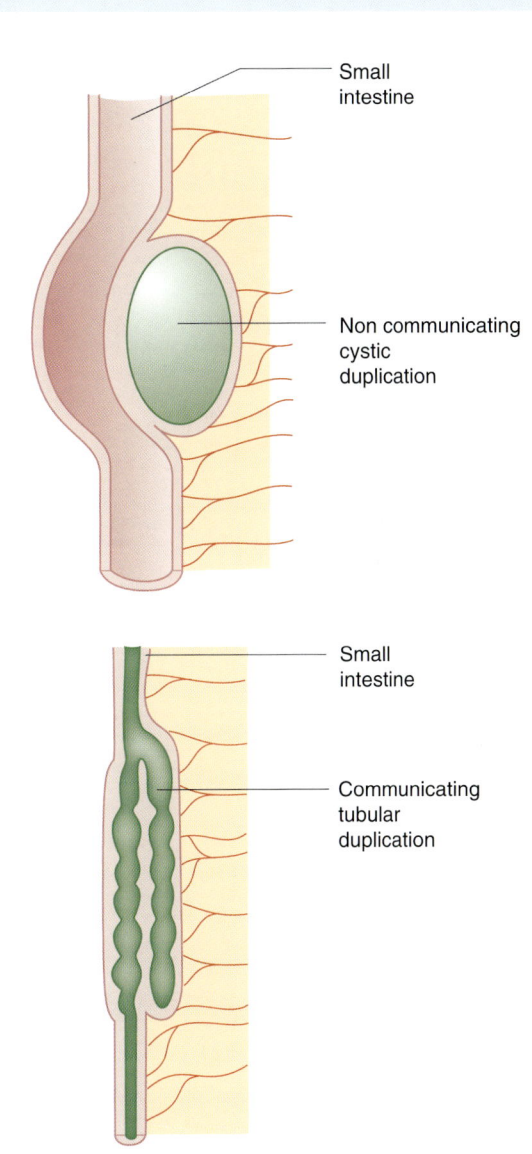

Figure 6.11 Duplication cysts of the bowel occur on the mesenteric border. Some are round and others tubular and they may or may not connect with the bowel lumen proper. They all have a clearly defined wall of mucosa and muscle which helps differentiate them from other cysts in the abdomen.

Intussusception

Intussusception occurs most commonly between the ages of 6 months and 3 years of age. A segment of bowel (usually ileum), the intussusceptum, telescopes into a more distal segment of bowel, the intussuscipiens. This is usually ileocolic but may also be ileo-ileocolic. Ultrasound is excellent in the diagnosis of intussusception, being up to 100% sensitive in some reported series. The incidence of intussusception is seasonal and related to mesenteric adenitis. In our practice ultrasound is the first

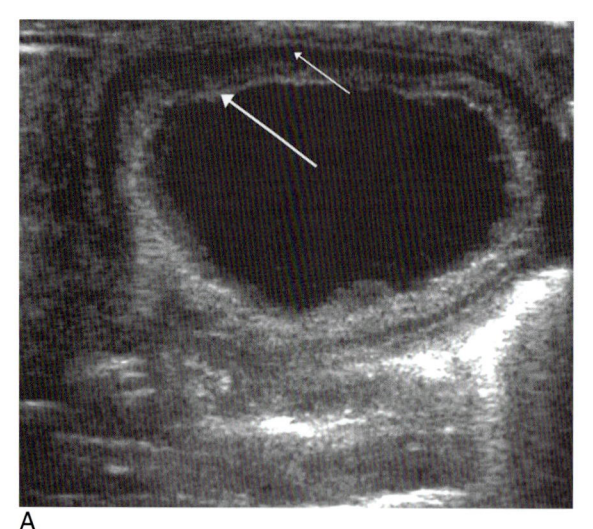

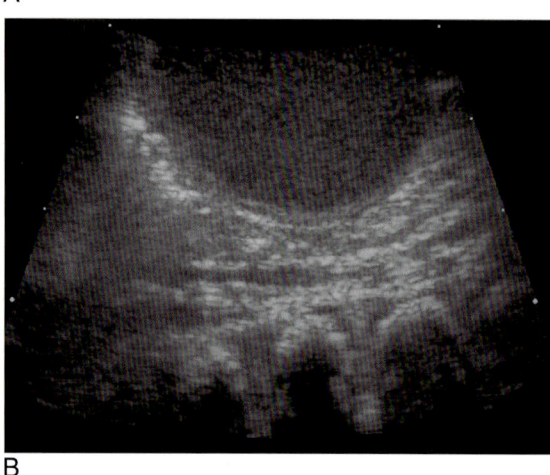

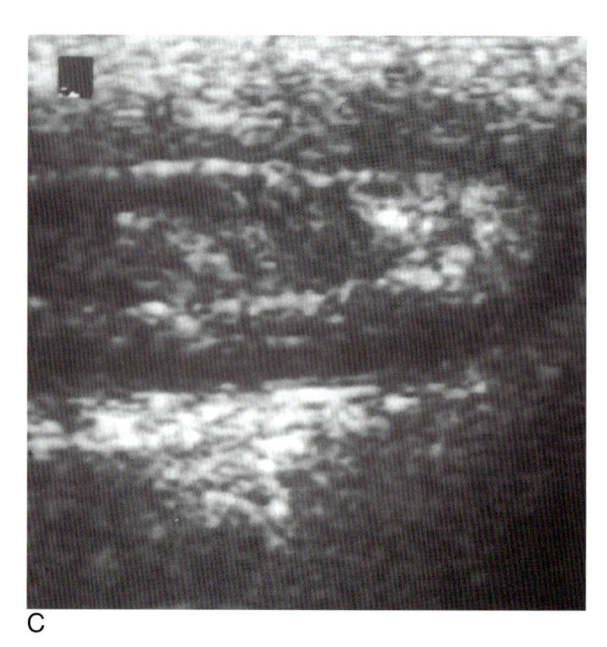

Figure 6.12 Duplication cysts. (A) Longitudinal scan of a cystic structure within the abdomen. The cyst has a well-defined muscle (short arrow) and mucosal layer (long arrow) which is typical of the appearances of a gut duplication cyst. (B) Magnified view of a duplication cyst anterior to the right kidney. There are multiple echoes within the cyst from hemorrhage. There is a clearly defined wall to this cyst. (C) Longitudinal sonogram of a right flank cyst. This duplication cyst is tubular in shape and contains multiple echoes from its communication with the bowel. These tubular bowel duplications occur more commonly in the large bowel.

investigation to confirm the diagnosis and assess viability before attempted air reduction.

If intussusception occurs outside the recognized age range, i.e. below 6 months and over 6 years of age, then lead points should be looked for. In the very young infant a Meckel diverticulum may intussuscept, and in the older child, lymphoma infiltrating the bowel wall is the commonest cause. There is an increased incidence of intussusception in children post-surgery with Peutz–Jaeger syndrome or with cystic fibrosis.

Children typically present with signs of intermittent obstruction and pain. Parents will describe drawing up the legs during attacks. A small percentage will have redcurrant jelly stool.

Technique of ultrasound examination

The child is examined supine and generally there is no specific preparation. Using a high frequency curvilinear probe, a careful initial preliminary examination of the whole of the abdomen should be performed. Attention should be focused on looking for a segment of solid-looking bowel which is non-peristaltic. The commonest site of the intussusception is in the region of the ascending and transverse colon underneath the liver, but the intussusceptions can occur anywhere along the route of the colon and, if severe, can even protrude from the rectum. Once the mass has been identified then the sonographer should change to a linear probe. Typical alternating hypo- and hyperechoic bands of mucosa and muscle can be seen. This has been described as the target, hamburger or doughnut appearance in cross section and as a pseudo-kidney in longitudinal section. Doppler examination should be used to evaluate the vascularity of the intussusceptum, as a poor vascularity may be associated with infarction of the bowel (Fig. 6.13). In addition, the presence of free fluid trapped between the colon and intussusceptum has been shown in several studies to be associated with a significantly lower success rate of reduction and with ischemia of the bowel. The presence of lymph nodes in the intussusceptum also reportedly reduces the success rate. Peritonitis is the one major contraindication to attempted reduction.

Intussusceptions are recognized to be intermittent, so that they may appear and disappear during the examination.

Occasionally diarrhea and vomiting may clinically mimic intussusception, and ultrasound has a role in excluding this diagnosis and thus avoiding an air enema.

The treatment of intussusception is to push the intussusceptum back, usually using air under pressure via a rectal catheter (Fig. 6.14). Reduction of the intussusception is generally performed in the prone position, as it is much easier to maintain a good seal of the tube in the rectum.

Ultrasound can be used to monitor pneumatic and hydrostatic reduction and has the advantage of not using radiation. However, reduction is sometimes a very rapid event, and most radiologists still feel more confident using fluoroscopy.[20-30]

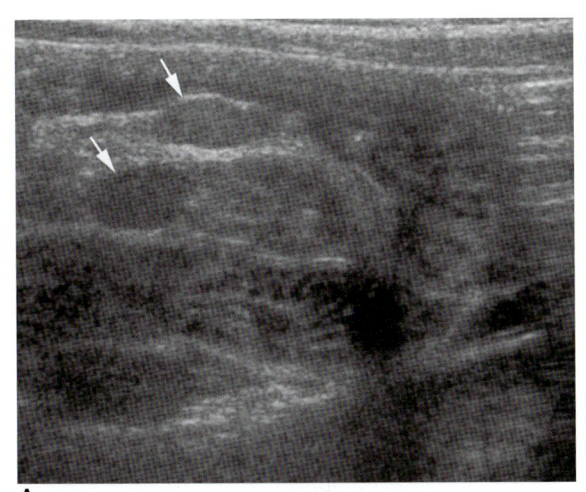

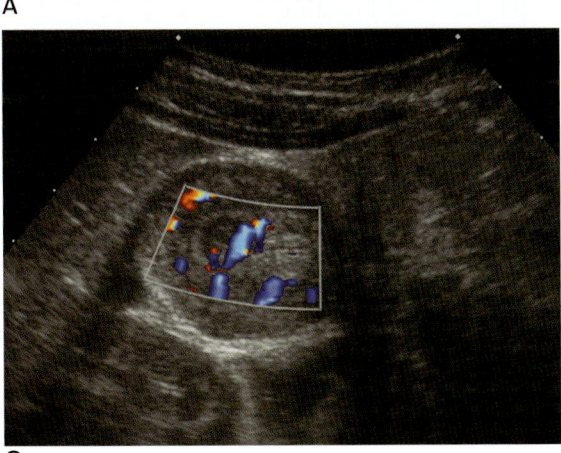

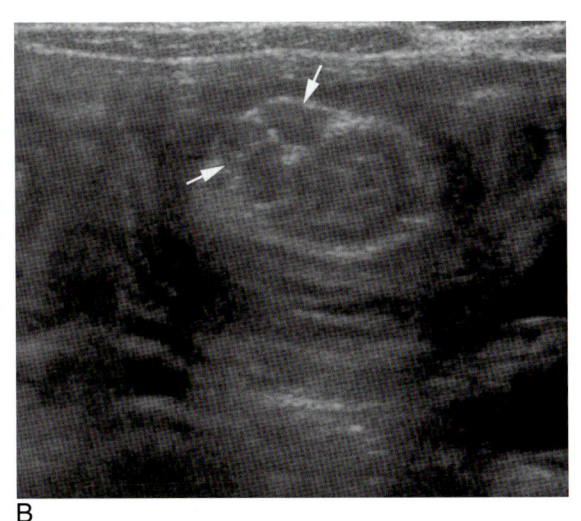

Figure 6.13 Intussusception. (A) Longitudinal sonogram of a child with the typical clinical presentation of intussusception. This is a longitudinal sonogram through the intussusception. There are multiple lymph nodes (arrows) in the intussusception. (B) Transverse sonogram of the intussusception showing the multiple lymph nodes (arrows) within the intussusception. If lymph nodes are seen within an intussusceptum it has been reported that it is more difficult to reduce the intussusception.
(C) Transverse sonogram of an intussusception showing the color flow within the intussusceptum. This indicates that the intussusception is still viable. When no color flow is seen on Doppler, suspicion must be raised that the intussusception is no longer viable and the risk of perforation is high.

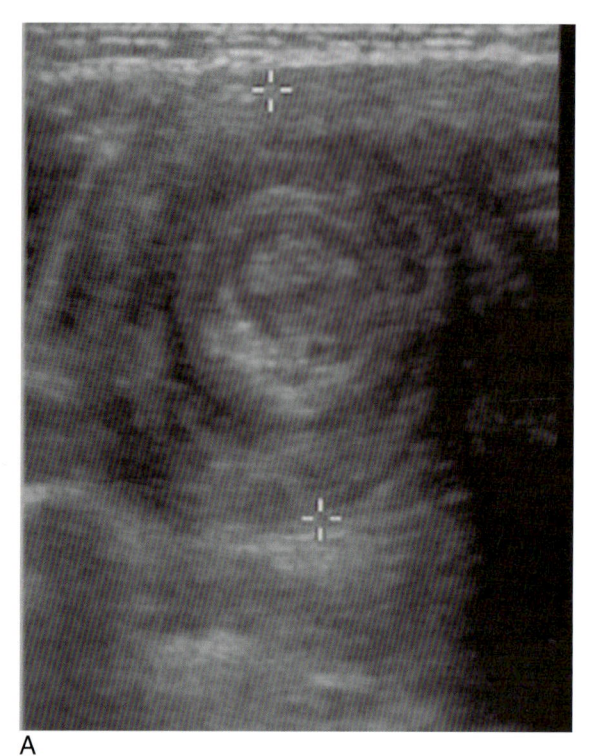

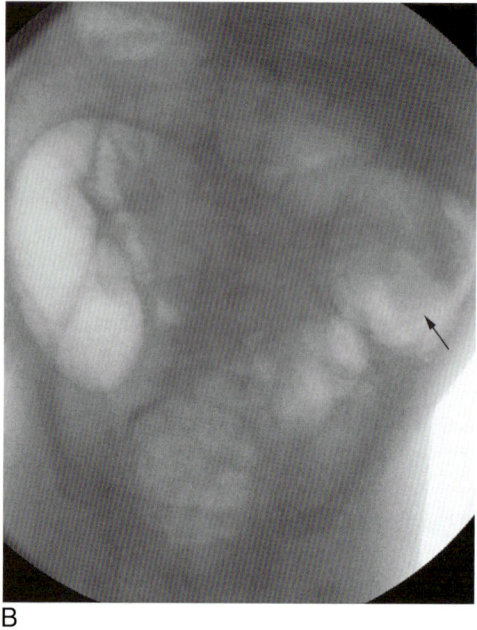

Figure 6.14 Air enema. The air enema is now the routine method for reduction of intussusception in many centers. Air is introduced into the rectum, and the intussusception is pushed back by this pressure of air. (A) Sonogram showing the intussusception (between calipers) in transverse section. (B) Air enema showing the intussusception is in the splenic flexure (arrow).

Appendicitis

Appendicitis is one of the common pediatric emergencies, occurring primarily in late childhood. While the clinical diagnosis may be straightforward in some cases, there are many other causes of an acute abdomen. Ultrasound is an excellent technique to aid diagnostic accuracy in the acute abdomen both to visualize the inflamed appendix and to exclude other conditions that may mimic appendicitis.

Typically in acute appendicitis the child will present clinically with initial periumbilical pain which moves to the right iliac fossa and with exquisite tenderness over the inflamed appendix.

Normal anatomy and technique of ultrasound examination

To the inexperienced sonographer the appendix may be difficult to identify. Practice and experience are essential, and with modern high resolution ultrasound scanners it is reported that the appendix is identifiable in most patients. However, the success rate for identifying the appendix varies widely in the reported literature and very much depends on the expertise of the sonographer.[31]

The normal appendix is a small tubular structure measuring no more than 7 mm in diameter and is easily compressible. It may contain air or fecal material as seen in the proximal bowel. There should be no fatty echogenic mesentery around the appendix. The normal appendix can be differentiated from small bowel by the absence of peristalsis, and it does not change its appearance over time. It should be distinguishable from ascending colon by its size. In children it is easier to visualize the normal appendix undergoing graded compression than in adults because the transducer is smaller and hence closer to the region of interest.

Technique The patient should preferably have a moderately full bladder and the examination started with a high frequency 7 MHz linear or curved array probe. First the whole of the abdomen should be carefully examined for pathology that may also present as an acute abdomen, and the normality of the liver, spleen, kidneys and pelvis confirmed. In particular subphrenic or pelvic collections should be excluded.

The main differential diagnoses to look for and exclude in children are: renal abnormalities, ovarian cysts, intussusception, inflammatory bowel disease and mesenteric lymphadenitis.

Then using a technique of what is called 'graded compression', start scanning over the right iliac fossa at the point of maximum tenderness (generally the site of the inflamed appendix). By gently and progressively compressing over the area, the surrounding bowel is displaced and the compressibility of the appendix assessed. Measurements of the appendix should be taken and should not be more than 6–7 mm. If the appendix is retrocecal, a lateral and posterior approach should be used.

The diagnosis of appendicitis lies in the identification of an abnormal inflamed appendix.

Box 6.1 Features of appendicitis

- The inflamed appendix is non-compressible
- The diameter of the appendix is over 6 mm and may even be up to 20 mm
- The surrounding mesentery and omentum become highly echogenic
- In 30% of cases a fecolith may be identified
- The appendix may have an irregular outline, and the bowel wall layers are not easily identified
- If the appendix is perforated there may be an associated pelvic mass which, in a female, usually accumulates in the pouch of Douglas
- On Doppler examination there is a marked increase in vascularity
- Enlarged lymph nodes may be noted within the abdomen
- An ileus may be present showing non-peristaltic fluid-filled loops of bowel
- There may be a para-appendiceal abscess and collection of pus

---

The abnormal appendix

Box 6.1 lists features to look for in appendicitis. Diagnostic accuracy is undoubtedly greatly improved if the sonographer is experienced. The presence of peritonitis and a rigid abdomen together with a large amount of gas in the bowel may make it difficult to scan and may obscure the inflamed appendix. The whole of the appendix should always be identified (Fig. 6.15). The appendix may have a thickened wall due to other conditions such as inflammatory bowel disease.[32-49]

Appendicoliths An appendicolith (a stone in the appendix) appears as an echogenic focus with acoustic shadowing. Appendicoliths vary in shape and size and may be seen within the lumen of the appendix or surrounded by an abscess after perforation, without the normal appendix landmarks (Fig. 6.16).

Abscesses When the appendix ruptures there may be a loculated collection of pus which is usually localized to the right iliac fossa or pelvis. Typically they may compress adjacent structures and have a mixed echogenicity. When there is free intraperitoneal fluid this may conform to the recesses in the peritoneum (Fig. 6.17).

A collection may also occur around the appendix which will be ill defined and may be associated with thickening of the adjacent bowel. The bowel loops in close proximity to the appendix may appear non-peristaltic. There may be pockets of fluid between the bowel loops.

Pericecal echogenicity Inflamed mesentery or omental fat may appear as an area of increased echogenicity around the cecum. This is a reliable finding and can be found in over 50% of children with appendicitis. It may also be seen in such other conditions as inflammatory colitis.

CT can provide further valuable information, but its routine use in children is controversial as the radiation dose is not insignificant. In Europe the diagnosis is generally made with ultrasound alone, and CT reserved for the more difficult, complex cases.

196 PEDIATRIC ULTRASOUND

A

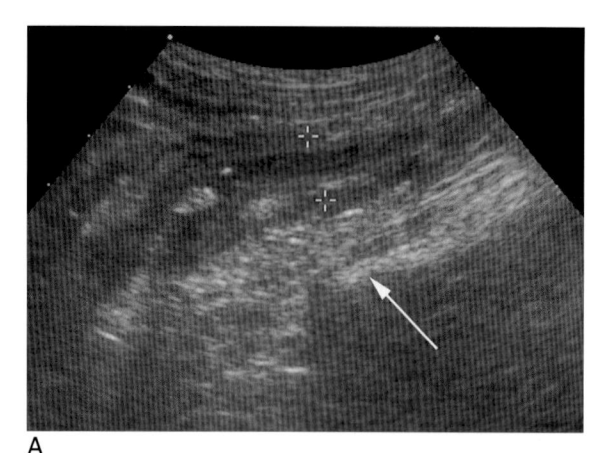

Figure 6.15 Appendicitis. (A) & (B) Longitudinal and transverse sonograms in a girl suspected of having appendicitis. There is an inflamed appendix (between calipers) in the right iliac fossa measuring over 1 cm and echogenic material within the appendix. It stands out in the echogenic inflamed omentum (arrow) surrounding it.

B

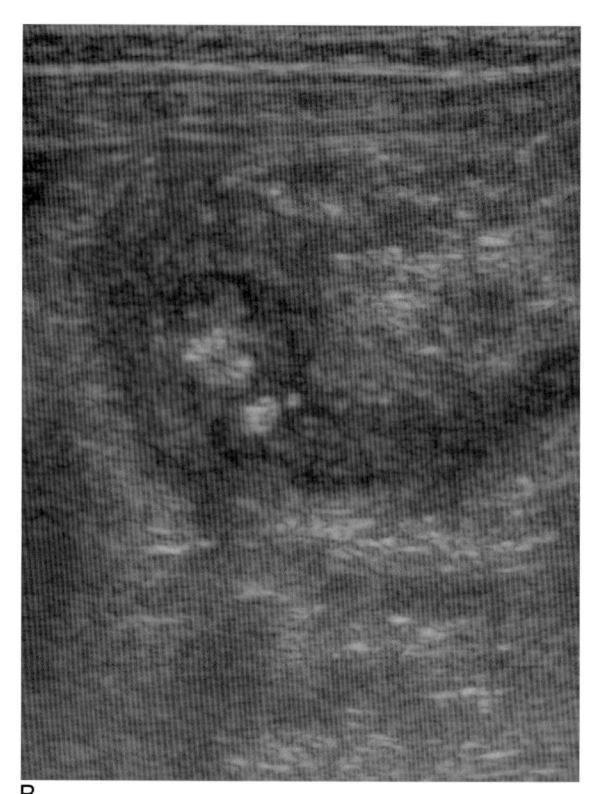

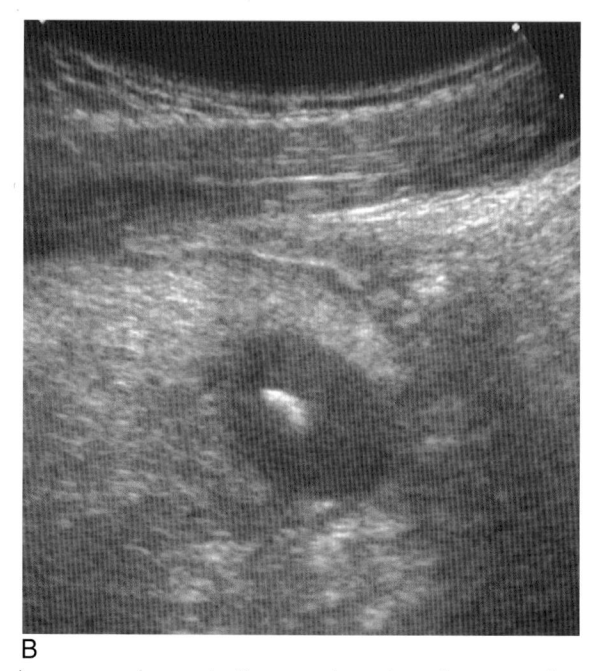

A B

Figure 6.16 Appendicitis and appendicolith. (A) Longitudinal sonogram demonstrating an enlarged swollen appendix (between calipers). It measured over 10 mm and there was thickening of the wall. The very echogenic omentum surrounding the appendix is typical when inflamed. (B) There was a localized abscess associated with this inflamed appendix containing an appendicolith.

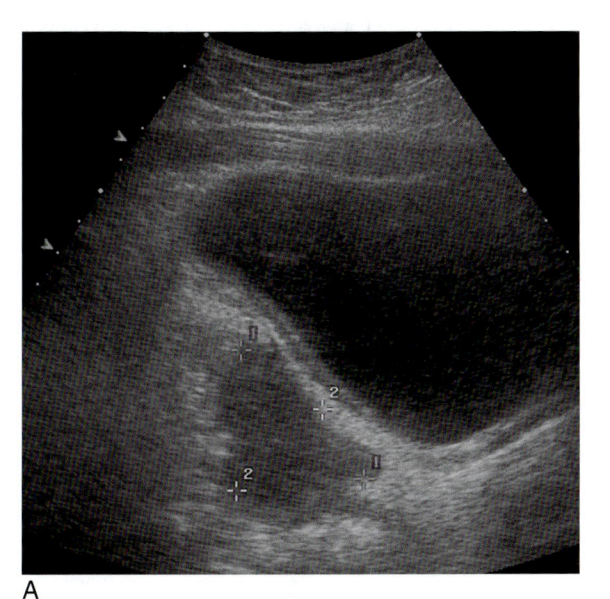

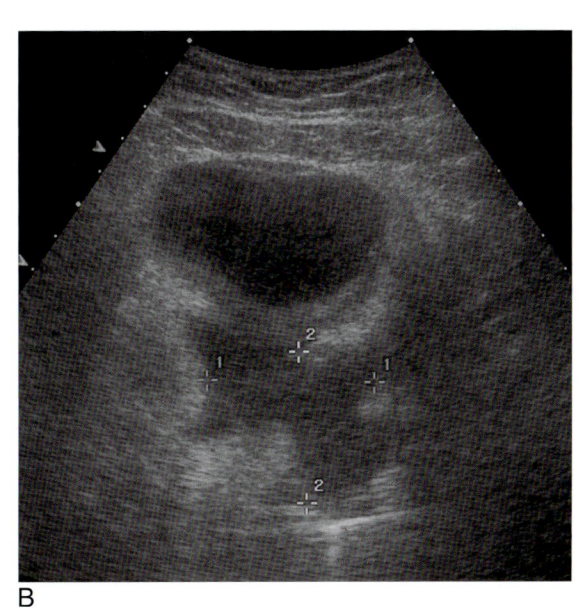

Figure 6.17 Appendix abscess. (A) & (B) Longitudinal and transverse scans of the pelvis in a boy with the typical clinical presentation of appendicitis. He has a large heterogeneous collection behind the bladder (between calipers) which is a result of his appendix rupturing. He was treated conservatively and recovered.

Mucocele A mucocele of the appendix is simply a collection of secretions within a chronically obstructed appendix. It may be a chance finding in a non-symptomatic patient. Ultrasonically a large fluid-filled sac-like structure will be identified in the right iliac fossa, often with a typical onion skin appearance. The treatment is surgery.

Solid appendix masses While rare, carcinoid tumors of the appendix can occur in children.

Bowel wall thickening/infiltrative disorders

The many causes of bowel wall thickening are listed in Table 6.2. Some additional helpful diagnostic features of each condition are also listed which can help narrow the differential diagnosis.[50–56]

Technique of ultrasound examination

No specific patient preparation is required. A high frequency linear probe 15L8 should be used to look at the bowel wall thickness and color flow within the wall. The distribution of the wall thickening should be assessed, and abnormalities elsewhere in the abdomen may be looked for to help identify the underlying diagnosis (see Table 6.2).

Bowel wall thickening can be suspected where measurement of the wall of the distended stomach, small or large bowel exceeds 3 mm. With measurements approaching 1 cm the observation can be made with certainty. The vascularity of the bowel wall may be increased (Fig. 6.18).

Anorectal anomalies

Anorectal anomalies are related to the embryologic development of the hindgut and include a wide range of disorders from an ectopic anus to a complete anorectal atresia. Anorectal atresias are classified as being either high, i.e. above the puborectalis muscle, or low, i.e. below the puborectalis sling. The importance of differentiating high or low anomalies lies in their treatment in that a high anomaly usually requires a colostomy and has an associated fistula whereas a low anomaly may simply require a cut-back from the anus to the low lying distal pouch.

Table 6.2 Causes of bowel wall thickening

Condition	Associated findings
Lymphoma	Bowel wall of low echogenicity and over 1 cm thick
	Mesenteric and para-aortic lymphadenopathy, hepatosplenomegaly
Crohn disease	Gallstones, mesenteric adenopathy
Necrotizing enterocolitis	Free fluid in abdomen
	Air seen within bowel wall
	Gas in portal vein and liver
Peptic ulcer disease	Ulcer crater demonstrated
Henoch–Schönlein purpura	Nephritis causes echogenic kidneys
	Hypervascular bowel wall seen on color flow imaging
Typhlitis	Seen in setting of chemotherapy-induced neutropenia
	Increased echogenicity of pericecal and appendix fat
Lymphangiectasia	Chylous ascites
	Chylous pleural effusions, lymphedema of a limb
	Mesentery very echogenic
Cystic fibrosis	Dilated bowel loops with echogenic contents
	Terminal ileum and cecal wall thickening result from therapy
Chronic granulomatous disease	Calcified hepatic and splenic granulomata, hepatosplenomegaly
	Gastric antrum wall most often affected
	Pseudotumoral cystitis in bladder

The use of ultrasound for determining whether these anomalies are high or low by measuring the distance from the skin surface to the distal colonic pouch has been reported. It is not used in routine clinical practice. The main role of ultrasound in children with these anomalies is to examine the renal tract, as there is a high association of anomalies of the kidneys, the commonest being single kidneys, cross-fused ectopia and vesicoureteric reflux. There is also an increased incidence of spinal abnormalities, so that all these children should routinely have both a renal and spinal ultrasound examination within the first 3 months of life.

Anorectal atresia

This is caused by an abnormal formation of the cloaca. There is a high, almost 100%, incidence of fistulas which usually occur to the posterior urethra in a male, or vagina or bladder in the female. These abnormalities form part of the VATER association.

Cystic abdominal masses

Cystic masses in the abdomen in children are not an uncommon finding. Diagnosis is not always easy, and Table 6.3 lists some of the more common cystic abdominal masses which have particular diagnostic features on ultrasound. The overlap among imaging features of cystic abdominal masses usually means that histology is necessary to make a diagnosis.

Mesenteric or omental cysts

The commonest type is a lymphangioma. This is a congenital malformation of the lymphatic vessels that occurs in the mesentery. It does not communicate with the small bowel lymphatics and results in a cystic mass. They are usually large, multiloculated and thin-walled. They may be intimately related with the bowel wall. Unusually they may hemorrhage into the mass. If very large they can fill the whole abdomen and may be mistaken for ascites. These cysts lie anterior to the bowel whereas ascites will accumulate around the kidneys and in the pelvis (Fig. 6.19).

THE ABDOMEN AND BOWEL   199

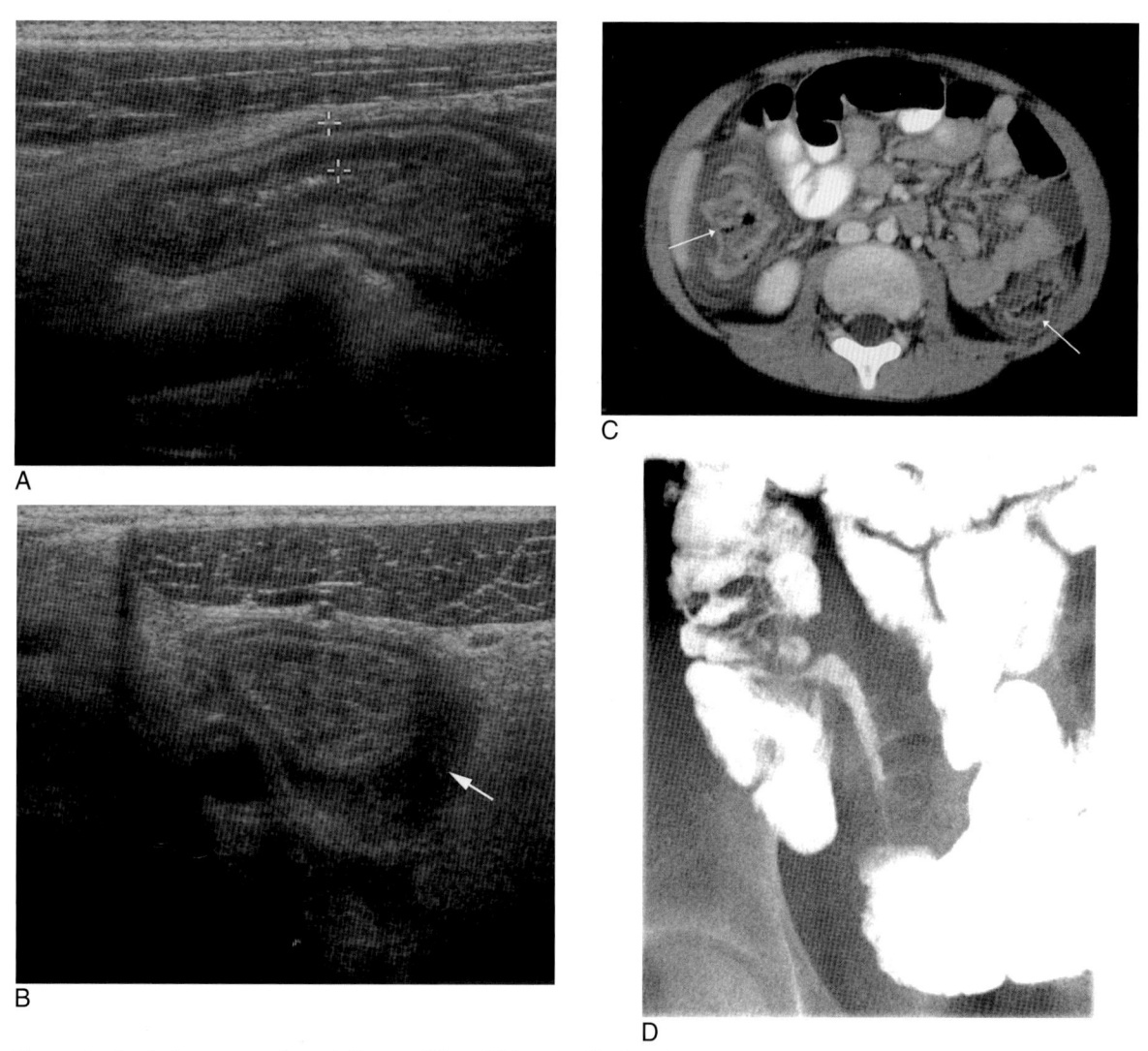

Figure 6.18 Inflammatory bowel disease. (A) & (B) Longitudinal and transverse sonogram of the bowel in the right iliac fossa. There is marked eccentric thickening of the bowel wall (arrow). This patient has inflammatory bowel disease. There were multiple areas of bowel wall thickening within the abdomen. (C) Contrast-enhanced CT examination just below the kidneys on the same child. There is marked thickening of the bowel wall, particularly in the right flank and left flank (arrows) with contrast enhancement. (D) Barium meal and follow-through examination demonstrating the marked narrowing and irregularity of the terminal ileum. This area corresponded to the abnormal bowel on ultrasound and on CT.

Non-pancreatic pseudocyst

These are cystic masses which are thought to be the sequelae of mesenteric or omental hematomas and are not related to pancreatitis. They are thick-walled, septated masses often with hemorrhagic contents. Often they may contain a fluid debris level.

MESENTERY, OMENTUM AND PERITONEUM

The peritoneal cavity is divided into different spaces by folds of peritoneum which in specific places become ligaments. The mesentery is a double layer of specialized peritoneum and connects

Table 6.3 Cystic abdominal masses

Diagnosis	Diagnostic features
Duplication cyst	Has a defined wall of echogenic mucosa and hypoechoic muscular wall. May be round or tubular and either be clear or contain internal echoes. Common situations are right iliac fossa or related to gastric antrum
Choledochal cyst	Related to head of pancreas and gastric antrum. May contain internal echoes of inspissated bile. No normal common bile duct demonstrated. May have dilated intrahepatic bile ducts
Ovarian cyst	May be situated anywhere within the abdomen, the so-called 'wandering tumor'. Wall not clearly defined. Typically has fluid debris level which changes on position of patient. Clumps of calcified hemorrhage may be detected internally or may be a clear cyst. Usually neonate. Occasionally bilateral
Mesenteric or omental cyst	Lies anteriorly within the abdomen compressing the bowel posteriorly. May be single large or multiple cysts. Thin internal septations (cyst wall). Wall identified by ultrasound. Sometimes mistaken for ascites
Cystic teratoma	May be found anywhere in the abdomen. May have solid components with very echogenic and calcified areas of fat and hair
Urinoma	May be large, displacing the kidney. In male infants posterior urethral valve should be excluded. Check for thick-walled bladder
Pancreatic pseudocyst	Collection predominantly related to pancreas but may occur anywhere. Irregular wall. Dilated pancreatic duct

the small bowel and colon to the posterior abdominal wall. The omentum is also a fold of peritoneum and it lies along the curvatures of the stomach. Peritoneum that covers the abdominal wall is called the parietal peritoneum, and peritoneum that covers the bowel and abdominal organs is called the visceral peritoneum.

During intrauterine development some of the bowel fuses to the dorsal body wall and becomes retroperitoneal, so that ultimately the duodenum, ascending and descending portions of the colon lie behind the peritoneum. The transverse colon and the sigmoid colon remain free.

The lesser omentum has two layers and connects the lesser curvature of the stomach to the liver via the hepatogastric ligament. It also attaches the liver to the duodenum via the hepatoduodenal ligament. The falciform ligament extends from the liver to the ventral abdominal wall and can be seen on ultrasound when ascites is present. The greater omentum has four layers of peritoneum and attaches to the greater curvature of the stomach and extends down to the colon. It also attaches via the gastrosplenic ligament to the hilum of the spleen.

The liver has a triangular area where it is not covered by the peritoneum, called the bare area.

The peritoneal cavity is divided into a number of spaces. Fluid can collect in these spaces and their positions need to be recognized by the sonographer.

The transverse colon separates the abdominal cavity into the supra- and infracolic compartments. The supracolic compartment is then further divided into the spaces around the liver and spleen called the perihepatic and perisplenic spaces. Morrison's pouch is an extension of the space around the liver and is the most dependent recess in the abdomen. It is also known as the subhepatic space. The lesser sac is a cavity bounded by the liver, stomach anteriorly, peritoneal reflections posteriorly, the hilum of the spleen to the left and the portocaval junction to the right. There is a communication to the lesser sac via the foramen of Winslow (Fig. 6.20).

Below the transverse colon the infracolic compartment can be divided into the left and right paracolic spaces (gutters), the lateral paravesical

THE ABDOMEN AND BOWEL   201

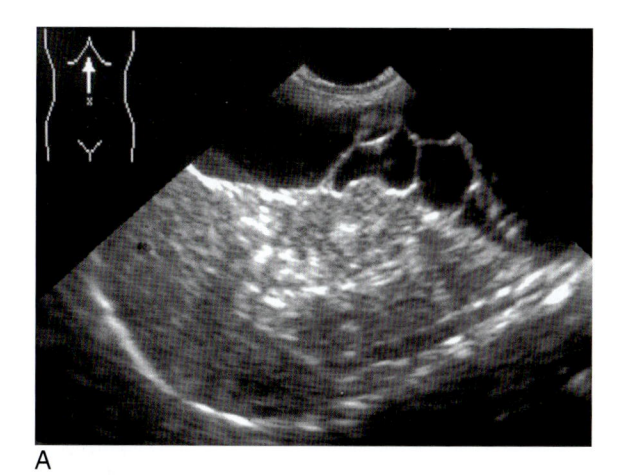

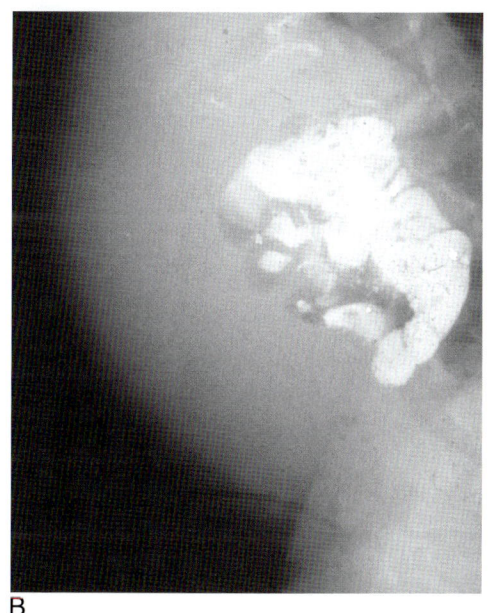

Figure 6.19 Mesenteric/omental cysts. (A) Longitudinal sonogram of the abdomen in a child presenting with an abdominal mass. There are multiple cysts located anteriorly in the abdomen with visible septations. The bowel is lying posteriorly. These are the typical appearances of omental cysts. (B) Barium study showing displacement of the gut posteriorly by the large omental cysts which were lying anterior in the abdomen. This is the classic position for omental cysts and they should not be mistaken for ascites.

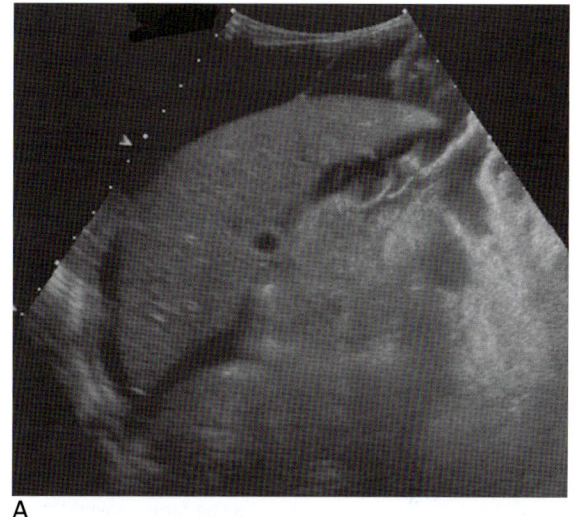

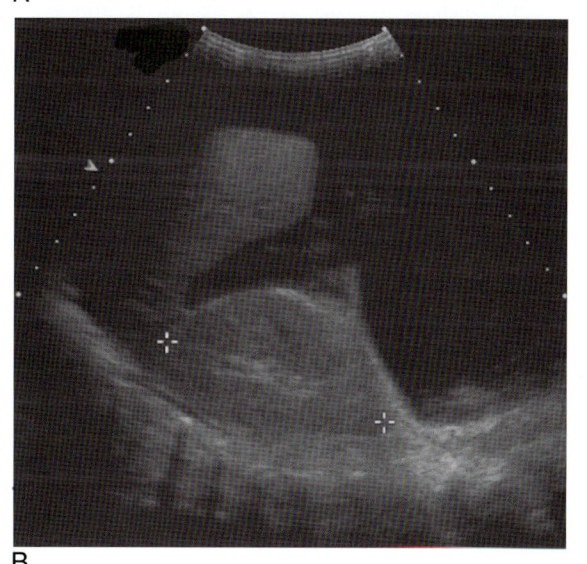

Figure 6.20 Perihepatic spaces. (A) Transverse sonogram of the liver in a child with a large amount of ascitic fluid in the abdomen. Notice the thin line of the ligamentum teres from the anterior surface of the liver. There is also fluid in the lesser sac and Morrison's pouch which is the most dependent portion next to the liver. (B) Longitudinal sonogram of the right kidney in the same child showing how the ascitic fluid collects anterior to the kidney, which is a retroperitoneal structure.

recesses on either side of the bladder, and the pouch of Douglas. The pouch of Douglas is midline and is the most dependent portion of this lower compartment in women. In men it is called the rectovesical space.

Peritoneal fluid

Peritoneal fluid can occasionally be seen in asymptomatic children. When present in larger quantities it generally accumulates in the most dependent recesses in the peritoneal cavity. Fluid initially accumulates in the pelvis behind the bladder, in the pouch of Douglas, and laterally in the paravesical recesses. The right and left paracolic spaces are the next most likely sites for fluid to collect. It is important to remember that the location of fluid collections in the abdomen does not always indicate where the fluid originated.

In the upper abdomen it is important for the sonographer to be able to differentiate between peritoneal fluid collections around the liver and spleen as opposed to pleural fluid. Pleural fluid collections are above the diaphragm and posterior to the crura.

Sometimes the sonographer can differentiate the different types of fluid collections within the abdomen, so that clear fluid such as urine is called urinary ascites, whereas blood and chyle may have an increased echogenicity with debris. Some collections of peritoneal fluid may become walled off by the mesentery and encysted and may behave as a cystic mass. This is not an uncommon finding in children treated with ventriculo-peritoneal shunts for hydrocephalus.

Infection

Generalized infection in the peritoneal cavity is known as peritonitis, whereas an abscess may be localized in the peritoneal cavity. Factors that affect whether the infection is generalized or localized depend on the site of infection and its association with the peritoneal sacs and gravity. In the infracolic compartment the commonest site of accumulation is in the pouch of Douglas and the commonest infection to cause this is a ruptured appendix. If the infecting organism is gas producing, then gas may be noted within the collection.

Peritonitis may be primary or secondary. Primary peritonitis is when the infecting organism is outside the abdominal cavity and is usually blood- or lymph-borne. Secondary peritonitis is secondary to a peritoneal origin such as an intraperitoneal abscess. Tuberculosis (TB) typically affects the mesentery and lies as an 'omental cake' anteriorly within the abdomen. This localized spread of infection is related to TB involving the lymph nodes.

Pneumoperitoneum is when free air is present in the peritoneal cavity, and this is usually related to a perforation of the bowel, post-surgery or from a pneumothorax tracking into the abdomen. In children a pneumoperitoneum can be seen for up to a week after surgery.

Free air rises to the top of the peritoneal cavity so that on erect radiographs it will lie underneath the diaphragms and on left decubitus views will come to lie underneath the liver. For sonographers scanning patients in the supine position it will be seen just underneath the anterior abdominal wall and generally anterior to the liver.

Trauma

After trauma fluid may be seen in the peritoneal cavity and is typically blood. Blood in the peritoneum is called a hemoperitoneum. If there is injury to the solid organs in the abdomen which extends beyond the capsule of the liver or spleen, at least 60% are associated with hemoperitoneum. CT is generally considered the examination of choice for any child suffering blunt abdominal trauma, particularly to delineate organ damage but also to demonstrate any intra-abdominal fluid collections. CT is also the superior modality when a bladder rupture is suspected. Contrast can be instilled into the bladder and with careful CT examination the site of leakage from the bladder demonstrated.

Mesenteric and omental abnormalities

Developmental abnormalities of the mesentery are generally related to malrotation of the bowel. In particular the mesentery between the duodeno-jejunal flexure and cecum may be shortened in children with malrotation, which will predispose them to volvulus. Abnormal peritoneal folds called Ladd's bands may also occur across the duodenum from the undersurface of the liver in malrotation. Other developmental defects in the mesentery may result in an internal herniation of the bowel. The bowel herniates through the hole in the mesentery and then accumulates in one of the peritoneal sacs. This may cause obstruction of the bowel.

If the lymph channels within the mesentery do not adequately develop, a lymphangioma may develop which is typically a multiseptated cystic mass.

Children generally have very little omental or mesenteric fat, which makes them good candidates for ultrasound examinations. There may be an increase in the omental fat in lymphangiectasia, obesity, treatment with steroids and Cushing syndrome.

Mesenteric lymphadenopathy

Mesenteric lymphadenopathy is a common finding when examining the abdomen in children and is generally reactive. It can be found in the folds of the small bowel mesentery around the superior mesenteric artery and vein and in the arteries supplying the jejunum and ileum. They are normally less than 5 mm in diameter (Figs 6.21 and 6.22).

Infections

Infections usually result in mesenteric lymphadenopathy. Children with immune disorders are particularly vulnerable to strange infections and lymphadenopathy. *Yersinia* enterocolitica or *Campylobacter* are particular infections which may give lymphadenopathy and bowel wall thickening. One of the most useful features to look for in appendicitis is an increased echogenicity of the peri-appendiceal mesentery.

Neoplasms

Primary neoplasms of the peritoneal cavity are rare. Most peritoneal involvement is metastatic spread and from tumor rupture. Wilms tumor is the commonest intra-abdominal solid tumor in which this occurs. Rupture of the tumor is either de novo through the capsule of the kidney or at the time of surgery.

Primary tumor involvement of the mesentery and omentum is mainly seen in lymphoma, which has a variety of different appearances. Lymphoma may infiltrate the bowel wall and mesentery or present as discrete rounded masses within the abdomen. Lymphomatous infiltration and masses are always hypoechoic. There is generally associated lymph node enlargement.

There are a number of other very rare tumors which may occur in the mesentery, the commonest of which is a fibroma.

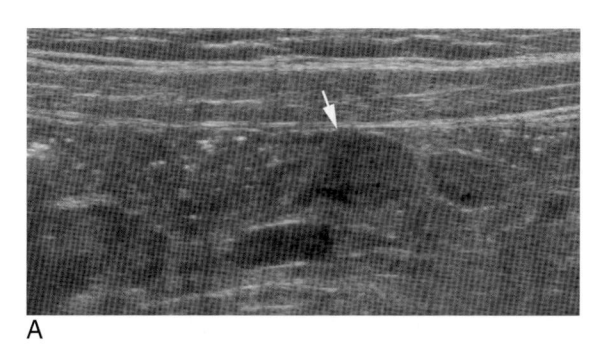

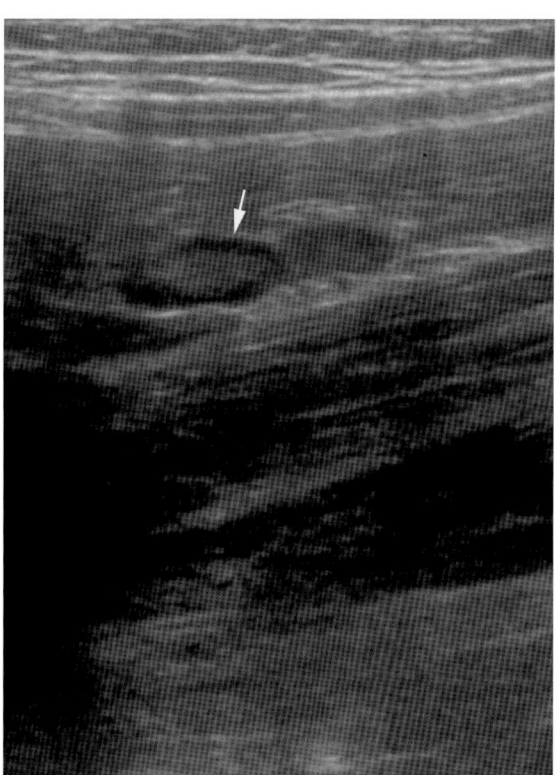

Figure 6.21 Mesenteric lymphadenopathy. (A) & (B) Two longitudinal scans in the right flank. There are multiple lymph nodes situated in the mesentery closely associated with the bowel (arrows). This is a common finding in children, in particular in association with intussusception.

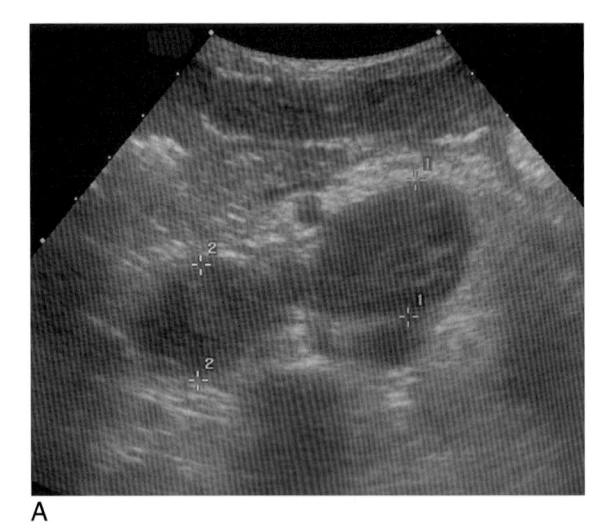

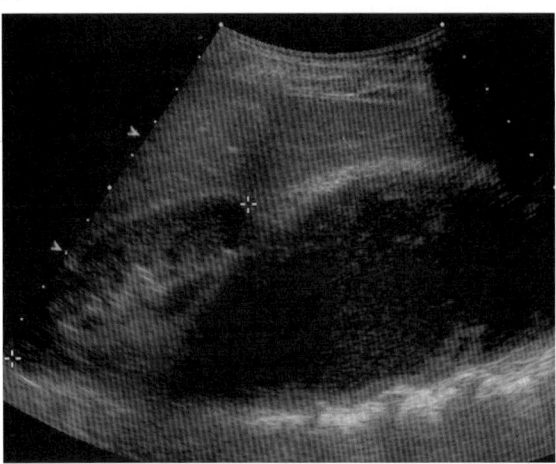

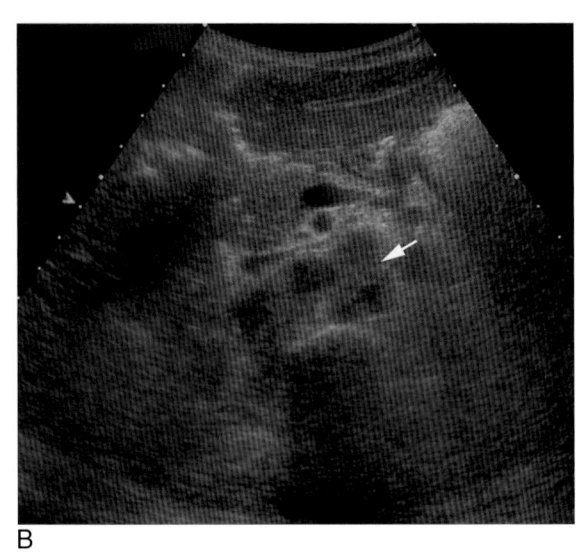

Figure 6.22 Lymphadenopathy in immune disorder and mycoplasma infection. (A) Transverse sonogram at the level of the superior mesentery artery. There is huge lymphadenopathy in the upper abdomen just anterior to the aorta and behind the superior mesenteric artery (nodes between calipers). This is a good position to look for upper abdominal lymphadenopathy. (B) Transverse sonogram at the same level 6 months later and after treatment. There are still lymph nodes in the upper abdomen but they are much smaller in size (arrow). (C) Longitudinal sonogram of the right kidney and flank. The right kidney is lying between the calipers. There is a large hypoechoic structure below the kidney which was a psoas abscess in this boy.

References

1. Hye Suk Jang, Joon Sung Lee, Gye Yeon Lim, et al. Correlation of color Doppler sonographic findings with pH measurements in gastro-oesophageal reflux in children. J Clin Ultrasound 2001; 29(4):212–217.
2. Bisset RAL, Gupta SC. Hypertrophic pyloric stenosis, ultrasonic appearances in a small baby. Pediatr Radiol 1988; 18:405.
3. Blumhagen JD, MacLin L, Krauter D, et al. Sonographic diagnosis of hypertrophic pyloric stenosis. AJR Am J Roentgenol 1988; 150:1367–1370.
4. Blumhagen JD, Noble HGS. Muscle thickness in hypertrophic pyloric stenosis: sonographic determination. AJR Am J Roentgenol 1983; 140:221–223.
5. Godbole P, Sprigg A, Dickson JA, et al. Ultrasound compared with clinical examination in infantile hypertrophic pyloric stenosis. Arch Dis Child 1996; 75:335–337.
6. Haider N, Spicer R, Grier D. Ultrasound diagnosis of infantile hypertrophic pyloric stenosis: determinants of pyloric length and the effect of prematurity. Clinical Radiol 2002; 57:136–139.
7. Haller JO, Cohen HL. Hypertrophic pyloric stenosis: diagnosis using US. Radiology 1986; 161:335–339.
8. Hernanz-Schulman M, Sells LL, Ambrosino MM, et al. Hypertrophic pyloric stenosis in the infant without a palpable olive: accuracy of sonographic diagnosis. Radiology 1994; 193:771–776.

9. Okorie NM, Dickson JAS, Carver RA, et al. What happens to the pylorus after pyloromyotomy? Arch Dis Child 1988; 63(11):1339–1341.
10. Rohrschneider WK, Mittnacht H, Darge K, et al. Pyloric muscle in asymptomatic infants: sonographic evaluation and discrimination from idiopathic hypertrophic pyloric stenosis. Pediatr Radiol 1998; 28(6):429–434.
11. Sargent SK, Foote SL, Mooney DP, et al. The posterior approach to pyloric sonography. Paediatr Radiol 2000; 30(4):256.
12. Teele RL, Smith EH. Ultrasound on the diagnosis of idiopathic hypertrophic pyloric stenosis. N Engl J Med 1977; 296:1149–1150.
13. Zerin JM, DiPietro MA. Superior mesenteric vascular anatomy at US in patients with surgically proved malrotation of the midgut. Radiology 1992; 183:693–694.
14. Smet MH, Marchal G, Ceulemans R, et al. The solitary hyperdynamic pulsating superior mesenteric artery: an additional dynamic sonographic feature of midgut volvulus. Pediatr Radiol 1991; 21:156–157.
15. Loyer E, Eggli KD. Sonographic evaluation of superior mesenteric vascular relationship in malrotation. Pediatr Radiol 1989; 19:173–175.
16. Leonidas JC, Magid N, Soberman N, et al. Midgut volvulus in infants: diagnosis with US. Radiology 1991, 179:491–493.
17. Hayden CK Jr, Boulden TF, Swischuk LE, et al. Sonographic demonstration of duodenal obstruction with midgut volvulus. AJR Am J Roentgenol 1984; 143:9–10.
18. Barr LL, Hayden CK Jr, Stansberry SD, et al. Enteric duplication cysts in children: are their ultrasonographic wall characteristics diagnostic? Pediatr Radiol 1990; 20:326–328.
19. Macpherson RI. Gastrointestinal tract duplications: clinical, pathologic, etiologic, and radiologic considerations. Radiographics 1993; 13:1063–1080.
20. Bowerman RA, Silver TM, Jaffe MH. Real-time ultrasound diagnosis of intussusception in children. Radiology 1982; 143:527–529.
21. Britton I, Wilkinson AG. Ultrasound features of intussusception predicting outcome of air enema. Paediatr Radiol 1999; 29(9):705–710.
22. Del-Pozo G, Gonzalez-Spinola J, Gomez-Arison B, et al. Intussusception: trapped peritoneal fluid detected with US – relationship to reducibility and ischaemia. Radiology 1996; 201(2):379–383.
23. Hadidi AT, El-Shal N. Childhood intussusception: a comparative study of nonsurgical management. J Pediatr Surg 1999; 34(2):304–307.
24. Hanquinet S, Anooshiravani M, Vunda A, et al. Reliability of colour Doppler and power Doppler sonography in the evaluation of intussuscepted bowel viability. Paediatr Surg Int 1998; 13(5–6):360–362.
25. Hu SC, Feeney MS, McNicholas M, et al. Ultrasonography to diagnose and exclude intussusception in Henoch–Schönlein purpura. Arch Dis Child 1991; 66(9):1065–1067.
26. Kenney IJ. Ultrasound in intussusception: a false cystic lead point. Pediatr Radiol 1990; 20(5):348.
27. Martinez-Frontanilla LA, Silverman L, Meagher DP Jr. Intussusception in Henoch–Schönlein purpura: diagnosis with ultrasound. J Pediatr Surg 1988; 23:375–376.
28. Stanley A, Logan H, Bate TW, et al. Ultrasound in the diagnosis and exclusion of intussusception. Ir Med J 1997; 90(2):64–65.
29. Stringer MD, Capps SN, Pablot SM. Sonographic detection of the lead point in intussusception. Arch Dis Child 1992; 67(4):529–530.
30. Tiao MM, Wan YL, Ng SH, et al. Sonographic features of small bowel intussusception in pediatric patients. Acad Emerg Med 2001; 8(4):368–373.
31. Sivit CJ, Applegate KE, Stallion A, et al. Imaging evaluation of suspected appendicitis in a pediatric population: effectiveness of sonography versus CT. AJR Am J Roentgenol 2000; 175(4):977–980.
32. Abu-Yousef MM, Bleicher JJ, Maher JW, et al. High-resolution sonography of acute appendicitis. AJR Am J Roentgenol 1987; 149:53–58.
33. Agha FP, Ghahremani GG, Panella JS, et al. Appendicitis as the initial manifestation of Crohn's disease: radiologic features and prognosis. AJR Am J Roentgenol 1987; 149:515–518.
34. Baker DE, Silver TM, Coran AG, et al. Postappendectomy fluid collections in children: incidence, nature and evolution evaluated using US. Radiology 1986; 161:341–344.
35. Borushok KF, Jeffrey RB Jr, Laing FC, et al. Sonographic diagnosis of perforation in patients with acute appendicitis. AJR Am J Roentgenol 1990; 154:275–279.
36. Ceres L, Alonso I, Lopez P, et al. Ultrasound study of acute appendicitis in children with emphasis upon the diagnosis of retrocecal appendicitis. Pediatr Radiol 1990; 20(4):258–261.
37. Douglas CD, Macpherson NE, Davidson PM, et al. Randomised controlled trial of ultrasonography in diagnosis of acute appendicitis, incorporating the Alvarado score. Br Med J 321; 919.
38. Garcia Peña BM, Mandl KD, Kraus SJ, et al. Ultrasonography and limited computed tomography

in the diagnosis and management of appendicitis in children. J Am Med Assoc 1999; 282(11):1041.
39. Hahn HB, Hoepner FU, Kalle T, et al. Sonography of acute appendicitis in children: 7 years experience. Pediatr Radiol 1998; 28(3):147–151.
40. Hayden CK Jr, Kuchelmeister J, Lipscomb TS. Sonography of acute appendicitis in childhood: perforation versus nonperforation. J Ultrasound Med 1992; 11:209–216.
41. Karakas SP, Guelfguat M, Leonidas JC, et al. Acute appendicitis in children: comparison of clinical diagnosis with ultrasound and CT imaging. Pediatr Radiol 2000; 30:94–98.
42. Pickuth D, Heywang-Kobrunner SH, Spielmann RP. Suspected acute appendicitis: Is ultrasonography or computed tomography the preferred imaging technique! Eur J Surg 2000; 166:315–319.
43. Puylaert JU. Acute appendicitis: U/S evaluation using graded compression. Radiology 1986; 158:355–360.
44. Quillin SP, Siegel MJ, Coffin CM. Acute appendicitis in children: value of sonography in detecting perforation. AJR Am J Roentgenol 1992; 159:1265–1268.
45. Quillin SP, Siegel MJ. Appendicitis: efficacy of color Doppler sonography. Radiology 1994; 191:557–560.
46. Quillin SP, Siegel MJ. Appendicitis in children: color Doppler sonography. Radiology 1992; 184:745–747.
47. Rao PM, Rhea JT, Novelline RA, et al. Helical CT technique for the diagnosis of appendicitis: prospective evaluation of a focused appendix CT examination. Radiology 1997; 202:139–144.
48. Vignault F, Filiatault D, Brandt M, et al. Acute appendicitis in children: evaluation with ultrasound. Radiology 1990; 176:501–504.
49. Warrel J, Drolshagen L, Kelly T, et al. Graded compression ultrasound in the diagnosis of appendicitis. J Ultrasound Med 1990; 9:145–150.
50. Alexander JE, Williamson SL, Seibert JJ, et al. The ultrasonographic diagnosis of typhlitis (neutropenic colitis). Pediatr Radiol 1988; 18:200–204.
51. Biller JA, Grand RJ, Harris BH. Abdominal abscesses in adolescents with Crohn's disease. J Pediatr Surg 1987; 22(9):873–876.
52. Dinkel E, Dittrich M, Peters H, et al. Real-time ultrasound in Crohn's disease: characteristic features and clinical implications. Pediatr Radiol 1986; 16:8–12.
53. Glasier CM, Siegel MJ, McAlister WH, et al. Henoch–Schönlein syndrome in children: gastrointestinal manifestations. AJR Am J Roentgenol 1981; 136:1081–1085.
54. Glass-Royal MC, Choyke PL, Gootenberg JE, et al. Sonography in the diagnosis of neutropenic colitis. J Ultrasound Med 1987; 6:671–673.
55. MacSweeney EJ, Oades PJ, Buchdahl R, et al. Relation of thickening of colon wall to pancreatic-enzyme treatment in cystic fibrosis. Lancet 1995; 345(8952):752–756.
56. Siegel MJ, Friedland JA, Hildebolt CF. Bowel wall thickening in children. Differentiation with US. Radiology 1997; 203:631–635.

Chapter 7

The female reproductive system

CHAPTER CONTENTS

Embryology   208
Normal appearances and ultrasound
      technique   210
   The ovaries   210
   The uterus   212
Congenital abnormalities   214
The female neonate   214
   Neonatal pelvic masses   214
   Ambiguous genitalia   218
   Ovarian cysts   219
Disorders of puberty   220
   Precocious puberty   221
   Isolated premature thelarche   223
   Isolated premature adrenarche   223
   Pubertal delay   224
   Menstrual dysfunction in adolescence   225
Ovarian neoplasms   228

Introduction

Investigation of the pediatric female genital tract has been revolutionized since the introduction of ultrasound, which is now the primary imaging modality in use today. Ultrasound is an ideal alternative to examination under anesthesia (EUA) and laparoscopy, with no radiation or anesthetic risk. Magnetic resonance imaging is gaining in importance, particularly for pelvic masses and complex genital abnormalities, but still the initial assessment lies with ultrasound.

Abnormalities of the genital tract are often accompanied by renal (in about 20%) and distal intestinal abnormalities, and these systems should always be examined as part of the ultrasound examination, particularly in neonates.

Successful sonographic examination and evaluation of anatomy and disorders of sexual development in girls, requires an accurate knowledge and assessment of both uterine and ovarian size and morphology as they grow and develop throughout childhood. It is essential that the sonographer is able to assess the normal appearance, because disorders related to premature or late pubertal development form the bulk of the workload related to the female genital tract in childhood. In the young infant with conditions such as ambiguous genitalia or intersex, ultrasound has an important and useful role, so an understanding of what to look for in these disorders is also very important.[1,2]

EMBRYOLOGY

The chromosomal and gonadal sex of an embryo is determined at fertilization by the kind of sperm that fertilizes the ovum, so that an X-bearing sperm gives rise to a chromosomal female and a Y-bearing sperm a male. The type of gonad that develops is determined by the sex chromosome complex (XX or XY). This is termed the gonadal sex, and differentiation occurs during the second month of development. Before the seventh week the gonads of the two sexes are identical in appearance and are called indifferent gonads.

Gonadal development occurs slowly in female embryos, and it is the X chromosome which bears the genes for ovarian development. Gonadal sex is then translated into body sex.

Development of the genital ducts

Both male and female embryos have two pairs of genital ducts. The mesonephric (Wolffian) ducts from the intermediate kidney play an important part in the development of the male reproductive system. The paramesonephric (Müllerian) ducts are those that develop lateral to the gonads and mesonephric duct system and have a leading role in the development of the female.

In male embryos (i.e. those with a 46XY chromosome complement) by 8 weeks, the fetal testes are producing two hormones which have a profound effect on the ultimate sexual and reproductive organs the fetus will have, i.e. its gonadal sex. Testosterone from the fetal Leydig cells stimulates the mesonephric ducts to form male genital ducts which then go on to develop into the epididymis, vas deferens and seminal vesicles. Müllerian inhibiting substance (MIS) also produced by testicular Sertoli cells causes the paramesonephric ducts to disappear, inhibiting the development of the female structures and causing their regression. If MIS is not present these female structures develop passively. So it is the presence of fully functioning testes that determines our reproductive organs or sexual development, in that testes are essential for male development whereas female development does not depend on the presence of ovaries.

In female embryos (i.e. those with a 46XX chromosome complement) the mesonephric ducts regress as there is no testosterone, and the paramesonephric ducts develop as there is no MIS.

The paramesonephric ducts develop into the fallopian tubes, uterus, cervix and upper vagina. The lower vagina develops separately from the urogenital sinus (Fig. 7.1).

In a 46XY (i.e. male) fetus with a female phenotype or appearance, there would have been no anti-Müllerian hormone active during intrauterine life, so that the female structures were able to develop passively. If the infant is 46XY and looks like a female but has no uterus (or an abnormal uterus) then there has been an abnormality of the androgen or male testosterone receptors so that the male ducts have not developed. This is otherwise known as testicular feminization.

Development of the ovary

The primary sex organ (gonad) in the female is the ovary. It contains germ cells derived from the yolk

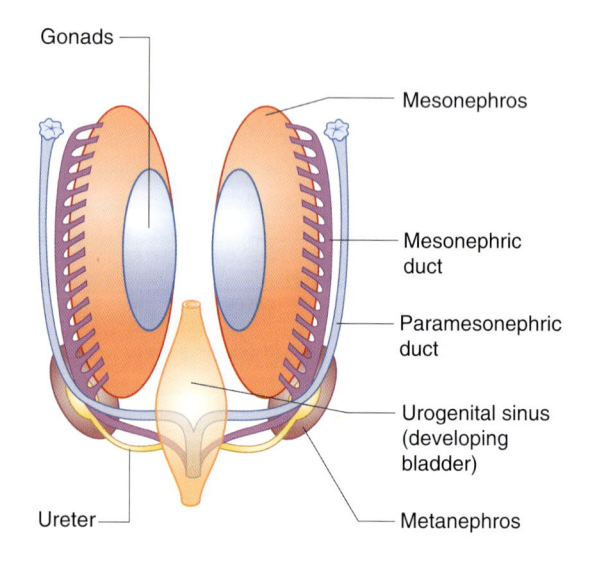

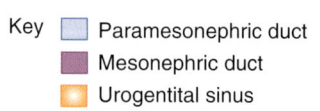

Figure 7.1 Normal development of the uterus. (A) Line diagram showing the development of the female genital tract from the paramesonephric duct or Müllerian duct system. The fallopian tubes and uterine body develop from the paired paramesonephric ducts. The vagina develops from the urogenital sinus.

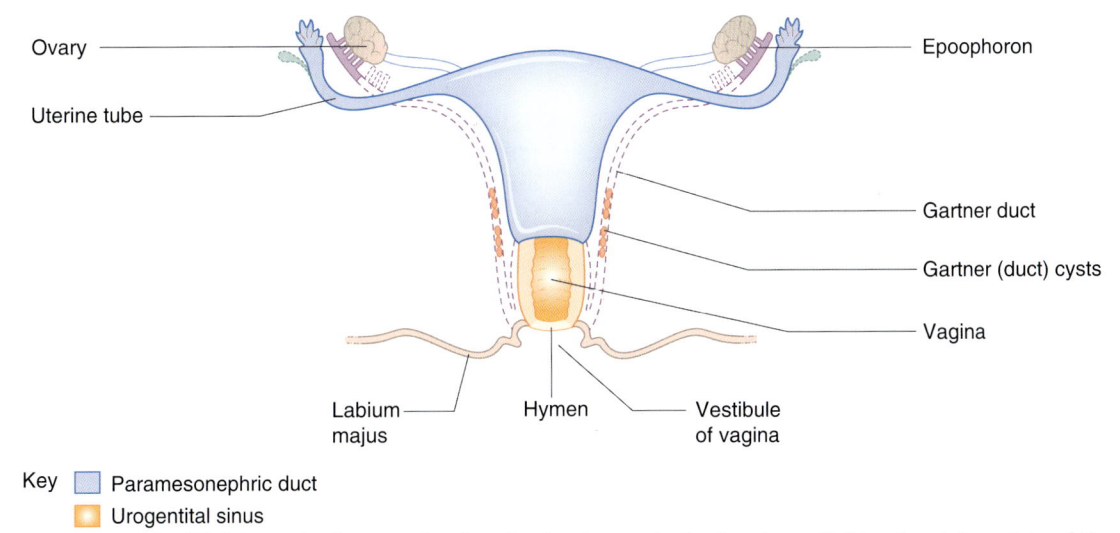

Figure 7.1, cont'd (B) Schematic diagram showing the development of a female genital tract and the origin of the fallopian tubes and uterus from the paramesonephric duct system and the vagina from the urogenital sinus.

sac and somatic cells derived from coelomic epithelium, mesenchyme and mesonephros.

In early fetal development the female germ cells, while migrating to the genital ridge from the yolk sac, undergo a series of mitotic divisions and then differentiate into oogonia. By 12 weeks of development, a proportion of the several million oogonia in the genital ridges enter the first phase of meiosis and then almost immediately become dormant, not completing the first meiosis until the onset of ovulation many years later. Before birth the offspring of the oogonias, with full chromosome complements, enlarge to become primary oocytes. The oocyte with a capsule of epithelium form the primordial follicle. The oocytes which are not incorporated into follicles undergo regression. By 5 months of gestation the number of primordial follicles peaks at about 7 million. Most of these follicles subsequently regress and degenerate before the follicle reaches any appreciable size. By birth only 1 million remain and by menarche less than half that number.

Growth of the ovary

In infancy and childhood follicles are present in the ovary in all stages of development but generally in the earlier stages of development than in later life.

The primordial follicles surrounded by their layer of flat cells start to grow. The flat cells become more spherical and are known as granulosa cells. As the coat becomes multilayered, an antrum appears and the Graafian follicle develops. The granulosa cells differentiate into two layers: the theca interna and theca externa.

The complete unruptured Graafian follicle may regress without expelling the ovum, first by the oocyte dying and then undergoing necrosis with eventual formation of the corpus restiforme; this vanishes without trace. In fetal and postnatal life this generally occurs before the follicle has reached an appreciable size. If the follicle expels the ovum (ovulation) then either a fully developed corpus luteum will result, or the remaining follicle will become luteinized and regress without the development of a corpus luteum. The distinguishing feature of the post-pubertal follicle is the ability of the follicle to liberate its ovum (ovulation) and be converted into a corpus luteum.[3]

The ovary is poorly vascularized in the infant and young child, but throughout childhood this vascularization slowly increases and by 6 to 8 years of age there is an identifiable medulla and cortex in the ovary. By 11 to 12 years of age primordial follicles are evenly distributed throughout the layers of the cortex. By 12 to 13 years ovulation begins and from then on, non-primordial ova containing follicles are present, with a gradual reduction of the primordial follicles until none remains in the mature ovary. After 14 years of age the ovary is essentially mature in the majority of females.

Endocrinology

Ovarian activity involves the production of gametes and hormones which determine sexual development and reproductive function. These two functions are closely related and under the control of the hypothalamic–pituitary axis. The hypothalamic–pituitary unit which is responsible for pubertal development is developed and potentially functional by mid-gestation in the fetus. During late gestation the placenta produces large quantities of sex hormones (i.e. estrogens and progesterone) which may inhibit fetal gonadotropin secretion. At birth and with maternal estrogen withdrawal, there is a rise in gonadotropin secretion which occurs at pubertal level for several months.

Gonadotropins fall to low levels in early childhood but start to rise again by 6 years of age. Concurrently, more mature antral follicles develop in the ovaries, producing a subsequent rise in estrogen levels.

In pre-puberty gonadotropin secretion can be measured but occurs in irregular bursts not linked to the night time. At about 7 to 8 years of age, pulsatile gonadotropin secretion becomes steadily linked to the night time and appears to be controlled primarily by the central nervous system. Throughout puberty the amplitude of gonadotropin pulses and gonadal sex steroid secretion gradually increases until late puberty, when adult levels are reached throughout the day. Although nocturnal pulsatility alone may permit menarche, usually anovulatory cycles, the development of diurnal and nocturnal high amplitude pulses is required for ovulatory cycles. Puberty ends with the final stage of ovarian maturation which is the establishment of regular ovulatory cycles. This reflects the maturation of the entire hypothalamic–pituitary–gonadal axis.[4]

NORMAL APPEARANCES AND ULTRASOUND TECHNIQUE

Recent advances in ultrasound equipment have resulted in small footprint, high frequency transducers, with the advantage of variable focus for deeper structures in the older child, which can produce images of superb resolution. This equipment is essential for scanning the pediatric pelvis in order to be able to measure small (1–2 mm) follicles and for careful measurement and recognition of the uterine endometrium. Generally, small footprint transducers of 5–7 MHz are best for young infants while curved linear transducers are good for an overall view of the pelvis in older children. Endovaginal scanning, while important in adult gynecology, can only be used in older girls who are sexually active, and is not used in routine pediatric practice. Endorectal scanning is also not routinely used in young girls for visualization of the ovaries. Clinically there are no conditions that can justify these forms of invasive scanning in young girls that cannot be achieved by other means.

A full bladder is needed as an acoustic window in all children. Infants and toddlers who are not potty-trained should be given a drink prior to the examination. Older children and adolescents should be well hydrated and given 300–500 ml of still fluid, preferably water, some 45 minutes before the examination is due. Timing is critical; an overfull bladder will distort the appearance of the uterus and displace or obscure the ovaries, while a partially empty bladder will result in inadequate visualization of these structures. We have found optimal bladder filling is best and most comfortably achieved at all ages if patients do this in the department and are scanned at regular intervals.

The ovaries are identified by scanning obliquely through the full bladder in the angle between the iliac vessels and bladder and then transversely, usually at the level of the uterine fundus. The ovaries are measured in three planes and the ovarian volume calculated according to the formula for a prolate ellipse. The number, size and distribution of the follicles is noted. The uterine length is measured in the longitudinal axis and the anteroposterior measurements taken at the cervix and fundus. If the endometrium is seen, the thickness is measured at the maximum depth of the body away from the cervix.

The ovaries

The ovaries are active throughout childhood, with continual follicular growth and atresia. Ovarian maturation continues throughout childhood.

There is continual growth in the size of the ovary with an increase in ovarian volume and an increase in number and size of the developing follicles as puberty approaches. It is often very surprising how follicular the ovaries of a child appear.[5]

Ovarian volume

Studies have shown the ovarian volume to be 0.8 cm^3 in the first 3 months of life, increasing in volume from a mean of 1 cm^3 at 2 years of age to 2 cm^3 at 12 years of age. Normal standards for ovarian volume in childhood and puberty are available.[6] The volume of the ovary is affected by the presence of large cysts, either primordial or ovulatory follicles, or a corpus luteal cyst, and cannot be reliably calculated when these structures are present.

There appear to be two particular periods of increased growth rate of the ovary. The first occurs at approximately 8 years of age, coinciding with the rise in androgen secretion from the adrenal cortex at adrenarche. The second growth spurt occurs immediately before and during puberty[6–13] (Fig. 7.2).

Follicles

In the neonate the size of the ovary and the number of visible follicles is variable although the follicles are often surprisingly numerous. This follicular activity in the infant is related to the maternal hormone influence. Occasionally a follicle may grow large so as to precipitate torsion of the ovary.

Throughout childhood the ovarian follicles increase in size and number. The size of the follicles varies and they may become atretic at any stage of their development. Pre-pubertally, the ovaries may appear quite active, with follicles of up to 9 mm in size. With the onset of high luteinizing hormone pulses at night, at about 8 to 9 years of age, the ovaries become 'multicystic' or multifollicular, defined on ultrasound appearances as more than six follicles of 4 mm diameter. This is a normal phase of development and is the herald of puberty.[14]

This coincides with breast development of Tanner stage 2. The follicles continue to increase in size with the progression through puberty. With the constant maturation and regression of the follicles there is a wide range of diameters seen at different pubertal stages. Also, lower levels of gonadotropin in prepubertal girls can result in larger follicles of up to 12 mm. This limits the value of follicular diameter in assessing pubertal status.

Menarche

The principal regulators of ovarian function are luteinizing hormone (LH) and follicle-stimulating hormone (FSH). In response to rising levels of FSH, between 5 and 12 primordial follicles commence to enlarge and are now called primary follicles. The ovarian follicles gradually enlarge until a follicle of at least 16 mm is attained. There is follicular secretion of estrogen which results in the development of an endometrium. Without ovulating (an anovulatory cycle) the follicle regresses, and the subsequent fall in estrogen results in a withdrawal bleed. Eventually, when a follicle diameter of over 20 mm is achieved, that follicle gains primacy, while the remainder of the other follicles recruited during the cycle degenerate. The remaining follicle is now known as a mature or dominant Graafian follicle. After ovulation the granulosa cells of the ruptured follicle wall begin to proliferate and give rise to the corpus luteum, which is an endocrine structure that secretes steroid hormones that maintain the uterine endometrium in readiness to receive an embryo. If no embryo implants

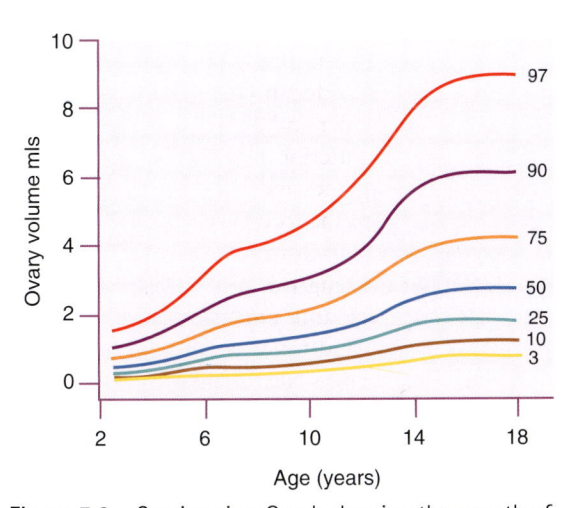

Figure 7.2 Ovarian size. Graph showing the growth of the ovary throughout childhood. There are two periods of acceleration: the first at adrenarche and the second around puberty.[6]

in the uterus the corpus luteum degenerates after about 14 days (Fig. 7.3).

The uterus

In the neonate, the uterus is still under the influence of maternal hormone stimulation and is large and plump. There is often a prominent endometrium, and uterine enlargement is predominantly of its corpus. Nussbaum et al found that the normal neonatal uterus was cylindrical in 58% and pear-shaped in 32%. The thin echogenic line of the endometrium can be identified in over 97% infants.[15] If present, the neonatal uterus can always be identified (Fig. 7.4).

After birth the uterus diminishes in size and assumes a normal pre-pubertal configuration with prominence of the cervix. This is termed the teardrop-shaped uterus. It reaches a minimum length at about 4 years before increasing again.[16]

During this early childhood period the cervix to body size ratio is approximately 2:1. After 4 years of age uterine growth begins, with some further increase at the time of adrenarche. There is a lengthening of the body, and then a growth in both the cervix and body to assume a tubular shape in the mid-childhood years, with the cervix and fundus being of the same size.

Pre-pubertally, the uterine length is generally up to 40 mm with an AP diameter at the cervix of 5–10 mm. As puberty approaches and follicle development matures, the increasing levels of

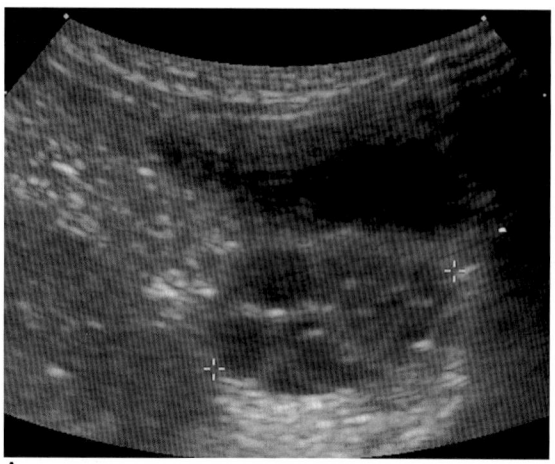

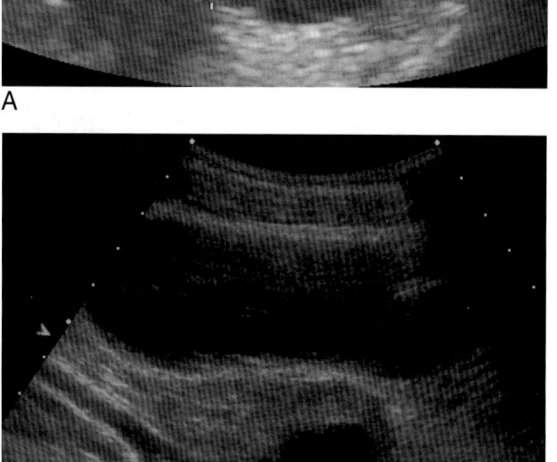

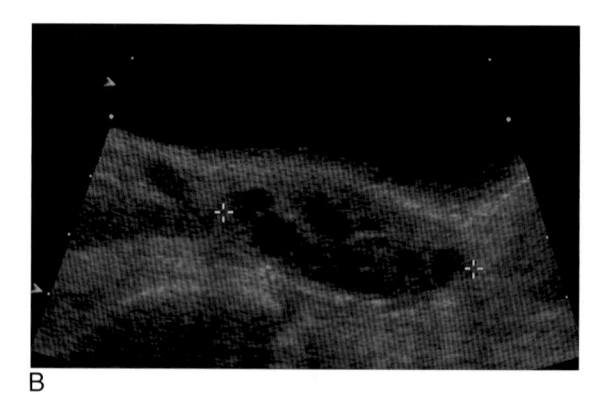

Figure 7.3 Normal ovarian appearance at different ages. (A) Oblique sonogram of the ovary in a neonate (between calipers). The ovary in a normal neonate can be very follicular and this, as in the uterus, is related to maternal hormone stimulation. (B) Oblique sonogram of the ovary (between calipers) in early pubertal development. The ovary appears very follicular. This multifollicular appearance is a normal stage of development and is the herald of puberty. (C) Oblique sonogram of the right ovary showing a dominant follicle. This is the last follicular change of the ovary as menarche begins. With the development of the dominant follicle, other follicular activity is suppressed.

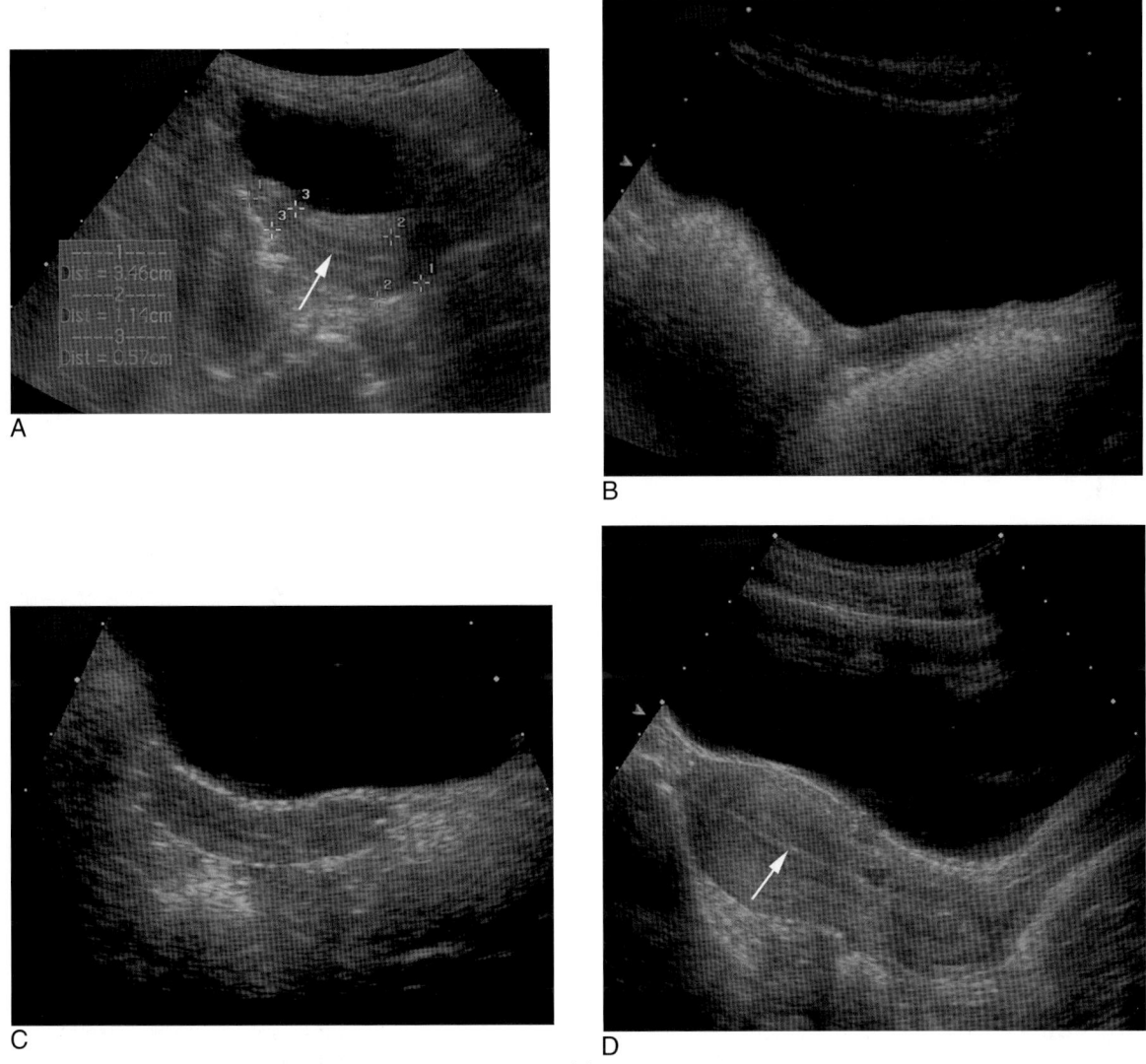

Figure 7.4 Normal uterine appearance at different ages. (A) Neonatal uterus. Longitudinal sonogram of the uterus in a neonate. The uterus is easily identified and is large and plump. The endometrial stripe is usually visible (arrow). The uterus length is measured, as is the cervix to fundal ratio (between calipers). (B) Prepubertal uterus. Longitudinal sonogram of the uterus in a young girl. The cervix is thicker than the fundus. (C) Tubular uterus. Longitudinal sonogram of the uterus when some growth has occurred around adrenarche. The uterus is now tubular. This is when the cervix and uterine body AP measurements are the same. (D) Adult uterus. Longitudinal sonogram of the uterus in a girl post-menarche. The uterus is now pear-shaped with an endometrium (arrow). There has been reversal of the cervix to fundal ratio seen in the pre-pubertal uterus.

estrogen result in both an increase in uterine size and in endometrial thickness. The uterus attains its adult 'pear-shaped' configuration with its body and fundus dominant.

The endometrium is seen as an echogenic midline echo. Uterine volumes are available but a better measure of uterine growth and development is a uterine length and an AP measure of the body and cervix with an evaluation of their ratio. A simple indication of uterine growth is an AP measurement of the cervix, and as a general rule of thumb a measurement over 8 mm indicates growth has started (Fig. 7.5).

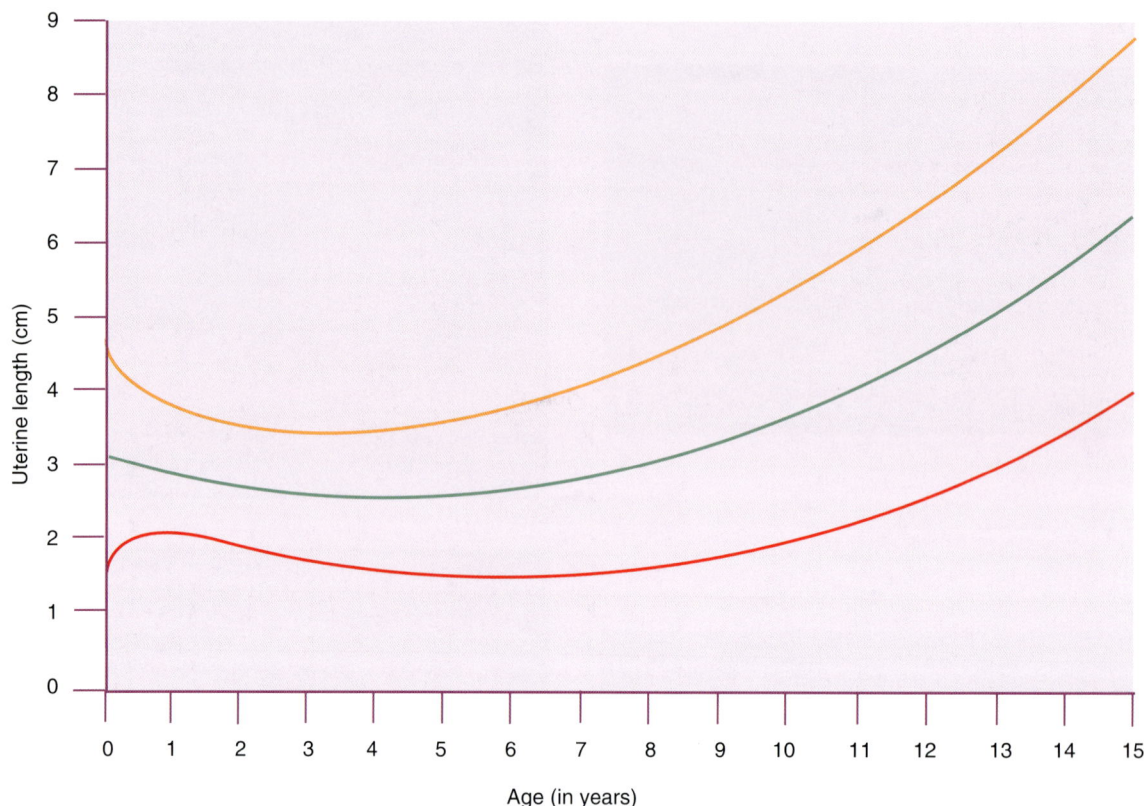

Figure 7.5 Uterine length versus age for the 3rd, 50th and 90th centile. (After Griffin et al.[8])

CONGENITAL ABNORMALITIES

Abnormal development of the female genital tract occurs either from Müllerian (paramesonephric) duct abnormalities or abnormalities of the urogenital sinus (Fig. 7.6). They may occur in isolation or together, resulting in a wide range of anomalies from failure of fusion of the paramesonephric (Müllerian) ducts (uterus didelphys—double uterus), to a persistent cloaca, where all orifices open into one perineal opening and are not separated. The ability of ultrasound to detect these fusion abnormalities lies in the recognition of two endometrial cavities, cervices and vaginas. They are difficult to diagnose in infants and may only be detected later in adolescence when the two endometriums are identifiable and are associated with an unusually wide fundal contour (Fig. 7.7).

THE FEMALE NEONATE

The sonographer is asked to evaluate the abdomen and pelvis of a female neonate mainly in three clinical settings:

- the evaluation of a pelvic mass
- the infant with ambiguous genitalia
- prenatally detected abdominal cyst.

Neonatal pelvic masses

In a female infant there is a limited differential diagnosis of pelvic masses, and the sonographer needs to be able to differentiate them. Solid masses are rare in the neonate and generally occur in the older child but are included here for completeness.

The important role of sonography is to determine whether the mass is arising *out* of the pelvis.

THE FEMALE REPRODUCTIVE SYSTEM   215

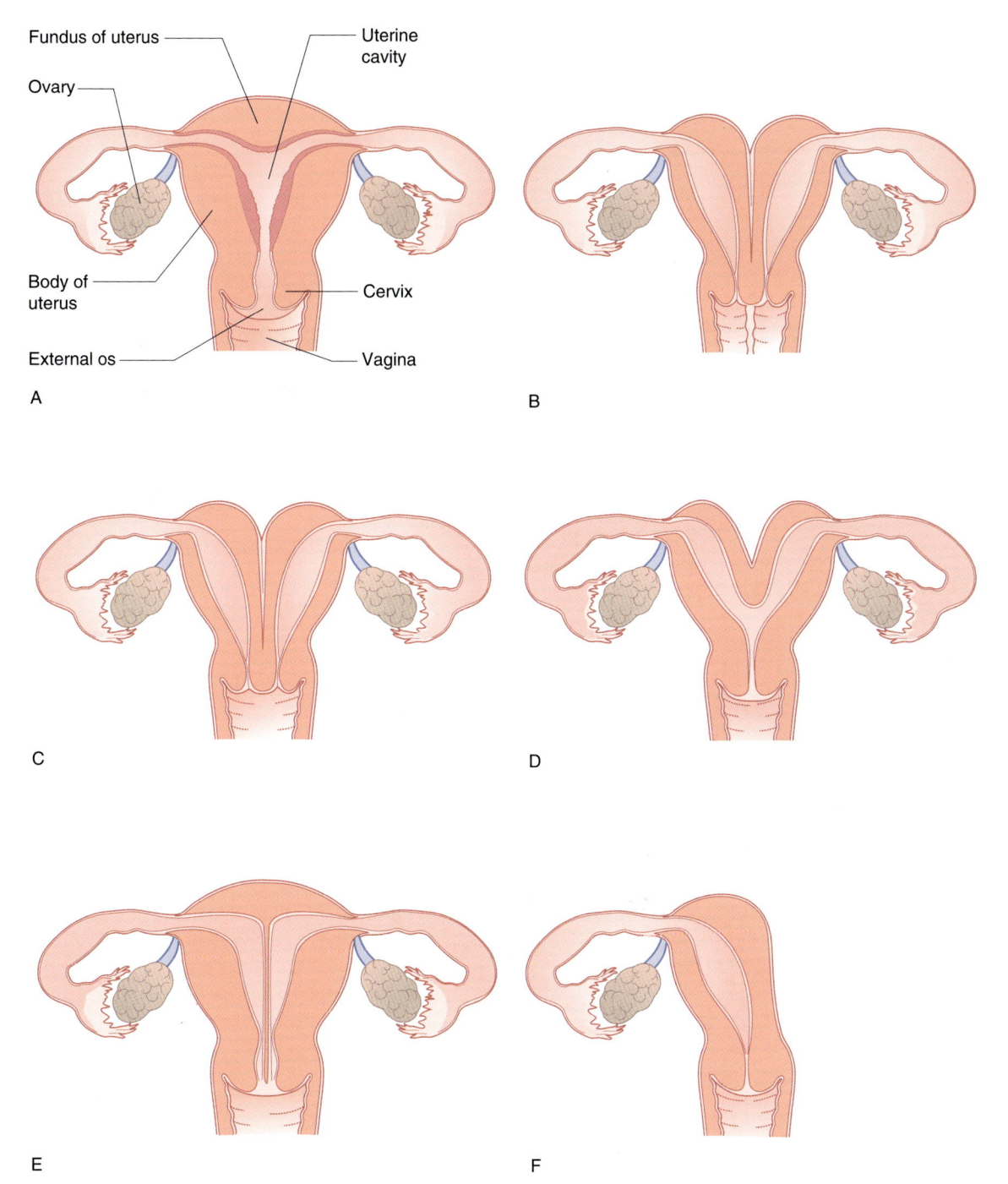

Figure 7.6 Congenital uterine abnormalities. (A) The normal configuration of the uterus and the ovaries. (B) & (C) Double uterus with a double vagina and single vagina. (D) Bicornuate uterus. (E) A uterus with a midline septum. (F) Unicornuate uterus.

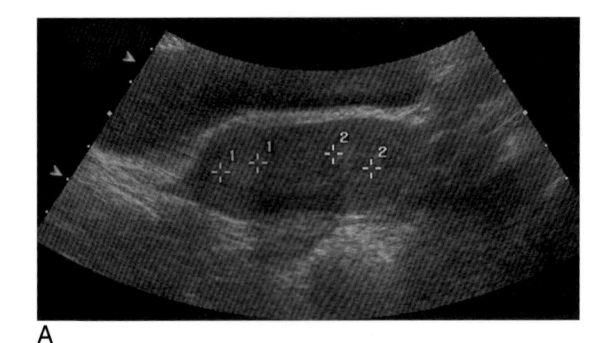

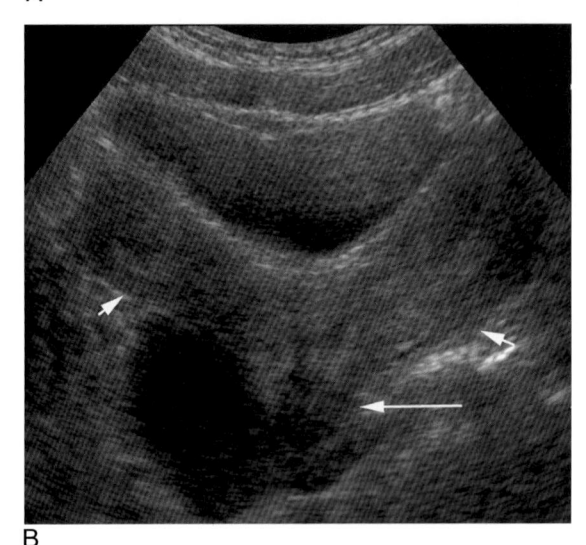

Figure 7.7 Double uterus. (A) Transverse sonogram at the level of the uterine fundus. Notice how wide the uterine body appears. There are two uterine bodies with a visible endometrium on both sides (between the calipers). The transverse sonogram is the best view to identify two uterine bodies. (B) Transverse sonogram on another menarchal girl showing the two uterine bodies (small arrows). These are tapered down to a single cervix and vagina (large arrow).

The appearance to look for is the shape of the mass, i.e. pear-shaped, and the inability to get below the mass. Masses going *into* the pelvis are generally teardrop-shaped, and ultrasound can generally show the lower extent of the mass. Ovarian masses go into the pelvis, as the ovaries in children lie high in the pelvis. A plain abdominal radiograph is always advised, as there may be classical calcification as in a teratoma or abnormalities of the spine as in an anterior meningocele (Table 7.1).

Genital tract obstruction

Genital tract obstruction presents in the neonate as an abdominal mass, or less commonly at puberty with amenorrhea and cyclical pain. One cause of the obstruction is an imperforate hymen, the membrane occurring at the junction between the upper (Müllerian duct) vagina and lower (urogenital sinus) vagina. This is an unusual cause in the neonate and is seen primarily in older girls. Other causes, particularly in the neonate, include vaginal stenosis or atresia or complex cloacal malformations and urogenital sinus abnormalities.

Hydrocolpos refers to vaginal obstruction alone. Hydrometrocolpos refers to both uterine and vaginal obstruction. If a pubertal girl is suspected of having started menarche, then the term hematometrocolpos to denote blood in the uterus and vagina is used.

In the neonate, ultrasound will reveal a predominantly pear-shaped cystic mass arising out of the pelvis and containing fluid and cellular debris sometimes with a sedimentation level. Often there is associated hydronephrosis of the kidneys as they become obstructed from the mass (Fig. 7.8).

In any neonatal cystic pelvic mass:

- The bladder must be carefully sought and clearly identified separate from the mass. It is usually empty and squashed anteriorly. Bladder catheterization is helpful, as the catheter can then be identified.
- The superior surface of the cystic mass must be examined for a small muscular uterine body. The uterus often has a distended cavity.
- The internal echoes give a clue to the diagnosis in that a hydrometrocolpos has multiple internal echoes, often with layering.

The major differential diagnosis is a sacrococcygeal teratoma arising deep in the sacrum and with a large intra-abdominal component. Sacral protrusion of the mass is usually evident which makes the diagnosis easier. It affects girls four times more commonly than boys. If removed immediately after birth over 90% are benign.

Other causes of cystic pelvic masses such as rectal duplications and anterior meningoceles are much rarer. Rectal duplications are usually tubular

Table 7.1 Mass arising out of the pelvis in a female neonate

Diagnosis	Ultrasound features	Clinical findings	Other
Cystic			
Hydrometrocolpos	Contains multiple echoes. Sometimes layering of the particulate matter can be seen. Muscular body of uterus above mass	Abdominal mass can be very large and arises out of the pelvis	Cloacal anomalies. Ambiguous genitalia
Duplication cyst of rectum	Clearly defined wall. Tubular shape may contain some echoes if hemorrhage has occurred	Pelvic mass	
Sacrococcygeal teratoma	Mixed cystic with very echogenic solid areas of fat, hair and teeth. Rarely purely cystic with septations	Swelling or mass on perineum from the sacrococcygeal origin	4F:1M. Must be removed because of malignant potential
Anterior meningocele	Cystic mass		Abnormalities of spine and sacrum, e.g. hemi-sacrum. Need radiograph, US, CT or MRI
Enlarged bladder	May be mistaken for a cystic mass arising out of the pelvis. Make sure bladder not obstructed by mass at bladder base, e.g. pelvic neuroblastoma	Mass arising out of pelvis	
Solid			
Pelvic neuroblastoma	Solid with typical fine calcification	Ill child. May present with retention of urine	Bone changes of neuroblastoma. Upper abdominal lymphadenopathy
Bladder rhabdomyosarcoma	Solid ± areas of necrosis. Liver metastases or upper abdominal lymphadenopathy	Abdominal mass. Older child	Metastases in liver and lungs
Pelvic kidney	Normal or hydronephrotic pelvic kidney	Abdominal mass	May be mistakenly removed

and have a clearly defined wall, while some anterior meningoceles will have a sacral defect.

A large bladder may also present as a fixed pelvic mass, in which case a careful search for a mass obstructing the bladder outlet must be made. A pelvic kidney is readily diagnosed but can some- times cause a diagnostic problem if it is grossly hydronephrotic. These kidneys are at risk of inadvertent removal, obstruction, hydronephrosis and vesicoureteric reflux.

An infant presenting with a presacral mass requires a full renal tract and spinal canal examination, as

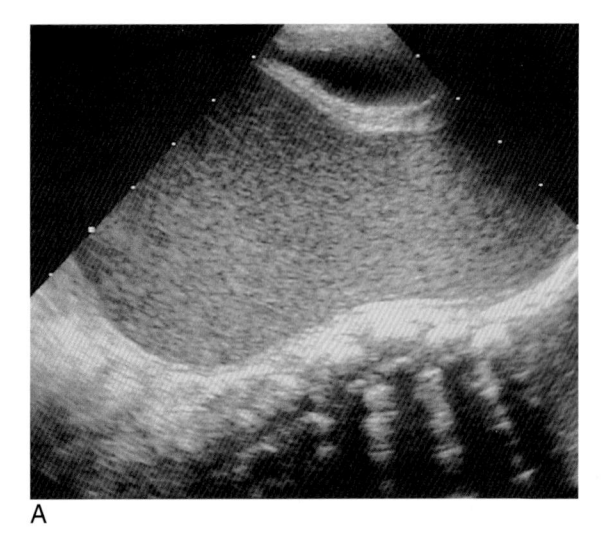

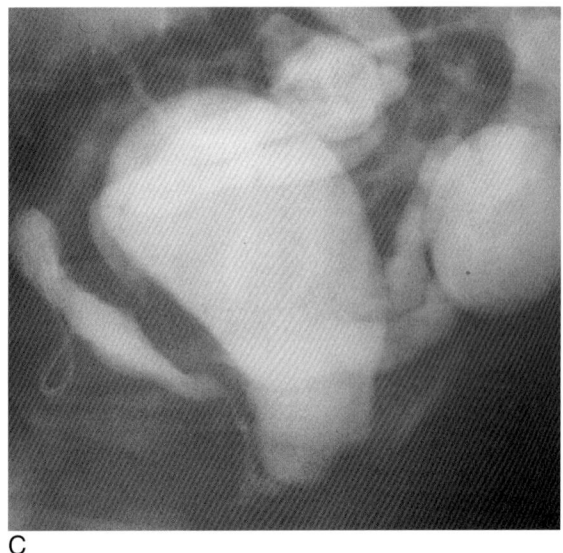

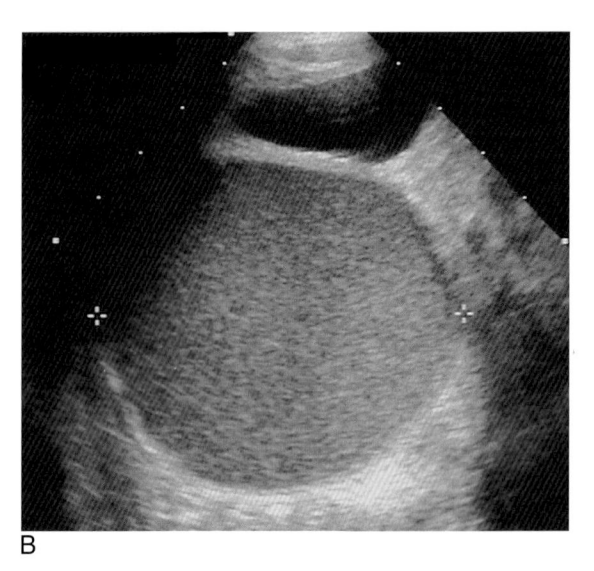

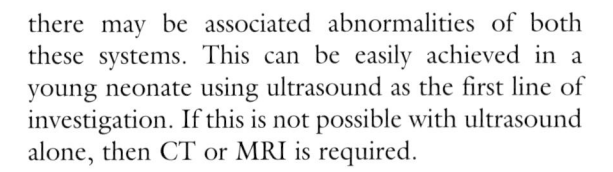

Figure 7.8 Hydrometrocolpos. (A) & (B) Longitudinal and transverse sonograms in a female infant with a large mass arising out of the pelvis. There is a large pear-shaped mass behind the bladder and anterior to the sacrum. It contains multiple echoes throughout. Sometimes layering of the echoes (particulate debris) occurs. These are the typical appearances of a hydrometrocolpos. (C) Contrast examination via a suprapubic bladder catheter in the same infant. The small bladder has filled and contrast has refluxed via the common channel into the large uterus and vagina. There is also reflux into the ureters. This infant had a cloacal abnormality.

there may be associated abnormalities of both these systems. This can be easily achieved in a young neonate using ultrasound as the first line of investigation. If this is not possible with ultrasound alone, then CT or MRI is required.

Ambiguous genitalia

The definition of ambiguous genitalia is a child born with a micropenis with no palpable gonads, or hypospadias without a palpable gonad or only one palpable gonad (Fig. 7.9). Hypospadias is a congenital abnormality of the penis that is caused by incomplete development of the anterior urethra. The meatal location can be anywhere along the ventral surface of the penis from the glans to the perineum.

The birth of a baby with ambiguous genitalia is hugely disturbing for parents, and sonographers should be sensitive to these anxieties and be extremely wary of making inadvertent remarks regarding the presence or absence of internal organs. Gender assignment can be a highly complex affair in these children and is dependent on the chromosomal, gonadal and phenotypic sex of the infant. All infants require an early assessment as there are many problems in delaying the assignation of gender, both in terms of parental bonding

THE FEMALE REPRODUCTIVE SYSTEM   219

androgens. Most are due to the adrenogenital syndrome, i.e. deficiencies in adrenal enzymes for cortisol synthesis. External appearances depend on the degree of virilization. All have a normal uterus, ovaries and vagina and should be raised as females.

In an infant with ambiguous genitalia the role of ultrasound is to:

- determine the presence of the uterus. The presence of a uterus and ovaries will point to a virilized female, whereas their absence suggests male pseudohermaphrodite.
- identify any gonads. Gonads palpable and visualized in the scrotum or lower inguinal canals below the inguinal crease have testicular tissue and are either testes or ovotestes. Ovaries are never this low unless in a hernia, in which case it will be palpable outside the inguinal ring. The presence of a gonad in this position rules out simple virilization of an otherwise normal female infant.
- identify adrenals and kidneys. In some but not all infants with CAH the adrenals may be enlarged.

Ultrasound is an excellent modality to identify the uterus, aided by sonography of the urogenital sinus to determine the anatomy of the vagina and uterus, when confronted with an infant with a single orifice (Fig. 7.11).

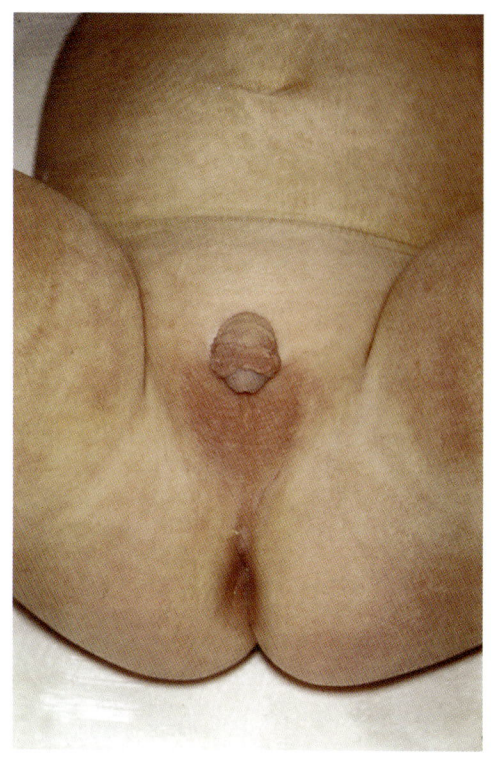

Figure 7.9 Ambiguous genitalia.

and attempting to register a birth without a sex being assigned.

An understanding of the terminology relating to sex and gender will help unravel what is often a very confusing subject. Genetic sex, i.e. the chromosomes a person has, is established when the egg is fertilized, with XX denoting a female and XY a male fetus. The gonads that develop in early fetal life are called gonadal sex, and this in turn later manifests in the body sex. A child with ambiguous genitalia is a hermaphrodite. A female hermaphrodite has ovaries while a male hermaphrodite has testes.

As mentioned earlier, testosterone from the testicular Sertoli cells induces the development of the mesonephric (Wolffian) ducts. Müllerian inhibiting substance (MIS) also produced by fetal Sertoli or testicular cells causes regression of the female structures such as the uterus and fallopian tubes (Table 7.2, Fig. 7.10).

The commonest cause of masculinization of the female is excess androgens. This results from excessive exposure of genetic females (46XX) in utero to

Ovarian cysts

Follicular ovarian cysts are commonly seen in girls and adolescents and are generally of no clinical significance. Ultrasonically they appear as uncomplicated cysts and are considered to be physiological. Rarely they may secrete estrogens and present as isosexual precocious puberty.[17] The majority will involute with time, and all that is required is serial scanning to document their involution. The endocrine changes will disappear with the cyst. Occasionally if large, they may hemorrhage or undergo torsion and then present as an acute abdomen. The mass may then appear solid on ultrasound, and differentiation from an ovarian tumor may be difficult.

Neonatal ovarian cysts

Large ovarian cysts may be seen in the neonatal period presenting as an abdominal mass. Most

Table 7.2 Findings in common conditions causing ambiguous genitalia

Name	Chromosomes	Problem	Structures
Congenital adrenal hyperplasia (CAH) (female pseudohermaphrodite)	46XX (genetic girl)	Masculinized female from excess androgens produced by the fetal adrenal gland	Uterus Ovaries Clitoromegaly Partial fusion of the labia Urogenital sinus
Androgen insensitivity syndrome (AIS) (testicular feminization syndrome)	46XY (genetic boy)	Resistence to androgens during development of sexual structures at a cellular level so that only small testes-like structures may be present MIS active so there is no uterus	Phenotypically girls Testes in abdomen, inguinal canals or labia majora No penis or scrotum No or rudimentary uterus Blind ending vagina Women with AIS are female in their orientation. At puberty develop normal female characteristics but fail to menstruate
Male pseudohermaphrodite	46XY (genetic boy)	Genetic defect in the synthesis of testosterone by the fetal testis	Rudimentary to normal testicular development Inadequate virilization of the male fetus
XY gonadal dysgenesis	46XY (genetic boy)	No gonads No testosterone so no testes No anti-Müllerian hormone in fetal life	Phenotypically girl No ovaries Uterus present

MIS, Müllerian inhibiting substance.

commonly, however, they are detected prenatally, usually around 26 weeks' gestation. Ultrasonically they have a mixed appearance: either simple, containing no internal echoes, or classically they may contain a fluid/debris level. There is virtually no other abdominal cystic mass in a female infant that produces this fluid debris level, and a confident diagnosis of an ovarian cyst can usually be made (Fig. 7.12).

The fluid debris level is considered to be a sign of preceding ovarian torsion. Such cysts are known as 'wandering' tumors and may be found anywhere in the abdomen after becoming detached from the fallopian tube. Rarely the wall or hemorrhagic contents may calcify. The important differential diagnosis is enteric duplications, which can be differentiated by the presence of a well-defined wall and which will not disappear with serial ultrasound examinations. Sometimes, ovarian cysts may be bilateral.[18]

The management of neonatal ovarian cysts is conservative, with only serial ultrasound examinations required. The cysts may take a long time to spontaneously involute—up to a year in the author's experience. Rarely is surgical intervention needed. If large (generally over 5 cm) and simple, i.e. transonic and causing pressure effects, for example respiratory difficulty, they may be aspirated under ultrasound guidance. The aspirated fluid will be high in estrogens.

DISORDERS OF PUBERTY

Puberty is the time when the body undergoes the complex transition from childhood to maturity,

THE FEMALE REPRODUCTIVE SYSTEM   221

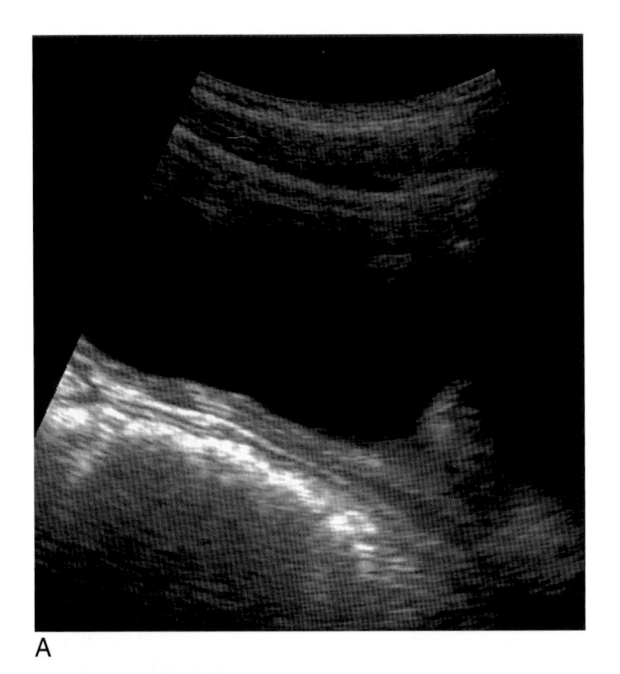

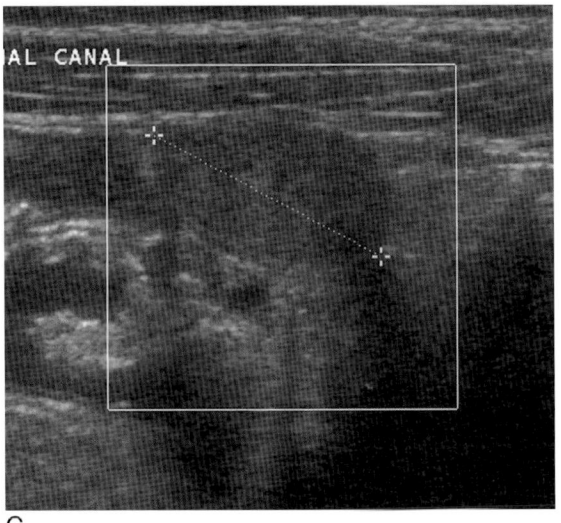

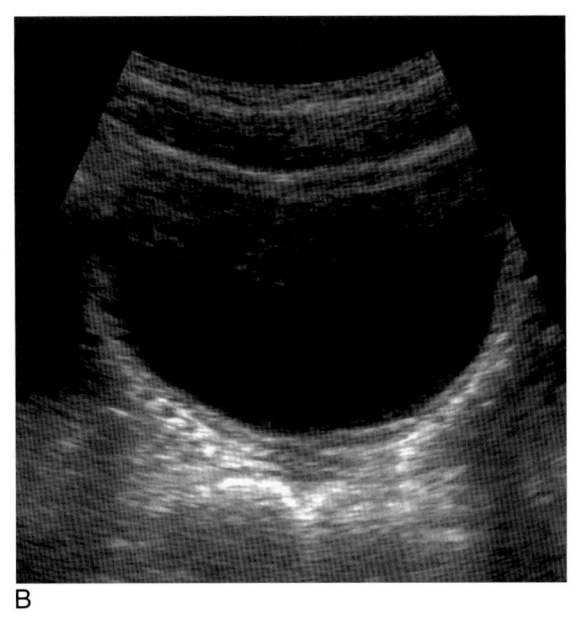

Figure 7.10 Ambiguous genitalia in a neonate. This infant presented with ambiguous genitalia. The clinical question was whether the infant had any female internal organs. (A) & (B) The longitudinal and transverse sonogram of the bladder demonstrates that there is no uterus. If present, a plump neonatal uterus should always be identifiable behind the bladder. (C) In the right iliac fossa a gonad was found which was a testicle.

and it is generally accepted to be the period between 10 and 16 years. For about 2 years before overt puberty, biochemical changes take place, particularly from the adrenal gland (Table 7.3). In a girl, breast enlargement is usually the first sign of normal puberty and is followed by the appearance of pubic hair. Menarche does not occur until breast stage four or five.

Pubertal development is abnormal if this normal sequence does not occur, or if it occurs at the wrong time, either too early (precocious puberty) or too late (delayed puberty) (Figs 7.13 and 7.14).

Precocious puberty

Precocious puberty in a girl is defined as the development of secondary sexual characteristics before the age of 8 years. Precocious puberty may be central (gonadotropin dependent) and is identical to normal puberty but occurs early because of the

222 PEDIATRIC ULTRASOUND

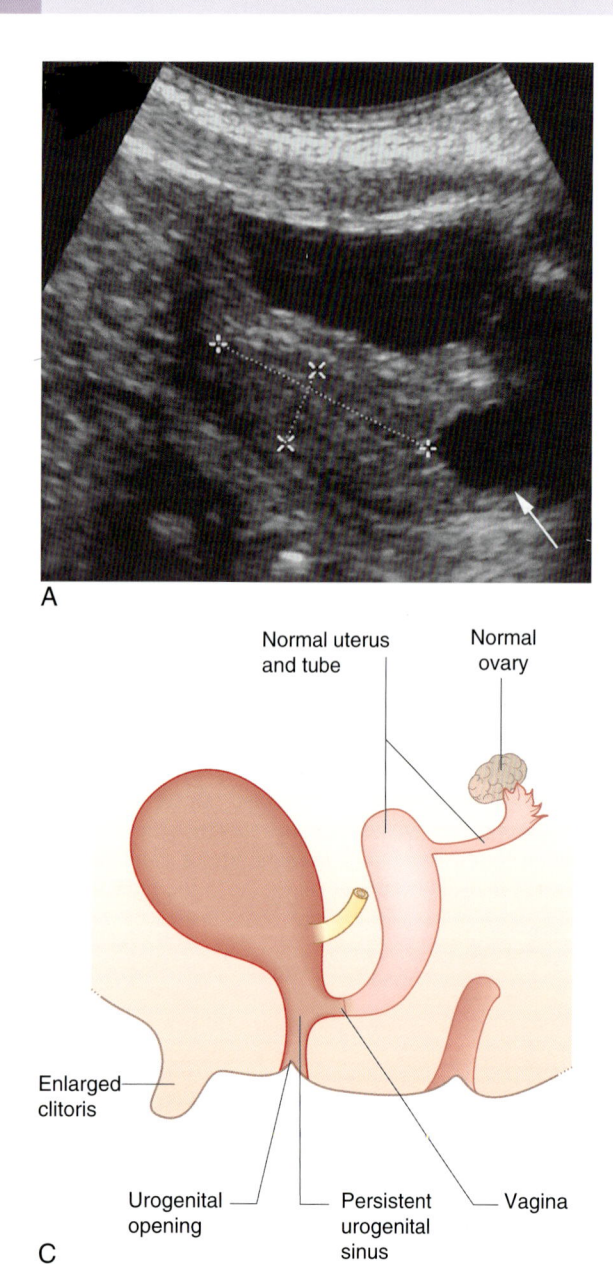

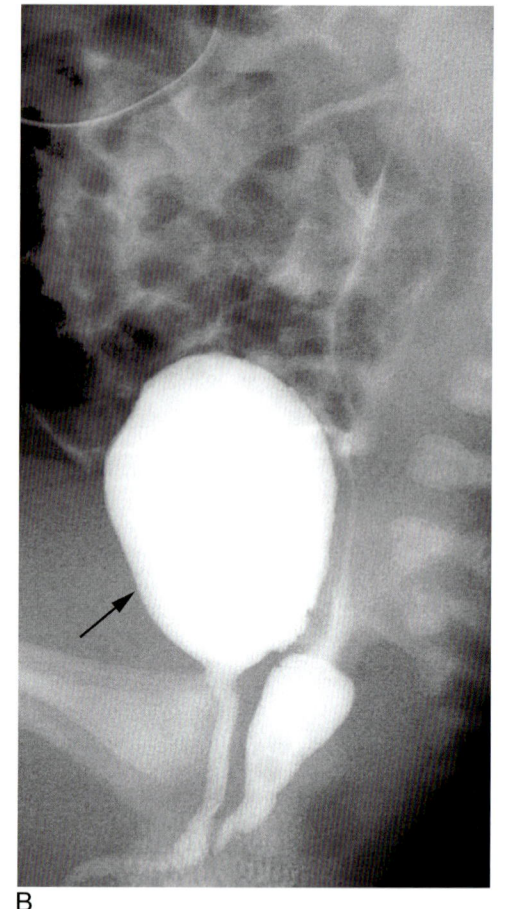

Figure 7.11 Urogenital sinus. (A) Longitudinal sonogram of the pelvis in an infant presenting with ambiguous genitalia. Behind the bladder a uterus can be seen (between calipers) with fluid in the vagina (arrow). (B) Contrast sinogram on the infant showing the distended vagina and its communication with the urethra. The bladder is also full of contrast (arrow). (C) Line diagram showing the anomaly of the persistent urogenital sinus. In clinical practice this is most commonly seen in congenital adrenal hyperplasia.

premature activation of the hypothalamic–pituitary–gonadal axis. Sonography in central precocious puberty shows large multifollicular ovaries. Because of the gonadal production of estrogen the uterus is large and there is endometrial proliferation.

Pseudoprecocious puberty may be caused by an ovarian or adrenal tumor. It is described as 'dissonant', i.e. when the sequence is abnormal: for example, isolated pubic hair with virilization from excess androgens due to congenital adrenal hypertrophy (CAH) or tumor. It is characterized by a rapid onset and sometimes associated with neurological symptoms, e.g. neurofibromatosis. In pseudoprecocious puberty, secondary sexual characteristics are present but not regular ovulation.

Ultrasound may also detect large follicular ovarian cysts which are functional and therefore cause

THE FEMALE REPRODUCTIVE SYSTEM

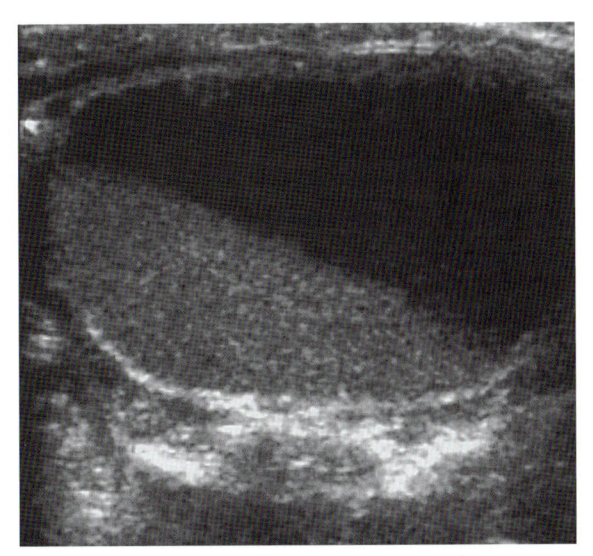

Figure 7.12 Neonatal ovarian cyst torsion. Sonogram of a cyst found in a female neonate. This is the typical appearance of an ovarian cyst that has undergone torsion. There is a fluid debris level in the cyst. This type of cyst has been referred to as the 'wandering tumor' as it detaches from the fallopian tube and wanders round the abdomen.

transient breast development.[16,17,19,20] Also ultrasound will readily distinguish solid or mixed echogenic tumors. Granulosa theca cell tumors of the ovary are the ovarian tumors which are most commonly present with isosexual precocious puberty (Fig. 7.15).

Table 7.3 The major events of female puberty

Event	Age	Effect
Adrenarche	8–10 years	Prepubertal adrenal function
Pubertal growth spurt	10–13 years	Starts at 10 and reaches peak rate at 12–13 years
Thelarche	10–12 years	Breast development
Pubarche	10–13 years	Pubic hair growth
Menarche	10–16 years	First menstrual period
Growth of axillary hair	>12 years	

Causes of precocious puberty

Gonadotropin-dependent causes are characterized by high LH and FSH levels ('central'):

- idiopathic/familial
- CNS abnormalities
  - —congenital, e.g. hydrocephalus
  - —acquired, e.g. post-irradiation/infection/surgery
  - —tumors, e.g. microscopic hamartomas.

Gonadotropin-independent causes are characterized by low FSH and LH levels ('pseudoprecocious puberty'):

- adrenal disorders, e.g. CAH, tumors
- ovarian, e.g. tumor (granulosa cell)
- exogenous sex hormone.

Box 7.1 lists tips for assessing the maturity of the uterus and ovaries.

Isolated premature thelarche

Isolated premature thelarche is isolated breast development without progression through puberty (Fig. 7.16).[21] The main features are:[16]

- females between 6 months and 2 years of age
- breast enlargement may be asymmetrical
- different from precocious puberty: absence of axillary and pubic hair and no growth spurt
- self-limiting.

Ultrasound may show fewer but larger ovarian follicles which wax and wane with breast enlargement, usually in 6-weekly cycles. The uterus is usually normal. No investigations are required.

Isolated premature adrenarche

Premature adrenarche is the premature development of pubic or axillary hair with no other signs of puberty. The uterus and ovaries are generally normal. Interestingly, Adams[1] has observed polycystic ovary morphology in eight out of twelve girls examined with premature adrenarche.

The main features are:

- before 8 years in a female and 9 years in a male
- more common in Asian and Afro-Caribbean children

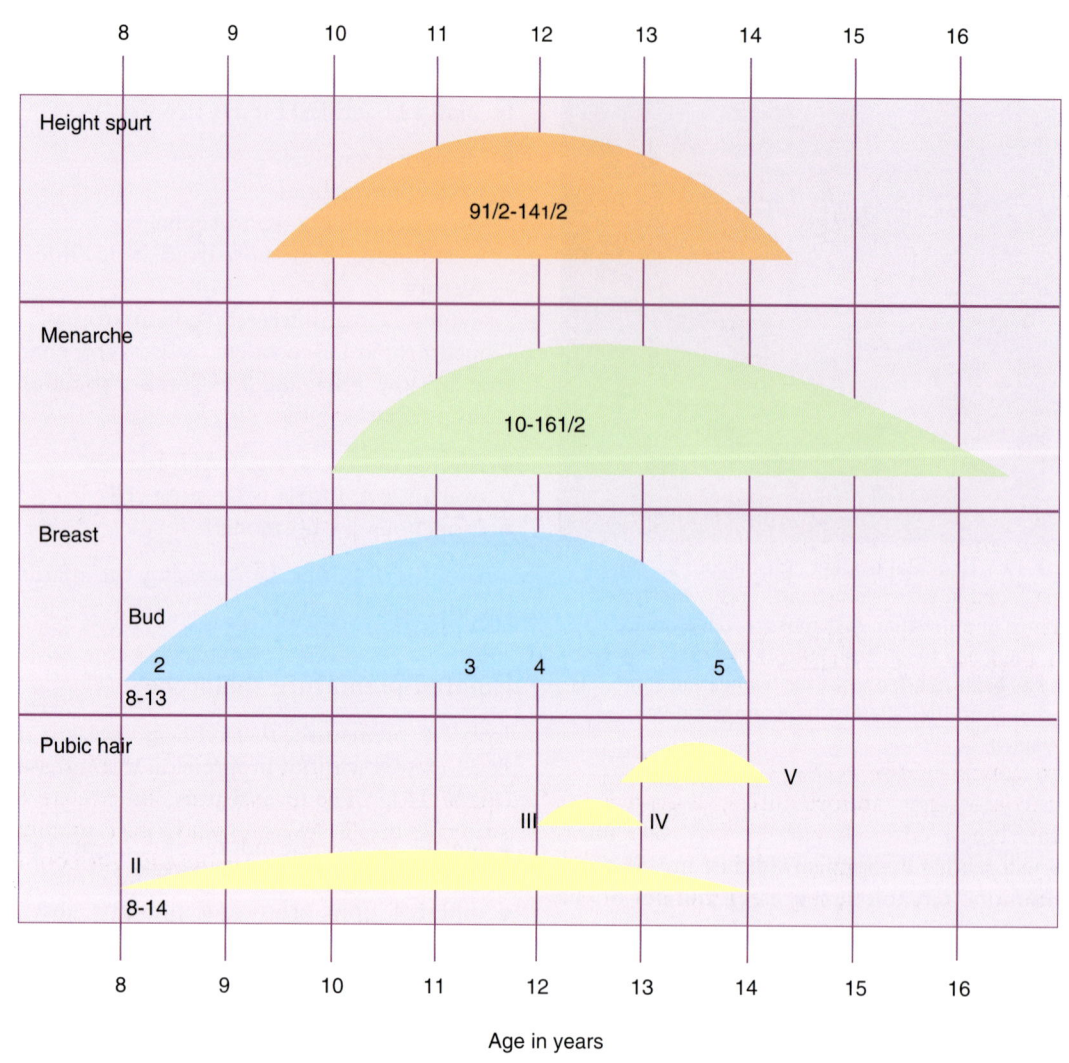

Figure 7.13 Example of the normal sequence of events at puberty in a girl. Menarche occurs only after stage 4 breast development has been attained. (After Tanner JM: Growth at adolescence, 2nd edn; Oxford: Blackwell Scientific; 1962.)

- slight increase in growth rate
- self-limiting
- ultrasound will show no accelerated development of uterus or ovaries.

Pubertal delay

This is defined as the absence of pubertal development by 14 years in females and 15 years in males. This is more common in males and it is usually constitutional. Affected boys are usually short in childhood, and there is a family history of a late puberty in the father. If pubertal delay is found in girls then they should be karotyped for Turner syndrome and their thyroid and sex hormones measured.

Causes of delayed puberty are:

- constitutional delay
- low gonadotropin secretion
  —systemic disease, e.g. CF, asthma, Crohn, anorexia nervosa
  —hypothalamo-pituitary disorders, e.g. growth hormone deficiency
  —acquired hypothyroidism

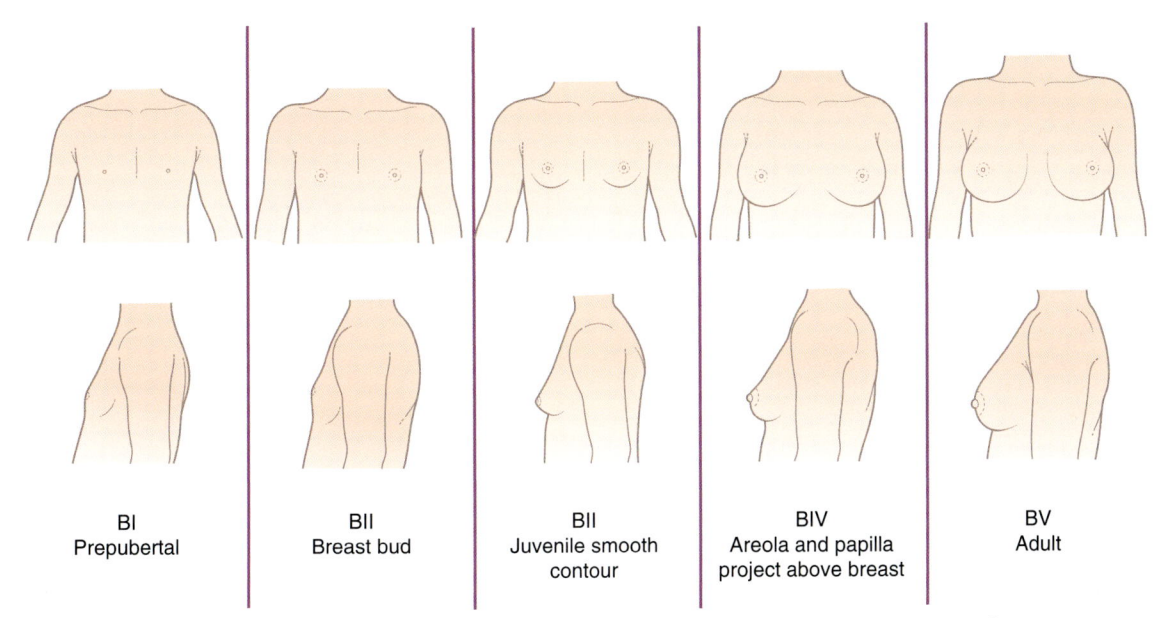

BI	BII	BII	BIV	BV
Prepubertal	Breast bud	Juvenile smooth contour	Areola and papilla project above breast	Adult

Figure 7.14 Breast development. The normal standards of breast development during adolescence. (After Tanner JM: Growth at adolescence, 2nd edn; Oxford: Blackwell Scientific; 1962.)

high gonadotropin secretion
—chromosomal abnormalities, e.g. Turner, Klinefelter
—steroid hormone enzyme deficiency
—acquired, e.g. chemo/radiotherapy, post-surgery.

Ultrasound will demonstrate the presence of normal (usually multifollicular) ovaries and uterus in a girl who is constitutionally delayed. In primary gonadal failure, for example Turner syndrome, ultrasound will also show the small 'streak' ovaries and prepubertal uterine development (Fig. 7.17).[22]

Amenorrhea, either primary or secondary, is an integral part of the diagnosis of anorexia nervosa. Patients with primary amenorrhoea show the prepubertal appearance of the uterus and ovaries, while those who become ill and lose weight after menses has commenced show a marked regression in the size of the uterus and ovaries. In particular, the ovaries become quiescent and show no follicular activity. Ultrasound now plays a major clinical role in predicting when an 'ideal' (i.e. healthy) target weight has been achieved for the resumption of menses.[23,24]

Interestingly, polycystic ovaries (PCO) has been reported in bulimia nervosa. The reason for the higher incidence of PCO in this eating disorder is unknown, but is thought to be related to the swings in insulin levels resulting from the bingeing and vomiting which is a feature of this condition.

Menstrual dysfunction in adolescence

Maturation of the hypothalamic–pituitary–ovarian axis which is responsible for cyclical activity during menstrual cycles is a gradual and slow process. It is recognized that up to 80% of menstrual cycles after menarche are anovulatory.

The major symptoms of adolescent menstrual dysfunction are:

- secondary amenorrhea
- primary amenorrhea
- dysfunctional bleeding
- oligomenorrhea.

A significant number of these girls will have PCO.

Polycystic ovaries

Until recently PCO was considered to be a problem confined to adult women; however it is increasingly recognized that the onset may take place in adolescence.

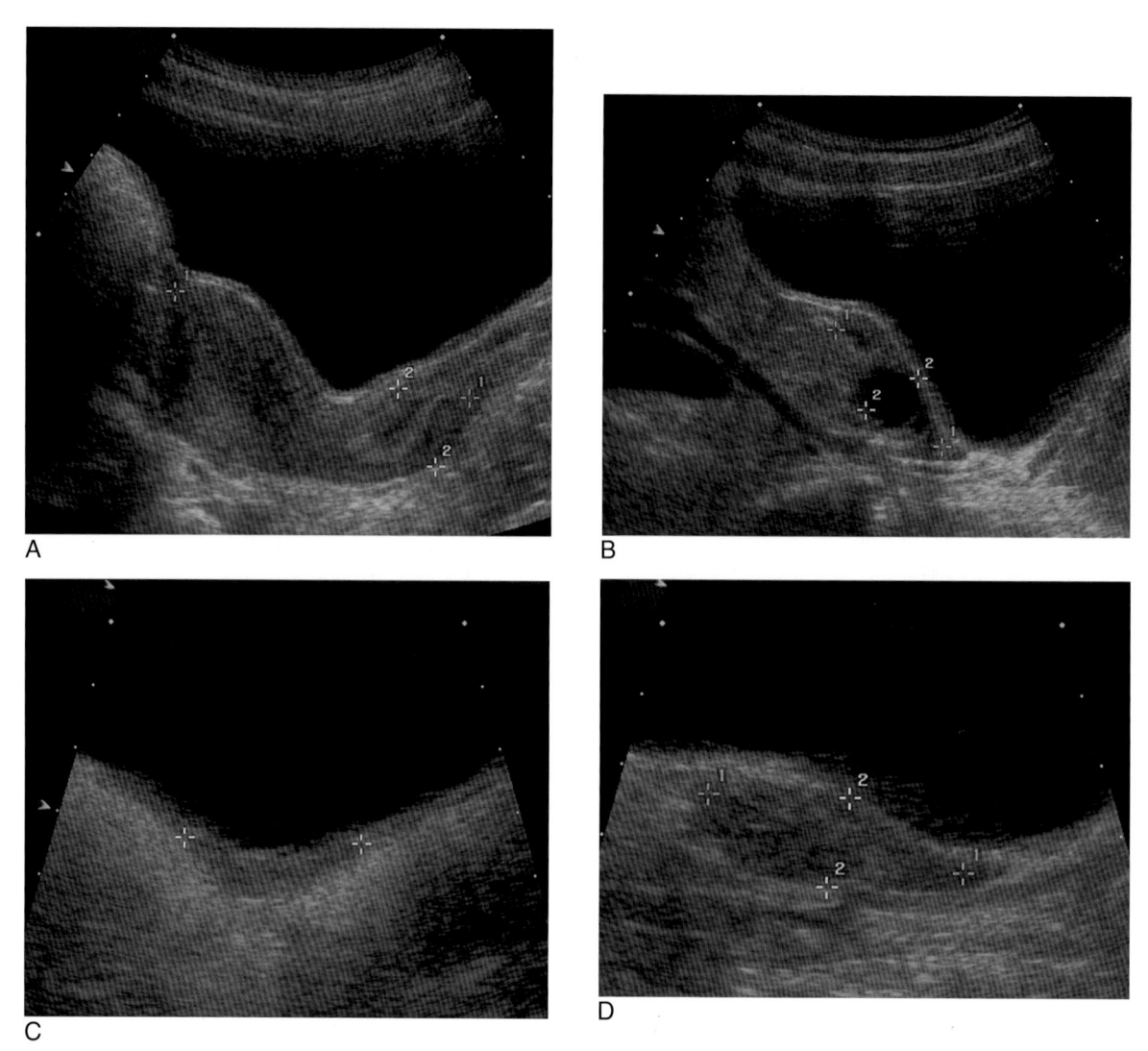

Figure 7.15 Precocious puberty. Ultrasound evaluation of two girls of 8 years, both presenting clinically with precocious puberty. (A) Girl 1. This shows the uterus is large and adult in configuration and has grown and developed. This uterus is truly precocious for the girl's age. (B) Oblique sonogram of the right ovary in the same girl (between calipers). The ovary contains a single large dominant follicle. This girl clearly has precocious development for her age. (C) Girl 2. Longitudinal sonogram of the uterus (between calipers) in this 8-year old girl showed that the uterus had not developed and has a prepubertal appearance. (D) The right ovary in this girl (between calipers) with no uterine development shows that it is not active and follicular and that she does not have precocious uterine or ovarian development.

THE FEMALE REPRODUCTIVE SYSTEM

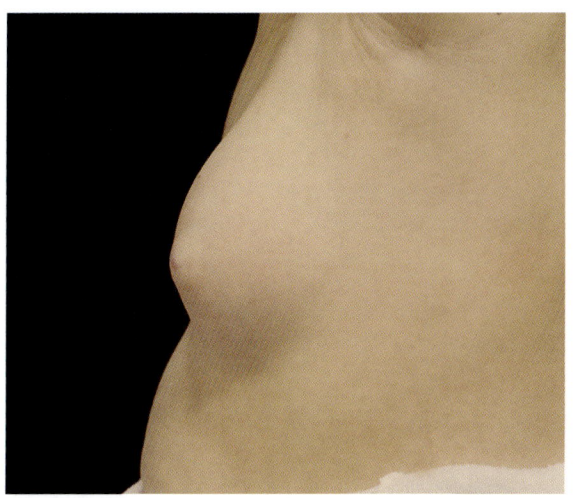

Figure 7.16 Isolated premature thelarche. Clinical picture of an 18-month old girl who presented with cyclical enlarging breasts.

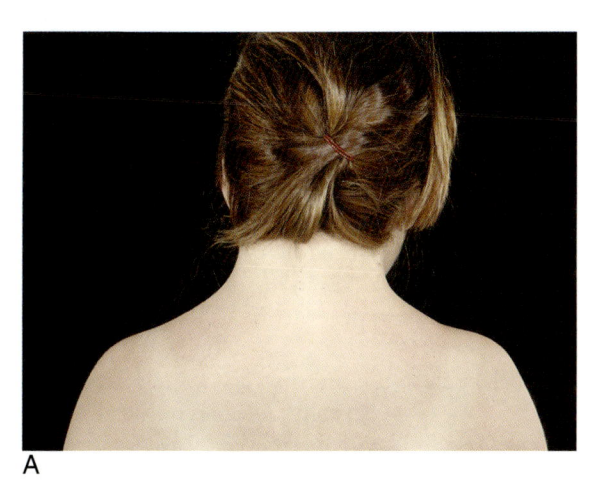

> **Box 7.1 Tips for assessing the maturity of the uterus and ovaries**
>
> - Ovaries can normally be very follicular throughout childhood
> - Uterine length and configuration of AP cervix and AP fundus together with ovarian volume are the best parameters to use
> - Active ovaries are those with a lot of follicular activity, and this generally indicates that they are stimulated
> - In true precocious puberty, enlarged active follicular ovaries are accompanied by concomitant growth of the uterus
> - A single large functioning ovarian follicle can stimulate the uterus. Regression will cause a withdrawal bleed
> - Menarche does not occur until breast stage 4 development
> - If the endometrial stripe is < 5 mm, menarche is not imminent

Polycystic ovaries are a distinct morphological entity and should not be confused with the polycystic ovarian syndrome (PCOS)—that is, the association of PCO, hirsuitism, obesity, oligo-amenorrhea and infertility as originally described by Stein and Leventhal in 1935. Prior to recent developments in pelvic ultrasound the morphological diagnosis was based on typical laparoscopic and histological findings on ovarian biopsy. Typical appearances of the ovary on ultrasound are now an important criterion for the diagnosis of PCOS in girls with suggestive clinical features, although these may not be present in all such girls.

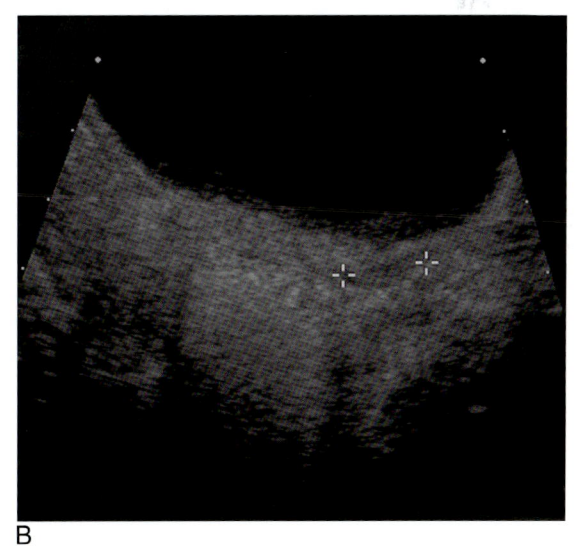

Figure 7.17 Turner syndrome. (A) This young girl with Turner sundrome has a web-shaped neck and a low hairline. (B) Sonogram of the ovary in a girl with Turner syndrome showing the small 'streak' ovary with virtually no follicular activity.

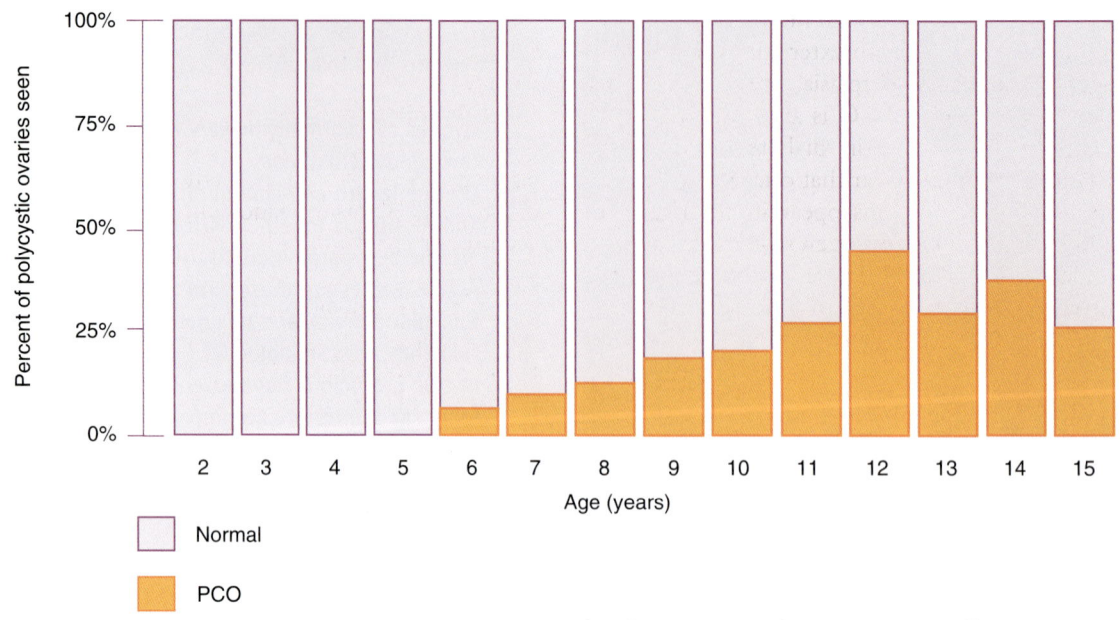

Figure 7.18 Chart showing occurrence of polycystic ovaries (PCO) in childhood. (After Bridges et al.[6])

Polycystic ovaries are defined on ultrasound as:

- ovaries with an increased ovarian volume (although they may be normal volume). In the adult PCO population studied by Polson et al[25] the mean ovarian volume was > 10 ml, which is at the maximum size of normal ovaries; however, some were diagnosed as PCO morphology at a volume of 4 ml
- a necklace of follicles with at least 8–10 follicles around the periphery of the ovary measuring 2–8 mm
- an increase in the echodense central stroma.

Studies have reported the incidence of PCO in the normal adult population to be 22–25%. Bridges et al[6] reported the morphological appearance of PCO as early as 6 years in their study of normal girls, with a peak incidence at puberty corresponding to the rise in insulin-like growth factor I and insulin at this time (Figs 7.18 and 7.19).[25–29]

The etiology of PCO is unknown, but that PCO is linked to puberty is well recognized. Women with PCOS have a family history of relatives with PCO, and there appears to be a strong hereditary component.

It has been suggested that PCOS may be caused by early or exaggerated adrenarche leading to increased anabolism (obesity), increased androgen stimulation (acne and hirsuitism) and inadequate feedback (chronic anovulation), presenting with various menstrual disorders.

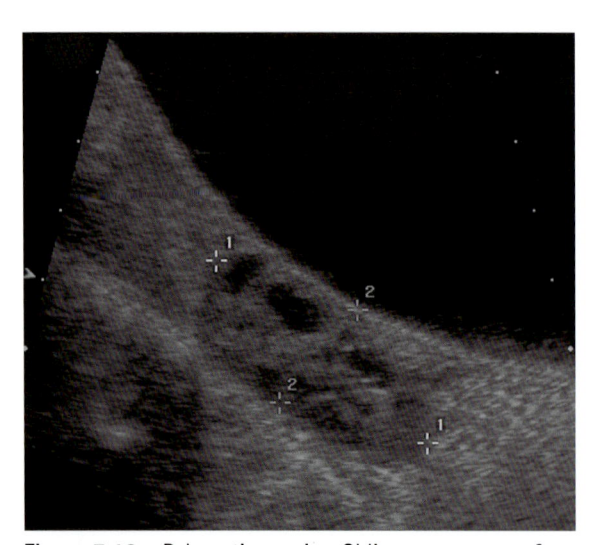

Figure 7.19 Polycystic ovaries. Oblique sonogram of the right ovary (between calipers) in an adolescent girl showing the underlying morphology of PCO. The ovary is large with multiple small follicles on the surface of the ovary, with an increase in the central stroma.

Conditions associated with high levels of androgen that originate from an external source, such as congenital adrenal hyperplasia, are known to be associated with PCO. PCO is also associated with low insulin levels (e.g. in diabetes) and insulin resistance. It would appear that once present, PCO morphology does not disappear in the ovary. In children it is found in glycogen storage disease and in older girls bulimia. These diverse conditions both clinically have swings in glucose levels. It is thought this is the cause of PCO.

OVARIAN NEOPLASMS

Ovarian neoplasms are extremely rare and account for less than 1% of all pediatric tumors. The majority are benign, with an overall malignancy rate of about 15–30%. The common presenting complaint is that of abdominal pain and a palpable abdominal mass. Some may undergo torsion.

Rarely, ovarian tumors may secrete hormones and the child will present with precocious puberty, typically with granulosa theca cell tumors. Andrenoblastoma is associated with virilization.

Ultrasonically a complex ovarian mass cannot be reliably differentiated from an ovarian cyst torsion, hemorrhage or tumor and, apart from the teratoma, none of the ovarian tumors can be reliably differentiated.

Once ultrasound has established the potential diagnosis of an ovarian or vaginal mass, further cross-sectional imaging such as CT or MRI is undertaken as this is more reliable in accurately staging the disease, local invasion of tissues, lymph nodes and distal metastases to the liver.

Ovarian tumors are classified according to their organ of origin, e.g. germ cell, epithelial or mesenchymal cells.

Germ cell tumors

Germ cell tumors predominate, and the commonest is a teratoma. Dermoids or teratomas make up nearly a half of all benign ovarian tumors. The age range is late childhood to early adolescence.

Teratomas Benign cystic teratomas are the commonest ovarian tumors. However, the younger the child, the more likely they are to have a malignant teratoma. They arise from all three germ layers, so that fat, teeth and fragments of bone may be found.

Ultrasonically they have a characteristic appearance due to their composition, with highly echogenic areas of calcification, teeth, bone and fat, and cystic areas. Acoustic shadowing from a nodule on the wall or central mass, or a fat fluid level may be present.

Thirty percent of teratomas are malignant, and these are associated with raised alfa-fetoprotein levels in the blood (Fig. 7.20).

Some infants may present with sacrococcygeal teratomas, which is the differential diagnosis of a pelvic mass if it extends into the pelvis (Fig 7.21).

Malignant ovarian masses

Malignant ovarian lesions usually occur in postpubertal girls. They present like any other pelvic mass, with pain, distension and evidence of lower gastrointestinal obstruction.

Sonography generally cannot differentiate such a mass from other pelvic masses, but the role of ultrasound is to determine the site of origin (Fig. 7.22). Characteristic appearances to look for would include:

- an ill-defined margin
- a more solid element
- fluid in the pouch of Douglas
- ascites
- lymphadenopathy
- liver secondaries.

Secondary ovarian neoplasms

These are most commonly lymphoma and leukemia, in which case the whole of the ovary appears large and hypoechoic. Neuroblastoma may also rarely metastasize.

Other genital tumors

Embryonal (botyroid) rhabdomyosarcoma of the vagina is seen in very young girls. They arise from the vaginal wall and present with a hemorrhagic

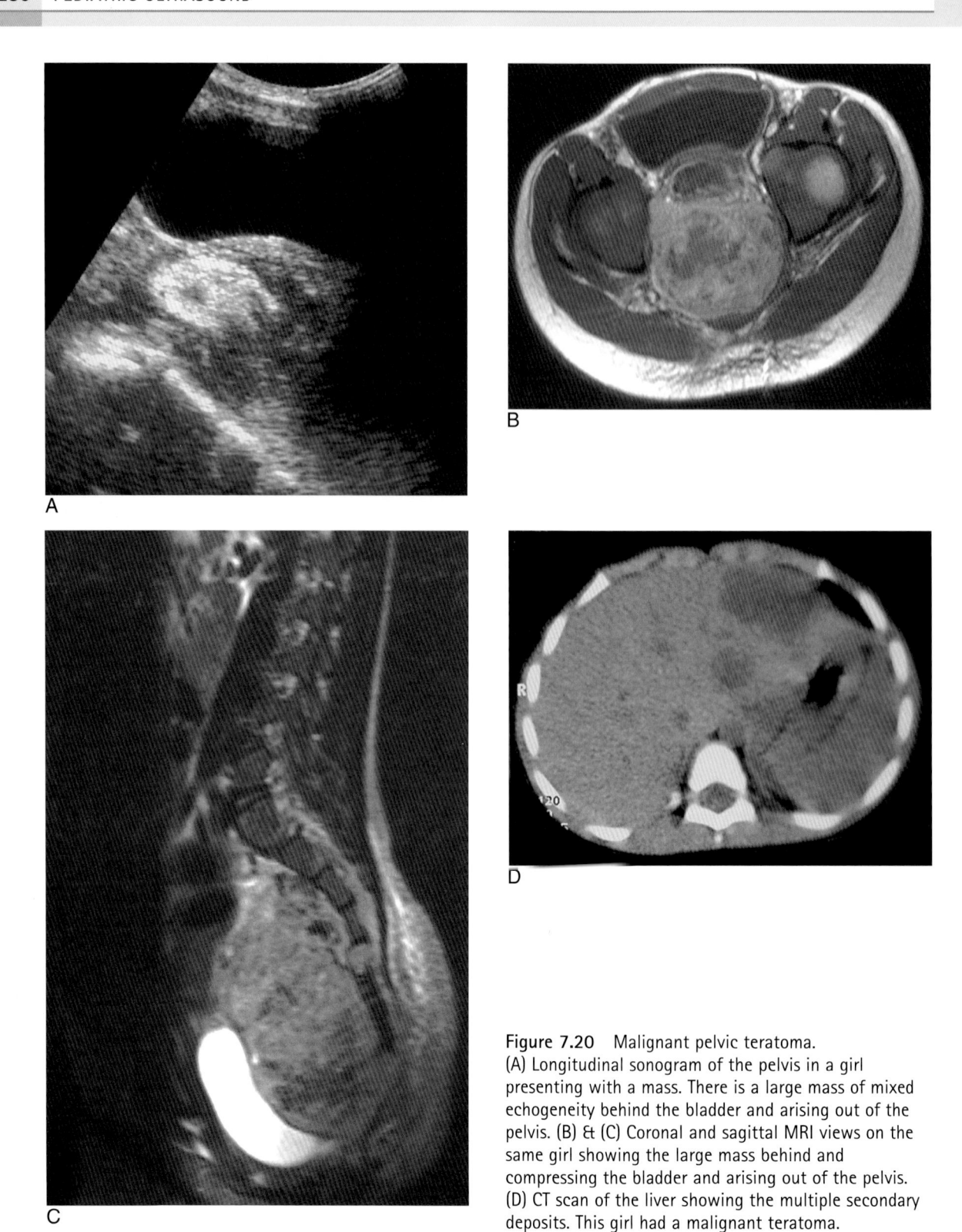

Figure 7.20 Malignant pelvic teratoma. (A) Longitudinal sonogram of the pelvis in a girl presenting with a mass. There is a large mass of mixed echogeneity behind the bladder and arising out of the pelvis. (B) & (C) Coronal and sagittal MRI views on the same girl showing the large mass behind and compressing the bladder and arising out of the pelvis. (D) CT scan of the liver showing the multiple secondary deposits. This girl had a malignant teratoma.

THE FEMALE REPRODUCTIVE SYSTEM   231

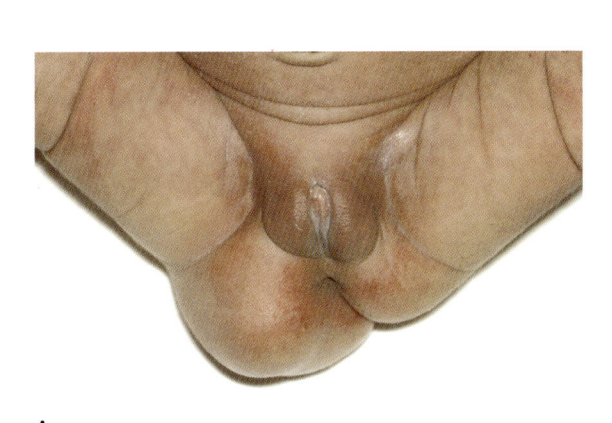

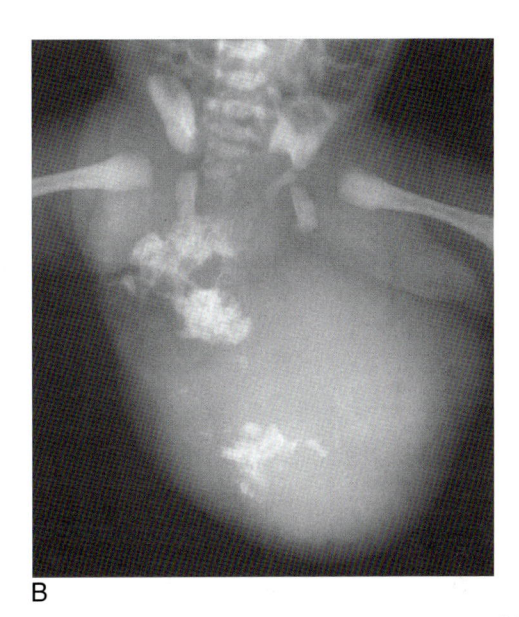

Figure 7.21 Sacrococcygeal teratoma. (A) This infant presented with a large lump protruding from the perineum. (B) Plain abdominal radiograph in another infant with a similar mass reveals the typical dense areas of calcification seen in sacrococcygeal teratomas. The pelvic bones appear widely splayed.

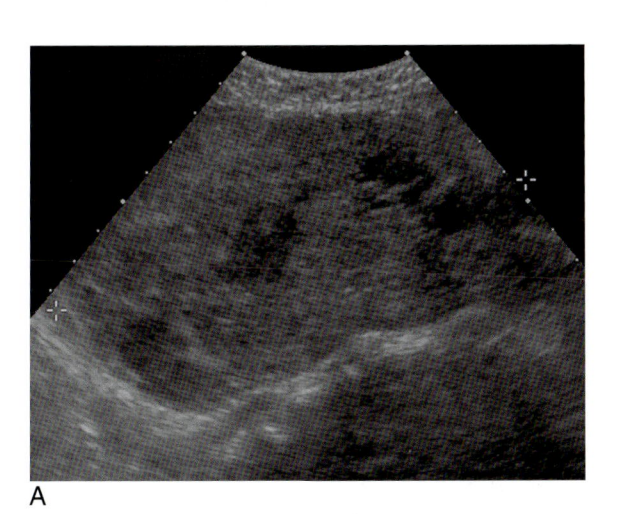

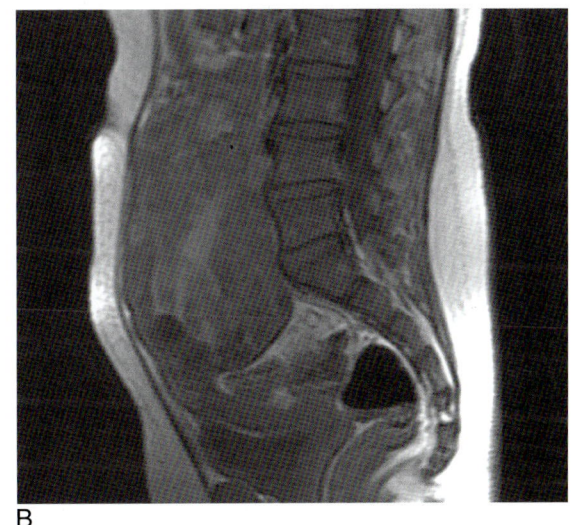

Figure 7.22 Ovarian mass. (A) This girl presented with a lower abdominal mass. The ultrasound examination revealed a well-defined mass of mixed echogenicity which at biopsy was found to be ovarian. The different types of ovarian masses cannot be differentiated on imaging. (B) Sagittal MRI scan on the same girl. This clearly shows how an ovarian mass enters the pelvis rather than arising out of the pelvis. This is a feature to look for when differentiating pelvic masses sonographically.

discharge, extrusion of the mass from the vagina (sarcoma botryoides) or an abdominal mass.

The role of ultrasound is to:

- define the origin of the mass
- note any complications such as hydrocolpos
- detect local nodal spread
- detect distal hepatic spread
- determine if there is obstruction to the urinary tract.

SUMMARY

Ultrasound is the imaging modality of choice in the pediatric female genital system. It is essential that the sonographer is familiar with the normal range of appearances throughout childhood and adolescence. MRI is a valuable adjunct in pelvic masses and to help delineate structural abnormalities of the genital system.

References

1. Adams J. The role of pelvic ultrasound in the management of paediatric endocrine disorders. In: Brook CDG, ed. Clinical paediatric endocrinology. 2nd edn. Oxford: Blackwell Scientific; 1993:675–691.
2. Currarino G. Caffey's pediatric X-ray diagnosis: the genitourinary tract. Chicago: Year Book; 1984:1719–1732.
3. Rosenfield RL. The ovary and female sexual maturation, In: Kaplan SA, ed. Clinical paediatric and adolescent endocrinology. Philadelphia: WB Saunders; 1982:217–288.
4. Boyar R, Finkelstein J, Roffwarg H, et al. Synchronization of augmented secretion of luteinizing hormone secretion with sleep during puberty. N Engl J Med 1972; 287:582.
5. Hackeloer BJ, Nitschke-Dabelstein S. Ovarian imaging by ultrasound: an attempt to define a reference plane. J Clin Ultrasound 1980; 8:497–500.
6. Bridges NA, Cooke A, Healy MJR, et al. Standards for ovarian volume in childhood and puberty. Fertility & Sterility 1993; 60:456–460.
7. Cohen HL, Tice HM, Mandel FS. Ovarian volumes measures by ultrasound: bigger than we think. Radiology 1990; 177:189.
8. Griffin IJ, Cole TJ, Duncan KA, et al. Pelvic ultrasound measurements in normal girls. Acta Paediatr 1995; 84:536–543.
9. Haller J, Friedman AP, Schaffer R, et al. The normal and abnormal ovary in childhood and adolescence. Semin Ultrasound 1984; 4(3):206–255.
10. Orsini LP, Salardi SS, Pia G, et al. Pelvic organs in premenarchal girls; real-time ultrasonography. Radiology 1984; 153:113–116.
11. Peters H, Himmelstein-Graw, Faber M. The normal development of the ovary in childhood. Acta Endocrinol 1976; 82:617–630.
12. Polhemus DW. Ovarian maturation and cyst formation in children. Paediatrics 1953; 11:588–594.
13. Salardi S, Orsini L, Cacciari E, et al. Pelvic ultrasonography in premenarchal girls: relation to puberty and sex hormone concentrations. Arch Dis Child 1985; 60:120–125.
14. Adams J, Polson DW, Abulwahid N, et al. Multifollicular ovaries: clinical and endocrine features and response to pulsatile gonadotrophin releasing hormone. Lancet 1985; ii:1375–1379.
15. Nussbaum AR, Sanders RC, Jones MD. Neonatal uterine morphology as seen on real-time US. Radiology 1986; 160:641–643.
16. Griffin IJ, Cole TJ, Duncan KA, et al. Pelvic ultrasound findings in different forms of sexual precocity. Acta Paediatr 1995; 84:544–549.
17. Lyon AJ, de Bruyn R, Grant DB. Transient sexual precocity and ovarian cysts. Arch Dis Child 1985; 60:819–822.
18. Nussbaum AR, Sanders RC, Hartman DS, et al. Neonatal ovarian cysts: sonographic–pathologic correlation. Radiology 1988; 168:817–821.
19. Salardi S, Orsini LF, Cacciari E, et al. Pelvic ultrasonography in girls with precocious puberty, congenital adrenal hyperplasia, obesity or hirsutism. J Paediatr 1988; 112:880–887.
20. Stanhope R, Adams J, Jacobs HS, et al. Ovarian ultrasound assessment in normal children, idiopathic precocious puberty and during low dose pulsatile GnRH treatment of hypogonadotrophic hypogonadism. Arch Dis Child 1985; 60: 116–119.
21. Stanhope R, Adams J, Brook CGD. Fluctuation of breast size in isolated premature thelarche. Acta Paediatr Scand 1985; 74:454–455.

22. Wood DF, Franks S. Delayed puberty. Br J Hosp Med 1989; 4:223–230.
23. Treasure JL, Gordon PAL, King EA, et al. Cystic ovaries; a phase of anorexia nervosa. Lancet 1985; ii:1379–1381.
24. Lai YCL, de Bruyn R, Lask B, et al. Use of pelvic ultrasound to monitor ovarian and uterine maturity in childhood onset anorexia nervosa. Arch Dis Child 1994; 71:228–231.
25. Polson DW, Adams J, Wadsworth J, et al. Polycystic ovaries: a common finding in normal women. Lancet 1988; i:870–872.
26. Clayton RN, Ogden V, Hodgkinson J, et al. How common are polycystic ovaries in normal women and what is their significance for fertility of the population? Clin Endocrinol 1992; 37:127–134.
27. Eden JA, Jones J, Carter GD, et al. Follicular fluid concentrations of insulin like growth factor, transforming growth factor alpha and sex steroids in volume matched normal and polycystic human follicles. Clin Endocrinol 1990; 32(4):395–405.
28. Hague WM, Adams J, Rodda C, et al. The prevalence of polycystic ovaries in patients with congenital adrenal hyperplasia and their close relatives. Clin Endocrinol 1990; 33:501–510.
29. McCluskey S, Evans C, Lacey JH, et al. Polycystic ovary syndrome and bulimia. Fertility & Sterility 1991; 55:287–291.

Chapter 8

The scrotum and testes

CHAPTER CONTENTS

Embryology 235
    Abnormalities of position of the testis 237
Normal anatomy 238
Ultrasound technique 240
Congenital anomalies 241
    Cryptorchidism 241
    Hernias and hydroceles 241
    Varicocele 242
Acutely painful scrotum 243
    Testicular torsion 243
    Epididymo-orchitis and epididymitis 246
    Torsion of the appendix testis 246
Microlithiasis 246
Testicular tumors 247
    Primary testicular tumors 248
    Secondary neoplasms 248
    Benign testicular masses 248
Extratesticular masses 248
    Cystic extratesticular masses 248
    Solid extratesticular masses 249
    Paratesticular rhabdomyosarcoma 249
Scrotal trauma 249

Ultrasound is the prime imaging modality of choice when examining the testes and scrotum in boys. High resolution ultrasound using a linear array transducer of 10–15 MHz is an excellent, extremely accurate, non-invasive technique for the detection and evaluation of scrotal pathology. Doppler is an essential part of the examination, particularly in suspected torsion. A gel stand-off is generally not required with these modern high frequency probes.

MRI has been used successfully to identify undescended testes in the abdomen and inguinal canal that ultrasound has failed to identify. CT plays little routine role in the scrotum except in malignant masses when the abdomen needs to be further evaluated.

EMBRYOLOGY

Duct system

The Sertoli cells of the developing fetal testes produce masculinizing hormones, such as testosterone, which stimulate the mesonephric (old kidney) ducts to form male genital ducts. Some mesonephric tubules persist and are transformed into efferent ductules. These ductules open into the mesonephric duct which has become the ductus epididymis. Just beyond the epididymis the mesonephric duct develops a thick covering of smooth muscle and becomes the ductus deferens. Lateral outgrowths from the caudal end of each mesonephric duct give rise to the seminal vesicles, glands that produce a secretion that provides nourishment for the sperm. The part of the mesonephric duct between the seminal vesicle ducts and the urethra becomes the ejaculatory duct (Fig. 8.1).

The prostate develops from multiple outgrowths from the prostatic part of the urethra, which grow into the surrounding mesenchyme. The appendix testis is a vestigial remnant of the paramesonephric duct system and is attached to the head of the epididymis.

Descent of the testes

The testes need to descend into the scrotum so that viable spermatozoa can develop. The scrotum is outside the thermal regulation of the body and is a cooler environment. Failure to descend can result in infertility or even malignancy.

The inguinal canals are the pathways for the testes to descend from their intra-abdominal location through the anterior abdominal wall into the scrotum. A ligament called the gubernaculum is attached at its upper or cranial end to the inferior pole of each gonad. It descends on either side of the abdomen and passes obliquely through the developing anterior abdominal wall at the site of the future inguinal canal (Fig. 8.2). The gubernaculum attaches caudally to the internal surface of the labioscrotal swellings and later serves to anchor the testes in the scrotum. The processus vaginalis is an evagination of the peritoneum and follows the gubernaculum. It herniates through the abdominal wall along the path formed by the gubernaculum and also serves to help guide the testis into the scrotum. The processus vaginalis carries the layers of the abdominal wall before it and goes on to form the walls of the inguinal canal. In males these layers are the coverings of the spermatic cord and testes.

Testicular descent is associated with enlargement of the testes and atrophy of the intermediate or mesonephric kidneys. This atrophy allows the movement of testes caudally along the posterior abdominal wall. Little is known about the cause of testicular descent through the inguinal canals into the scrotum, but the process is controlled by androgens produced by the fetal testes. Conditions associated with

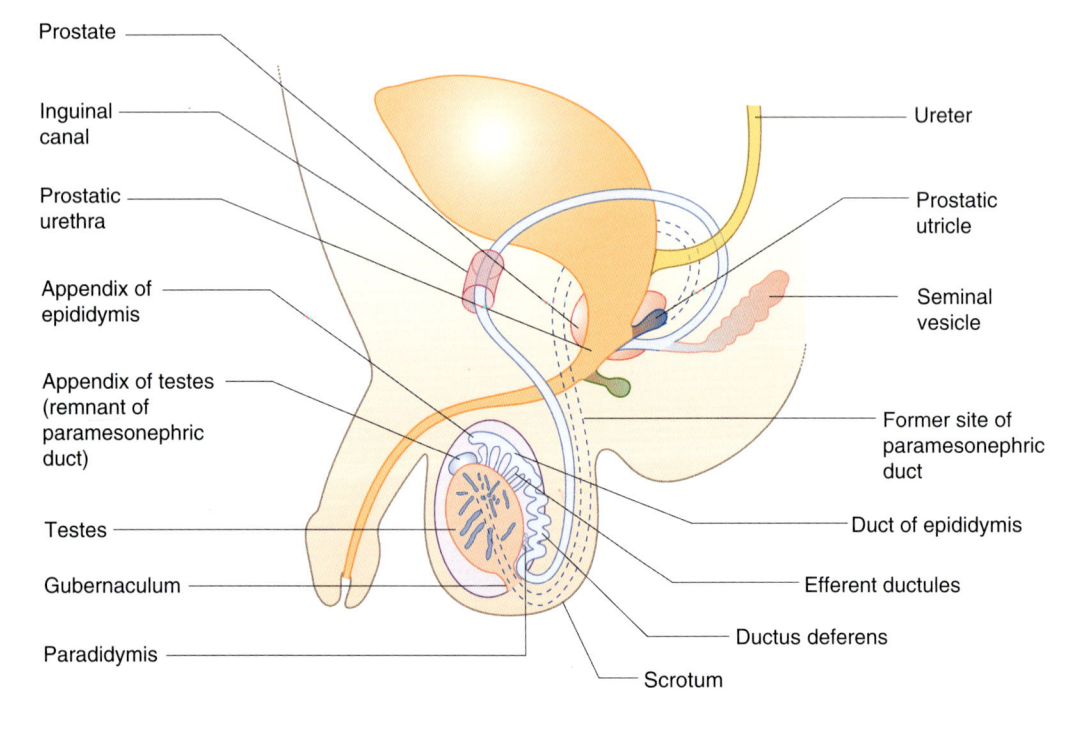

Figure 8.1 Male embryology. The origin of the male genital tract from the mesonephric duct system and from the urogenital sinus.

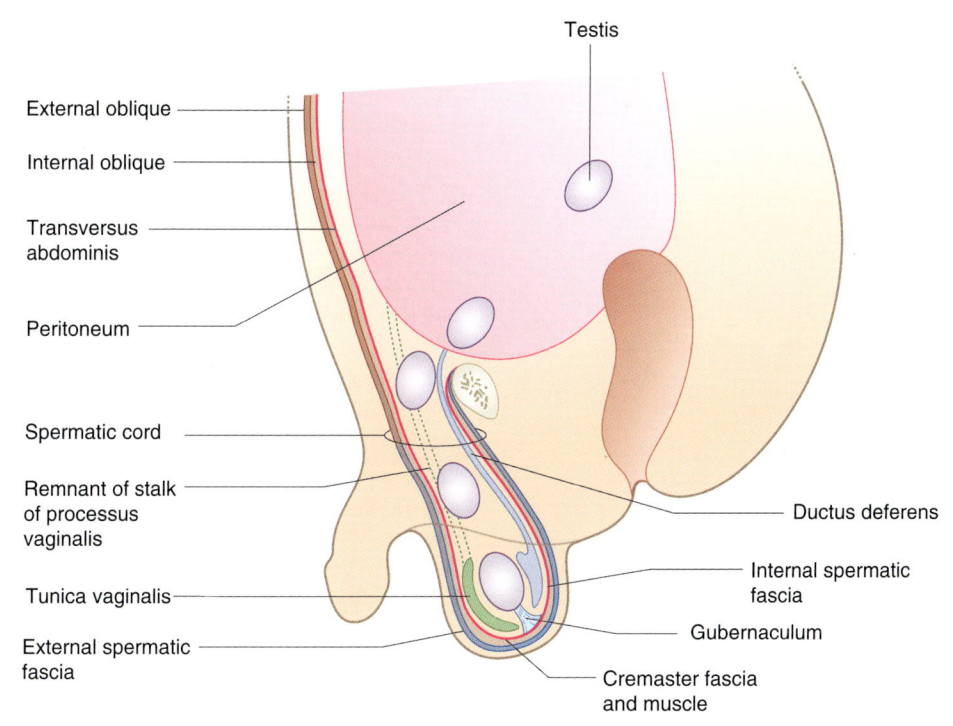

Figure 8.2 The path of descent of the normal testis into the scrotum.

diminished gonadotropins are associated with cryptorchidism such as the Prader–Willi syndrome.

The initial descent of the testes in the transabdominal phase is androgen independent and usually takes place before the 26th week of intrauterine life. After that the testes enter the scrotum from the internal inguinal ring, and this phase appears to be androgen dependent. The inguinal canal then contracts around the spermatic cord.

During the first 3 months after birth most undescended testes descend into the scrotum. Spontaneous testicular descent does not occur after the age of 1 year.

During the perinatal period, the connecting stalk of the processus normally obliterates, isolating the tunica vaginalis as a peritoneal sac related to the testes.

Abnormalities of position of the testis

Cryptorchidism, or undescended testes

Cryptorchidism occurs in up to 30% of premature males and in about 3–4% of full-term males. It is the commonest genitourinary abnormality in males. Cryptorchidism may be unilateral in about 65% of males or bilateral in about 10%, but in most cases the testes descend into the scrotum by the end of the first year. If testes remain in the abdominal cavity they fail to mature and sterility is common. Cryptorchid testes may be in the abdominal cavity or anywhere along the usual path of descent but they are usually in the inguinal canal.

The cause of cryptorchidism is unknown, but a deficiency of androgen is an important factor. There is a higher incidence of cryptorchidism in prune belly syndrome and abdominal wall defects. Men with a history of cryptorchidism have a 20–44% increase in risk of developing testicular cancer.

Ectopic testes

After traversing the inguinal canal, the testes may deviate from their usual path of descent and lodge in various abnormal locations (Fig. 8.3). They may be present in the contralateral scrotum, the perineum, the superficial inguinal pouch, the femoral

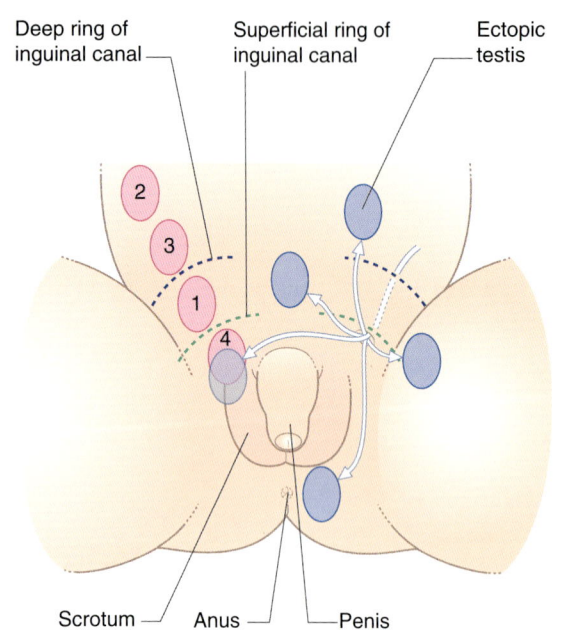

Figure 8.3 Common positions where an ectopic (right) or undescended testis (left, numbered) may be found.

NORMAL ANATOMY

At birth the testes are oval shaped and normally 1.5 cm in length increasing to 2 cm by the age of 3 months. At adrenarche around about 7 years they slightly increase in size again, and at puberty they again increase in size to measure approximately 3–5 cm in length and 2–3 cm in width. Both sides are normally of similar size. The testis is enclosed in a tough fibrous membrane, the tunica albuginea, which is visible as a linear structure at the mediastinum. The tunica albuginea is not usually identified unless the testis is surrounded by fluid. Fibrous septae divide the testis into lobules centered on the hilum which are also not seen on a normal ultrasound. The 200–300 lobules contain tightly coiled seminiferous tubules. The rete testis is the massing together at the testicular hilum of the seminiferous tubules. The normal testis appears as a homogeneous granular structure of medium echogenicity. The mediastinum testis is seen as a highly echogenic line along the superior–inferior axis of the testis (Fig. 8.6).

The epididymis is the echogenic curved structure which lies posterolateral to the testis and has three segments: the head, the body and the tail. It consists of the ductus epididymis, which is a tightly coiled tube. The efferent duct from the head and body drain into the tail as the vas deferens which then passes through the inguinal ring as the spermatic cord. In patients with a hydrocele the extra testicular structures may be seen more clearly. The appendix testis is a separate structure and can be seen usually when a hydrocele is present in about a third of patients.

The scrotum and its contents are supplied by three arteries which can be identified passing through the inguinal canal. The testicular artery arising from the aorta supplies the testes and epididymis. The small cremasteric artery arising from the vesical artery provides part of the blood supply to the scrotal wall and extratesticular structures. Next the deferential artery arising from the inferior epigastric artery supplies the vas deferens. There are anastomoses between these three arteries. The testicular artery penetrates the tunica albuginea towards the head of the testes and branches into capsular arteries that course around the testes. Distally the testicular artery supplies the tunica vas-

canal or suprapubically. Ectopic testes occur when a part of the gubernaculum passes to an abnormal location and the testes follow it. Ectopic testes do not have a higher incidence of malignancy but should be placed in a normal position before the age of 2 years.

Retractile testis

A retractile testis is one that is fully descended but can move freely from its intrascrotal position to the groin because of a hyperactive cremasteric reflex. It occurs in the older boy once the cremasteric reflex develops, and descends spontaneously at puberty. There is no increase in infertility in these boys.

Hydrocele

Occasionally the abdominal end of the processus vaginalis remains open but is too small to permit herniation of intestine. Peritoneal fluid passes into the patent processus vaginalis and forms a hydrocele of the testes. If the middle part of the processus vaginalis canal remains open, fluid may accumulate and give rise to a hydrocele of the spermatic cord (Figs 8.4 and 8.5).

THE SCROTUM AND TESTES 239

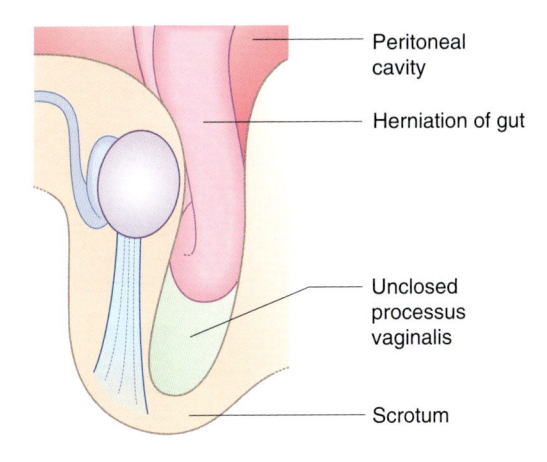

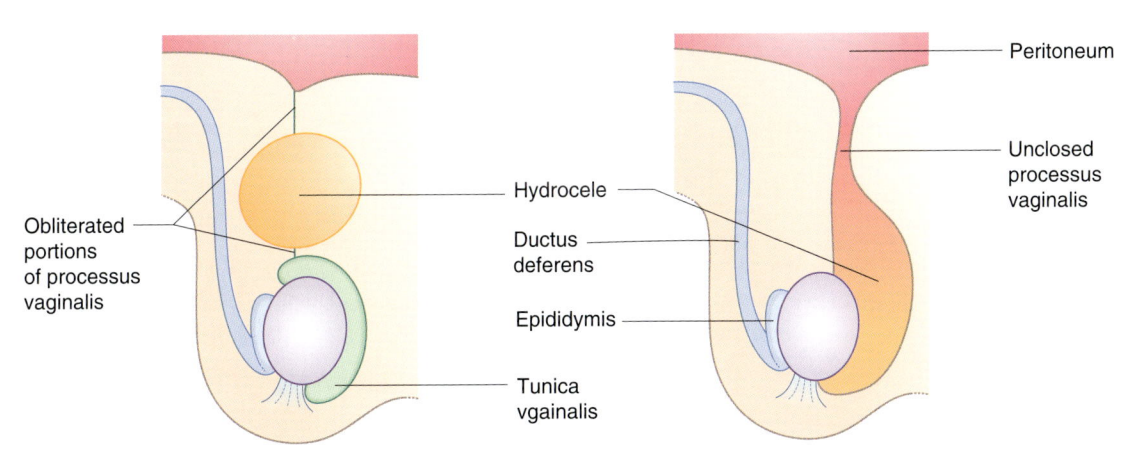

Figure 8.4 Positions of hydroceles in the inguinal canal and scrotum. The diagram shows the positions of hydroceles and herniations related to the inguinal canal and testis, depending on the patency of the processus vaginalis.

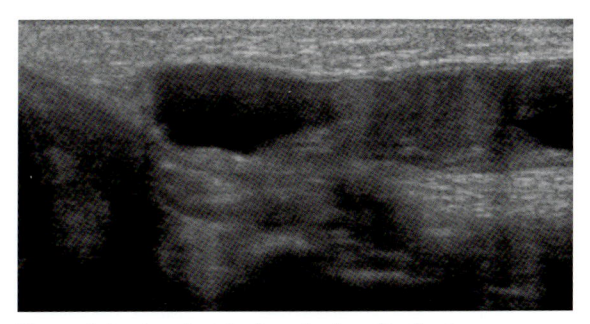

Figure 8.5 Inguinal hydrocele. Longitudinal sonogram of the inguinal canal. There is a hydrocele within the canal, and the testis can also be seen lying ectopically high in the inguinal canal.

culosa, a network of blood vessels that surround the testes. The testicular artery is an important artery to learn to identify, particularly in the region of the inguinal canal.

The testicular veins run in similar planes to the arteries. They emerge from the back of the testes where, with branches from the epididymis, they form the pampiniform plexus which passes as part of the spermatic cord through the inguinal canal. This plexus is closely related to the epididymis, and it is difficult to separate the two structures. Enlarged veins or a varicocele may be readily identified on

240 PEDIATRIC ULTRASOUND

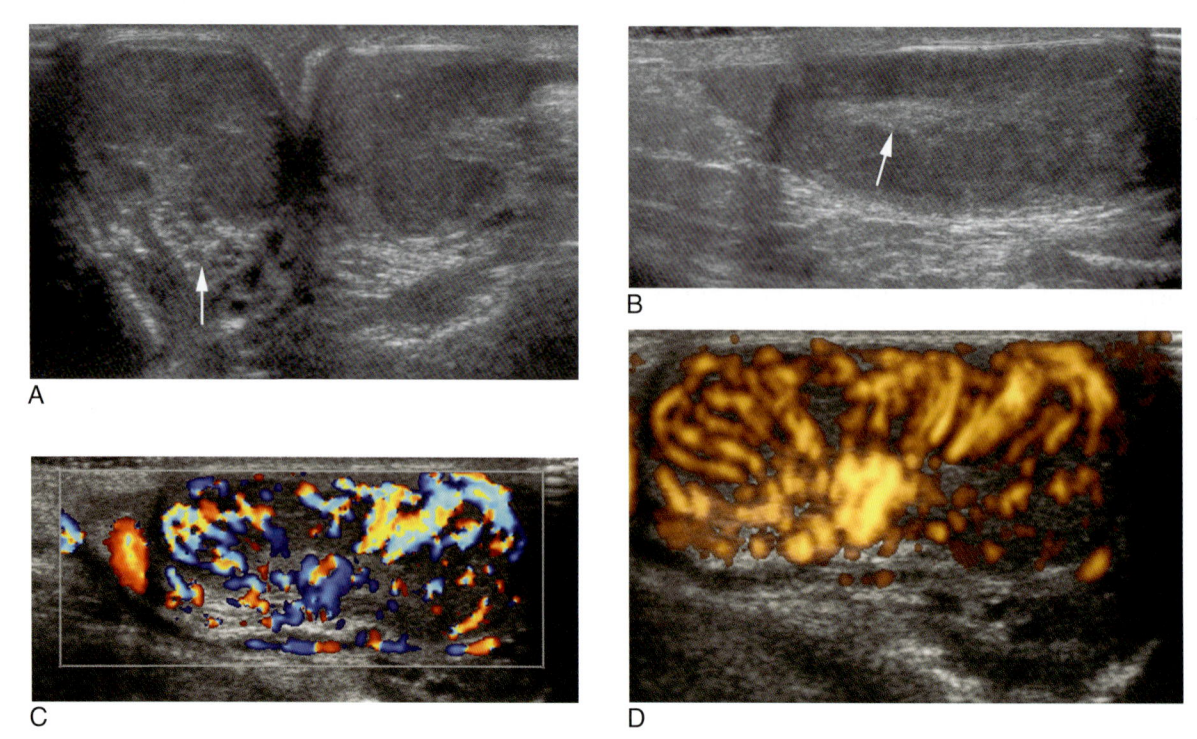

Figure 8.6 Normal testicular appearances. (A) Transverse sonogram of the scrotum showing two normal testes. This view usefully compares the echogenicity and size of both testes. The pampiniform plexus (arrow) can be seen behind the testis on the right. Most commonly this cannot be separated from the body of the epididymis. (B) Longitudinal sonogram of the normal testis showing the testicular hilum (arrow) and the normal epididymis and epididymal head. (C) & (D) Color Doppler and color Doppler energy of the testis showing excellent blood flow within the normal testis.

Doppler examination. The pampiniform plexus drains into the testicular veins on the right emptying into the inferior vena cava, and on the left into the left renal vein. It is for this reason that pathologies affecting the left renal vein may be reflected as a varicocele in the left testis, hence the reason for scanning the kidneys when this is found.

The appendix testis is a testicular appendage which is a remnant of the Müllerian duct (see Fig. 8.1). It is important because it may undergo torsion. Unless there is a hydrocele present it is not normally identified.

ULTRASOUND TECHNIQUE

The examination is usually carried out with the patient supine. Gel stand-offs are not usually necessary with modern high resolution transducers. In the young infant the legs should either be in the neutral position or the knees flexed and abducted so the baby is in a frog-legged position to allow better access to the scrotum. In an adolescent boy the sonographer should be sensitive to the patient's modesty and either perform the examination in a private area or provide sufficient covering with sheets or inco pads so that he does not feel uncomfortably exposed and naked. The young boy should be asked to hold the penis in place over the pubis for better access to the perineum. This is not needed in an infant. If necessary, folded sheets or foam pads can be used for support. If a small scrotal or testicular mass is present, it is best to ask the patient to demonstrate the mass. If the scrotum is tense and tender, care should be taken not to hurt the child.[1]

Transducer

The scrotum is best examined with a high frequency linear 15L8 probe, with the testes being testis and can often be indistinguishable from a lymph node. Ultrasound is the initial imaging modality of choice, although MRI is recommended for locating testes within the abdomen or pelvis which are not seen with ultrasound.

A renal examination should always be included when looking for an undescended testis, because of the association with renal anomalies.

Hernias and hydroceles

Hernias and hydroceles are the commonest causes of a painless scrotal mass in childhood. The following terms should be understood when examining the inguinal canals and scrotum.

- A hernia is the protrusion of a portion of an organ or tissue through the wall normally containing it.
- A hydrocele is a collection of fluid surrounding the testes, which may or may not communicate with the abdomen via the processus vaginalis (Fig. 8.7).

Virtually all hydroceles in infants represent collections of peritoneal fluid that have entered the scrotal sac via a patent processus vaginalis (Fig. 8.8). Most non-communicating hydroceles disappear within 1 year.

Prematurity and low birth-weight are associated with an increased risk of hernias. Bilateral hernias are more frequent in this population. Other associations of hernias are:

- hydrops
- meconium peritonitis
- ascites
- ambiguous genitalia
- cryptorchidism
- ventriculoperitoneal shunts
- abdominal peritoneal dialysis
- mucopolysaccharidosis.

They are more frequent on the right (60%) than on the left and bilateral in 10% (because the right testis descends later). Consequently, if the child has a left-sided hernia there is a high frequency of occult right-sided hernia. There is an association between inguinal hernias and undescended testes.

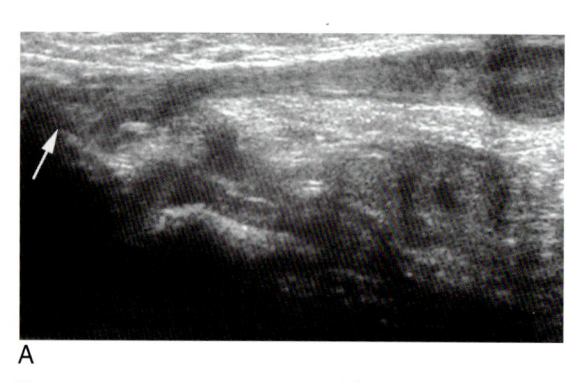

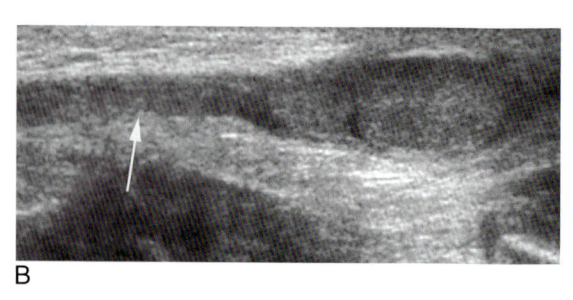

Figure 8.7 Processus vaginalis. (A) This is a scan of the inguinal canal showing the entry of the processus into the peritoneum (arrow). The processus must be carefully examined in infant males because this is the position in which hydroceles or hernias occur, and the vascular supply to the testis can be seen with Doppler. (B) Longitudinal sonogram of the inguinal canal lower down, showing the processus vaginalis (arrow). The testis and epididymis are lying low in the canal.

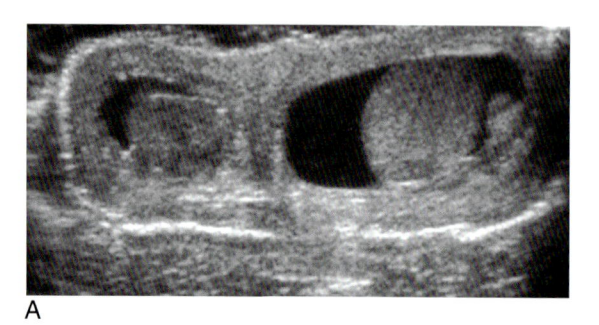

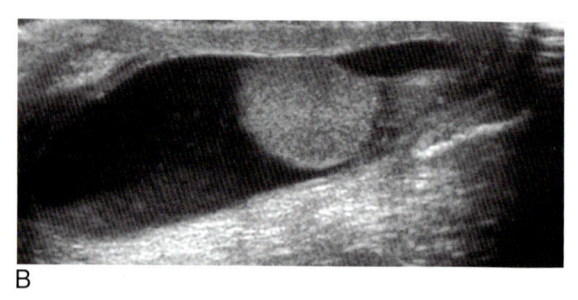

Figure 8.8 Hydroceles. (A) Transverse sonogram of the scrotum of a male neonate. There is a large amount of fluid around the testis on the left and a smaller hydrocele on the right. (B) Longitudinal sonogram of the left scrotum showing the large hydrocele and testis lying in the scrotum.

Clinical features

It can occasionally be difficult to determine an inguinal hernia from a tense hydrocele or testicular torsion. Incarceration of the hernia may result in small bowel obstruction, perforation and peritonitis and is most common in the first 6 months of life. Ultrasound is valuable in differentiating these entities: an irreducible incarcerated hernia and a testicular torsion are both surgical emergencies (Fig. 8.9).

Varicocele

This is an acquired dilation of the veins of the pampiniform plexus (see Fig 8.6A). When this condition is suspected, Doppler examination must always be used. In addition a full pelvic and abdominal scan should be undertaken, as the underlying cause may be pelvic or renal pathology such as renal vein thrombosis, a renal tumor or a retroperitoneal tumor. The majority, however, are caused by incompetent valves.

On ultrasound they appear as tortuous tubular structures and are located superiorly and posterolaterally within the scrotum as they extend up the spermatic cord. Doppler examination can be used to demonstrate the dilated veins, although it may be difficult to evaluate as blood flow is usually slow and may even appear absent. For this reason Doppler using the low flow presets should be used. It is ideally assessed in the erect position or during Valsalva maneuver in cooperative boys. Veins measuring more than 2 mm are generally considered to be abnormal in the supine position.

THE SCROTUM AND TESTES 243

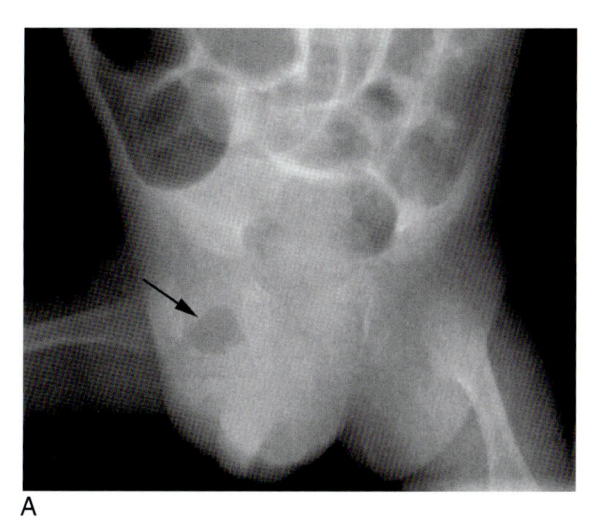

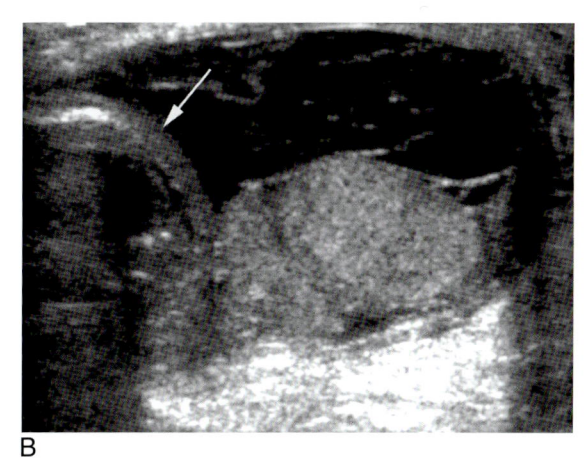

Figure 8.9 Inguinal hernia. (A) Plain abdominal radiograph of the abdomen in an infant presenting with a tense, swollen right inguinal canal and scrotum. The radiograph reveals an abnormal air collection in the right groin (arrow). (B) Longitudinal sonogram of the right groin revealed an undescended right testis surrounded by a hydrocele and herniation of the bowel (arrow).

Varicoceles are most commonly seen between 10 and 15 years of age. They are rare under 10 years, and 85–90% occur on the left.

Testicular growth arrest is recognized in adolescents with varicoceles, as is infertility with a decreased sperm count. This is related to the increase in temperature in the scrotum with the increased venous blood flow. Growth arrest is reversible in 80% if the varicocele is corrected. Testicular volume should be measured if a varicocele is identified.

Clinical features

Varicoceles are usually asymptomatic but may present with a dull ache in the scrotum. Ultrasound with Doppler is more reliable than clinical examination in the identification of varicoceles.

ACUTELY PAINFUL SCROTUM

Causes of an acutely painful enlarged scrotum in a child include:

- trauma
- testicular torsion
- torsion of the appendix testis
- epididymitis
- epididymo-orchitis
- acute hydrocele
- incarcerated hernia
- tumor
- vasculitis
- idiopathic scrotal edema.

The main clinical dilemma of a child presenting with an acutely painful swollen testis is a distinction between testicular torsion and acute epididymo-orchitis. Clinically this can be difficult to diagnose in over half of the patients, as fever and pyuria may occur in both. The painful scrotal mass is a surgical emergency and is considered to be testicular torsion until proven otherwise. It is surgical dictum that surgery has to take place within 24 hours of the onset of symptoms if the testis is to remain viable and saved.[4]

Testicular torsion

The peak incidence of testicular torsion is in the prepubertal and pubertal boy. Testicular torsion occurs when the spermatic cord is twisted. There are two types: extravaginal and intravaginal.

Extravaginal (or neonatal) torsion occurs in utero, in the newborn or, less commonly, during the neonatal period. It occurs when there is absent fixation of the testis in the scrotum by a flimsy gubernaculum. Torsion occurs at the level of the external ring. Extravaginal torsion is where the entire testis, epididymis and tunica vaginalis twist. At presentation there is usually irreversible testicular damage, and the clinical approach is not to operate on these neonates.

Intravaginal (or pubertal) torsion is the more common type, and the peak incidence is between 12 and 18 years. In intravaginal torsion the gubernaculum is fixed to the scrotal wall. However, there is an anomalous suspension of the testis on a long stalk of spermatic cord with investment of the testis and the epididymis by the tunica vaginalis. The tunica vaginalis inserts high on the cord instead of the lower pole of the testis, so that the testis can rotate freely within the tunica: the so called 'bell and clapper deformity'. The degree of torsion can vary from 90° to three complete turns of the vascular pedicle. Initially the venous return and lymphatics are obstructed and compromised and venous infarction tends to occur earlier with lesser torsion. It begins about 2 hours after complete occlusion of the testicular artery. After 6 hours the ischemia is irreversible. This need for urgent surgery is related to the testicular viability.

Torsion of the spermatic cord occurs most commonly (65%) in and around adolescence but anytime between the ages of 3 and 20. Clinically boys present with acute unilateral scrotal pain, often with nausea and vomiting and the diagnosis is usually obvious from the history. There may also be a history of prior episodes, and a history of trauma is also important. Acute torsion is a surgical emergency since, if the testis is to be salvaged, surgery must occur within 24 hours of onset of the symptoms. Patients are often taken directly for surgery without imaging, but if there is a suspicion of epididymo-orchitis then ultrasound examination may be requested in order to prevent unnecessary surgery.[5]

Ultrasound appearances and technique

With this clinical diagnosis and history, in addition to the standard ultrasound examination, Doppler is essential in order to demonstrate the absence of blood flow in the testes. The contralateral testis should always be examined and used as a baseline for the color Doppler parameters and assessment. Testicular volume has been shown to be a more reliable indicator of flow, with testes of less than 1 ml only demonstrating flow in 32%. However, newer machines, high resolution transducers and better Doppler sensitivity will undoubtedly improve ability to detect blood flow.

Sonographic findings The primary abnormality in testicular torsion is at the spermatic cord, so accurate examination of the inguinal canal and scrotum is essential. On high resolution ultrasound the cord can normally be seen as a straight tubular structure with well-defined and hyperechoic margins. On transverse scans it can be identified as an ovoid structure slightly medial to the head of the epididymis. With power and color Doppler the spermatic artery is seen as a structure of sinuous course connected to the capsular artery (Fig. 8.10).

When torsion is present there may be:

- a rotation of the spermatic cord. Doppler flow may be seen within the rotation with a corkscrew appearance. This is best seen in the transverse view. The torsed testis may lie high within the hemiscrotum because of the shortening of the spermatic cord secondary to twisting
- venous engorgement of the cord distal to the rotation
- a small amount of intrascrotal fluid with scrotal wall thickening
- no blood flow in the testis on Doppler.

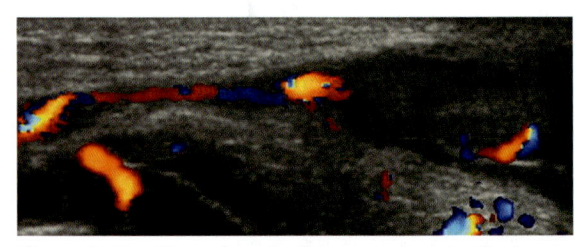

Figure 8.10 Normal testicular artery. Longitudinal sonogram of the normal right testis with Doppler showing the normal blood flow to the testis from the testicular artery in the inguinal canal. It is important to examine the vessels in the inguinal canal when torsion is suspected.

Factors affecting diagnostic accuracy

- Experience of the operator is critical and the ability to identify Doppler flow in the testicular artery and testis is important.
- The examiner must be familiar with the technical characteristics and settings of the equipment in order to use the Doppler settings optimally.
- Initial torsion and incomplete torsion may show relatively normal intratesticular flow.
- Torsion–detorsion phenomenon may represent increased flow mimicking epididymo-orchitis.
- The patient's age is a factor. Flow may be difficult to detect in a prepubertal testis even with optimal operator technique and equipment.

Change in appearances with time Appearances change with time as follows.

- *Early.* The ultrasound image may be unimpressive and the appearances normal. This may progress to a swollen testis with thickening of the epididymis, but the appearances are non-specific. There may be a small reactive hydrocele and a thickened scrotal wall.
- *After 24 hours.* The testicular appearances change to a mixed echogenicity, indicating areas of infarction and hemorrhage. The most characteristic sign is the hyperechoic epididymis, which is not always present or easy to appreciate (Fig. 8.11).
- *Late appearance.* Missed torsion is a term used to describe a testis that has been untreated for 48 hours or more. Ultrasound will give a homogeneous hypoechoic or mixed echogenic appearance due to the areas of hemorrhage in the testis, often with a characteristic hyperechoic rim around the periphery of the testis which ultimately will go on to calcify. There may be a small reactive hydrocele, and the epididymis will appear enlarged and hyperechoic.
- *Long-term.* The testes will atrophy, often with a small calcified rim.

Doppler examination Doppler settings must be those for low flow, as velocity of blood in the small testicular vessels is low. If Doppler settings are too high then blood flow at lower velocities will not be detected.[6]

It must be remembered that in 10% of normal neonates, it may be impossible to detect blood flow in the normal testes. It is essential to differentiate intra- from extratesticular blood flow. Seeing blood flow in the epididymis is not enough, and intratesticular flow must be seen. In addition the inguinal canal must be examined and, if torsion is present, the twisted artery may be demonstrated similar to the whirlpool sign seen in malrotation and volvulus of the bowel. It is important to realize that torsion of a cord may occlude the veins but not the artery. Initially,

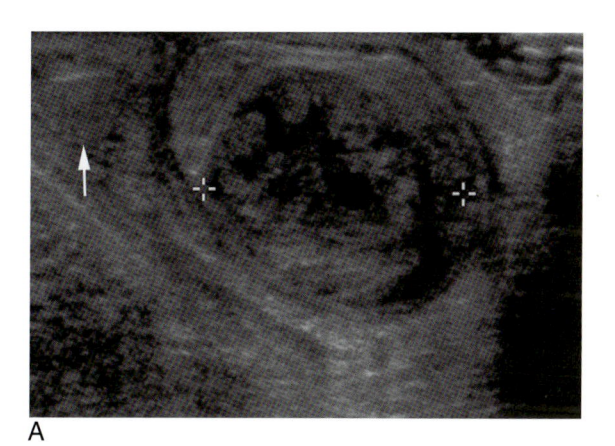

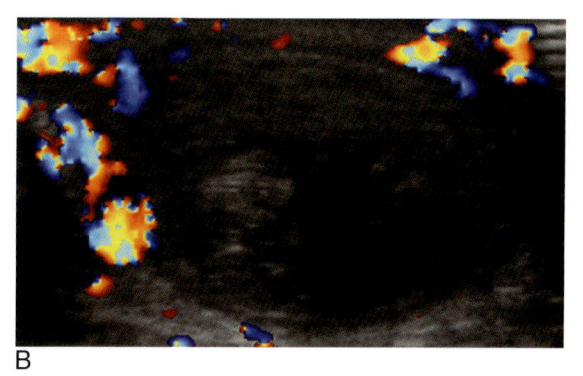

Figure 8.11 Torsion of the testis. (A) Transverse sonogram of the scrotum in an adolescent boy with a painful, swollen left testis. The ultrasound examination revealed the left testis (between calipers) to have a heterogeneous appearance and to be much larger than the right testis (arrow). (B) Longitudinal sonogram with Doppler of the enlarged testis showing no Doppler flow within the testis and only in the surrounding epididymis.

therefore, there may be arterial flow as far as the testis although there is no flow within the parenchyma. There may be reversed diastolic flow in the testicular artery. In a few cases torsion may be incomplete, in which case there may be reduced flow in the testis. It is for this reason that it is essential that the contralateral testis is examined for comparison and, in particular, to set the Doppler settings.

Epididymo-orchitis and epididymitis

The main differential diagnosis of testicular torsion is epididymo-orchitis, which is caused by an inflammation of the epididymis and testis as a result of infection. The commonest infections affecting the epididymis and testis are those of pyogenic, viral or mycotic origin. Clinically the presentation may be identical with a painful swollen scrotum except the child may have a fever and pyuria. Epididymitis can occur in children with acute urinary tract infections, in particular those with genitourinary abnormalities. The treatment is very different from that of testicular torsion. Torsion, if the testis is still viable, requires an orchidopexy—that is the surgical fixation of the testis in the scrotum so that it cannot twist. In addition, the contralateral testis is usually fixed at the same time. By contrast, epididymo-orchitis is treated with antibiotics.

Ultrasound appearances

Doppler examination is essential to differentiate these two conditions, and gray scale ultrasound may not be sufficient. The Doppler signal is markedly enhanced in orchitis because the testis is hyperemic. The testis is also usually enlarged and has a hypoechoic appearance. Hyperemia or normal flow in the testis excludes torsion. Also there is a markedly increased vascular flow detected in the epididymis in epididymitis, so that the whole of the scrotum is awash with color. Epididymo-orchitis may go on to abscess formation in the testis.

However, it is also important to recognize that testicular ischemia may be secondary to epididymitis because of swelling of the spermatic cord. This is a relatively late complication.

Torsion of the appendix testis

Torsion of the appendix testis presents with acute or gradual scrotal pain and presents difficulties in differential diagnosis. The appendix testis is the commonest appendage to twist on its base, developing venous congestion, swelling, arterial occlusion and necrosis. Clinically the pain is localized to the superior pole of the testis, and there may be a blue dot on the scrotal wall. If it can be reliably differentiated clinically from testicular torsion the treatment is analgesics and ice packs for the scrotum.

Ultrasound

The appendix testis cannot be seen on a normal sonogram but, when it has undergone torsion, it becomes swollen and appears as a mass superior to the testis, with a variable echogenicity. There may be a small hydrocele present.

MICROLITHIASIS

Testicular microlithiasis is a well-known but rare finding in the pediatric age group. The typical ultrasound appearance consists of diffuse intratesticular non-shadowing echogenic foci occasionally with comet tail artifacts. This is from calcium deposits forming in the lumen of the seminiferous tubules from atrophy and degeneration of the tubular cells. They may be distributed focally within a testis or be diffuse in both testes. The etiology is uncertain, but it is now well recognized that there is an association with germ cell tumors. In adults, reports indicate up to a 40% association and the tumor most commonly seen is seminoma. All patients should be regularly followed (Fig. 8.12).[7]

Testicular calcification is found in cryptorchidism, infertility, subfertility, varicocele, epididymitis, torsion of the testes or appendix testis, and testicular intraepithelial neoplasia. Some authors have reported tumor development 4–6 years after the diagnosis of testicular microlithiasis in the pediatric age group. When found in children, close clinical follow-up and annual ultrasound until the age of peak incidence of germ cell tumors is indicated.[8]

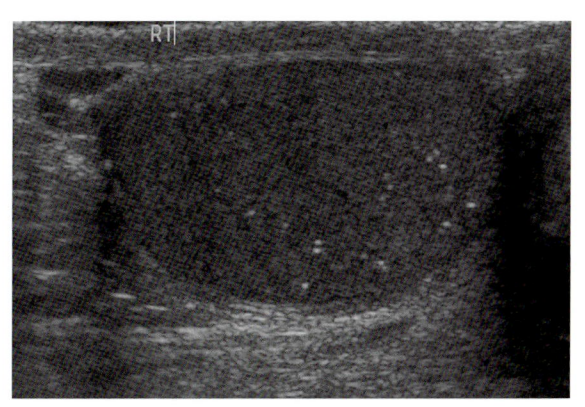

Figure 8.12 Microlithiasis. Longitudinal sonogram of the left testis showing the multiple small punctate areas of calcification within the testis typical of microlithiasis.

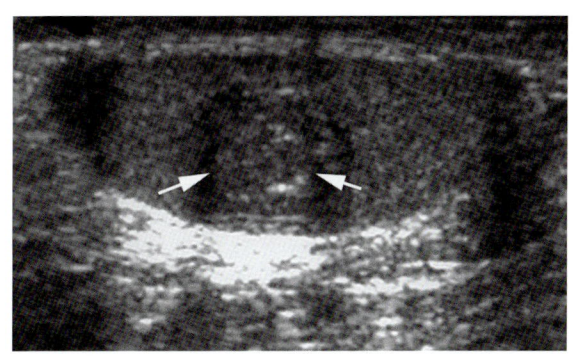

Figure 8.13 Dermoid of the testis. Longitudinal sonogram of the left testis. There is a well-defined mass within the testis which at surgery was a dermoid (between arrows).

TESTICULAR TUMORS

The most valuable role of ultrasound in evaluating scrotal masses is to differentiate intratesticular from extratesticular masses. Extratesticular lesions are usually benign and, even when solid, are rarely malignant. Intratesticular masses may be malignant or benign. Malignant tumors are usually focal, and although the appearance is variable, some normal testicular tissue may be apparent. In non-malignant conditions such as orchitis or hematoma, no normal testis is usually visible. Scrotal wall swelling as well as hydroceles also suggest a benign condition.

Most testicular solid masses are malignant and usually present with painless unilateral testicular enlargement. Testicular tumors account for 1% of all childhood malignancies, and approximately 70% are germ cell in origin.

Testicular tumors may be primary or non-primary. The non-primary tumors include lymphoma and leukemia.

Primary testicular tumors may be classified into germ cell tumors and non-germ cell tumors. The most common germ cell tumor seen in childhood is the infantile embryonal cell carcinoma (yolk sac tumor).

Ultrasound appearance

It is not possible on ultrasound to differentiate the different histological types of primary tumor nor between primary and secondary tumors. It is important to have an excellent clinical history, otherwise distinguishing between tumor, hematoma, orchitis, abscess or infections may be difficult. (Fig. 8.13) All children with a solid testicular mass should have a full blood count and measurement of alfa-fetoprotein levels.

Most testicular tumors are hypoechoic compared with the normal testicular tissue and are usually solid, well-defined masses varying in appearances depending upon whether they have undergone hemorrhage or necrosis. Areas of increased echogenicity may represent areas of calcification or fat. Sometimes by the time of diagnosis the whole of the normal testis may be replaced by tumor. An associated hydrocele may be present.[9] Abscess, infarction or orchitis may all have similar appearances to a tumor.

Teratomas are typically heterogeneous complex tumors which are usually well defined. They may contain hyperechoic areas representing hematoma, calcification, cartilage or bone and may also contain cystic spaces. Teratomas have a peak in early childhood when they are usually benign and again in the third decade when they are usually malignant.

Typically, focal areas of increased echogenicity due to calcium deposits may be found in teratocarcinomas. Ultrasound may not be able to differentiate between any of these solid masses. The treatment of all solid suspected malignant lesions of the testes is removal.

Primary testicular tumors

Germ cell tumors

Seventy percent of germ cell tumors are yolk sac tumors, and the remainder are usually benign teratomas. These tumors usually occur in prepubescent boys. This is the commonest tumor to occur in undescended testes. In older children after puberty, germ cell tumors are more likely to be embryonal cell carcinomas, seminomas, choriocarcinomas and teratocarcinomas.

Non-germ cell tumors

These account for 30% of all testicular tumors in childhood. Leydig cell tumors account for 42%, Sertoli cell tumors 20% and paratesticular rhabdomyosarcomas 38%. Leydig cell tumors usually present in children 3–6 years of age with precocious puberty and gynecomastia.

Secondary neoplasms

Lymphoma and leukemia are the most common malignant diseases to involve the testis. Although primary testicular leukemia is rare, the testis is a frequent site of relapse after bone marrow transplantation and acts as a sanctuary site for leukemic blasts during chemotherapy and remission. This testicular 'sanctuary' is thought to be protection from the 'blood–gonad barrier'. Although leukemic infiltrates are present in 60–90% of such children at autopsy, they are rarely clinically apparent.

Ultrasound usually demonstrates a diffuse testicular enlargement with homogenous or heterogeneous, mainly hypoechoic areas. Less commonly there may be focal areas of decreased echogenicity. In leukemia the testis is a common site for involvement in the acute phase and for relapse during remission.[10,11]

Other metastases that involve the testes include Wilms tumor, neuroblastoma, histiocytosis, retinoblastoma and rhabdomyosarcoma.

Benign testicular masses

Simple cysts These are uncommon. If the cyst is multiloculated a tumor should be suspected. They are well defined and thin walled and frequently occur near the mediastinum.[12]

Complex cysts Epidermoid cysts are benign tumors of germ cell origin. The sonographic appearances are variable. They are sometimes well-defined intratesticular lesions, sharply circumscribed, of low echogenicity with an echogenic fibrous or calcilfic rim. They occasionally have a 'whorled' appearance.[13]

Teratomas Teratomas may have a mixed solid and cystic appearance.

Liquefying hematoma and abscess These may have areas of central necrosis and appear cystic.

Echogenic masses The differential diagnosis includes granulomas such as TB, old hematoma or infarct, and testicular microlithiasis. Very rarely, ectopic rests of adrenal tissue may occur. These are thought to arise from aberrant adrenal cortical rests which migrate to the gonadal tissue in fetal life.

EXTRATESTICULAR MASSES

Extratesticular lesions may be solid or cystic.

Cystic extratesticular masses

Cystic lesions may arise from the tubules of the testes such as the rete testis and epididymis (Fig. 8.14). These lesions are usually superior and posterior to the testes. They are usually spermatoceles and epididymal cysts. A hydrocele may also present as an extratesticular cystic lesion. Ultrasound cannot differentiate the two.[14]

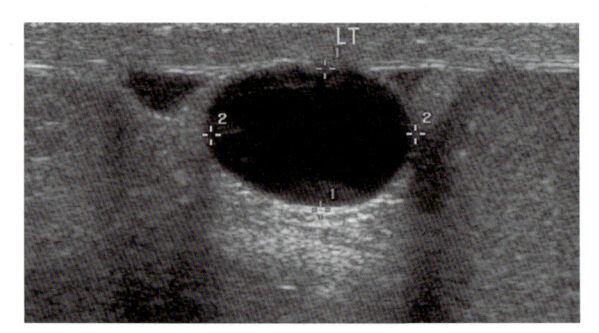

Figure 8.14 Epididymal cyst. Longitudinal sonogram showing the upper pole of the testis. There is a cyst within the epididymis (between calipers). Cysts in the epididymis are occasionally seen.

Solid extratesticular masses

Malignant solid extratesticular masses are more common than benign solid masses, accounting for 59% of scrotal lesions and representing 14% of all scrotal masses.

The most common malignant mass is a paratesticular rhabdomyosarcoma arising from the tunica of the testes or spermatic cord. Other malignant tumors include metastatic neuroblastoma, leiomyosarcoma and fibrosarcoma.

The benign lesions are usually cystic but benign solid lesions may represent a lipoma of the spermatic cord.

Paratesticular rhabdomyosarcoma

This is the primary site in 10% of those with rhabdomyosarcoma and is of the embryonal type in 97% of cases. It usually presents as a rapidly growing painless intrascrotal mass, and 40% have retroperitoneal nodes at presentation. Peak incidence is 2–5 years of age.

SCROTAL TRAUMA

Trauma to the scrotum is usually blunt injury as occurs in sporting or fighting injuries. This may result in a tender swollen scrotum and hematoma. Ultrasound examination may be requested in order to exclude a ruptured testis, while a hematoma of the testis or scrotal layer can be treated conservatively. However, the possibility of an underlying malignancy should always be borne in mind. Differentiation of a testicular tumor and hematoma may be extremely difficult on ultrasound, and serial examinations are required (Fig. 8.15).

Ultrasound appearances

Typical appearances are:

- swelling of the testis with echogenic areas due to intratesticular hemorrhage
- hematoma of the testis, epididymis or surrounding scrotal wall
- hematoceles, i.e. blood surrounding the testes in the scrotal cavity, may appear similar to a hydrocele but contain multiple echoes.

The major role of ultrasound is to exclude a fractured testis with rupture of the tunica albuginea. If an underlying tumor cannot be confidently excluded, as is often the case, then serial scanning is required to monitor the normally expected evolution of the hematoma.[15]

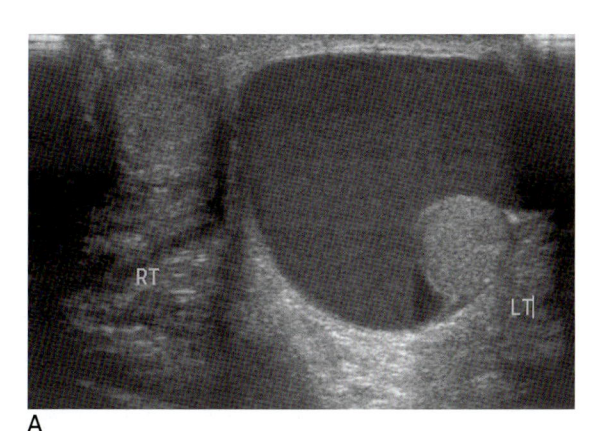

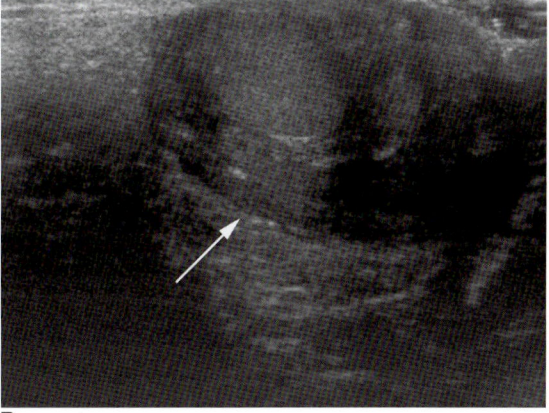

Figure 8.15 Scrotal hematocele. (A) Transverse sonogram of the scrotum in a boy who had recently had surgery for bilateral hydroceles. He presented with a painful, swollen discolored scrotum. There is still a large hydrocele on the left which contains multiple echoes in keeping with fresh blood. On the right there is echogenic material lying around the testis in the scrotum. (B) Longitudinal sonogram of the smaller right scrotum showing there is echogenic material lying around the testis in the scrotum (arrow).

References

1. Howlett DC, Marchbank NDP, Sallomi DF. Ultrasound of the testis. Clin Radiol 2000; 55:595–601.
2. Ingram S, Hollman AS, Azmy A. Testicular torsion: missed diagnosis on colour Doppler sonography. Pediatr Radiol 1993; 23(6):483–484.
3. Hollman AS, Ingram S, Carachi R, et al. Colour Doppler imaging of the acute paediatric scrotum. Pediatr Radiol 1993; 23(2):83–87.
4. Arce JD, Cortes M, Vargas JC. Sonographic diagnosis of acute spermatic cord torsion. Rotation of the cord: a key to the diagnosis. Pediatr Radiol 2002; 32:485–491.
5. Ingram S, Hollman AS. Colour Doppler sonography of the normal paediatric testis. Clin Radiol 1994; 49(4):266–267.
6. Furness PD, Husmann DA, Brock JW, et al. Multi-institutional study of testicular microlithiasis in childhood: a benign or premalignant condition? J Urol 1998; 160:1151–1154.
7. Leenen AS, Riebel T. Testicular microlithiasis in children: sonographic features and clinical implications. Paediatr Radiol 2002; 32:575–579.
8. Schwerk WB, Schwerk WNM, Rodeck G. Testicular tumours: prospective analysis of real-time ultrasound patterns and abdominal staging. Radiology 1987; 164:369–374.
9. Rayor RA, Scheible W, Brock WA, et al. High-resolution ultrasonography in the diagnosis of testicular relapse in patients with lymphoblastic leukaemia. J Urol 1982; 128:602–603.
10. Doll DC, Weiss RB. Malignant lymphoma of the testis. Am J Med 1986; 81:515–523.
11. Harm B, Fobbe F, Loy V. Testicular cysts: differentiation with ultrasound and clinical findings. Radiology 1998; 168:19–23.
12. Eisenmenger M, Lang S, Donner G, et al. Epidermoid cysts of the testis: organ-preserving surgery following diagnosis by ultrasonography. Br J Urol 1993; 72:955–957.
13. Malvica R. Epidermoid cyst of the testicle: an unusual sonographic finding. AJR Am J Roentgenol 1993; 160:1047–1048.
14. Cross JJL, Berman LH, Elliott PG, et al. Scrotal trauma: a cause of testicular atrophy. Clin Radiol 1999; 54:317–320.

Chapter 9

The head, neck and spine

CHAPTER CONTENTS

Head 251
Ultrasound technique 252
 Measurements 252
 Normal anatomy 253
Intracranial hemorrhage 258
 Types of intracranial hemorrhage 258
 Classification 262
Periventricular leukomalacia 263
Hemorrhage in term neonates 268
Common congenital cystic abnormalities 268
Other congenital abnormalities 271
Trauma 272
 Non-accidental injury 272
Hydrocephalus 274
Vascular abnormalities 275
Neck 276
The thyroid gland 276
 Normal anatomy of the thyroid 276
 Embryology and congenital
  anomalies 276
 Ultrasound technique for examination of the
  neck 277
 Diffuse thyroid enlargement 277
 Thyroid malignancy 278
Parathyroid glands 280
Neck masses 280
 Thyroglossal duct cysts 280
 Branchial cleft anomaly 282
 Cystic hygroma 282
 Congenital torticollis (fibromatosis colli) 283
 Cervical lymphadenopathy 284

The thymus 285
Salivary glands 286
 Parotid—normal appearances and ultrasound
  technique 287
 Parotid enlargement 287
Tumors of the head and neck 287
Spine 291
Ultrasound technique and normal
 anatomy 291
Indications for spinal ultrasound 293
Classification of common types of occult spinal
 dysraphism 293
 Sacral pit 293
 Dorsal dermal sinus 294
 Diastematomyelia 295
 Spinal lipomas 295
 Tight filum terminale 296
Meningocele and myelomeningocele 296
Caudal regression syndrome 297
Traumatic spinal cord lesions in newborns 297

HEAD

The acoustic window provided by the unossified anterior fontanelle in the newborn makes ultrasound an ideal modality for examining the brain in the neonate. Cranial ultrasound is now firmly established in the pediatric ultrasound armamentarium and has been used in routine clinical practice for the past 20 years. During this time of improved obstetric and neonatal care the spectrum of abnormalities seen has changed. Now the major role of ultrasound is in screening those newborn, usually premature infants, at high risk of intracerebral hemorrhage and for following up infants who have sustained hemorrhage. Ultrasound is also used in the initial diagnosis of infants suspected of having hydrocephalus and in some suspected congenital malformations. It is of particular value in the intensive care setting, so that any equipment chosen should be portable and easily maneuvered at the bedside.

ULTRASOUND TECHNIQUE

The routine cranial ultrasound examination for visualization of the intracranial contents in neonates is via the acoustic window created by the anterior fontanelle. This is the 'soft area' of the cranium and is generally only usefully open before the sutures have fused and the fontanelle becomes ossified at about 6–9 months. In conditions such as hydrocephalus where the sutures and therefore the anterior fontanelle remain open longer, the examination can be undertaken in an older infant.

The best transducers to use are those that can fit snugly into the access provided by the anterior fontanelle, and generally for an overall view of the intracranial contents a vector 8V5 is best, but a small curvilinear transducer of high frequency is also very acceptable. Overriding sutures and thick hair can sometimes be a problem, and this is best overcome using a small transducer with copious gel. A high frequency linear probe is very useful to examine the subarachnoid space. With new high frequency linear transducers a stand-off pad is not necessary, but gain settings have to be adjusted to avoid the increase in echogenicity in the near field. It is important to use a transducer with sufficient power to be able to visualize the posterior fossa. The convention for orienting the images coronally is the same as that for other cross-sectional imaging, such that the right hemisphere is on the left of the image. Sagittal scans should be oriented so that the face is on the left and the occiput on the right. Higher frequency transducers are needed for older children and when accessing the intracranial structures via the squamous bone.

In the intensive care setting infants often have an endotracheal tube and lines in position. Nowadays they are usually secured in position by tying them to the bonnet. It is essential not to disturb these tubes; access to the anterior fontanelle should then be gained via a hole in the bonnet. Newborns are vulnerable to becoming cold so it is best to examine them via the access holes in incubators and always to ensure that exposed infants remain warm.

A minimum of five coronal and five sagittal views are required for a standard examination, with additional views of the brain surface or any pathology found as required.

Doppler is extremely useful for the routine cranial examination. This is particularly true when trying to differentiate subdural from subarachnoid fluid in the subarachnoid spaces and in any suspected vascular lesion such as a vein of Galen anomaly. It has also been used in assessing vascular malformations post-embolization.[1] Doppler ultrasound has been used to monitor the neonatal brain, in particular in birth asphyxia, brain injury, hydrocephalus and brain death, with varying results. Transcranial Doppler in children with a closed fontanelle has been used in a limited way. The use of Doppler has been reported in children with sickle cell anemia and to determine brain death.[2]

Measurements

There is a large range of ventricular size both antenatally and in the newborn. Reliable measurements are needed to:

- define enlargement of the ventricles
- monitor hydrocephalus
- minimize interobserver variations
- provide proper and adequate documentation.

An integral part of the cranial ultrasound examination, in particular when ventricles are dilated, is a measure of the degree of dilation. There are many coronal and sagittal measurements quoted in the literature, presenting a confusing array to the uninitiated. It is important to have a standard technique and measurement within a department so that it is consistently reproducible between sonographers undertaking the examinations and so that

THE HEAD, NECK AND SPINE

the clinicians clearly understand the figures produced. There is still no consensus as to which is best, but the most widely accepted measure is the ventricular index as described by Levene.[3] This chart is for preterm infants. The index measures the distance from the falx to the lateral border of the lateral ventricle. This is measured coronally in the plane of the third ventricle posterior to the foramen of Monro (Fig. 9.1A). The measure is easy to understand and is reproducible. Clear visualization of the lateral ventricles can be obtained and landmarks clearly identified. It shows little interobserver error. A centile chart expressing the 3rd, 50th and 97th centiles from 26–42 weeks is shown in Figure 9.1B. The only problem with Levene's ventricular index occurs when there is midline shift. Observed values of various brain measures (Fig. 9.2) in term babies are shown in Table 9.1.[4] The author (Virkola) has also published similar charts for preterm babies.

Some practitioners also use the measure of the lateral ventricle at the foramen of Monro as a reliable, reproducible and easily identifiable landmark. The width of the ventricles may be expressed as a ratio of the total width of the cranium. The ventricles may be measured directly and now with 3D techniques and volumetric measurements have been been reported. Using measurements expressed as a ratio does not reliably monitor growth, and measurements of both ventricles and cortex may not produce an abnormality when expressed as a ratio. Direct measurement of the ventricles is still the simplest, most reproducible and easy to teach technique.

The occipital poles enlarge before the body of the lateral ventricles, but measurements are unreliable and impractical because of the wide range of size and shape of the occipital horns. Measuring the biventricular diameter is also not reliable, as one ventricle may enlarge more rapidly than another.

Tips for cranial ultrasound examination are given in Box 9.1.

Normal anatomy

Cranial ultrasound examinations are performed in coronal and sagittal planes (Figs 9.3 and 9.4).

Coronal section
Coronal planes are:

- through the frontal lobes
- through the frontal horns of the lateral ventricles
- foramen of Munro and third ventricle
- lateral ventricles and choroid plexus
- occipital lobes.

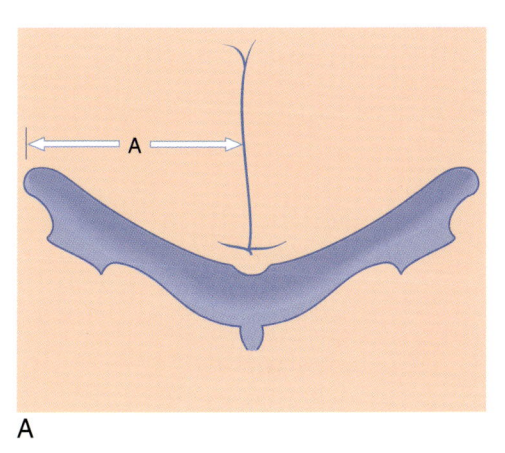

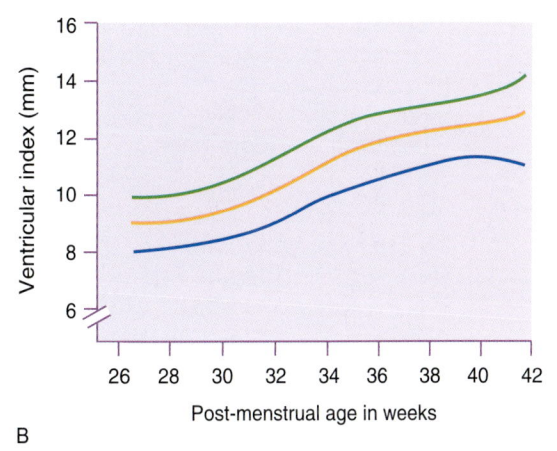

Figure 9.1 Ventricular index (Levene[3]). (A) Diagram showing how the measurement is taken for the ventricular index of Levene on a coronal view. Measurement is from the midline to the lateral wall of the anterior horn of the lateral ventricle. (B) Ventricular index measurements for infants from 26 to 42 weeks. This centile chart expresses the values of the 3rd, 50th and 97th centiles.

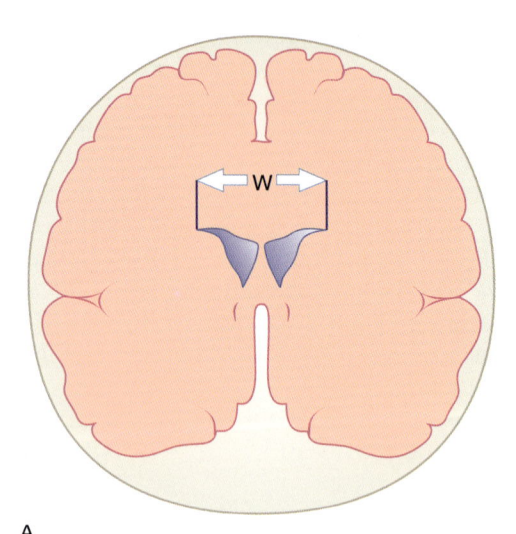

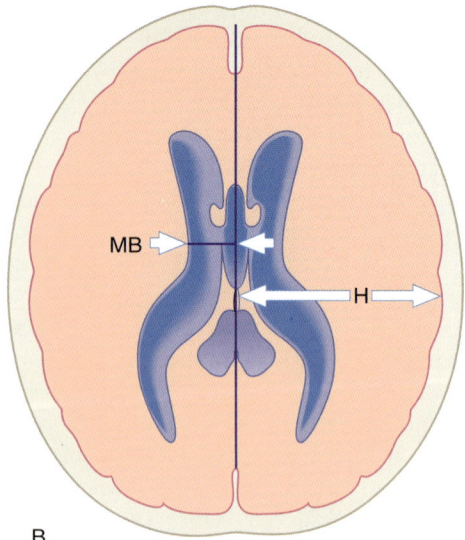

Figure 9.2 Measures of the lateral ventricles in full-term infants: H, hemisphere width; MB, ventricular midbody width; W, combined coronal ventricular width. (After Virkola.[4])

Sagittal planes Rotate the transducer 90° from the coronal section. Angle the beam approximately 20° from the midline, both right and left, to obtain the full length of the lateral ventricles:

- midline through the third ventricle aqueduct, fourth ventricle and cerebellum
- right lateral ventricle
- right parietal lobe
- left lateral ventricle
- left parietal lobe
- additional views if necessary.

Axial planes Axial planes are not routinely used but can be extremely useful if subdural or extra axial fluid is suspected. Axial sections can be diffi-

Table 9.1 Normal ranges (−2 SD to +2 SD) for different ultrasonographic measures[a] of the neonatal and infant brain in healthy full-term infants

Age (months)	Midbody width (mm)	Hemispheric width (mm)	Combined coronal ventricular width (mm)
0	11.5–14.1	39.0–46.4	21.6–27.9
1	11.9–14.8	40.6–48.2	22.4–29.0
2	12.3–15.4	42.1–50.0	23.2–30.1
3	12.7–16.1	43.7–51.9	24.0–31.1
4	13.1–16.7	45.2–53.7	24.8–32.2
5	13.5–17.3	46.8–55.6	25.6–33.3
6	13.9–18.0	48.3–57.4	26.4–34.3
7	14.3–18.6	49.8–59.2	27.1–35.4
8	14.7–19.3	51.4–61.1	27.9–36.5
9	15.1–19.9	52.9–62.9	28.7–37.5

[a]See Figure 9.2 for definitions of measures.
After Virkola.[4]

> **Box 9.1 Tips for cranial ultrasound examination**
>
> - If monitoring equipment in situ, ensure it is well secured
> - Get parent or helper to immobilize the head
> - Use a high frequency transducer that fits snugly onto the anterior fontanelle
> - Start in the coronal plane and look for symmetry of the right and left cerebral hemispheres and intracranial structures
> - Increased echogenicity usually signifies fresh blood or ischemia
> - Confirm suspected abnormality in the sagittal plane
> - Asymmetric echogenic areas are usually abnormal
> - Evaluate the subarachnoid space and fissures
> - Asymmetry in ventricular size can be normal
> - Occipital flare is a normal finding
> - Slit-like ventricles in the absence of other changes can be normal

cult to understand, so the plane is best taken at the body of the lateral ventricles, where anatomy is easily recognized.

The ventricular system

The ventricular system of the brain consists of two lateral ventricles, a third ventricle, aqueduct of Sylvius and a fourth ventricle. The lateral ventricles are the largest and consist of the frontal horn, the body, the temporal horn and the occipital horn. They communicate with the third ventricle via the foramen of Monro and with the fourth ventricle via the aqueduct of Sylvius. In addition they communicate with the subarachnoid spaces. The third ventricle is not easy to see on the coronal scan, as it is a slit-like structure, neither is the aqueduct on the sagittal scan. The fourth ventricle has a typical rhomboid 'Napoleon's hat shape' and extends into the cerebellar vermis (Fig. 9.5).

Coarctation of the lateral ventricles is a normal variant, where there are cystic areas adjacent to the superolateral angle of the lateral ventricle at the level of the foramen of Monro. These cysts appear as a string of beads along the floor of the lateral ventricle. In some of the literature these are called subependymal pseudocysts. It is important not to confuse these with periventricular leukomalacia (Fig. 9.6).[5]

Choroid plexus

The choroid plexus comprises the two paired echogenic structures which lie in the floors of the lateral ventricles. They are best seen in the sagittal scans extending anteriorly from the caudothalamic groove extending around the thalamus in the body of the lateral ventricle. When scanned coronally they can be seen in the floor of the lateral ventricles in the region of the foramen of Monro. Choroid plexus cysts are often seen as incidental findings.

Cavum septum pellucidum and cavum vergi

The lateral ventricles are separated by the septum pellucidum. Occasionally and in particular in preterm infants, a cavity is seen between the two leaves as a result of incomplete fusion. The cavum septum pellucidum lies anteriorly and the cavum vergi posteriorly. They are almost always seen in the preterm and obliterated by term. They vary in size and do not communicate with the ventricular system.

The basal ganglia

The basal ganglia is the area seen best at the level of the foramen of Monro and consists of the caudate nucleus and thalamus. They are separated by the caudothalamic groove, an important landmark when assessing for germinal matrix hemorrhages. The two thalami are connected via the massa intermedia which can be seen in a pathologically dilated third ventricle (see Fig. 9.5).[6]

Cerebellum

The cerebellum is a rounded echogenic structure seen in the posterior fossa. It lies behind the pons in the fourth ventricle, and the vermis is a particularly echogenic central structure.

256　PEDIATRIC ULTRASOUND

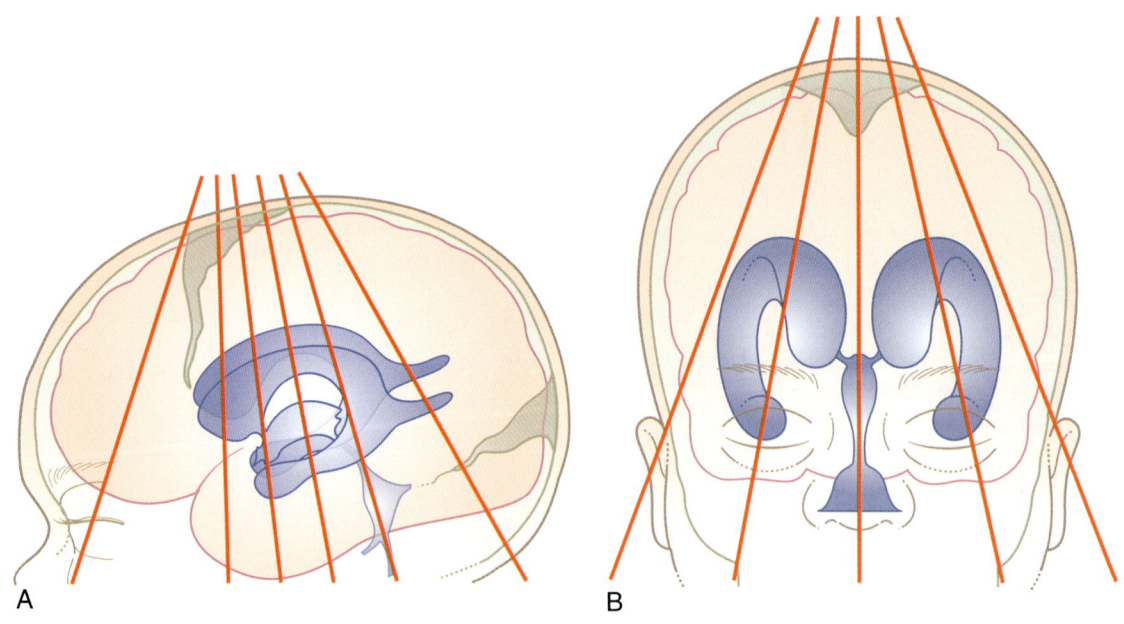

Figure 9.3　Technique of intracranial scanning: (A) coronal planes; (B) sagittal planes.

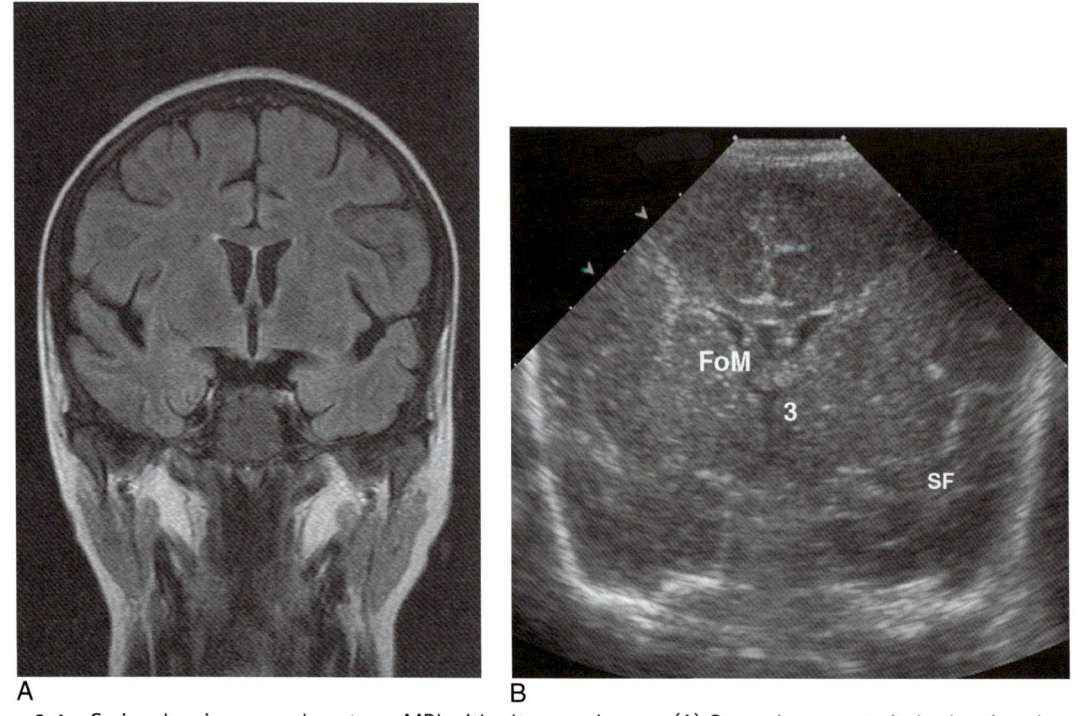

Figure 9.4　Series showing normal anatomy MRI with ultrasound scans. (A) Coronal scan anteriorly showing the frontal horns of the lateral ventricles. There is a small cavum centrally and some echogenic choroid plexus in the floor of the lateral ventricles. (B) &

Continued

THE HEAD, NECK AND SPINE   257

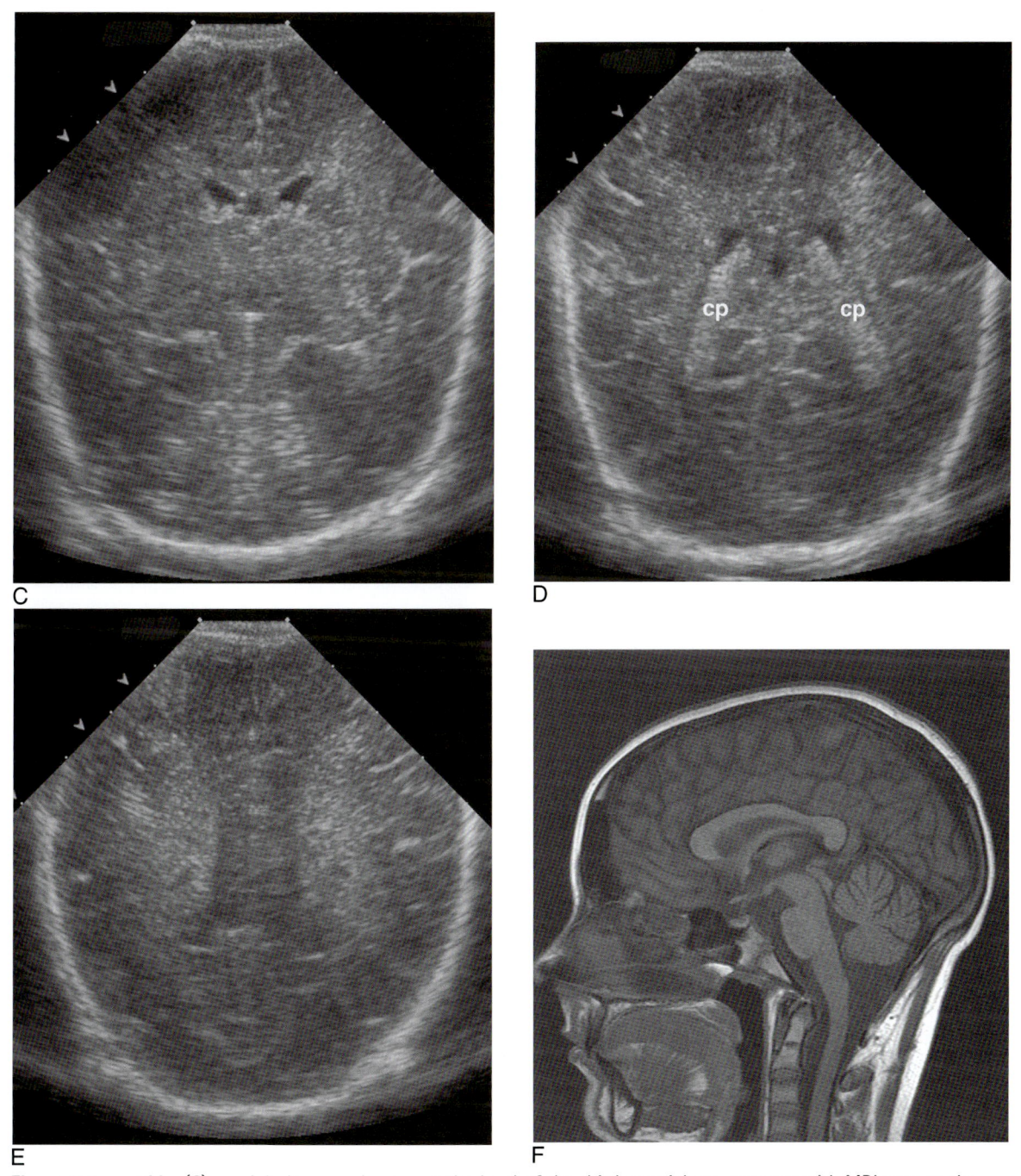

Figure 9.4, cont'd (C) cranial ultrasound scans at the level of the third ventricle to compare with MRI scan at the same level. The third ventricle (3) is a small slit-like structure in the midline below and between lateral ventricles. The connection with the lateral ventricles at the foramen of Monro (FoM) can be clearly seen and is an important landmark. The sylvian fissure (SF) is an important landmark laterally and becomes deeper the more posterior the scan. (D) Moving the transducer posteriorly the lateral ventricles can be seen containing the echogenic choroid plexus (cp). Symmetry of the choroid can be assessed in this view. (E) Coronal section posteriorly over the sulci and gyri of the occipital lobes. The surface of the brain must be examined to assess for fluid collections and gyral pattern. (F) &

Continued

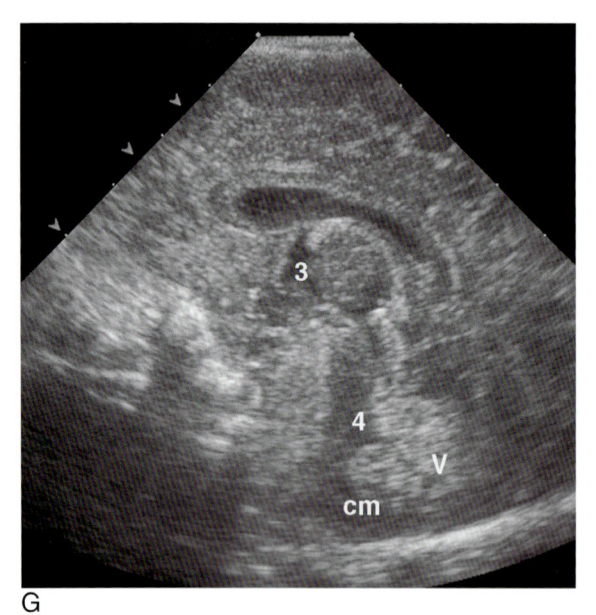

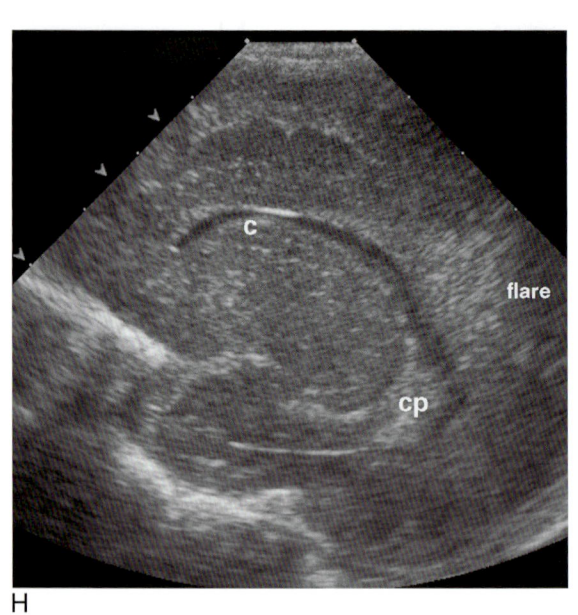

Figure 9.4, cont'd (G) Midline sagittal MRI and ultrasound scans to compare the normal anatomy. This is a very useful image and can clearly demonstrate the echogenic cerebellar vermis (v), fourth ventricle (4) and third ventricle (3). The corpus callosum can be seen as a C-shaped structure just above the third ventricle. (H) Parasagittal section through the lateral ventricle. The caudate nucleus ('c') lies in the floor of the lateral ventricle, and the caudothalamic groove is the landmark from which the choroid plexus (cp) inserts posteriorly. The caudate nucleus is more echogenic than the thalamus. The echogenic flare in the occipital white matter can be normal.

INTRACRANIAL HEMORRHAGE

The major cause of intracranial hemorrhage used to be trauma during delivery. Nowadays the major cause is prematurity, since the brain of the premature infant is highly susceptible to ischemia and hypoxia. Other causes include hypothermia, coagulopathy and pneumothoraces. One of the major roles of intracranial ultrasound is in the detection of hemorrhage, and the intracranial sites of hemorrhage are different depending on the etiology and age of the infant. The optimal time for scanning is 72 hours after birth. All periventricular hemorrhages occur after birth and within the first week of life, and the incidence of hemorrhage is directly related to prematurity.

All at risk infants should have a scan by 7 days, repeated at 14, as a small percentage will be missed on the first scan. All infants under 34 weeks should be routinely scanned.

Bleeding may occur in a number of places related to the skull and intracranial contents. Fresh blood always appears highly echogenic. After a few weeks these intraparenchymal hemorrhagic areas may liquefy and become cystic.

The following should always be assessed:

- basal ganglia, particularly the area of the germinal matrix in the floor of the lateral ventricles
- ventricles for size and intraventricular hemorrhage
- cerebral parenchyma, particularly periventricular region for flares
- choroid plexus for symmetry
- cerebellum
- extra-axial fluid such as subdural and subarachnoid collections (Fig. 9.7).

Types of intracranial hemorrhage

Germinal matrix

This is a small area of brain occurring in the floors of the lateral ventricles and is best seen on anterior

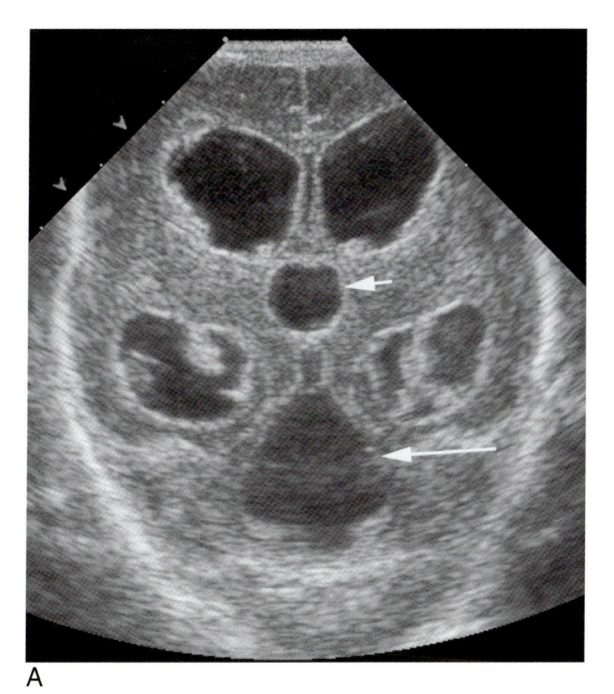

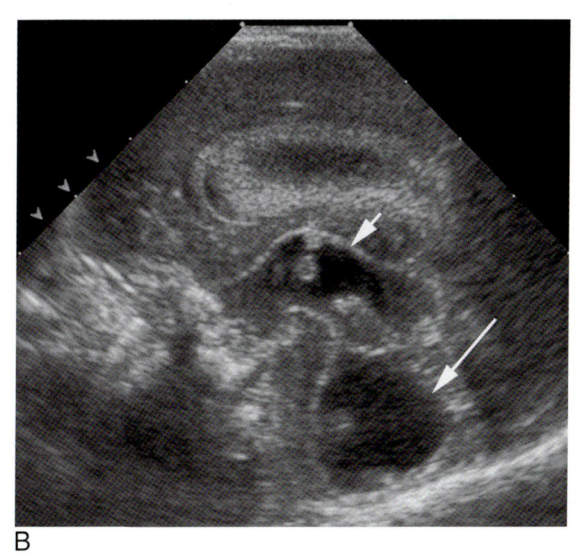

Figure 9.5 Ventricular dilation. (A) Coronal scan in an infant who had had an intraventricular hemorrhage. There is dilation of the lateral ventricles with blood clot lying in the occipital horns. There is quite marked dilation of the third ventricle (short arrow) and the fourth ventricle (long arrow). (B) Midline sagittal scan on the same infant showing the dilated third ventricle (short arrow) with the massa intermedia and dilation of the fourth ventricle (long arrow). The cerebellum is compressed posteriorly and there are echogenic areas of blood clot within the dilated ventricles.

coronal scans. This area is very vascular in the premature infant, and hence these hemorrhages occur primarily in premature infants. It has a rich matrix of fragile capillaries, and alterations in cerebral blood flow cause vasodilation of these tiny vessels, leading to hemorrhage. This may be an isolated finding but they occasionally will rupture into the ventricle and in a small percentage will rupture into the parenchyma through the roof of the lateral ventricle. By term the subependymal plate has almost completely disappeared. There is almost universally a good prognosis, with only a very small number (2%) reportedly resulting in neurological sequelae.[7]

Small germinal matrix hemorrhages, if they are fresh, appear echogenic. They may occasionally be mistaken for choroid in the floor of the lateral ventricle. Hemorrhages need to be confirmed in the sagittal view and occur anterior to the caudothalamic groove (Fig. 9.8). There is no distortion of the ventricular system, and after a number of weeks they may become cystic and eventually disappear as the brain grows.

Periventricular hemorrhage

Periventricular hemorrhage (PVH) is the commonest parenchymal hemorrhage to occur. It is a loose term and encompasses germinal matrix hemorrhages (subependymal hemorrhage, SEH) and intraventricular rupture with parenchymal extension.

Choroid plexus hemorrhage

Choroid plexus hemorrhage is not common and tends to be more of a term event. Fresh hemorrhage and blood in the choroid plexus may be missed because of the similar echogenicity of the paired choroid plexus structures. In association there may be fluid blood in the ventricles, which can sometimes adhere to the choroid. Hemorrhage should be diagnosed when the choroid plexus

260 PEDIATRIC ULTRASOUND

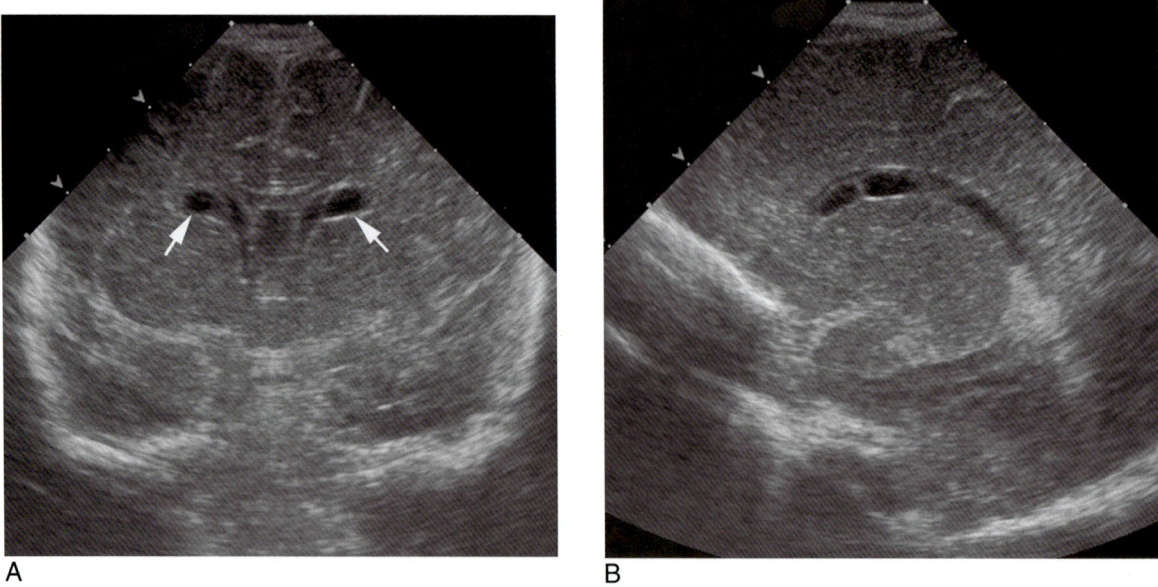

Figure 9.6 Coarctation of the ventricles. (A) Coronal scan showing the anterior horns of the lateral ventricles. There are cystic areas lateral to this (arrows). This is not periventricular leukomalacia but rather a normal appearance called coarctation of the ventricles. (B) Sagittal scan through the right lateral ventricle. There are two cystic areas just beneath and lateral to the anterior horns of the lateral ventricles. Echogenic choroid is lying posteriorly within the ventricle.

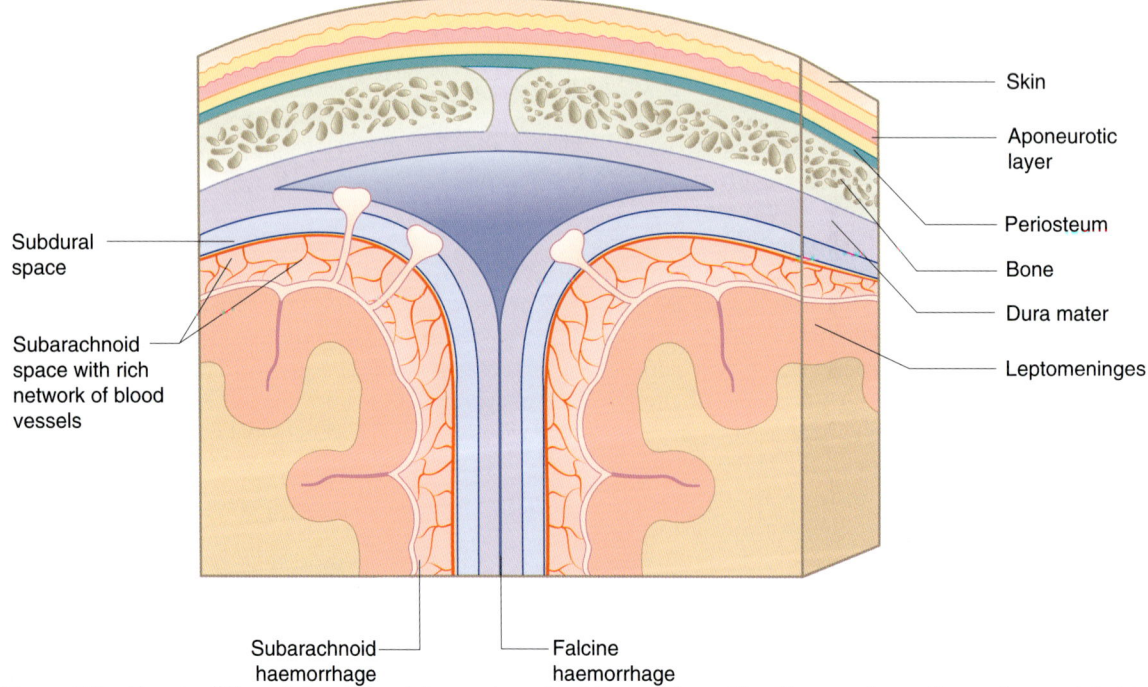

Figure 9.7 How to differentiate subdural from subarachnoid hemorrhage. The diagram shows the anatomy related to the subarachnoid and subdural spaces. This demonstrates the rich network of blood vessels in the subarachnoid space. If there is an increase in fluid in this space, using Doppler one can demonstrate small vessels crossing, whereas with subdural fluid these small vessels are compressed on the surface of the brain.

THE HEAD, NECK AND SPINE 261

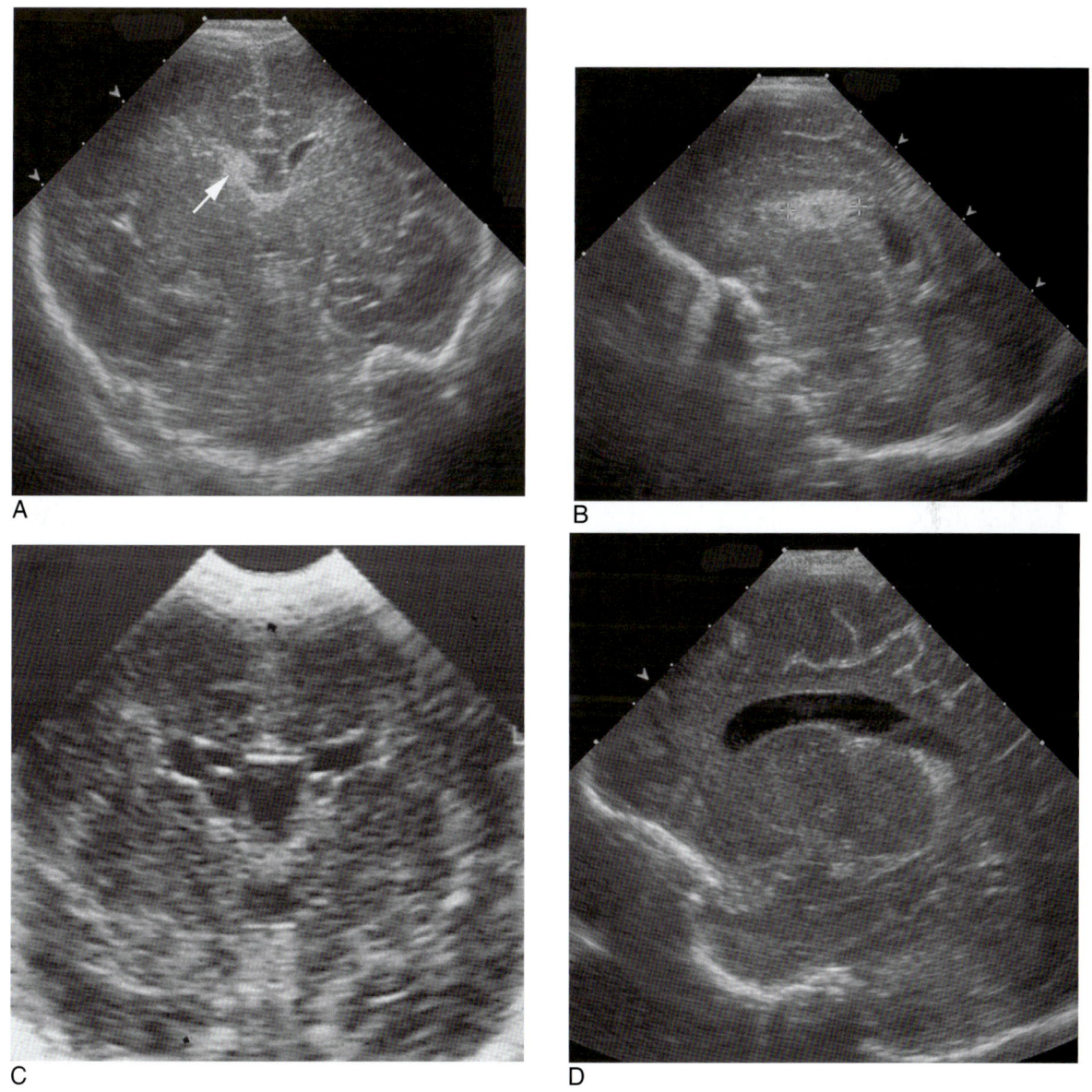

Figure 9.8 Germinal matrix hemorrhage. (A) Coronal scan through the anterior horns of the lateral ventricle. There is an echogenic area in the region of the germinal matrix on the right (arrow). (B) Sagittal scan through the right lateral ventricle showing the echogenic area in the region of the thalamus (between calipers). This is a fresh germinal matrix hemorrhage. On the sagittal view a germinal matrix hemorrhage always occurs anterior to the caudothalamic groove. (C) Coronal scan anteriorly showing the anterior horns of the lateral ventricles. There is a large cavum centrally and cystic areas in the floors of the lateral ventricles on both the right and left side. This is the appearance of bilateral old germinal matrix hemorrhages with residual cystic change. (D) Sagittal scan through the lateral ventricle in a normal child, showing the caudothalamic groove. This is an important landmark as no increase in echogenicity should be seen anterior to this groove in the basal ganglia.

appears enlarged, asymmetrical or irregular in outline. Associated occipital horn dilation is sometimes seen. Generally there is no subarachnoid blood seen. Choroid plexus diameters of 12 mm or more are suggestive of hemorrhage.

Intracerebellar hemorrhage

Cerebellar hemorrhage is well described and may occur in the preterm and term infant. Hemorrhage may occur due to a bleeding disorder or trauma, and has been associated with tight fitting face masks.[8] The cerebellum is normally echogenic but hemorrhage may increase the echogenicity. It may be unilateral with an irregular outline.

Ultrasound is not a reliable method of making this diagnosis, as blood around the tent may be confusing.

Thalamic hemorrhages

Primary thalamic hemorrhages are extremely rare.

Subdural hemorrhages

Subdural hemorrhages are caused by trauma at birth, non-accidental injury, and bleeding disorders. Bleeding results from dural tears.[9-11]

Subarachnoid hemorrhages

Subarachnoid hemorrhages may be due to blood in the ventricular system as a result of an intraventricular hemorrhage or a bleeding diathesis causing bleeding from the blood vessels. Other causes include passive dilation of the subarachnoid space, which may be due to brain atrophy, subdural effusion or to an abscess which may develop as a result of meningitis or subdural hemorrhages at various stages. Visualization of the cortical veins and their branches within fluid collections around the brain suggest that the pericerebral collection is caused by an enlarged subarachnoid space and not a subdural. This is best demonstrated with color Doppler to show the flow in superficial cortical vessels which lie along the superficial gyri and sulci.

Differentiation of subdural and subarachnoid hemorrhages can be difficult on ultrasound (Fig. 9.9 and Box 9.2).

Classification

There is no internationally accepted grading system for germinal matrix hemorrhage/intraventricular hemorrhage (GMH–IVH). Boxes 9.3 and 9.4 outline the grading systems for periventricular hemorrhage used for ultrasound scanning. The advantage of Papille's grading system is that it is simple and easy to understand.[8] Levene's grading system has also gained some acceptance but it is more complicated, and neither takes account of periventricular leukomalacia.[12,13]

It is far better to document the site and size of the hemorrhage and, if there is ventricular dilation, to measure it (Fig. 9.10).

Grade 1 hemorrhage These are small hemorrhages in the germinal matrix region.

Grade 2 hemorrhage This is when there is intraventricular blood. The ventricles show mild or no dilation. Fresh blood in the ventricles may not cause dilation initially, and the only evidence later may be fibrin stranding in the ventricles. If the intraventricular hemorrhage is large, the ventricle may dilate with echogenic blood within the whole of the ventricle.

Grade 3 hemorrhage This is when the whole of the ventricle dilates with large intraventricular hemorrhages. This large amount of blood within the ventricular system may obstruct the foramina and may interfere with the reabsorption of CSF by the arachnoid granulations. An echogenic halo around the ventricles, similar to that in ventriculitis, may be apparent. These dilated ventricles need regular ultrasound monitoring until the dilation either resolves or the treatment regimen is secured. Some will require shunting.

Grade 4 hemorrhage This is the most severe form of hemorrhage and is the result of a germinal matrix hemorrhage extending into the ventricles and into the parenchyma of the brain. This is typically into the frontoparietal region. In time the intraparenchymal hemorrhage liquefies and the child is left with a cystic cavity communicating with the ventricle. This is thought to be the origin of a porencephalic cyst.

In those infants suffering a grade 3 or 4 hemorrhage, the neurological sequelae are severe, with over 50%, and in some series up to 90%, being left

THE HEAD, NECK AND SPINE 263

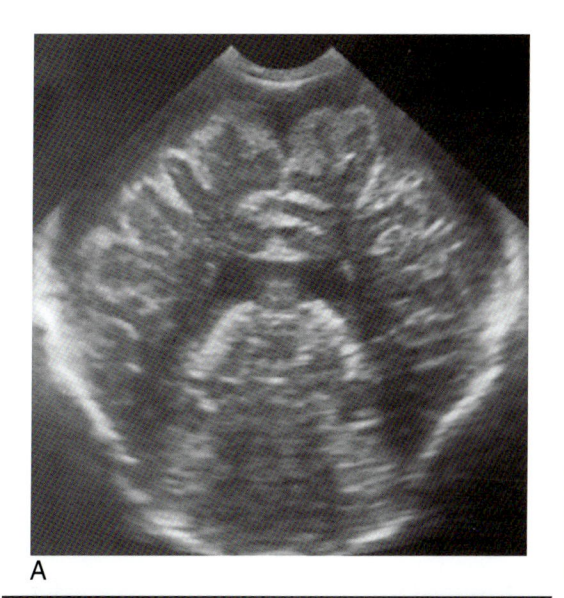

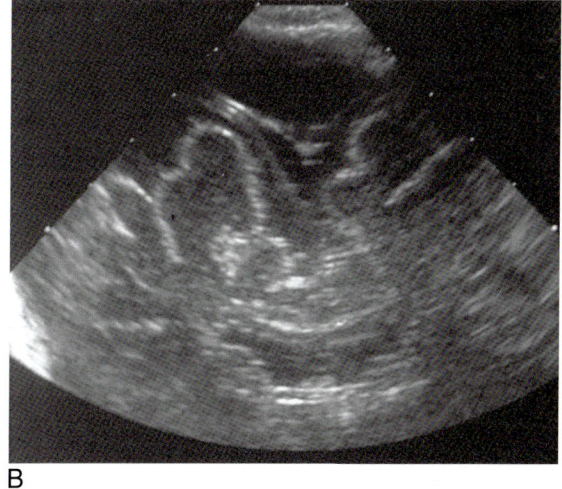

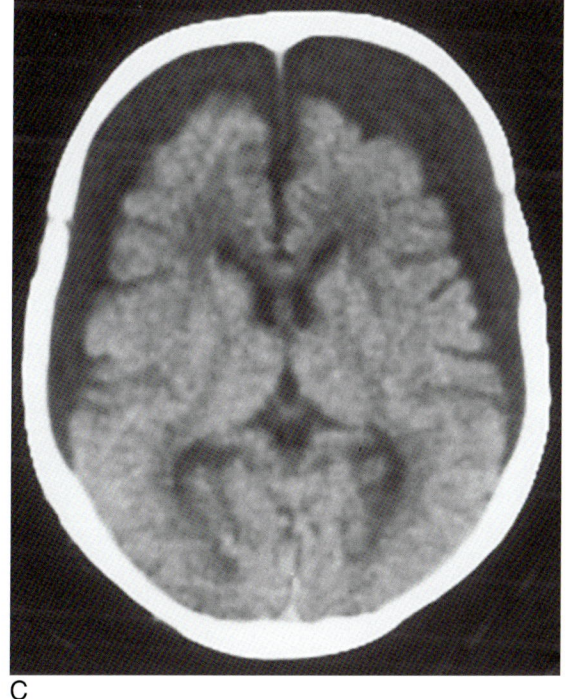

Figure 9.9 Extra-axial fluid. (A) Coronal scan posteriorly, showing the echogenic choroid plexus in the lateral ventricles. Notice the extra-axial fluid enhancing the gyri of the brain. (B) Magnified view anteriorly in the same infant. There is a combination of subarachnoid and subdural fluid. The line of the elevated dura can be identified. (C) CT scan of the same infant showing the large amount of fluid predominantly over the frontal lobes.

with motor abnormalities such as poor tone, spastic diplegia and cognitive abnormalities.

PERIVENTRICULAR LEUKOMALACIA (PVL)

This is a condition primarily occurring in the premature infant and is associated with hypoxic-ischemic brain insult. During weeks 32–34 there are many changes in the cerebral vasculature with disappearance of the germinal matrix and rapid growth of the cortex and white matter. There is a marked increase in the vascular and oxygen requirement to these areas. PVL is related to a lack of oxygen (hypoxia) or a reduction in cerebral perfusion (ischemia).

> **Box 9.2 Differentiation of subdural and subarachnoid hemorrhages**
>
> **Subdural**
> - If large may have midline shift
> - Look for linear elevation of dura
> - Does not follow convolution of gyri
> - Compressed, flattened gyri
> - May be hyperechoic if fresh blood and hypoechoic if old
> - May be localized to one area and not lying diffusely over cerebral cortex
>
> **Subarachnoid**
> - Either hyper- or hypoechoic depending on age of blood
> - Doppler will show vessels crossing the subarachnoid space
> - Usually follows the line of the gyri
> - Look for blood in the Sylvian fissure

> **Box 9.3 Grading system for periventricular hemorrhage[8] used or adapted for use with ultrasound brain scanning**
>
> | | |
> |---|---|
> | Grade I | Isolated SEH |
> | Grade II | Rupture into ventricle, but no dilation |
> | Grade III | Rupture into ventricle with dilation |
> | Grade IV | IVH with parenchymal extension |
>
> IVH, intraventricular hemorrhage; SEH, subependymal hemorrhage.

> **Box 9.4 A modification of the grading system for periventricular hemorrhage and ventricular dilation[13]**
>
> *Hemorrhage*
> 0 No hemorrhage
> 1 Localized hemorrhage < 1 cm in its largest measurement
> 2 Hemorrhage > 1 cm in its largest measurement but not extending beyond the atrium of the lateral ventricle
> 3 Blood clot forming a cast of the lateral ventricle and extending beyond the atrium
> 4 Intraparenchymal hemorrhage
>
> *Ventricular dilation*
> 0 No dilation
> 1 Transient dilation
> 2 Persistent but stable dilation
> 3 Progressive ventricular dilation requiring treatment
> 4 Persistent asymmetrical ventricular dilation

PVL may occur some time after birth and in some reported series up to 11 weeks. The causes of PVL are primarily prenatal events such as abruptio placenta, twin-to-twin transfusion and perinatal birth asphyxia, recurrent apnea, cardiac arrest and shock, severe respiratory distress syndrome (RDS) in the premature, and perinatal asphyxia in the newborn.

PVL is characterized by multiple periventricular infarcts and necrosis affecting the white matter and sparing the gray matter. It describes the cystic changes that affect the white matter typically in the watershed areas which are affected by ischemia. The white matter usually affected is anterior to the frontal horns, the external angle of the lateral ventricles and the lateral surface of the occipital horns.

Ultrasound examination

The earliest appearances are echogenic areas around the anterior horns of the lateral ventricles, with a triangular shape, the tip pointing towards the cranium. These areas correspond to necrosis and hemorrhage (Fig. 9.11).[13,14]

Serial scanning will demonstrate that these areas of increased echogenicity become cystic within about 2–6 weeks, with no communication with the ventricular system. The cysts may remain for a

THE HEAD, NECK AND SPINE   265

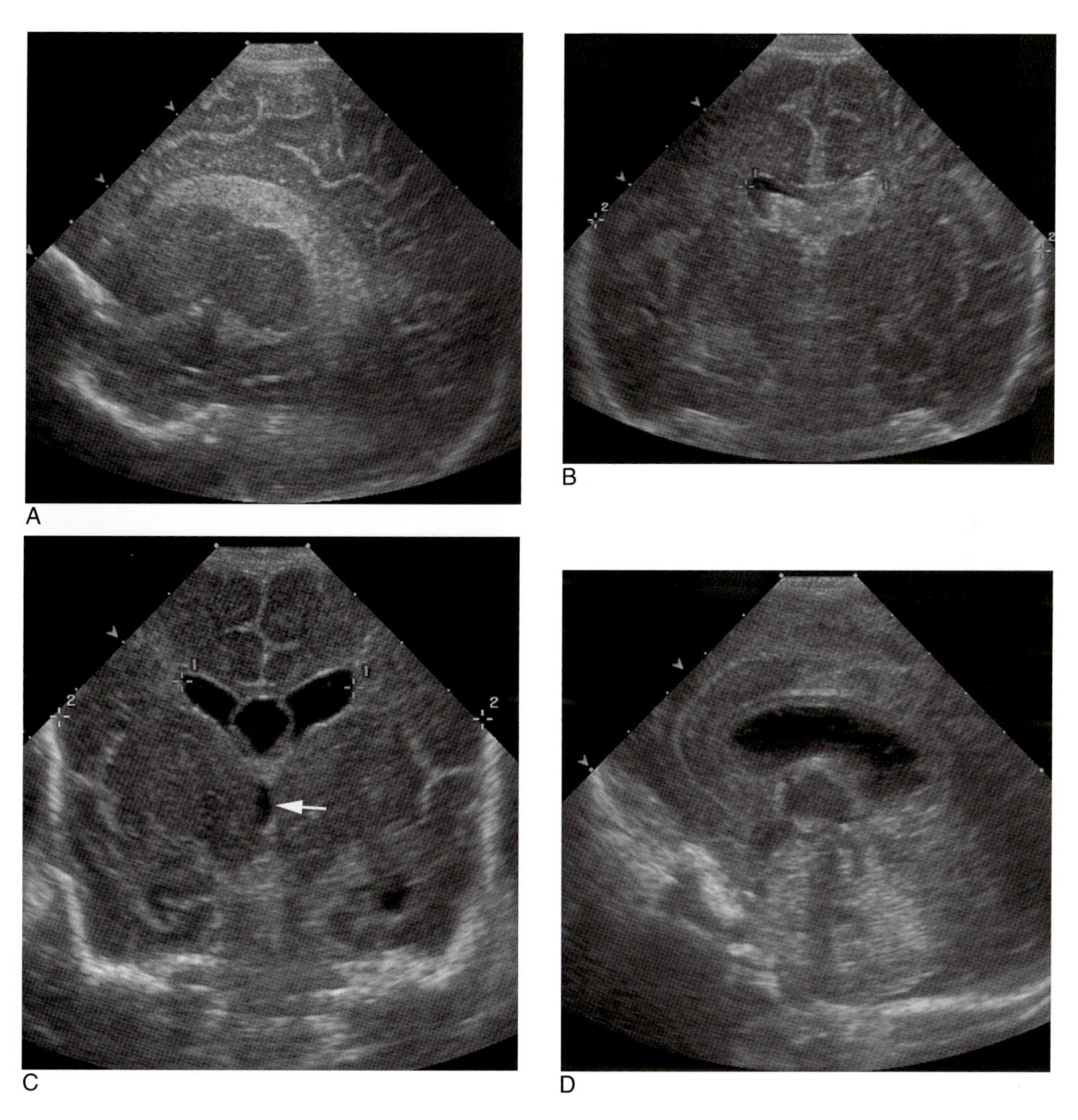

Figure 9.10 Severe intraventricular hemorrhage with hydrocephalus. (A) & (B) Grade 2 hemorrhage. This is intraventricular hemorrhage without ventricular dilation. Sagittal and coronal scan on a baby with a fresh intraventricular hemorrhage. The ventricles are filled with echogenic blood clot. (C) Grade 3 hemorrhage, with ventricular dilation. There is asymmetric dilation of the lateral ventricles with a very prominent cavum septum pellucidum centrally. Notice that it lies anterior to the third ventricle (arrow) and should not be confused with the third ventricle. (D) Midline sagittal scan on the same infant showing the dilated cavum above the third ventricle. This was a premature infant, and the brain gyri and sulci are not yet fully developed.

Continued

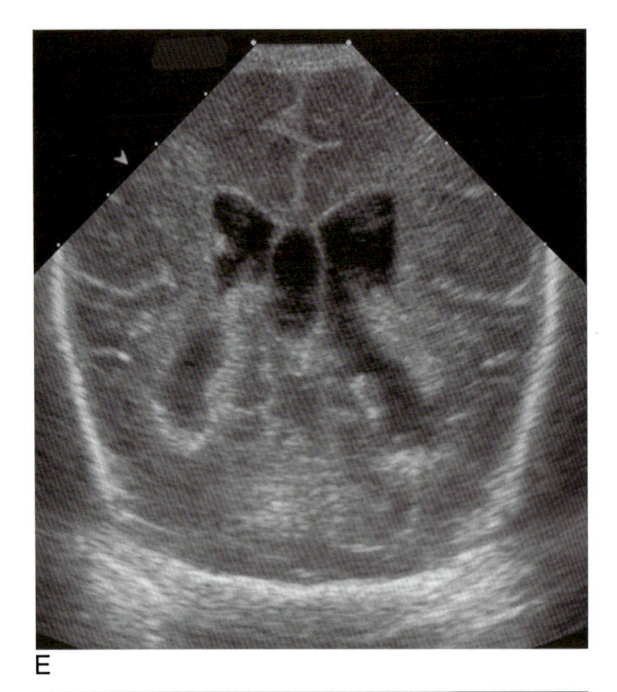

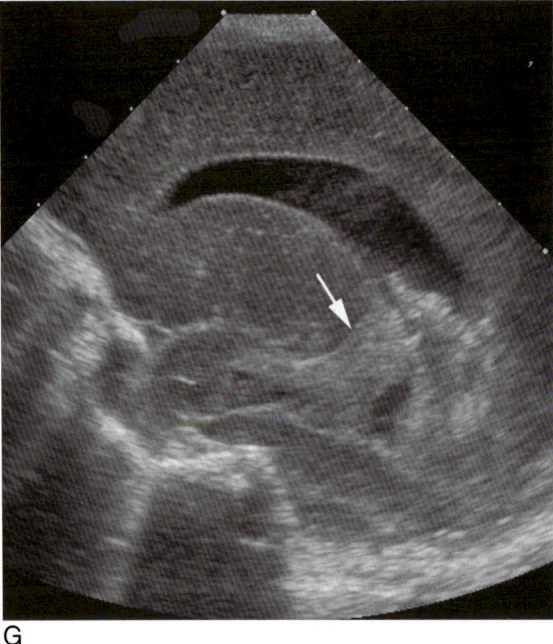

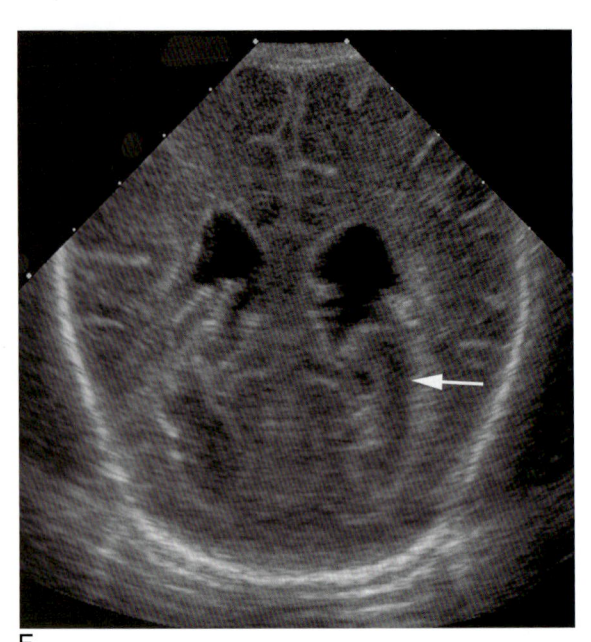

Figure 9.10, cont'd (E) Coronal scan posteriorly showing the dilation of the lateral ventricles and the very prominent midline cavum. Notice the echogenic material lying in the ventricles, which was clotted blood. (F) Coronal scan in the same infant posteriorly. The lateral ventricles are dilated and there is a large amount of intraventricular hemorrhage which, on the right, is taking the shape of the ventricle (arrow). (G) Sagittal scan of the left lateral ventricle in the same infant. The blood clot has settled posteriorly and is lying primarily in the occipital horn of the lateral ventricle. The echogenic choroid plexus can be seen separate and anterior to this (arrow).

number of weeks. They enlarge, coalesce and eventually break through into the ventricle. They may result in an abnormal contour to the ventricular outline. The extent and severity of these lesions is variable. They will eventually disappear, sometimes leaving an echogenic glial scar. The neurological damage is severe, sometimes fatal, and with the ultimate outcome dependent on the area of the brain affected (Fig. 9.12).

There is no universally accepted grading system but the system described by Devries et al in 1992[15] is useful (Box 9.5 and Fig. 9.13).

THE HEAD, NECK AND SPINE 267

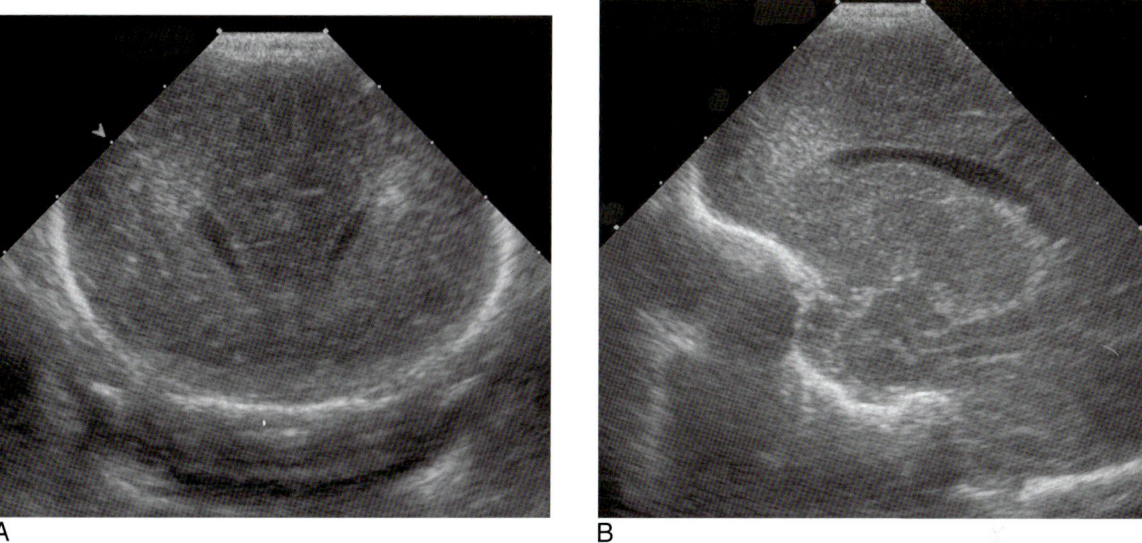

Figure 9.11 Early periventricular leukomalacia. (A) This premature infant had suffered a severe ischemic event. Coronal scan anteriorly showing the anterior horns of the lateral ventricles and the marked echogenic areas anterior to this extending in a triangular shape out towards the skull. (B) Sagittal scan showing the right ventricle and the echogenic area anteriorly around the anterior horn of the lateral ventricle.

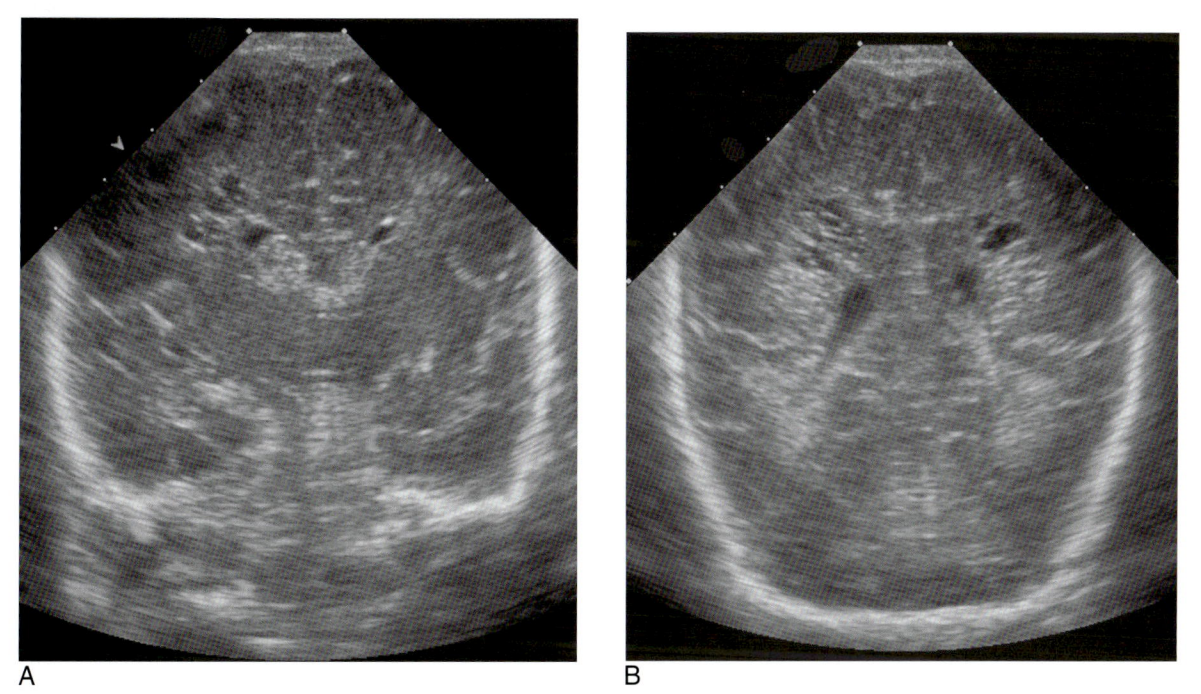

Figure 9.12 Germinal matrix hemorrhage and periventricular leukomalacia. (A) Coronal scan anteriorly, demonstrating cystic areas around the anterior horns of the lateral ventricle. There are also fresh germinal matrix hemorrhages on both sides. (B) Coronal posterior scan showing the two lateral ventricles containing the choroid plexus. There are small cystic areas around the lateral ventricles in keeping with periventricular leukomalacia.

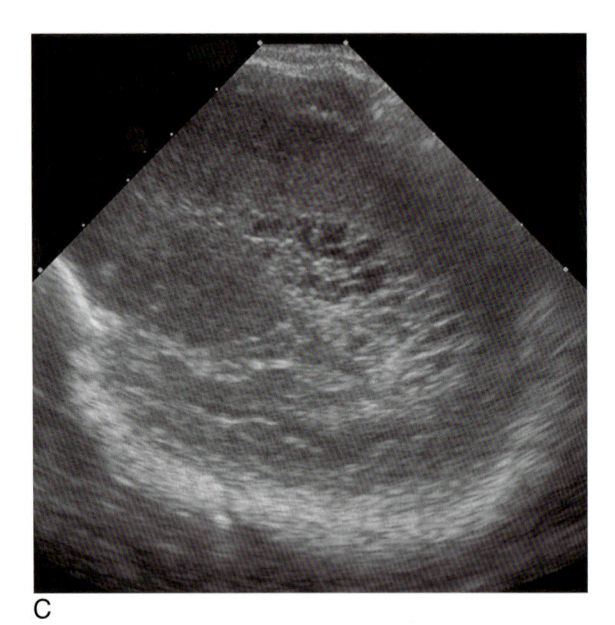

Figure 9.12, cont'd (C) Sagittal scan lateral to the lateral ventricle on the right. Notice that there are a large number of cystic spaces surrounding the right lateral ventricle.

Distinguishing features of PVL   Features are:

- early phase—echogenic
- late phase—cystic
- bilateral and symmetrical
- can be seen in coronal and sagittal planes separate from the ventricles
- cortical sparing.

HEMORRHAGE IN TERM NEONATES

Term infants are at risk from hemorrhage, particularly because of perinatal events such as assisted deliveries. They may sustain subdural hemorrhages which may be detected over the surface of the brain. Infratentorial hemorrhages are more difficult for ultrasound to diagnose, because of the normally high echogenicity of the cerebellum. Any infant having a difficult traumatic delivery should be monitored with ultrasound.

Extracorporeal membrane oxygenation (ECMO), which is used for the treatment of young infants with severe respiratory problems, is another cause of intracranial hemorrhage. Catheters are placed in the internal carotid artery and internal jugular vein in a system similar to that used in bypass surgery, so that the lungs are 'rested' and allowed time to recover. These infants are anticoagulated, and it is this that increases the risk of hemorrhage, which may occur anywhere but particularly intracerebrally, intraventricularly and in the subarachnoid spaces (Fig. 9.14).

Any bleeding disorder in the neonatal period may predispose the infant to intracranial hemorrhage.

COMMON CONGENITAL CYSTIC ABNORMALITIES

Congenital malformations are increasingly being diagnosed prenatally (see Ch. 2). Postnatally intracranial abnormalities may be suspected from facial appearances ('the face mirrors the brain'). Ultrasound is particularly good at detecting the fluid-filled abnormalities such as hydrocephalus and the cystic abnormalities of the brain. A normal ultrasound examination can exclude these abnormalities.

Box 9.5	Grading system for periventricular leukomalacia[15]
Grades I and II	Echogenic flares which either resolve or persist, evolving into small cysts. Multiple cysts in the parieto-occipital white matter. There is no known neurological outcome
Grade III	Multiple white matter cysts
Grade IV	Severe periventricular leukomalacia in the term infant, affecting the deep white matter and evolving into multiple subcortical cysts

THE HEAD, NECK AND SPINE   269

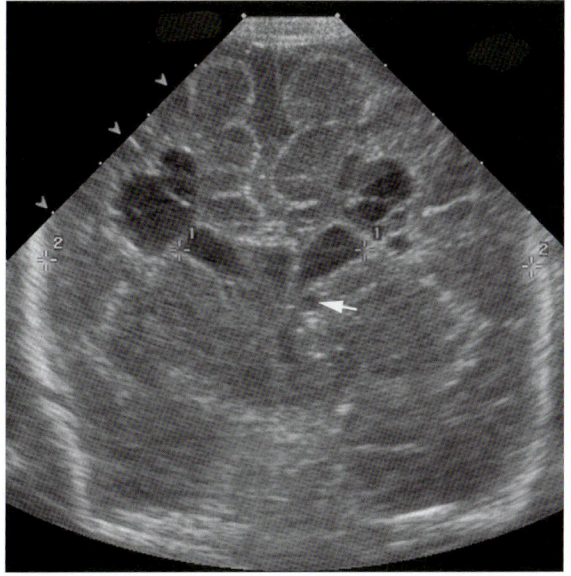

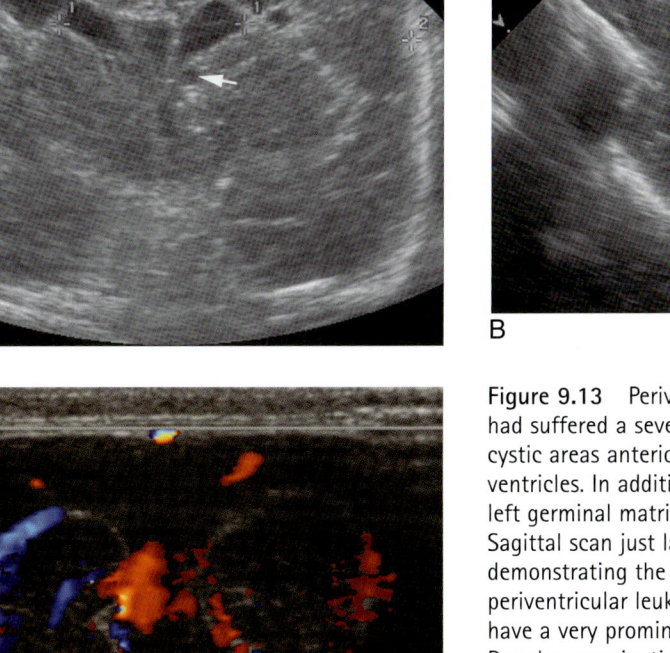

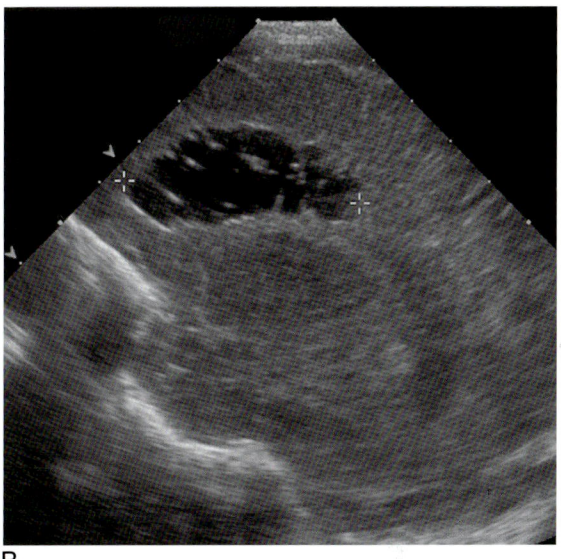

Figure 9.13 Periventricular leukomalacia. (A) This baby had suffered a severe ischemic episode. There are large cystic areas anterior to the anterior horns of the lateral ventricles. In addition there is a small cystic area in the left germinal matrix from an old hemorrhage (arrow). (B) Sagittal scan just lateral to the left ventricle demonstrating the large cystic spaces of the severe periventricular leukomalacia. (C) This baby was noted to have a very prominent amount of extra-axial fluid. This Doppler examination demonstrates blood vessels crossing this fluid in the subarachnoid space, which helps to differentiate it from subdural fluid.

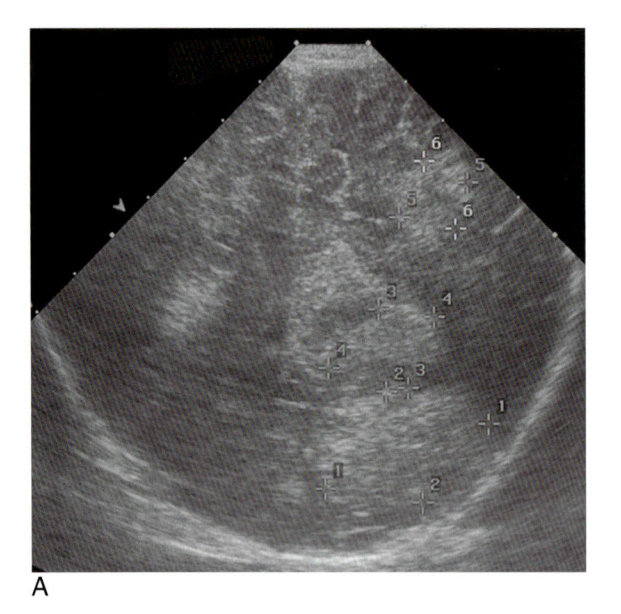

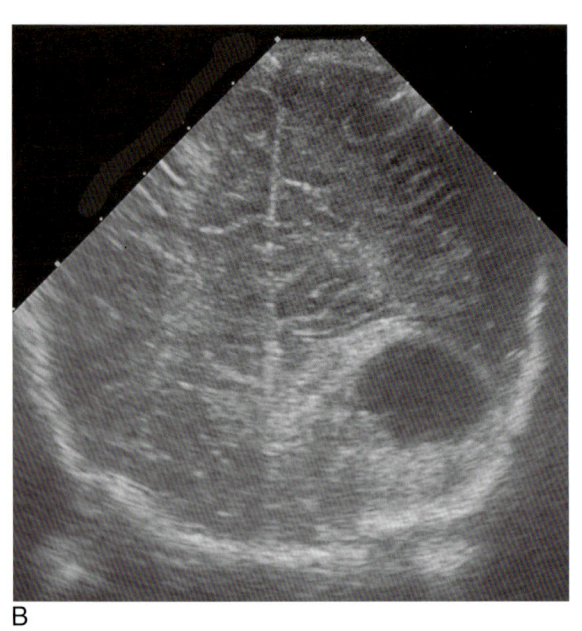

Figure 9.14 Consequences of extracorporeal membrane oxygenation. (A) Coronal scan showing three marked areas of hemorrhage resulting from the anticoagulation given in ECMO (between the calipers). There is an anterior mid and a posterior hemorrhage on the left side. (B) Coronal scan posteriorly in the same infant 2 weeks later showing the posterior hemorrhage has started to liquefy with a large cystic area centrally.

Porencephalic cysts

Porencephalic cysts are most commonly the result of acquired focal parenchymal lesions. This may be due to infarction, hemorrhage, trauma or infection that causes localized brain destruction. The cysts contain CSF and usually communicate with the ventricles or the subarachnoid spaces. There may be associated ventricular enlargement. The evolution of a porencephalic cyst may be seen with initially a highly echogenic area which in time evolves with central liquefaction and eventual cyst formation.

Dandy–Walker cysts (complex)

Dandy–Walker malformation is a result of atresia of the foramen of Magendie and sometimes the foramen of Luschka. There is also partial agenesis of the cerebellar vermis. The appearances are those of a large posterior fossa with massive dilation of the fourth ventricle and to a lesser extent of the third and lateral ventricles (Fig. 9.15). This malformation is commonly diagnosed in utero (see Ch. 2). It has been reported in association with agenesis of the corpus callosum and holoprosencephaly.

The Dandy–Walker variant has a very similar appearance but there is a lesser degree of hypoplasia of the cerebellar vermis. The foramen of Magendie is, however, patent. The fourth ventricle is less dilated.

Holoprosencephaly

This is an anomaly which results from the failure of the cerebral hemispheres to divide in early brain development and is a wide spectrum of abnormalities.

The most severe form of holoprosencephaly has a typical facial appearance. The facial abnormalities may be hypotelorism (close set eyes) of varying degrees, a single nostril of the nose or even a proboscis. Other midline defects include clefting of the lip and palate. There is a single common ventricle which lies centrally. Holoprosencephaly may be a feature of trisomy 13 or 15 (Fig. 9.16).

THE HEAD, NECK AND SPINE 271

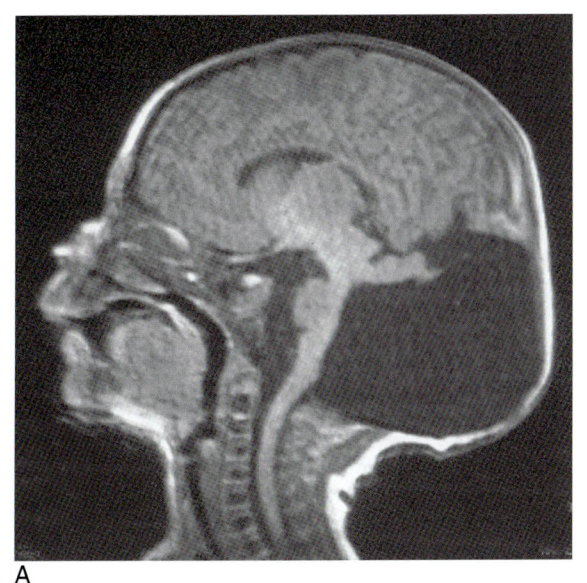

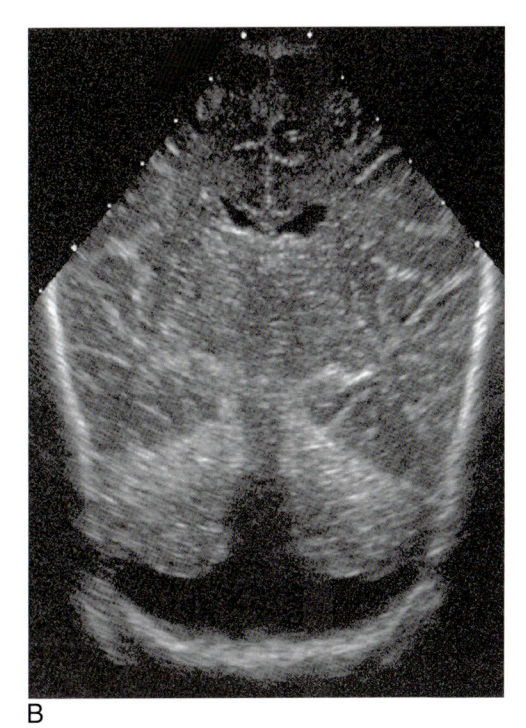

Figure 9.15 Dandy–Walker malformation. (A) MRI scan on an infant showing a large cystic area in the posterior fossa. The cerebellum is hypoplastic and there is complete absence of the cerebellar vermis. (B) Coronal ultrasound scan showing the hypoplasia of the cerebellar hemispheres and absence of the cerebellar vermis. There is a large amount of fluid surrounding the cerebellar hemispheres.

Choroid plexus cysts

Choroid plexus cysts are commonly seen prenatally. It is now generally accepted that they are not a marker of any chromosomal abnormality and are of no significance.

Arachnoid cysts

Arachnoid cysts are developmental cysts that contain CSF and are usually incidental findings. They are found particularly in the middle and posterior cranial fossa. They may cause no intracerebral effect or may cause pressure symptoms if large, or obstruct the ventricular system.

OTHER CONGENITAL ABNORMALITIES

Agenesis of the corpus callosum

The normal corpus callosum is usually easily visible in the midline and is best seen in sagittal scans.

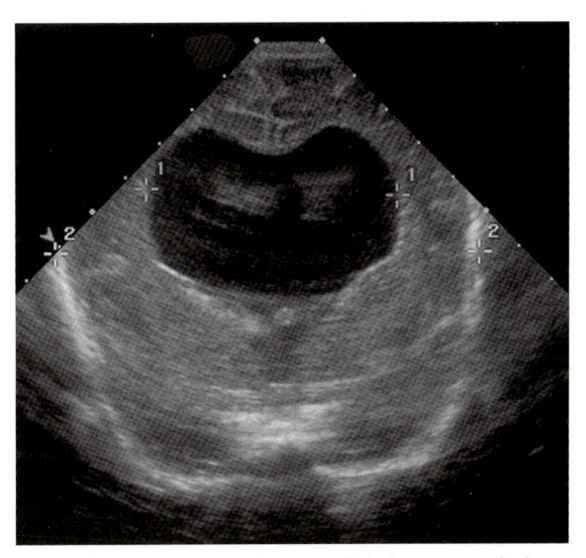

Figure 9.16 Holoprosencephaly. This is a congenital abnormality where there is a single ventricle. Coronal ultrasound scans anteriorly demonstrating the single midline ventricle. Posteriorly the monoventricle becomes enlarged and sac-like. The septum pellucidum is always absent.

When the corpus callosum is absent, the third ventricle is high, riding between the two lateral ventricles, and the lateral ventricles assume a typical shape. In the coronal plane they may lie parallel, with prominence of the occipital horns and flattening of the anterior horns of the lateral ventricles in the sagittal plane. There are variable degrees of agenesis of the corpus callosum which are not all detectable with ultrasonography. The importance lies in its association with other abnormalities such as the Dandy–Walker malformation, Arnold–Chiari II malformation and midline defects such as encephalocele and holoprosencephaly (Fig. 9.17).

Thalamostriate vessels

Linear echogenicities in the thalamus and basal ganglia are occasionally encountered. The causes include congenital infections such as in TORCH, Down syndrome, trisomy 13, congenital HIV, asphyxia, fetal alcohol syndrome and hydrops (Fig. 9.18).

TRAUMA

CT and MRI are the investigations of choice for accidental trauma and those infants suspected of having non-accidental injury. Another form of injury is hypoxic ischemic encephalopathy secondary to very severe birth asphyxia.

Non-accidental injury

Non-accidental injury (NAI) is a deliberate injury to a child, and intracranial injury is a major source of mortality and physical disability. It has been reported that 95% of severe head injuries in the first year of life result from physical abuse, and head injury is the commonest cause of death in these children. Young babies are particularly at risk because of their large heads and poor neck control. There are also a number of other contributing factors such as the mobility of the brain in the high volume of CSF, and open sutures. The mechanism

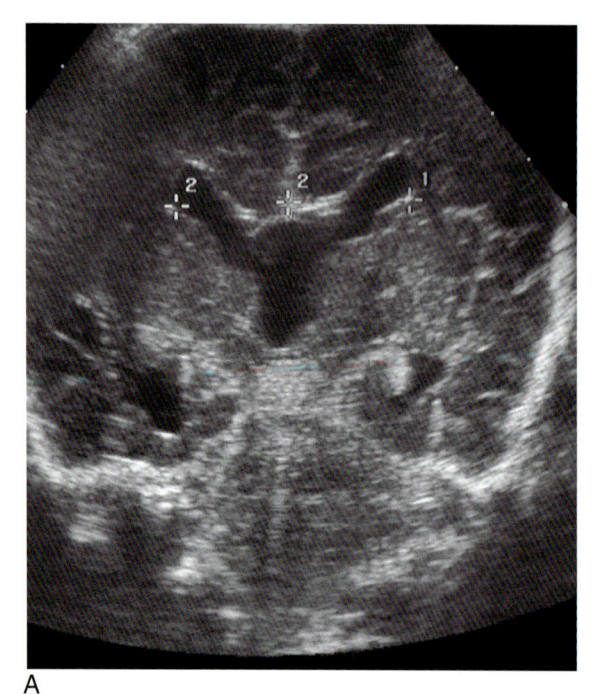

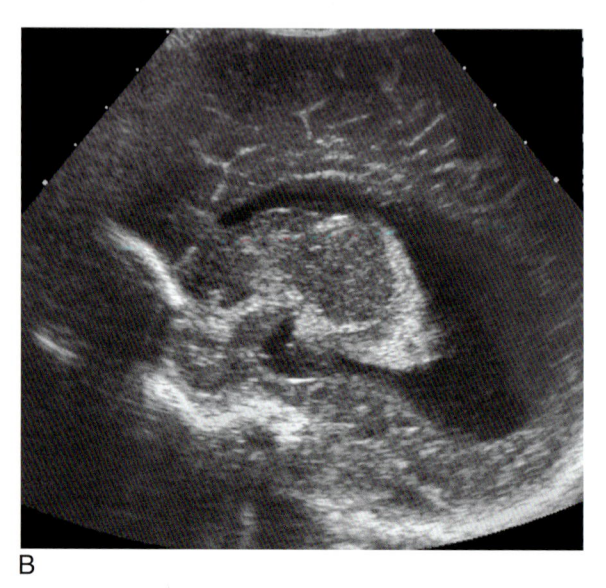

Figure 9.17 Agenesis of the corpus callosum. (A) Coronal scan on an infant suspected of having absence of the corpus callosum. The lateral ventricles are lying parallel to one another and the third ventricle is high riding. (B) Sagittal scan through the right lateral ventricle showing the unusual configuration of the lateral ventricle which is typical of this condition. There is prominence of the occipital horn and tapering of the anterior horns of the lateral ventricle.

THE HEAD, NECK AND SPINE   273

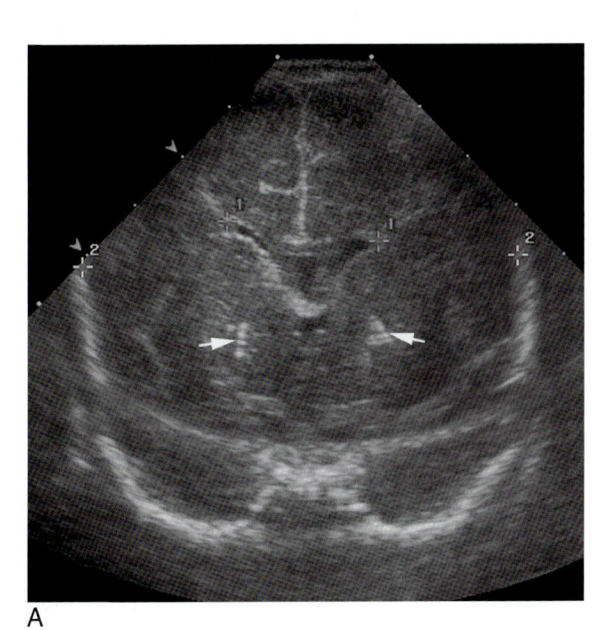

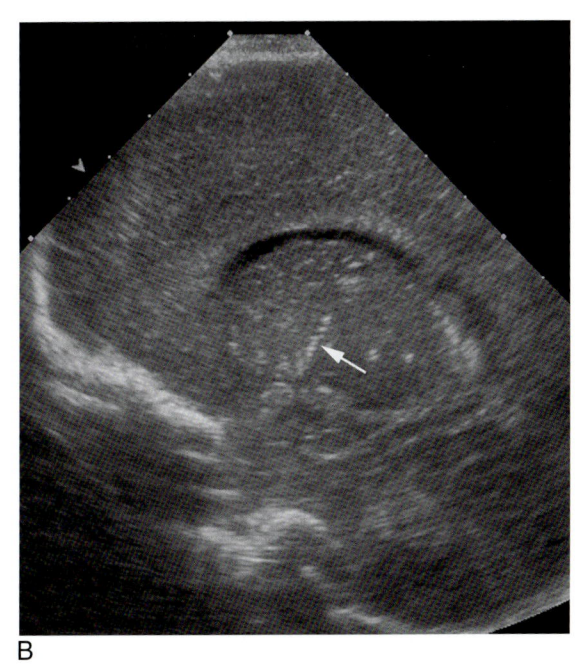

Figure 9.18 Linear echogenicity in the thalamus. (A) Anterior coronal scan through the anterior horns of the lateral ventricles. This demonstrates linear echogenic areas bilaterally in the basal ganglia (arrows). (B) Sagittal scan through the right basal ganglia showing the echogenic linear thalamostriate vessels (arrow). This is most commonly associated with congenital infections.

of injury is usually severe shaking (the shaken baby syndrome). This is sometimes associated with blunt trauma against a hard surface, for example a wall, or a combination of both shaking and hitting.

Other typical non-accidental injuries include unexplained fractures, bruises or burn marks, periorbital hemorrhages, retinal hemorrhages, rib fractures (typically posteriorly or laterally from squeezing the chest), metaphyseal fractures and fractures of different ages in the long bones. In any child suspected of having NAI, a cranial CT should be performed as soon as possible. There is no universally accepted protocol for imaging these children, because physical abuse often goes undetected for many months, and health workers have only a superficial awareness of the pediatric neuroradiology. Recently a full imaging strategy has been proposed.[16]

The ultrasound findings in NAI have been well described, but currently its use still lies in the hands of the interested expert. It has a limited role in the overall picture of non-accidental brain injury, but the sonographer undertaking cranial examinations should be aware of the main sonographic appearances because ultrasound is particularly suited to examination in the intensive care scenario in a severely injured child. High quality equipment is essential.

The ultrasound examination needs to be focused on a number of areas where useful information can be obtained, such as extra-axial hematomas and parenchymal injury, particularly contusional shearing tears at the corticomedullary junction (Fig. 9.19).[16,17]

The severely injured child may have scalp wounds and bruising with a fractured skull and subarachnoid and subdural hemorrhages. High frequency linear transducers should always be used to examine particularly the interhemispheric region.

Complex subdural hemorrhages containing membranes may reflect fresh and old blood. Fresh echogenic blood can be found overlying the cerebral hemispheres and in the midline falx region.

Parenchymal abnormalities such as contusional injuries are seen best at the gray/white matter interface in the frontoparietal region. They appear as echo-free linear branching areas and are also best seen using a linear transducer. Other acute injuries such as hemorrhagic contusions, lobar disruption and transcerebral lacerations can also be seen.

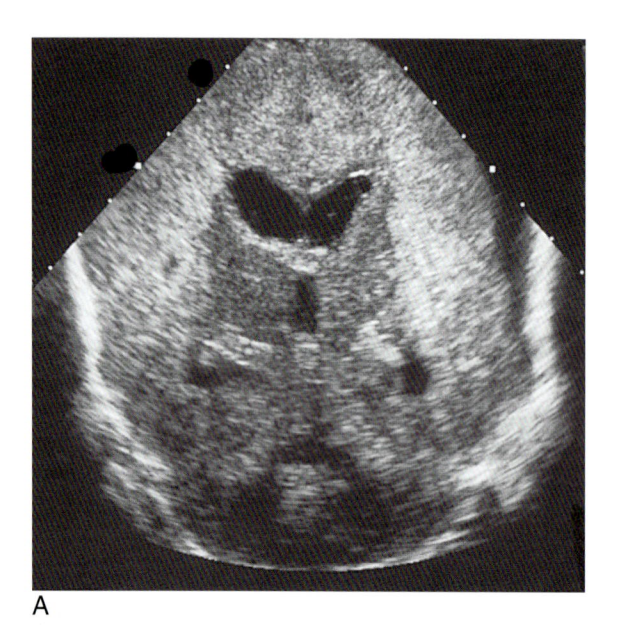

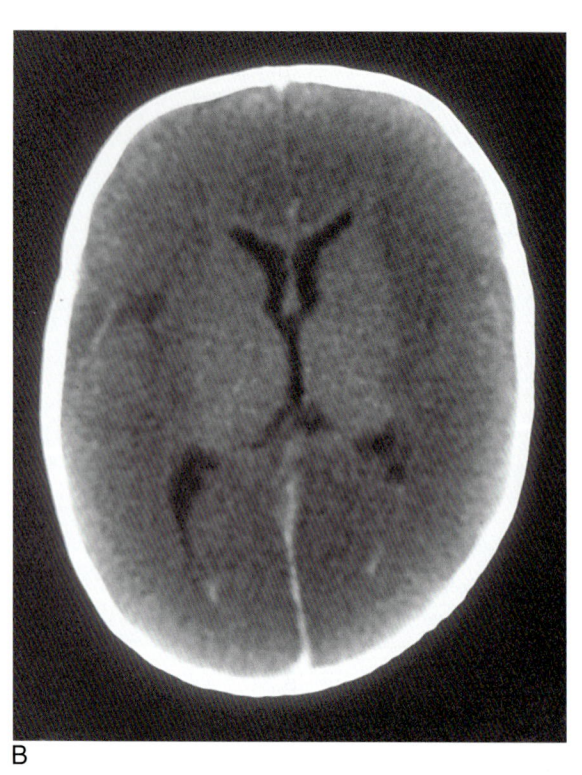

Figure 9.19 Non-accidental brain injury. (A) This child had suffered a severe brain injury. Coronal scan in the midplane showing mild dilation of the lateral ventricles. The most striking feature is the echogenic parenchyma and the different echogenicity of the basal ganglia. (B) CT scan of the same infant showing the difference in attenuation between the basal ganglia and the brain parenchyma. Such infants have had such a severe anoxic event that only the blood supply to the areas undertaking the primary function of the brain is preserved, accounting for the difference in attenuation.

Secondary damage to the brain is a result of the primary injury and may appear within hours of the original injury. Cerebral edema with swelling of the brain produces a typical 'bright brain' appearance. This may be focal or diffuse depending on the severity of the injury. The brain has a featureless appearance and the normal landmarks are lost. In very severe hypoxic ischemic injury there may be preservation of the vital centers with blood selectively diverted to these areas so that the 'central' areas around the caudate and thalamus, pons and medulla are spared. The cerebral cortex is particularly vulnerable as the blood is shunted away from these areas. If edema is very severe, death may result.

HYDROCEPHALUS

Any infant found to have a large head or a head that is enlarging should have an ultrasound examination. Ultrasound is the imaging method of choice for monitoring ventricular dilation and the response to treatment of hydrocephalus. Hydrocephalus and enlarged ventricles may be due to excess CSF, an obstruction of the ventricular system or failure of reabsorption of the CSF. Cerebrospinal fluid is produced by the choroid plexus. Increase in the amount of CSF results in raised intracranial pressure, dilation of the ventricles and compression of the brain parenchyma.

Cerebral atrophy as a cause of ventriculomegaly is associated with loss of brain parenchyma, irregular dilation of the ventricles and/or cystic changes in the brain substance. There are no symptoms or signs of increased intracranial pressure with bulging of the fontanelle. The head circumference is not enlarged.

Raised intracranial pressure causing hydrocephalus results in bulging of the anterior fontanelle, enlarging cranial circumference and 'sunset' eyes. The infant may also be vomiting with irritability and convulsions.

Causes of hydrocephalus include:

- congenital—aqueduct stenosis, Dandy–Walker malformation, Vein of Galen aneurysm
- acquired in fetal life—infection such as TORCH, intracranial hemorrhage
- acquired as a neonate—meningitis, post-hemorrhagic, abnormal skull development
- cerebral atrophy with loss of white matter such as in twin-to-twin transfusion, maternal collapse.

Hydrocephalus may be obstructive in that there is no communication in the ventricular system, or non-obstructive in which case there is no obstruction but an increase in CSF production. Doppler examination can be used to demonstrate flow through and, therefore, patency of the ventricular system in communicating hydrocephalus. A characteristic sinusoidal waveform is detected.

Treatment of hydrocephalus is surgical by inserting either a ventriculo-peritoneal shunt or a ventriculo-atrial shunt. Ultrasound can be used to monitor the degree of ventricular dilation and position of the intraventricular shunt. In addition, if a peritoneal shunt is placed and the tip of the shunt becomes 'walled off', ultrasound can demonstrate the collection related to the tip of the tube in the abdomen. Radiography is generally performed to demonstrate an intact shunt system.

VASCULAR ABNORMALITIES

Aneurysm of the Vein of Galen

These infants usually present in extreme heart failure. Clinically they have a loud bruit if the cranium is auscultated. An aneurysm of the Vein of Galen is essentially an AV malformation that causes shunting of the blood from the arteries to the deep veins, resulting in massive heart failure.

Ultrasound examination reveals a cystic structure behind the third ventricle which on Doppler examination, demonstrates blood flow. These infants all used to die in early infancy but now, with interventional radiology and improved catheter technology and embolization techniques, their survival is much improved. All require further imaging with MRI and interventional angiography in expert hands if considered suitable for treatment (Fig. 9.20).

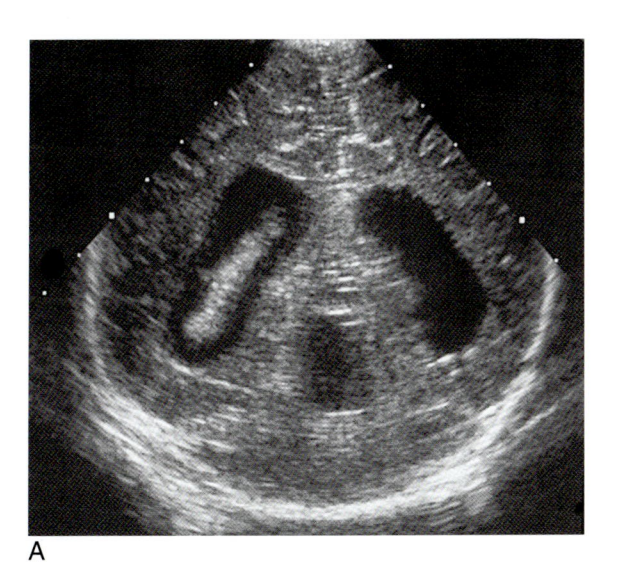

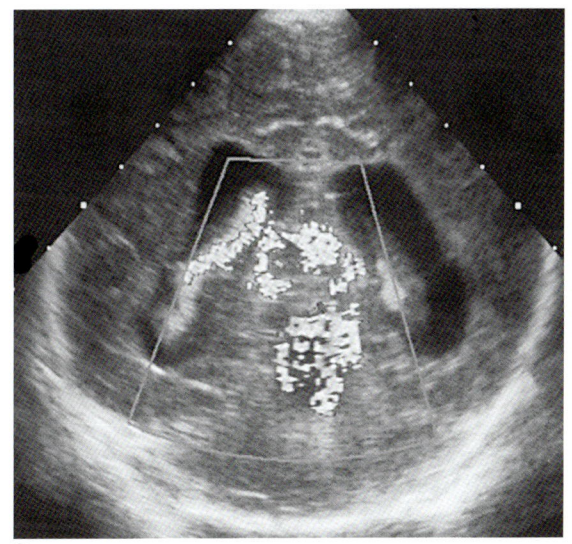

Figure 9.20 Aneurysm of the vein of Galen. (A) Coronal scan in the mid-plane showing the dilation of the lateral ventricles and a cystic structure lying posterior to the third ventricle. (B) Doppler examination at the same level shows that the cystic structure is vascular.

Continued

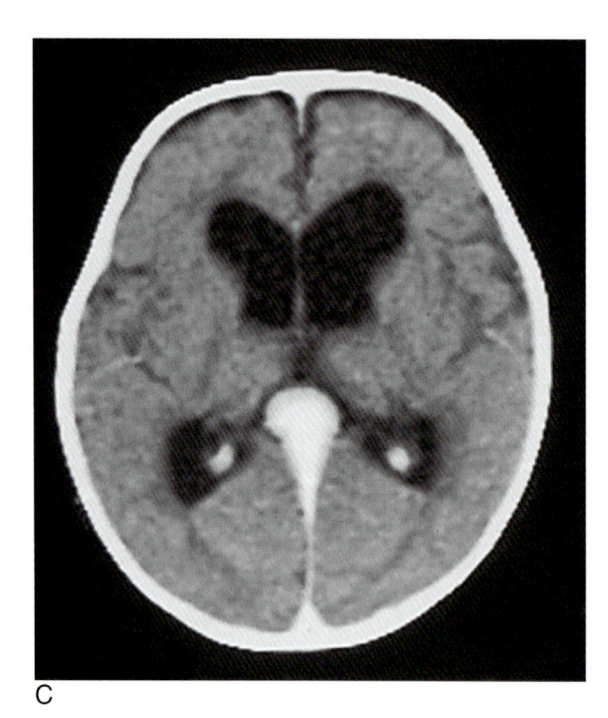

Figure 9.20 Cont'd (C) Contrast-enhanced CT scan showing the midline vein of Galen aneurysm. The echogenic areas in the lateral ventricles are choroid.

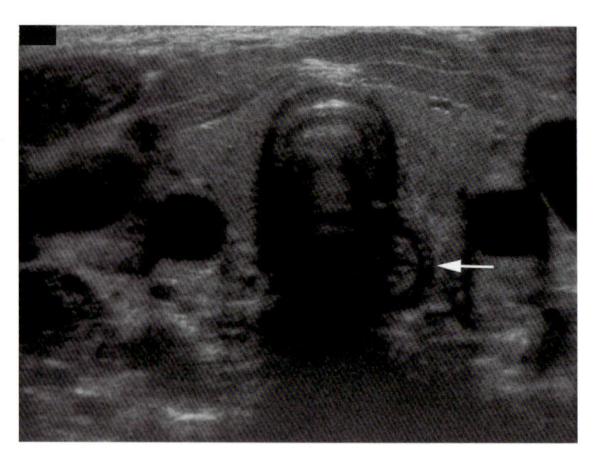

Figure 9.21 Normal thyroid. The thyroid has a homogeneous echogenicity. In this transverse scan the esophagus can be clearly seen next to the air shadow from the trachea and behind the left lobe of the thyroid (arrow).

NECK

THE THYROID GLAND

Normal anatomy of the thyroid

The thyroid gland normally lies just below the thyroid cartilage in the neck. It consists of a right and left lobe and an isthmus across the midline joining the two. A pyramidal lobe may be present extending from the isthmus up to the hyoid bone.

The normal thyroid has a homogeneous echo texture throughout. It is bounded anteriorly by the more hypoechoic neck muscles and posteriorly by the jugular and carotid vessels. The esophagus can be seen immediately posteriorly on the left as an air-containing structure with a muscular wall. The thyroid is highly vascular with prominent Doppler signals throughout. The normal parathyroid gland is not identified in a child (Fig. 9.21).[18–22]

Embryology and congenital anomalies

The thyroid gland starts developing early in the floor of the pharynx (base of the tongue) and then later descends into the neck. For a short time the developing thyroid gland is connected to the tongue by a narrow tube, the thyroglossal duct. The thyroglossal duct normally then degenerates and disappears. The pyramidal lobe of the thyroid represents a persistence of the inferior portion of the thyroglossal duct.

Congenital hypothyroidism

These infants are generally detected in countries using the Guthrie test soon after birth. It is a common disorder of pediatrics and is usually related to a developmental anomaly such as ectopia or enzyme defects such as dyshormonogenesis.

The role of imaging in these infants is debatable as it does not affect treatment and thyroid replacement therapy. Ultrasound on the other hand is most definitely indicated in an infant with a midline neck mass prior to surgery, in order to determine if there is thyroid tissue in the normal position. The use of ultrasound has been reported in hypothyroidism but does not really play a role in these infants. Nuclear medicine imaging is preferable in order to detect any ectopic thyroid tissue.

There are a number of causes of hypothyroidism in the neonate, ranging from a small ectopic thyroid, often in the base of the tongue, to an enlarged thyroid (a neonatal goiter) resulting from dyshormonogenesis due to an enzymatic defect. Ultrasound may be used to show the enlarged neonatal thyroid.

Ectopic thyroid gland

An ectopic thyroid gland is an infrequent congenital anomaly, and it is usually located along the normal route of its descent from the tongue. A lingual thyroid is the most common ectopic thyroid tissue. Incomplete descent of the thyroid gland results in the sublingual thyroid gland appearing high in the neck.

It is important when scanning midline masses in the neck to ensure that the normal thyroid gland is present, as this may be the only functioning thyroid tissue. This will prevent inadvertent surgical removal of the thyroid gland. Failure to do so may leave the child permanently dependent on thyroid medication.

Accessory thyroid gland tissue

Accessory thyroid gland tissue may also appear in the thymus inferior to the thyroid gland. Although this tissue may be functional, it is often of insufficient size to maintain normal thyroid function if the thyroid gland is removed. An accessory thyroid gland may develop in the neck lateral to the thyroid cartilage. It usually lies on the thyrohyoid muscle and originates from remnant of the thyroglossal ducts.

Ultrasound technique for examination of the neck

Use a high resolution linear probe such as a 15L8 with good near field visualization. Gel standoffs are not used in young children, as access to the neck is limited by their small size and short necks.

The sonographer can improve access by positioning the infant or child with their shoulders on a pillow and their head extended over the edge.

An examination of the neck should include all the structures from the base of the tongue superiorly to the thymus in the upper mediastinum. This is because the majority of requests for examination are related to masses in the neck and it is very important to clearly identify all the normal structures. In addition, ultrasound may demonstrate whether the thyroid gland is present and will demonstrate focal or diffuse abnormalities. Some conditions of the thyroid are associated with lymphadenopathy, so lymph nodes should always be looked for and their normality commented upon. Lymphadenopathy is one of the commonest findings in the neck. Always examine the whole of the neck.

Diffuse thyroid enlargement

Thyroid problems in children are not common. Table 9.2 summarizes the features of conditions causing diffuse thyroid enlargement.

Thyroiditis

Graves disease is a disorder of hyperplasia and hyperfunction and is seen predominantly in adolescent girls. They present with all the clinical signs and symptoms of hyperthyroidism such as tachycardia, exophthalmos and an enlarged thyroid. Graves disease may be associated with myasthenia gravis, pernicious anemia and adrenal insufficiency.

On ultrasound the gland will appear enlarged with a lobulated contour. The general texture of the gland may be heterogeneous and echo-poor due to the infiltration of lymphocytes and the multiple blood vessels. On Doppler examination there is an extremely hypervascular thyroid, often referred to as the 'thyroid inferno', and often associated diffuse lymphadenopathy in the neck. The appearances are very similar to those of Hashimoto disease (Fig. 9.22).

Hashimoto thyroiditis is a chronic autoimmune condition with lymphocyte infiltration of the gland. The thyroid is diffusely enlarged with a coarse parenchymal echo texture. When the child becomes hypothyroid there is an increasing vascularity on Doppler examination. The gland eventually becomes small and atrophied (Fig. 9.23).

Bacterial thyroiditis is extremely rare and seen most commonly in association with a fourth branchial arch anomaly on the left.

Table 9.2 Diffuse thyroid enlargement in children

Diagnosis	Clinical presentation	Ultrasound features	Nuclear medicine appearances
Hashimoto thyroiditis	Autoimmune disease Mainly affecting adolescent girls Euthyroid	Diffuse thyroid enlargement Coarse hypoechoic texture but may be normal Lymphadenopathy	
Graves disease	Goiter, tachycardia, exophthalmos	Diffuse thyroid enlargement Hypoechoic gland Lymphadenopathy	Not usually indicated Homogenous high uptake
Simple goiter	Neonatal congenital dyshormonogenesis or iodine deficiency in older children	Heterogeneous gland	
Multinodular goiter		Solid or cystic areas or both Hypoechoic areas (colloid cysts) may become hemorrhagic with necrosis and calcification	Endocrine active nodule and uptake on imaging likely to be benign
Lymphoma	Swelling in neck May obstruct the airways	Focal lesions but more commonly diffuse enlargement of the thyroid gland Hypoechoic parenchyma Lymphadenopathy	

Goiter

Goiter is a non-specific general term used to describe an enlarged thyroid gland. There are many causes of this enlargement, and affected children are most commonly euthyroid but may be hypothyroid in dyshormonogenesis. Ultrasound and nuclear medicine are two techniques which are used and are generally considered to be complementary.

Ultrasound technique The ultrasound examination should be according to the standard technique. Generally, there will be a diffuse enlargement in a simple goiter, with a homogeneous echo texture. The goiter may also be multinodular. Doppler examination is essential in order to show the hypervascular gland, as in Graves disease or other inflammatory conditions.

Thyroid malignancy

Carcinoma of the thyroid is also uncommon but very closely related to irradiation of the head and neck. The Chernobyl disaster resulted in a major increase in thyroid malignancy in children exposed to this radiation.

Papillary carcinoma accounts for the majority of thyroid carcinomas in children. The outstanding feature of papillary carcinoma is the presence of microcalcification, both in the primary thyroid tumor and lymph node metastases, which occurs in over 85% of cases. Lymph nodes in the neck are present in over 50%. Spread is by the lymphatics, and when secondary deposits are present in the lungs they are typically miliary. The primary thyroid tumor is usually well defined and echo poor.

The other form of thyroid carcinoma is medullary carcinoma which is part of the genetic disorder known as multiple endocrine neoplasia and may be associated with pheochromocytoma and parathyroid hyperplasia. These children require a total thyroidectomy, as this tumor tends to metastasize early.

Lymphoma of the thyroid is seen in children and produces an enlarged hypoechoic gland. The majority are seen in conditions causing chronic thyroiditis.

THE HEAD, NECK AND SPINE 279

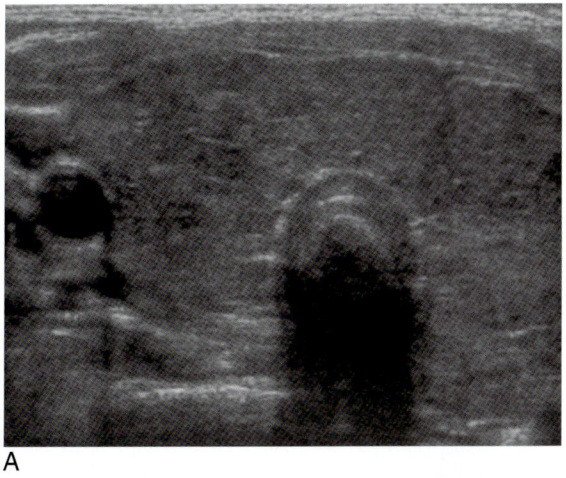

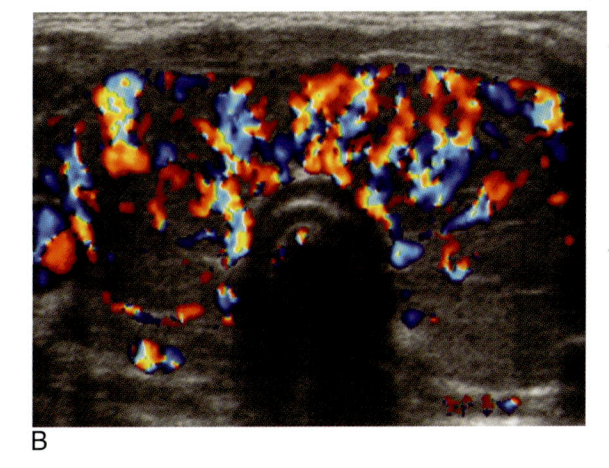

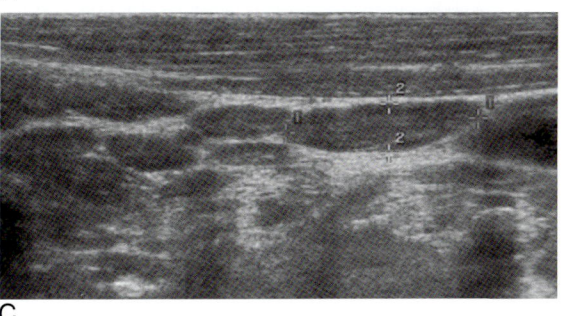

Figure 9.22 Graves disease. (A) Transverse sonogram of the thyroid in a child presenting with hyperthyroidism. The thyroid gland is enlarged and heterogeneous. (B) Doppler examination showing that the thyroid is hypervascular. (C) This child also had associated lymphadenopathy in the neck, which is a common association.

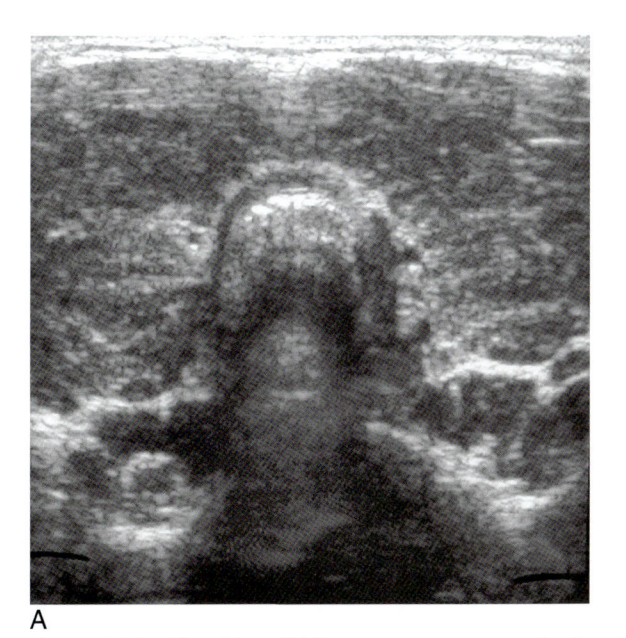

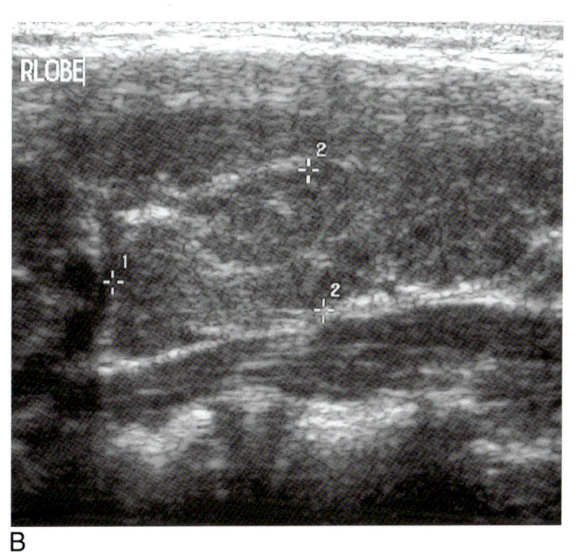

Figure 9.23 Thyroiditis. (A) Transverse sonogram of a thyroid in an adolescent girl. Notice the thyroid is heterogeneous throughout. (B) Longitudinal sonogram of the thyroid in the same patient demonstrating the heterogeneity of the thyroid and nodules (between calipers). These appearances are typical of thyroiditis.

Table 9.3 summarizes the features of focal thyroid lesions.

PARATHYROID GLANDS

The parathyroid glands are two paired structures occurring superiorly and inferiorly in the thyroid lobes. The normal parathyroid glands cannot be detected in children on ultrasound.

Ultrasound may be used to detect parathyroid adenomas in children with hyperparathyroidism. This is an extremely rare condition and is usually secondary to severe renal disease in children.

Parathyroid cysts can occur (Fig. 9.24).

NECK MASSES

Masses related to the head and neck are commonly encountered in children. There are basically three types of lesions: congenital, inflammatory and neoplastic. The role of ultrasound is to define the masses and give an indication of their origin.

It is important that the sonographer has a good understanding of the embryological origin and differentiation of the structures in order to accurately diagnose these masses and give direction to any further imaging as required. The vast majority of head and neck lesions are benign.

Congenital cystic masses of the neck include:

- thyroglossal duct cysts
- branchial cleft cysts

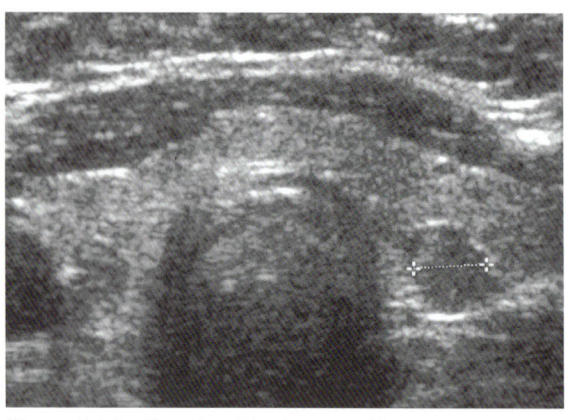

Figure 9.24 Parathyroid adenomas. Transverse sonogram of the thyroid showing the hypoechoic parathyroid adenomas (between calipers). This patient had severe renal disease.

- cystic hygroma
- dermoid and epidermoid cysts
- thymic and bronchogenic cysts
- laryngoceles.

Thyroglossal duct cysts

Normally the thyroglossal duct atrophies and disappears, but a remnant of it may persist and form a cyst in the base of the tongue or anywhere along the course followed by the duct (Fig. 9.25). Thyroglossal duct cysts are the commonest congenital neck masses and second only to benign lymphadenopathy of the neck. About 50% occur under the age of 10 years. Most thyroglossal duct

Table 9.3 Focal thyroid lesions

Diagnosis	Clinical presentation	Ultrasound features	Nuclear medicine appearances
Simple cysts	Lump	Well-defined cyst Rare Lesion should be aspirated	Photon deficient
Benign thyroid nodule (adenoma)	Thyroid lump	Well-defined solid nodule Hypoechoic rim	If active may take up isotope
Hemorrhagic cyst	Discovered following trauma	Evolving echogenic to central necrosis and internal echoes Fluid level	Photon deficient
Papillary carcinoma	History of neck irradiation Thyroid nodule	Focal hypoechoic nodule Microcalcification in primary and lymph nodes Miliary lung metastases	Photon deficient area suggestive of malignancy

THE HEAD, NECK AND SPINE   281

Foramen cecum of tongue
Lingual thyroglossal duct cyst
Cervical thyroglossal duct cyst
Hyoid bone
Opening of thyroglossal duct sinus
Pyramidal lobe of thyroid gland

A

B

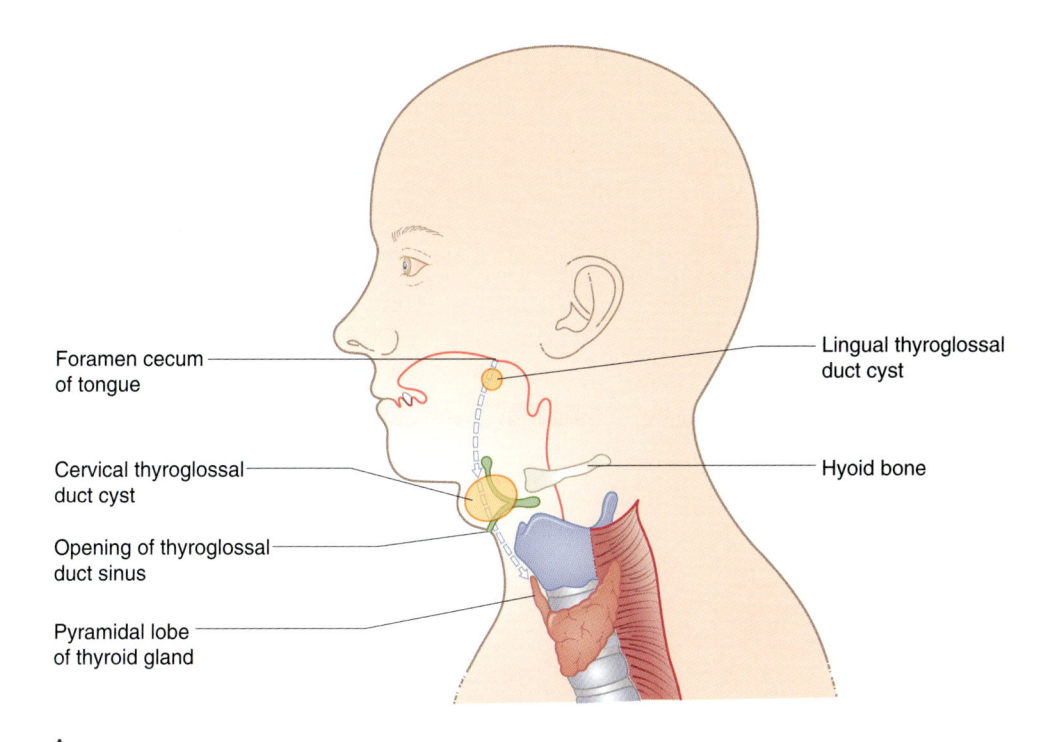

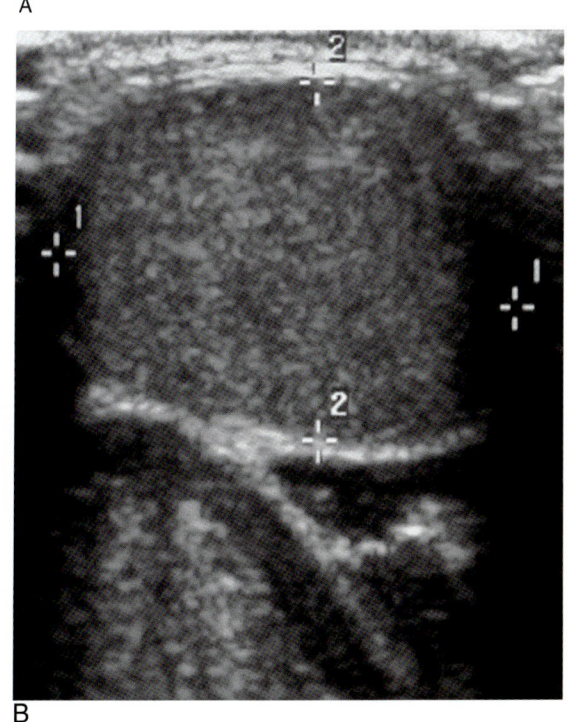

Figure 9.25 Thyroglossal duct cyst. (A) The descent of the thyroid in embryological life from the foramen cecum at the base of the tongue to its normal position in the neck. Its relationship to the hyoid bone is shown. The vast majority of thyroglossal duct cysts occur in this region. They are midline and typically move with protrusion of the tongue. (B) Longitudinal sonogram through a thyroglossal duct cyst (between calipers). There are multiple echoes within the cyst, related to the thick sebaceous material. Sometimes these may be purely cystic.

cysts are observed by the age of five years and unless the lesions become infected, the majority are asymptomatic. The swelling is painless, progressively enlarging and moveable. If the cyst becomes infected it may perforate the skin forming a thyroglossal duct sinus. Some may improve after antibiotics but frequently recur.

Cysts are usually found just inferior to the hyoid bone. Above the hyoid bone these lesions are midline but may deviate from the midline below the hyoid. Sixty-five percent of these cysts occur just below, 15% at the hyoid, and 20% above. It should be confirmed that a normal thyroid is present, as sometimes these cysts contain the only functioning thyroid tissue. Ultrasound is generally sufficient, as the clinical picture is often diagnostic. Ultrasound may show an anechoic discrete cyst, but the content does vary depending on infection, hemorrhage, post-aspiration or proteinaceous fluid (Fig. 9.26).

The treatment is to completely resect the cyst, resect the hyoid bone and trace the course of the thyroglossal cyst to the base of the tongue. Simple excision and drainage will result in recurrence and a sinus track.

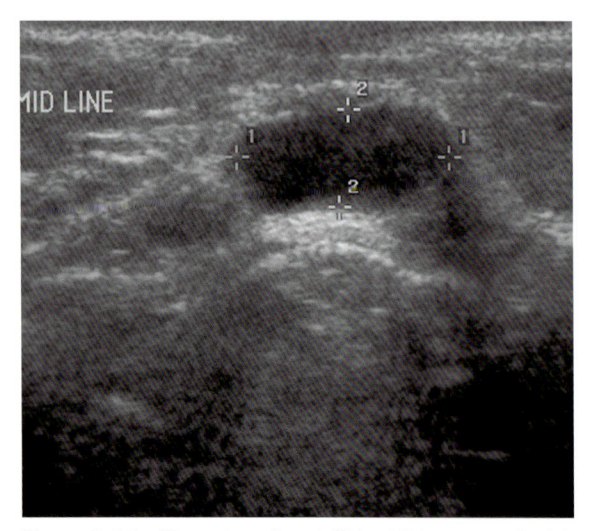

Figure 9.26 Thyroglossal cyst. This child presented with a midline cystic nodule. The ultrasound revealed a well-defined cyst (between calipers), and this was found to be a thyroglossal duct cyst at surgery.

Branchial cleft anomaly

There are four paired branchial clefts and pouches, all giving rise to different structures in the head and neck (Fig. 9.27). The first branchial arch gives rise to the eustachian tube, tympanic membrane, external auditory canal and middle ear. The second to the fourth pouches give rise to the tonsil, tonsillar fossa, thymus, inferior parathyroid gland, superior parathyroid gland and pyriform sinus. The clefts involute, and failure to involute leaves branchial cysts, sinus tracks or fistulas. All these branchial cleft anomalies may manifest as a culmination of cyst, sinus or fistula.[23,24] (A sinus opens externally through the skin whereas a fistula connects the skin with an internal structure such as a tonsil.)

There are four types of branchial cleft cysts:

- The second is by far the commonest (95%) and involves a track from the lower border of the sternocleidomastoid muscle to the palatine tonsil, passing between the internal and external carotid arteries.
- First cleft cysts involve the parotid gland and external ear and may present as repeated parotid abscesses. A skin opening may be present at birth around the angle of the mandible.
- The third and fourth are lower in the neck and both involve the piriform fossa. The fourth cyst is a classic cause of recurrent suppurative thyroiditis and is usually found on the left.

All of these branchial cleft cysts present clinically with a fluctuant mass. On ultrasound there is a well-defined cyst which may or may not be filled with material usually due to hemorrhage or infection. The cyst is usually intimately related to the sternocleidomastoid muscle. Further imaging is generally required, such as CT or MRI. MRI is generally better because it will be able to demonstrate inflammation and a sinus or fistula if it is present.

Complete surgical excision is required to prevent recurrent reinfection.

Cystic hygroma

The commonly accepted theory regarding the development of cystic hygromas is that they arise from a failure of developing lymphatics to drain

THE HEAD, NECK AND SPINE

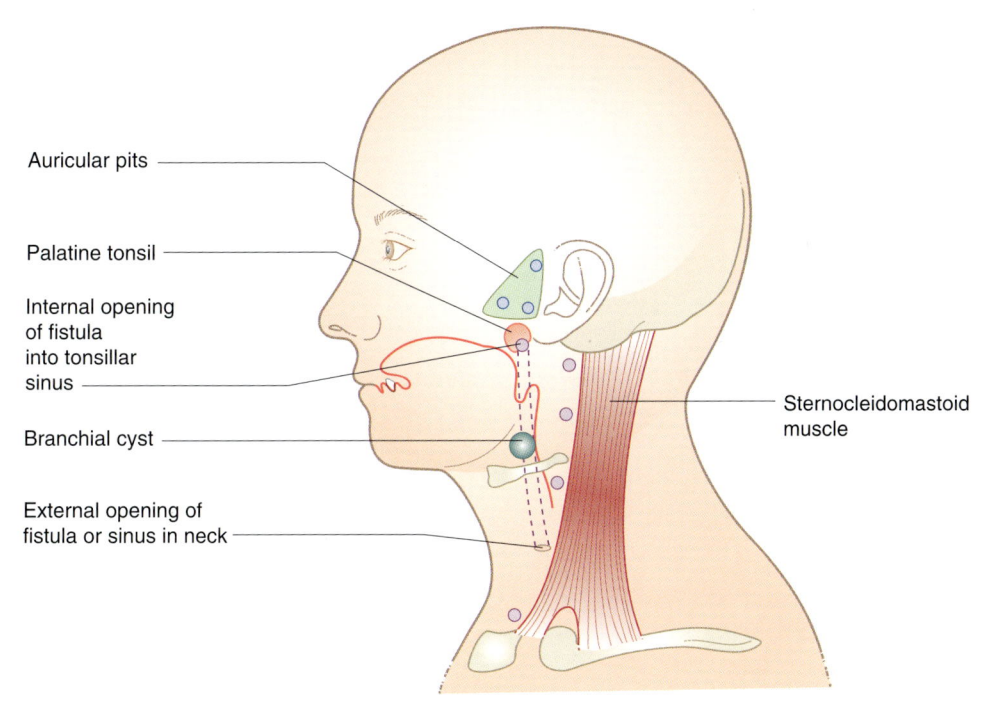

Figure 9.27 Branchial arch remnants. Notice the position of the branchial cyst and the fistula or sinus track from the palatine tonsil to the skin.

into veins, in particular the jugulo-axillary lymphatic sac to drain into the jugular vein. This produces a congenital obstruction of the lymphatic drainage. This is a spectrum of anomalies and it varies from the cystic hygroma (large spaces) to a cavernous lymphangioma (smaller spaces) to a capillary (simplex lymphangioma).[25]

The large cystic hygromas are the most common, with over 50% presenting at birth with some association with Down syndrome and Turner syndrome. About 70% of all cystic hygromas involve the neck and lower face. They may also occur in the axilla and in the mediastinum. They are painless and compressible unless there has been bleeding into them, in which case they become tense and distended. Most contain multiple cysts of varying sizes, and the interconnecting stroma may be variable in appearance depending on the hemangiomatous component. They are often very complex, making it difficult on ultrasound to clearly delineate the normal structures as they infiltrate and insinuate the surrounding tissues.

The role of ultrasound is to define the extent of the mass and give some indication of the contents such as lymph channels and hemangiomatous components (Fig. 9.28).

The treatment is either surgery or sclerosing agents under ultrasound control.

Congenital torticollis (fibromatosis colli)

The cause of fibromatosis colli remains unclear but results from shortening and fibrosis, with mature dense fibroblasts deposited and found in the sternocleidomastoid muscle. This typically pulls the head and neck to the affected side causing torticollis. The mass is usually noted a couple of weeks after birth and is not thought to be related to birth difficulties or trauma. There is a known association with developmental dysplasia of the hip and tibial torsion.

Without treatment of the torticollis the infant will develop marked facial asymmetry. Treatment consists of massage and stretching exercises.

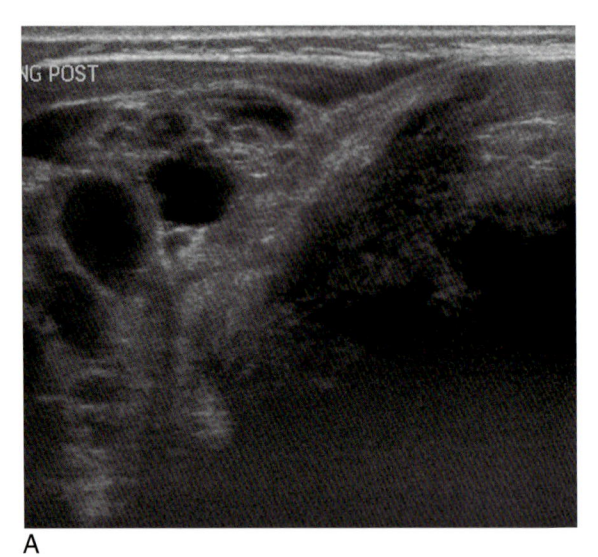

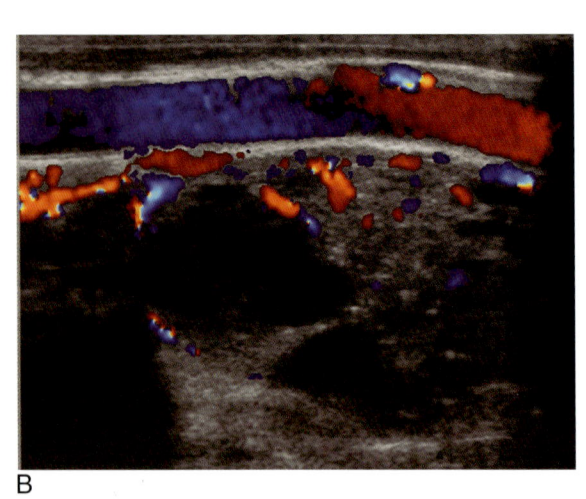

Figure 9.28 Cystic hygroma. (A) Longitudinal scan over a large mass in the neck. It shows multiple cystic areas which are ill defined. (B) Color Doppler of the mass demonstrates that the stroma is very vascular. There are also cystic spaces in relation to the carotid vessels which are lying anteriorly. This mass was a mixture of lymph and hemangiomatous elements.

Ultrasound will reveal a dense mass of tissue within the belly of the sternocleidomastoid muscle (Fig. 9.29).

Cervical lymphadenopathy

Cervical lymphadenopathy may be a normal finding in children and is commonly seen in routine neck ultrasound examinations. In infants, however, they are rare and much more likely to be significant. If lymphadenopathy occurs in the supraclavicular region it must be considered to be abnormal. Any upper respiratory tract infection and scalp lesions can result in lymphadenopathy, and most are reactive.

Acute suppurative lymphadenopathy is one of the commonest reasons for an ultrasound request.

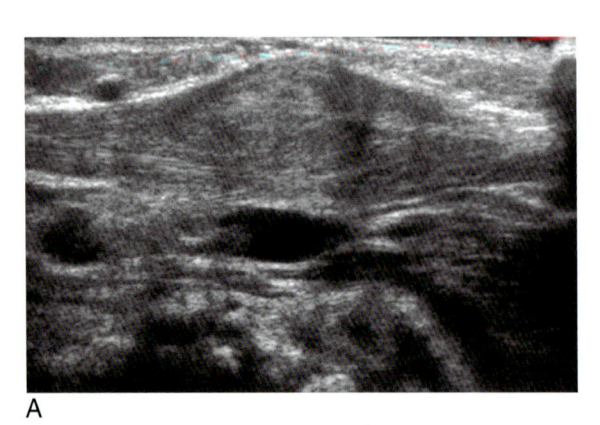

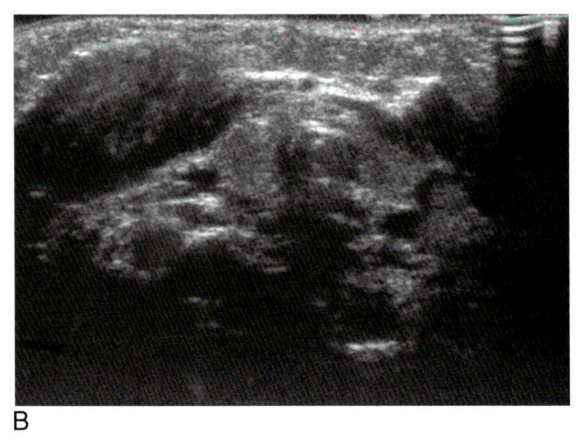

Figure 9.29 Fibromatosis colli. (A) Longitudinal sonogram of the right sternocleidomastoid muscle. There is a mass arising in the belly of the muscle. This results in a contraction of the muscle by fibromatous tissue, causing a torticollis. (B) Transverse scan at the level of the thyroid, showing marked enlargement of the right sternocleidomastoid belly.

The ultrasound is sometimes needed in order to detect breakdown of the nodal mass as an indication for drainage. On ultrasound this will show the disruption of the normal lymph node architecture and swirling debris indicative of breakdown of the nodes. If lymphadenopathy does not resolve after treatment in a timely way then a biopsy is indicated in order to exclude lymphoma (Fig. 9.30).

THE THYMUS

The thymus is a gland which lies anterior to the aortic arch and is commonly visualized in children up to 2 years of age in the superior mediastinum. It has a typical radiological appearance of a 'sail' when seen on a chest X-ray. In later childhood it atrophies.

Ultrasound evaluation can be done via the suprasternal notch, and the thymus is commonly seen in children undergoing echocardiography. There is quite a wide variation in size of the thymus.

In all patients the thymus has a smooth margin which is sharply defined. The echogenicity is homogeneous, and the sonographic appearance is similar to that of the liver. The thymus is deformable and normally moulds to underlying structures such as the great vessels and should never cause obstruction to the structures in the superior mediastinum. Longitudinally the right lobe has an inverted teardrop shape whereas the left lobe is triangular in shape. Ultrasound is extremely valuable as a quick, non-invasive means of identifying a normal thymus and can be used

A

B

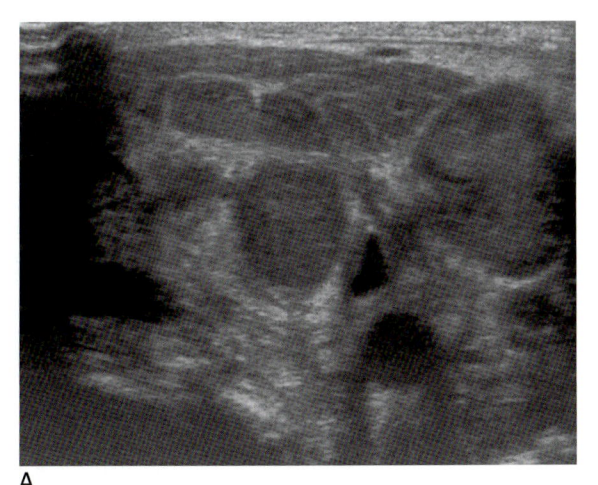

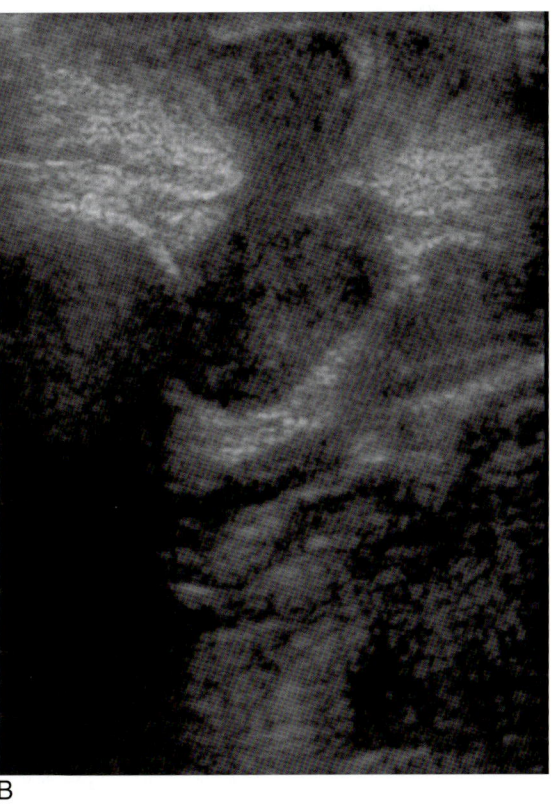

Figure 9.30 Neck abscess and lymph nodes. (A) Longitudinal sonogram of the neck of a child presenting with a large swelling. There are multiple lobulated lymph nodes. This child had a severe ear infection with secondary reactive cervical lymphadenopathy. (B) This child presented with a mass in the neck. Ultrasound examination revealed a subcutaneous mass connecting with a group of necrotic lymph nodes. There was swirling debris within the collection. This is the typical appearance of an abscess resulting from the breakdown of the lymph nodes, and it required surgical drainage.

particularly effectively in the anterior superior mediastinum (Fig. 9.31).

Thymic cysts

Thymic cysts are extremely uncommon and may occur anywhere from the path of the thymopharyngeal duct from the angle of the mandible to the thoracic inlet. Sixty percent are discovered within the first decade and may present with hoarseness, dysphagia, stridor and respiratory distress in newborns.

On ultrasound they are usually unilocular and there may be thymic tissue present in the cyst wall.

SALIVARY GLANDS

There are three salivary glands: the parotid (just anterior to the ear), the submandibular and the

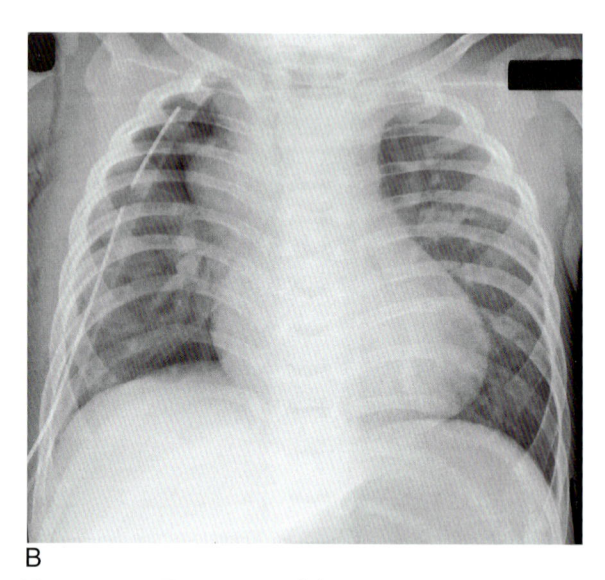

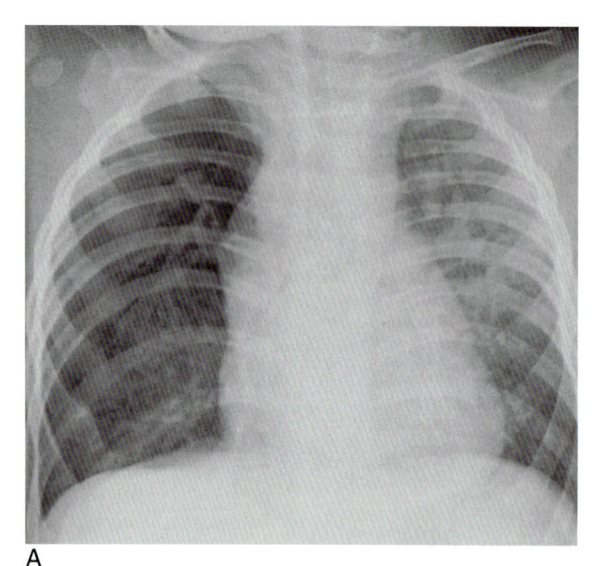

Figure 9.31 Thymic mass. (A) Chest X-ray on a child before cardiac surgery. (B) Chest radiograph after cardiac surgery, showing a right intercostal drain. There is widening of the superior mediastinum and what appears to be a mass. Clinically this child was thought to have an aneurysm. (C) Transverse sonogram at the level of the mass and aortic branches demonstrates that this is all thymic tissue. This is a simple examination to perform and should always be done in the first instance.

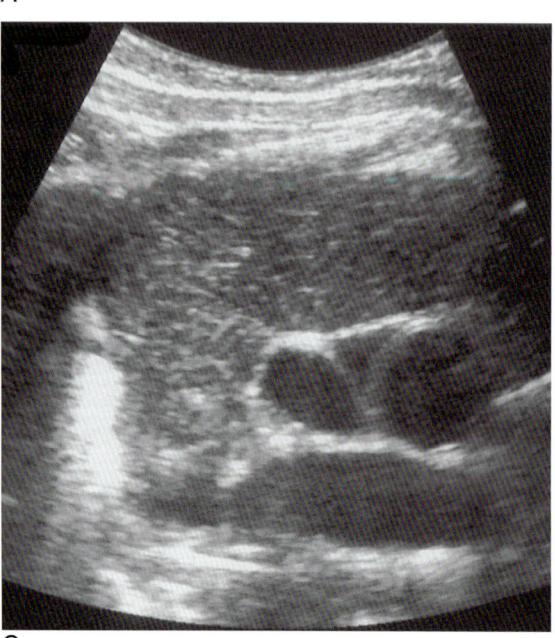

sublingual. The parotid gland is most commonly involved in disease in children.

Swelling at the angle of the mandible is not an uncommon pediatric complaint, and ultrasound is well suited to the initial examination. Clinical history and age important information when coming to a diagnosis.

Embryology

The parotid gland is composed of secretory tissue and stromal tissue, and secretions begin by the 18th week in utero. It is unusual in that it becomes encapsulated and contains intraparotid lymph nodes. It also encircles the facial nerve, which is then incorporated into the parenchyma.

Parotid—normal appearances and ultrasound technique

Ultrasound technique

A high frequency linear probe such as 15L8 with excellent near field visualization should be used. Both right and left glands should be examined for comparison, particularly if the lesion is unilateral.

Scan longitudinally and transversely over the glands and use Doppler to identify the normal vasculature. The parotid gland is intimately related to the external carotid and facial artery.

Normal appearances

The normal parotid gland appears echogenic and homogeneous. It can generally be clearly differentiated from the adjacent muscle. As the child grows older the parotid is replaced with fat. Highly reflective parallel lines of the normal ducts can be distinguished within the parenchyma. The normal parotid wraps around the angle of the mandible, so that the deeper retropharyngeal portion is not visualized on ultrasound because it is obscured by the bone.

On Doppler examination the parotid gland is intimately related to the neck vasculature but is not hypervascular in its appearance. Lymph nodes can sometimes be identified in the gland.

The submandibular glands are also quite easily seen below the jaw on either side of the midline.[26]

The sublingual glands are difficult to identify on ultrasound in children.

Parotid enlargement

The differential diagnosis of parotid enlargement is:

- inflammatory
    —parotitis
    —lymphadenitis
- neoplastic
    —benign
        –hemangioma
        –cystic hygroma
    —malignant
        –rhabdomyosarcoma
        –lymphoma.

Infection

Parotitis is one of the most common parotid diseases in children. The causes of parotitis are mumps and acute bacterial infection such as *Staphylococcus aureus*. Immunocompromised children such as the premature and HIV-infected are most susceptible to these infections. On ultrasound the appearances are those of a large swollen heterogeneous gland with increased blood flow on Doppler. There may be hypoechoic foci in keeping with local abscesses and associated reactive lymphadenopathy in the neck. The treatment is antibiotics and drainage if there is a fluctuant abscess. TB can also occur in the parotid.

Sialectasis is occasionally seen in children and is due to chronic infection.

Ultrasound appearance is an enlarged gland which may be heterogeneous and contain small cystic spaces of the dilated ducts. A stone occluding the duct may be seen. Plain radiographs, both intra-oral and tangential views of the gland, should be performed in order to exclude stones.[27] Small reactive lymph nodes may be seen in the neck.

TUMORS OF THE HEAD AND NECK

Hemangioma

Tumors of the salivary glands are uncommon in children, but most occur in the parotid. The majority are also benign. Hemangiomas are the most common parotid gland tumor and predominantly occur in females.

Hemangioendothelioma or hemangioma is a benign tumor that presents in infancy as a rapidly growing mass that is small and unnoticed at birth but soon becomes large and readily apparent within the first couple of months of life. The parotid hemangioma may be associated with a cutaneous strawberry lesion. Confirmation using MRI is generally performed primarily to show the deeper extent, which is not possible with ultrasound. However, a careful Doppler ultrasound examination should give the diagnosis in the first instance. Ultrasound should also obviate the need for biopsy, as it will give a clear indication that the mass is vascular in origin (Fig. 9.32).[28-30]

The natural history of these parotid hemangiomas is to rapidly enlarge in early infancy. They then undergo a spontaneous involution which continues for up to about 18 months. Complications such as cardiac failure are not common. Treatment is with oral steroids. Surgical resection need not be performed, as these lesions regress with time naturally and there is the huge risk of causing damage to the facial nerve.

The most widely quoted paper is that by Mulliken & Glowacki[29] where they describe two types of major vascular lesions (Box 9.6 and Table 9.4):

- masses with a history of rapid neonatal growth and involution which are characterized by hypercellularity during the proliferating phase and fibrosis and diminished cellularity during the involuting phase (hemangiomas)
- those masses which were present at birth and grow with the child and which are characterized by a normal endothelial cell turnover (malformations). They may have any combination of capillary, venous, arterial and lymphatic components.

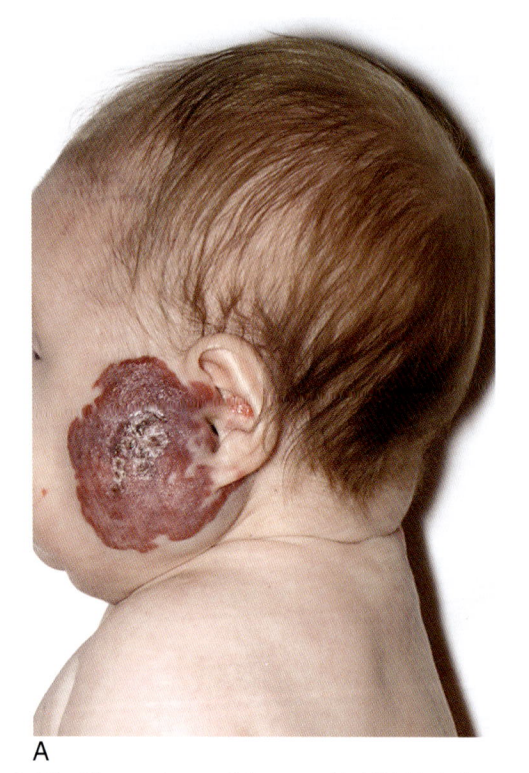

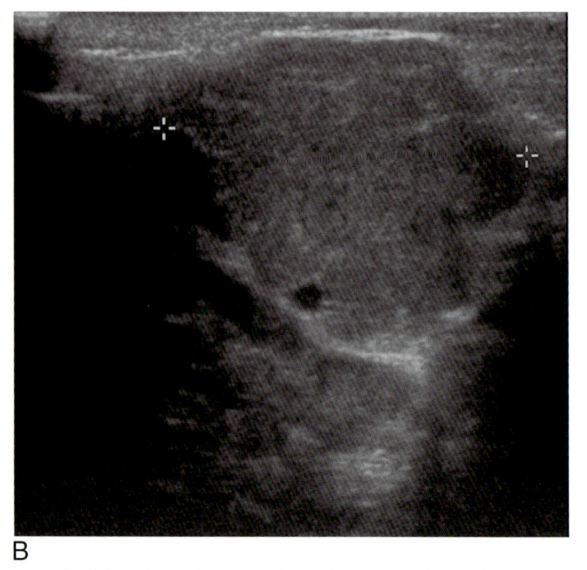

Figure 9.32 Hemangioma of the parotid. (A) This infant presented with a large hemangioma in the region of the parotid. This is accompanied by a skin hemangioma. Sometimes these hemangiomas are small and are merely a lump in relation to the parotid. (B) Longitudinal sonogram. The lump in the parotid is between the calipers. There is a heterogeneous echo texture and no normal parotid tissue can be identified.

Continued

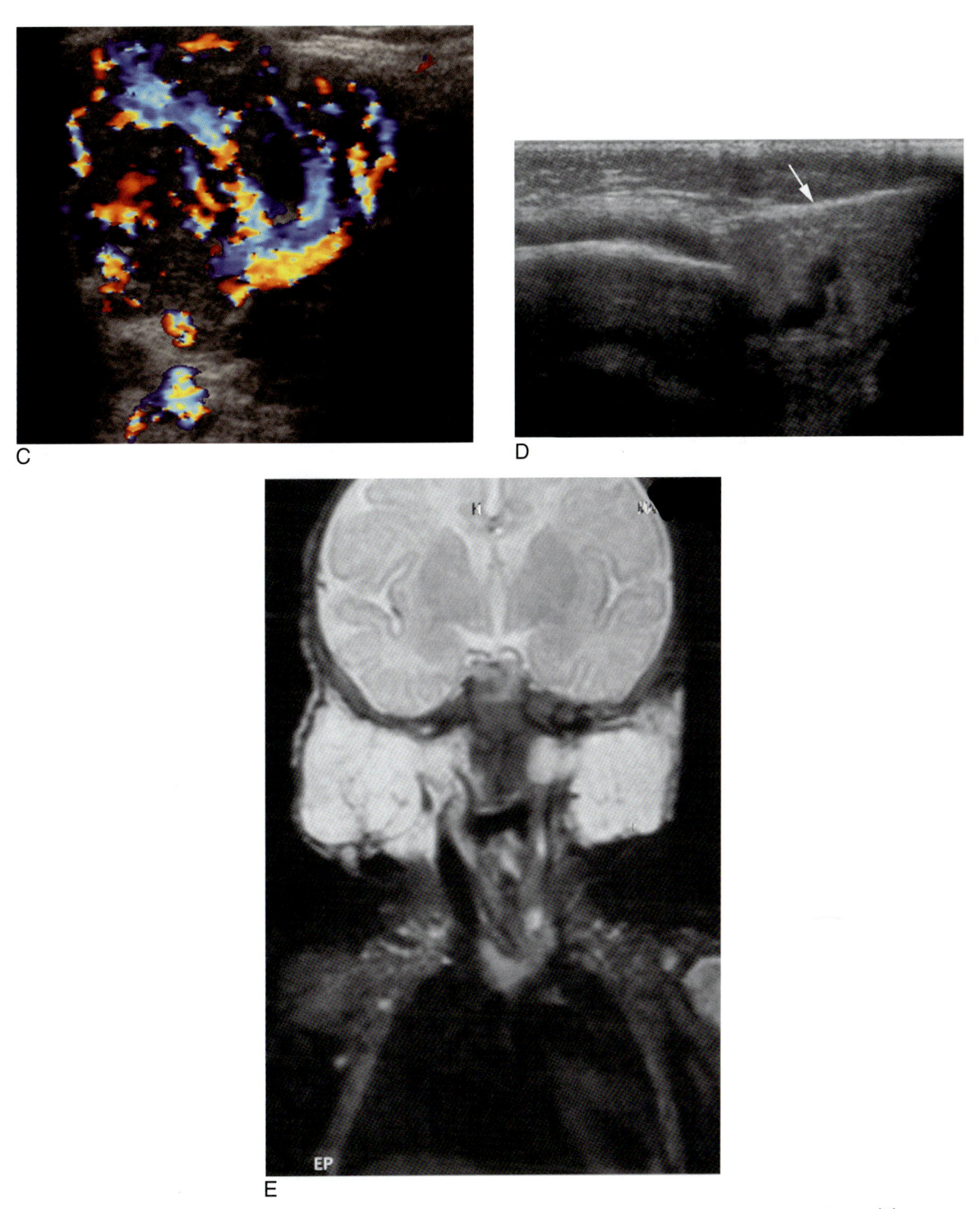

Figure 9.32, cont'd (C) On color Doppler imaging this was a very vascular mass typical of a hemangioma. (D) Ultrasound examination of the normal parotid shows a heterogeneous structure (arrow). It is very easy to identify when it is normal. (E) MRI examination on another baby who presented with bilateral parotid hemangiomas. A T2-weighted image produces the typical hyperintense signal of a hemangioma.

> **Box 9.6 Classification of vascular lesions in infants and children**
>
> **Hemangiomas**
> - Proliferating phase
> - Involuting phase
>
> **Malformations**
> - Capillary
> - Venous
> - Arterial
> - Lymphatic
> - Fistulae

Lymphangiomas

Lymphangiomas are congenital malformations of the lymphatic system. A significant proportion are present at birth and manifest as a soft asymptomatic neck mass. Hemorrhage may complicate a lymphangioma.[31]

On ultrasound they typically appear cystic with multiple thin septations.

Rhabdomyosarcoma

Rhabdomyosarcoma is the commonest pediatric sarcoma, and approximately 40% originate in the head and neck. The parotid gland may be involved by direct extension. Rhabdomyosarcomas are typically small cell tumors and, while predominantly solid on ultrasound, may have a mixed appearance.

Neuroblastomas may also occur in the neck.

Lymphoma/leukemia

The involvement of the salivary glands, in particular the parotid, by primary lymphoma and leukemia is extremely rare. On ultrasound the gland may appear globally hypoechoic with diffuse enlargement. This may be indistinguishable from other causes of an enlarged parotid.

SPINE

Introduction

Ultrasound of the pediatric spine was described nearly twenty years ago but never really received widespread acceptance, as the technique was complicated and images not easily understood by clinicians. With new equipment and applications such as extended field of view and 3D, together with higher resolution linear probes, it is now a more widely used examination with images of the most exquisite quality and detail.

Ultrasound can detect the entire spectrum of spinal anatomy with a high degree of accuracy. It is most useful in the very young infant when the bony vertebral arches are incompletely ossified, up to about 3 months of age. The posterior spinal elements then start to ossify so that the acoustic window is not adequate and the intraspinal detail is obscured.

Ultrasound examination of the spinal cord in infants has many advantages. The infant does not need sedation or general anesthesia, ultrasound is readily available and can be performed in the intensive care unit at the bedside. It is cheap and, with some experience, easy to perform and is an excellent screening modality. While MRI is accepted as the imaging modality of choice, a carefully performed ultrasound examination can give a wealth of information.

Ultrasound can detect normal variants such as ventriculus terminalis and congenital abnormalities together with intraspinal disease occurring after birth trauma. Ultrasound is the initial imaging modality of choice for investigating the spinal cord

Table 9.4 Cellular and clinical features of pediatric vascular lesions[29]

Hemangiomas	Malformations
Endothelial cell proliferation	Normal endothelial cell cycle
Forty percent present at birth, usually as a small red mark	Ninety percent recognized at birth
Rapid postnatal growth and slow involution	Grow commensurately with child
Female:male = 5:1	Female:male = 1:1

in newborns, and the main indication is in screening for occult spinal dysraphism.[32–36]

Embryology

Brain and spinal cord arise at approximately 16 days of gestation from an area of ectoderm known as the neural plate. This neural plate thickens bilaterally to form the neural folds. The neural folds close in towards the midline, forming successively the neural groove and neural tube. The tube closes in a zipper-like fashion from the middle, which then extends cranially and caudally (Fig. 9.33).

The cranial or rostral neuropore closes at about 24 days and the caudal neuropore at about 26 days. If there are defects in the closure of the rostral neuropore there may be incomplete development of the brain or the cranial vault, resulting in conditions such as anencephaly. If there is a defect in the closure of a caudal neuropore there may be a resulting neural deficit and conditions such as spina bifida occulta and meningomyelocele. In addition by a separate process of retrogressive differentiation the caudal portion of spinal cord and cauda equina develops from an undifferentiated mass of cells known as the caudal cell mass. At this time differentiation of the cloaca into the urethra, vagina and rectum occurs, which is why conditions such as anorectal anomalies and bladder exstrophy are often associated with spinal abnormalities in this region.

ULTRASOUND TECHNIQUE AND NORMAL ANATOMY

A high frequency linear probe is required. The higher the frequency, such as a 15L8, the better the image quality, but a linear 5 transducer can also be used.

The infant must be lying prone, curved over a pillow, with the head elevated (Fig. 9.34). This allows CSF to accumulate low down in the spinal theca and optimizes visualization of any abnormal fluid filled sacs. Also good flexion allows a better acoustic window. No sedation is needed, just a well-fed and therefore quiet baby. The spinal canal must be scanned in the transverse and sagittal plane from the craniocervical junction down to the coccyx. Optimal images will be obtained by using extended field of view in the sagittal plane.

However, if this is not available, using a linear probe and splitting the image will produce diagnostic images, although they will not be as technically satisfying as the extended field of view (Figs 9.35 and 9.36).[37]

Start off by splitting the image into right and left. Scan sagittally over the sacrum and lower lumbar spine on the right hand image. Staying in exactly the same position, switch to the left hand image. On the split screen there will be two identical images. With the left image active, gradually move the transducer caudally so that the same vertebral body on the extreme left of both images overlaps. In so doing a combined image of the lumbosacral spine will be produced.

The key to success in this examination is identifying S1 which, on the sagittal image, is the first vertebral body that tilts posteriorly. Once this has been achieved, the level of the end of the conus can be identified, which usually lies at the level of L1–L2. If a sinus is present, using a gel stand-off may give better resolution of the immediate near field to identify the sinus tract and extension into the theca. The normal spinal cord is a tubular, hypoechoic structure with hyperechoic walls lying in the darker subarachnoid space surrounding it. The caudal end of the cord terminates in the conus medullaris, which then continues as the cauda equina or nerve roots. The cord generally lies centrally within the spinal canal, and the filum or nerve roots can be seen to be lying freely within the CSF and pulsating.[38] Box 9.7 lists some normal features to look for.

The cord should also be scanned axially and will be a round structure lying within the anechoic subarachnoid space. Below the end of the conus the nerve roots of the cauda equina can be seen.[39,40]

Ventriculus terminalis

This is a small cystic structure seen at the tip of the conus medullaris to the origin of the filum terminale and develops as a result of the embryological development of the lower cord. Longitudinally it can measure up to 10 mm and transversely up to 4 mm. It regresses in the first few weeks of life and has no clinical significance.

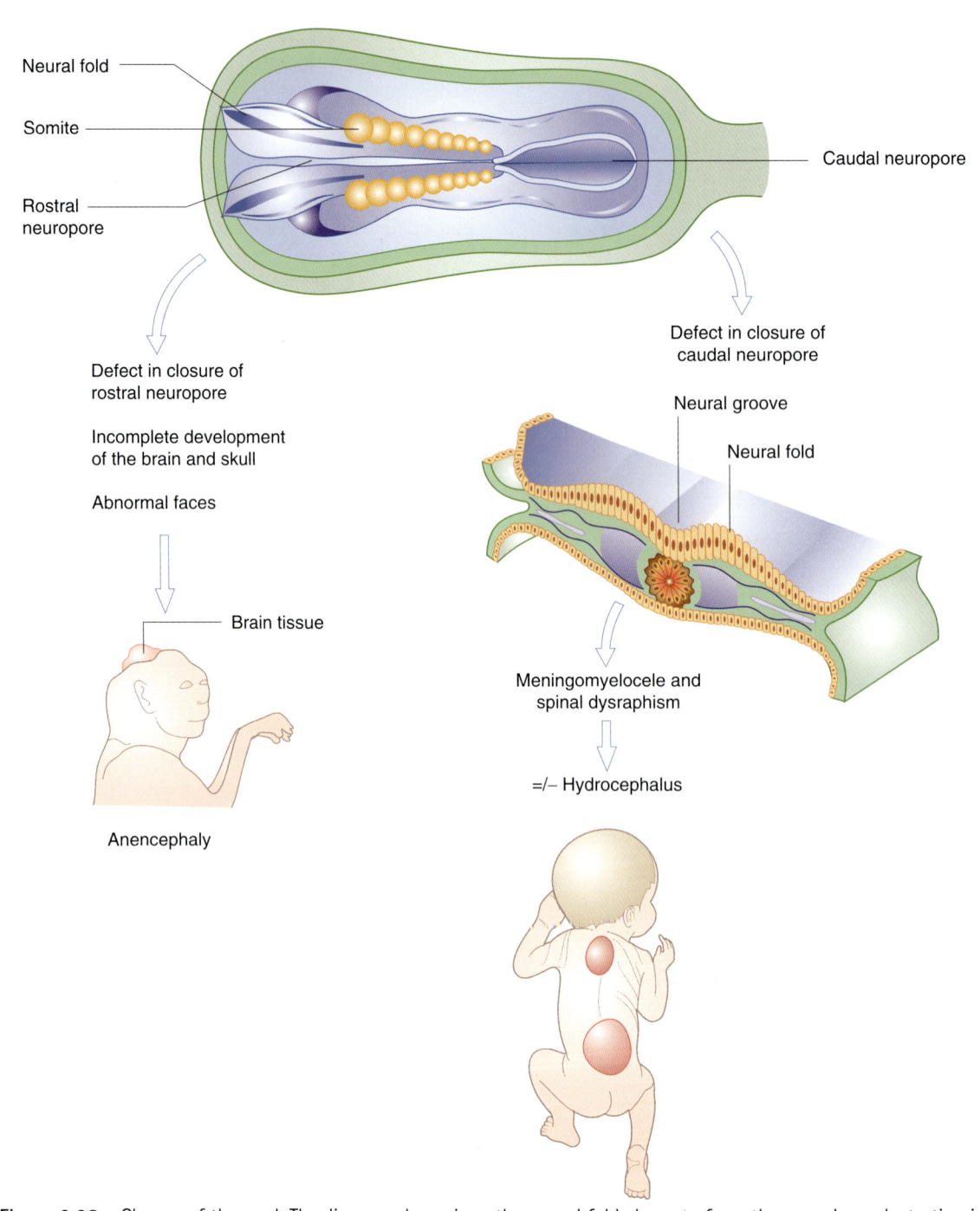

Figure 9.33 Closure of the cord. The diagram shows how the neural fold closes to form the neural canal, starting in the middle and extending cranially and caudally. Failure to close cranially will result in abnormalities of the head and neck such as anencephaly, while failure to close caudally will result in spinal dysraphism.

THE HEAD, NECK AND SPINE   293

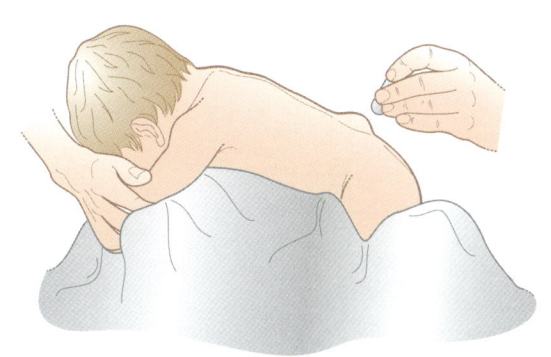

Figure 9.34 Position of the infant for examination of the spine.

- lower lumbar skin markers such as hairy patch, skin tag, cutaneous hemangioma or sinus
- closed lumbar mass
- congenital anomalies such as anorectal atresia and cloacal exstrophy.[43–46]

The major contraindication to ultrasound examination, because of the potential introduction of infection, is an 'open' defect where the spinal cord and nerve roots are exposed.

INDICATIONS FOR SPINAL ULTRASOUND

Spinal dysraphism is defined as incomplete or absent fusion in the midline of neural, mesenchymal and cutaneous structures. Spina bifida aperta are open defects and are not skin covered—these are not suitable for ultrasound. Occult spinal dysraphism is a heterogeneous group of skin-covered defects often associated with an overlying lumbar mass or skin stigmata.

The major indication for spinal ultrasound in the young infant is screening for occult spinal dysraphism. Ultrasound can also be used to visualize tumors, vascular malformations and for trauma, although this is really only for the enthusiasts and not widely applied in clinical practice.[41,42] Infants to be scanned are those with:

CLASSIFICATION OF COMMON TYPES OF OCCULT SPINAL DYSRAPHISM

Screening for suspected occult spinal dysraphism is probably the most useful role of ultrasound. Frequently, however, these 'occult' lesions are not entirely occult but associated with back masses or skin abnormalities such as a dorsal dermal sinus (a thin little track onto the skin with a dimple), a hairy patch or cutaneous nevus.[47–49]

Sacral pit

A sacral pit is one of the commonest referrals for an ultrasound examination of the spine. If the pit is associated with a hairy tuft or cutaneous nevus then a careful examination should be performed in case this is in fact a dorsal dermal sinus. If the pit is paramedian and low, this is invariably innocent, but ultrasound can be reassuring to parents and clinicians.[50,51]

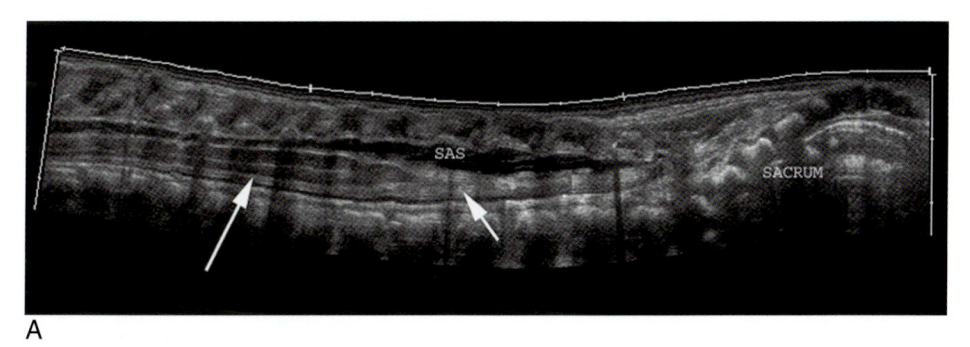

Figure 9.35 Normal spine. (A) Extended-field-of-view image of a normal spine in a neonate. The vertebral bodies are regularly arranged down the spine. The first vertebra that tilts posteriorly is S1. The coccyx is not ossified. The subarachnoid space (SAS) is the CSF-filled space around the cord. The spinal cord terminates at L1–L2 normally (long arrow). The central canal can be seen in the spinal cord as two parallel lines. The nerve roots (short arrow) can be seen extending down from the lower end of the cord.

Continued

294 PEDIATRIC ULTRASOUND

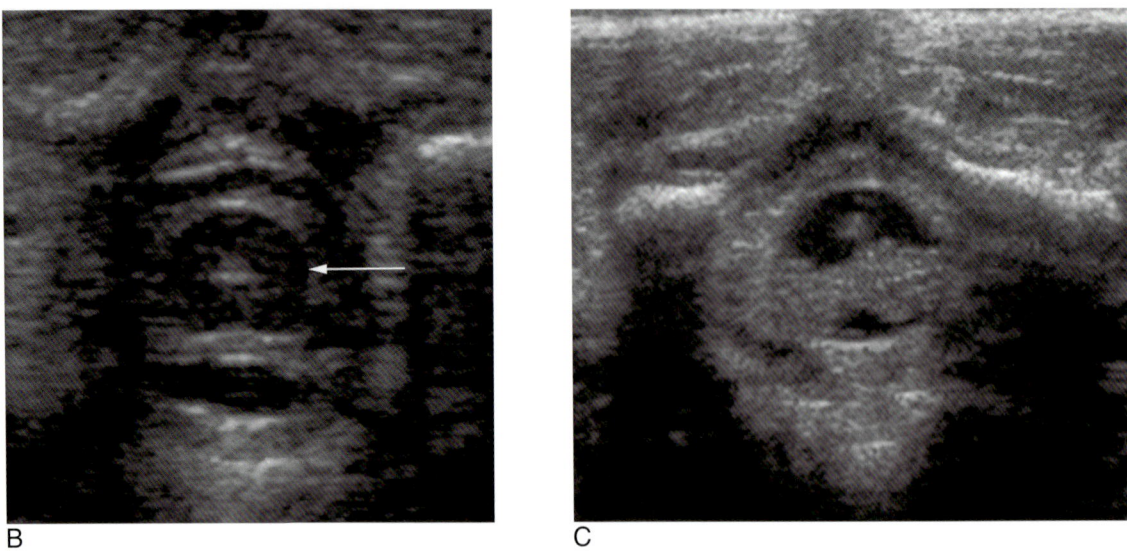

Figure 9.35 Cont'd (B) Transverse sonogram at the level of the spinal cord. The spinal cord lies centrally in the canal (arrow). (C) Transverse sonogram at the level of the nerve roots shows multiple nerve roots within the spinal canal.

Dorsal dermal sinus

A dorsal dermal sinus is different to a sacral pit in that it is an epithelium-lined tube extending inwards from the skin surface for varying distances. It is caused by an incomplete separation of the skin ectoderm from the neural ectoderm in a small localized area. As the spinal cord ascends in intrauterine life it stretches the area into a track. Half extend intraspinally and may be associated with a dermoid or epidermoid cyst, in particular if they are paramedian in location (Fig. 9.37). The majority are lumbosacral and often associated with skin angiomas, a hairy patch or skin thickening. They are almost always midline and only very rarely paramedian. They may present with meningitis or a spinal abscess because of the connection with the spinal canal. A meticulous ultrasound examination must be performed in these infants. The track must be carefully identified and will extend cranially. The echo-poor track can be very easy to miss in the

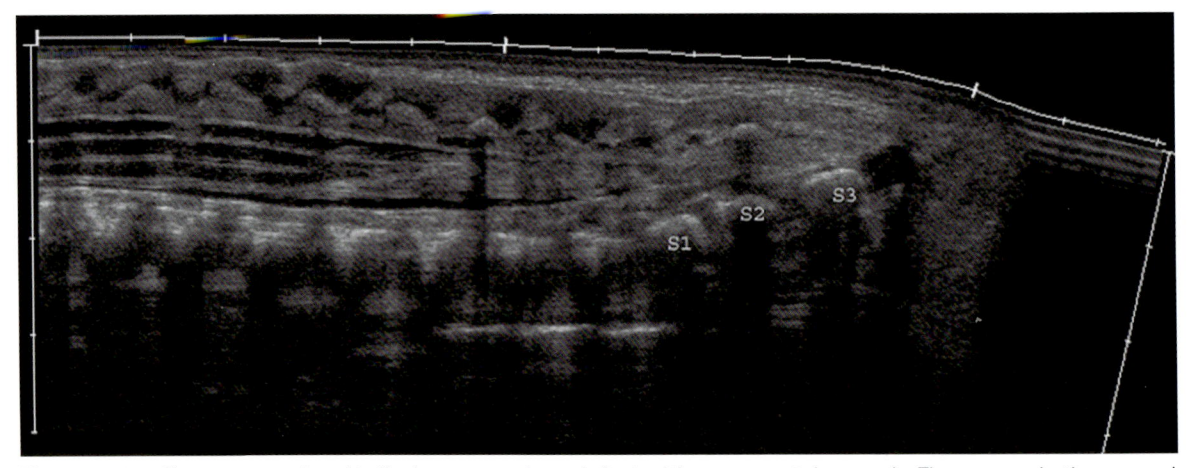

Figure 9.36 Short sacrum. Longitudinal sonogram in an infant with an anorectal anomaly. There are only three sacral segments, and the sacrum appears short with no identifiable coccyx.

THE HEAD, NECK AND SPINE

> **Box 9.7 Normal features to look for in sonography of the spine**
>
> - Normal level of the conus medullaris in a newborn is L1–L2
> - Spinal cord usually lies half way between the anterior and posterior walls of the spinal canal. If it lies posteriorly and appears fixed then tethering should be suspected
> - Spinal cord and nerve roots are normally freely mobile on dynamic real time scanning. M mode has also been used to assess for tethering
> - Thickness of the filum terminale is usually 2 mm or less
> - The central canal is seen as two parallel lines in the middle of the cord and is filled with CSF. There may be transient dilation in the newborn
> - All the lumbar vertebral bodies and sacrum should be counted and present
> - Always perform a cranial ultrasound examination, as posterior fossa abnormalities may be associated.

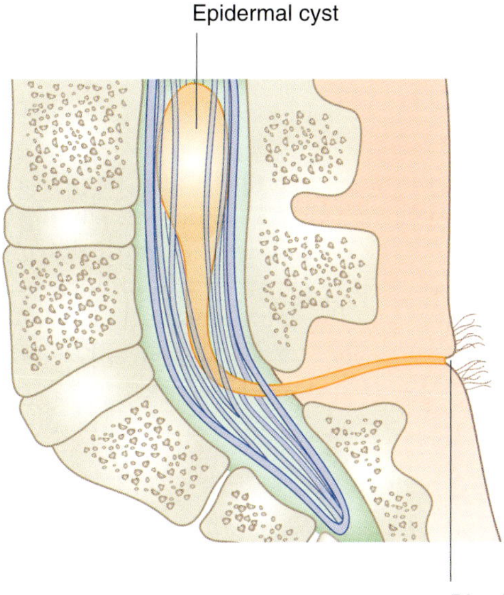

Figure 9.37 Diagram showing the track of a dorsal dermal sinus and an associated epidermoid.

uninitiated or inexperienced and sometimes it may be worth using a gel stand-off.

These patients all require an MRI examination.

Diastematomyelia

Diastematomyelia is a splitting of the spinal cord into two either symmetrical or asymmetrical hemicords which usually unite caudally. There may be a bony cartilaginous or fibrous septum. Each segment has a central canal and a single dorsal and ventral nerve root. This may be difficult to appreciate in the sagittal plane, and it is for this reason that axial scanning is essential. Hydromyelia, or dilation of the central canal, may be present above the lesion. This is associated with cutaneous nevi, scoliosis in 50–60% and vertebral anomalies in 85%. Congenital anomalies of the legs such as club foot are often associated. Tethering is present in 75% of patients, therefore all of these abnormalities must be looked for and excluded in the presence of diastematomyelia. Females are more commonly affected than males, and it is usually present in the lumbar region.

Spinal lipomas

These are the commonest type of occult spinal dysraphism, and the sonographer must learn to recognize them. The lipomas are distinct and encapsulated, and they connect directly to the posterior surface of the spinal cord.

To the uninitiated the diagnosis of spinal lipoma may be difficult, as the lipoma or fatty tumor is highly echogenic and may be disregarded. They are always dorsal to the cord, and there are three types to look for:

- intradural lipoma (4%)—the overlying skin is normal
- lipomyelomeningocele (84%)—this presents as a lumbosacral mass with neurological symptoms. The spinal cord lies in a low tethered position and posteriorly, and may herniate into the meningeal sac or may be displaced by an echogenic lipomatous mass. The lipoma may extend into the central canal of the cleft spinal cord (Fig. 9.38) Dorsally the lipomatous back mass may appear continuous with the intraspinal lipoma.

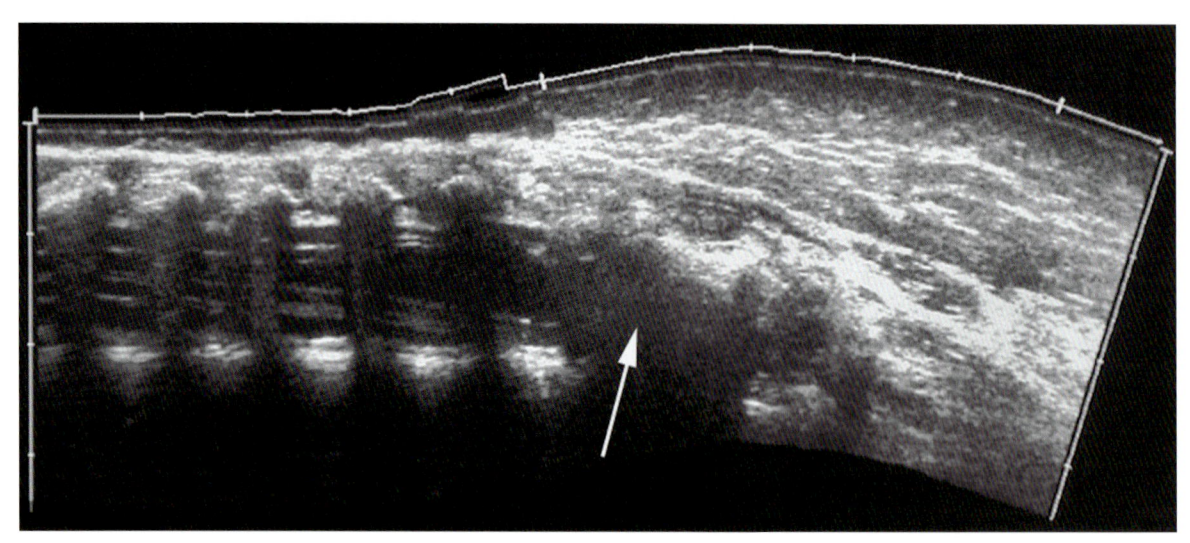

Figure 9.38 Spinal lipoma. Longitudinal sonogram in an infant with a large lump over the lower back. There is an echogenic subcutaneous lipoma. The spinal cord extends low down into the mass and is tethered by the lipoma (arrow). There is also some dilation centrally of the canal.

- fibrolipoma of the filum terminale (12%)—this may be incidental and may be identified by a low lying cord and a highly echogenic thickened filum terminale.

Tight filum terminale

This is most likely due to a failure of complete involution of the distal spinal cord during embryogenesis. The cord is always tethered and below L2–3. The filum is thickened, usually measuring more than 2 mm, because of the incomplete involution. In a significant number of cases there is a fibrolipoma present or a small cyst of the filum terminale.

MENINGOCELE AND MYELOMENINGOCELE

These are two of the commonest abnormalities seen and arise from localized failure of fusion of the neural folds. The open spinal cord causes abnormal development of the mesenchyme, mainly bony and ectoderm or skin structures. They occur in up to two in a thousand live births.

In a meningocele there is herniation of the meninges but no neural tissue, whereas in the myelomeningocele portions of the spinal cord and nerve roots lie within the sac. These anomalies most commonly occur at the lumbosacral level. Sonography should not be performed on open lesions. In closed lesions sonography shows an anechoic, lobulated meningocele in continuity with a tethered low-lying spinal cord. Both myelomeningoceles and myeloceles are associated with cord tethering and diastematomyelia. Hydromyelia or dilation of the central canal occurs in up to 80% of these infants.

Cranial ultrasound should always be performed in these infants, as there may be associated hydrocephalus. Chiari II malformation with downward displacement of the pons, medulla oblongata and cranial portion of the spinal cord is present in over 99%. The cerebellar vermis herniates through the foramen magnum (Fig. 9.39).

Lateral meningocele

This is a CSF sac that extends laterally through an intervertebral foramen. They may be thoracic or lumbar in position and present as masses in the paraspinal, intrathoracic or retroperitoneal loca-

THE HEAD, NECK AND SPINE 297

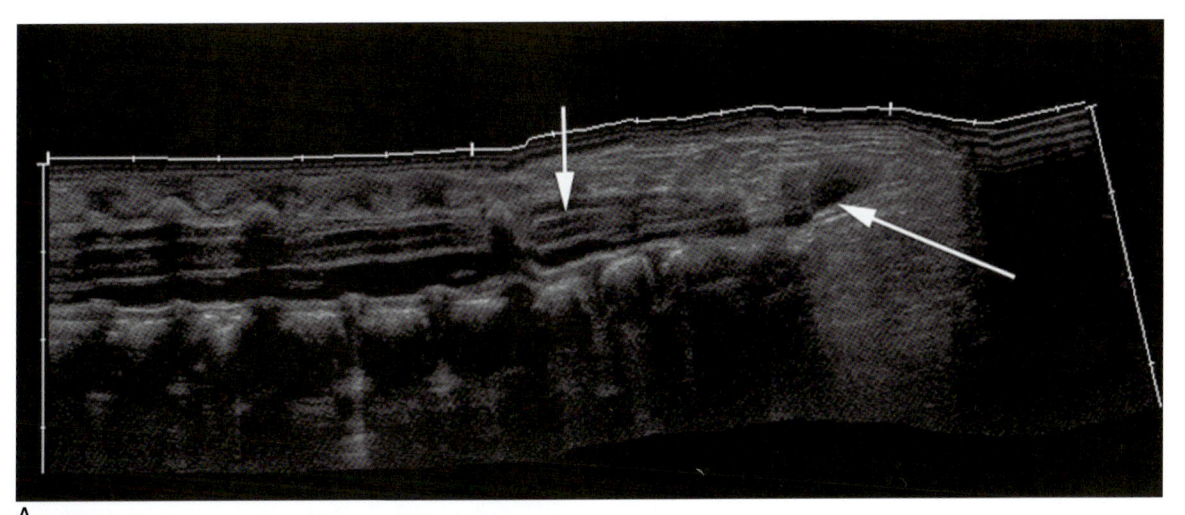

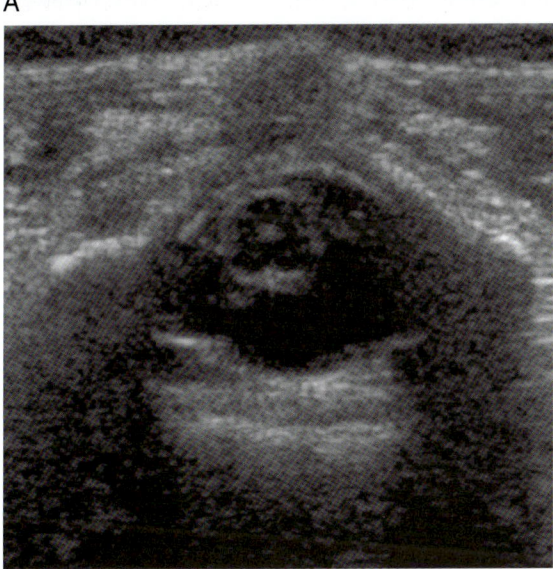

Figure 9.39 Meningomyelocele. (A) Longitudinal extended field of view image in an infant with a small skin-covered lump in the lumbar region. Notice the spinal cord is lying posteriorly in the canal and extends very low down (short arrow). The cord enters the small cystic meningomyelocele (long arrow). This is the typical appearance of a tethered cord, which is a common association with a meningomyelocele. (B) Transverse sonogram in the same infant. The cord is lying posteriorly in the canal.

tions. There is expansion of the spinal canal and displacement of the spinal cord. There is an association with Marfans and Ehlers–Danlos syndromes and neurofibromatosis.

CAUDAL REGRESSION SYNDROME

This syndrome has a wide spectrum of abnormalities of the caudal end of the trunk and is associated with having a diabetic mother. The abnormalities are related to abnormal retrogressive differentiation and failure of development of the lower spine and spinal cord. The spectrum ranges from a partial to complete sacral agenesis. There are associated abnormalities such as anorectal agenesis and genitourinary tract malformation.

TRAUMATIC SPINAL CORD LESIONS IN NEWBORNS

Injury to the spinal cord generally occurs through stretching and longitudinal traction of the cord during a difficult delivery. Breech presentations and transverse lie of the fetus requiring assisted delivery with forceps are predisposing factors.

The injuries to the cord that may occur are complete cord transection, laceration or avulsion of the spinal nerve roots and meningeal tears. Ultrasound will demonstrate the intraspinal hemorrhage and displacement of the cord. All infants suspected of having intraspinal trauma should have an MRI examination.[52,53]

SUMMARY

Ultrasound is an excellent screening modality for examining the neonatal spine. It is best performed under 3 months of age before the posterior vertebral elements have ossified and obscured the acoustic window. Ultrasound is indicated in suspected occult spinal dysraphism.

References

1. Babcock DS. Sonography of the brain in infants: role in evaluating neurologic abnormalities. AJR Am J Roentgenol 1995; 165:417–423.
2. Seibert JJ, Miller SF, Kirby RS, et al. Cerebrovascular disease in the symptomatic and asymptomatic patients with sickle cell anaemia: screening with duplex transcranial Doppler ultrasound – correlation with MR imaging and MR angiography. Radiology 1993; 189:457–466.
3. Levene MI. Measurement of the growth of the lateral ventricles in preterm infants with real-time ultrasound. Arch Dis Child 1981; 56:900–904.
4. Virkola K. The lateral ventricle in early infancy. Thesis, Helsinki, 1988 (ISBN: 952–90012–9–0).
5. Rosenfeld DL, Schonfeld SM, Underberg-Davis S. Coarctation of the lateral ventricles: an alternative explanation for subependymal pseudocysts. Pediatr Radiol 1997; 27:895–897.
6. Bowie JD, Kirks DR, Rosenberg ER, et al. Caudothalamic groove: value in identification of germinal matrix hemorrhage by sonography in preterm neonates. AJR Am J Roentgenol 1983; 141:1317–1320.
7. Levene MI. Diagnosis of sub-ependymal pseudocysts with cerebral ultrasound. Lancet 1980; ii:210–211.
8. Papille LA, Burstein J, Burstein R, et al. Incidence and evolution of subependymal and intraventricular haemorrhage: a study of infants with birth weight less than 1500gm. J Pediatr 1983; 102:281–287.
9. Chen C, Chou T, Zimmerman RA, et al. Pericerebral fluid collections: differentiation of enlarged subarachnoid spaces from subdural collections with colour Doppler US. Radiology 1996; 201:389–392.
10. Cohen MD, Slabaugh RD, Smith JA, et al. Neurosonographic identification of ventricular asymmetry in premature infants. Clin Radiol 1984; 35(1):29–31.
11. Libicher M, Troger J. US measurements of the subarachnoid space in infants: normal values. Radiology 1992; 184:749–751.
12. Levene MI, Starte DR. A longitudinal study of post-haemorrhagic ventricular dilatation in the newborn. Arch Dis Child 1981; 58:905–910.
13. Levene MI, de Crespigny L. Classification of intraventricular haemorrhage. Lancet 1983; i:643.
14. Levene MI, Fawer C-L, Lamont RF. Risk factors in the development of intraventricular haemorrhage in the preterm neonate. Arch Dis Child 1982; 57:410–417.
15. De Vries LS, Eken P, Dubowitz LMS. The spectrum of leucomalacia using cranial ultrasound. Behav Brain Res 1992; 49:1–6.
16. Jaspan T, Griffiths PD, McConaghie NS, et al. Neuroimaging for non-accidental head injury in children: a proposed protocol. Clin Radiol 2003; 58:44–53.
17. Jaspan T, Narborough G, Punt JAG, et al. Cerebral contusional tears as a marker of child abuse – detection by cranial sonography. Pediatr Radiol 1992; 22:237–245.
18. Knudsen N, Bols B, Bulow I, et al. Validation of ultrasonography of the thyroid gland for epidemiological purposes. Thyroid 1999; 9:1069.
19. Peterson S, Sanga A, Elklof B, et al. Classification of thyroid size by palpation and ultrasonography in field surveys. Lancet 2000; 355:106.
20. Vitti P, Martino E, Aghini-Lombardi F, et al. Thyroid volume measurement by ultrasound in children as a tool for the assessment of mild iodine deficiency. J Clin Endocrinol Metab 1994; 79:600.
21. World Health Organization / International Council for Control of Iodine Deficiency Disorders / UNICEF. Assessment of the iodine deficiency disorders and monitoring their elimination. Iodine Deficiency Disorders Newsletter 1999; 15(3):33.
22. Chanoine JP, Toppet V, Lagasse R, et al. Determination of thyroid volume by ultrasound from the neonatal period to late adolescence. Eur J Pediatr 1991; 150:395.
23. Lowe LH, Stokes LS, Johnson JE, et al. Swelling at the angle of the mandible: imaging of the paediatric

23. parotid gland and periparotid region. Radiographics 2001; 21:1211–1227.
24. Reynolds JH, Wolinski AP. Sonographic appearance of branchial cysts. Clin Radiol 1993; 48(2):109–110.
25. Kraus R, Han BK, Babcock DS, et al. Sonography of neck masses in children. AJR Am J Roentgenol 1986; 146:609–613.
26. Garcia CJ, Flores PA, Arce JD, et al. Ultrasonography in the study of salivary gland lesions in children. Pediatr Radiol 1998; 28:418–425.
27. Friedman AP, Haller JO, Goodman JD, et al. Sonographic evaluation of non-inflammatory neck masses in children. Radiology 1983; 147:693–697.
28. Koch BL, Myer CM. Presentation and diagnosis of unilateral maxillary swelling in children. Am J Otolaryngol 1999; 20:106–129.
29. Mulliken JB, Glowacki J. Hemangiomas and vascular malformations in infants and children: a classification based on endothelial characteristics. Plast Reconstr Surg 1982; 69(3):412–422.
30. Roebuck DJ, Ahuja AT. Hemangioendothelioma of the parotid gland in infants: Sonography and correlative MR imaging. AJNR Am J Neuroradiol 2000; 21:219–223.
31. Glasier CM, Seibert JJ, Williamson SL, et al. High resolution ultrasound characterization of soft tissue masses in children. Pediatr Radiol 1987; 17:233–237.
32. Dick EA, de Bruyn R. Ultrasound of the spinal cord in children: its role. Eur Radiol 2003; 13:552–562.
33. Unsinn KM, Geley T, Freund MC, et al. US of the spinal cord in newborns: spectrum of normal findings, variants, congenital anomalies and acquired diseases. RadioGraphics 2000; 20:923–938.
34. Scheible W, James HE, Leopold GR, et al. Occult spinal dysraphism in infants: screening with high-resolution real-time ultrasound. Radiology 1983; 146(3):743–746.
35. Toma P, Lucigrai G. Ultrasound assessment of spinal dysraphism. Riv Neuroradiol 1996; 9(6):679–683.
36. Rohrschneider WK, Forsting M, Darge K, et al. Diagnostic value of spinal US: comparative study with MR imaging in pediatric patients. Radiology 1996; 200(2):383–388.
37. Naidich TP, Fernbach SK, McLone DG. John Caffey Award. Sonography of the caudal spine and back: congenital anomalies in children. AJR Am J Roentgenol 1984; 142(6):1229–1242.
38. Hughes JA, De Bruyn R, Patel K, et al. Three-dimensional sonographic evaluation of the infant spine: preliminary findings. J Clin Ultrasound 2003; 31:9–20.
39. DiPetro MA. The conus medullaris: normal US findings throughout childhood. Radiology 1993; 188:149–153.
40. Wolf S, Schneble F, Troger J. The conus medullaris: time of ascendence to normal level. Pediatr Radiol 1992; 22(8):590–592.
41. Page LK. Occult spinal dysraphism and related disorders. In: Wilkins RH, Rengachary SS, eds. Neurosurgery. New York: McGraw-Hill; 1985:2053–2058.
42. Raghavendra BN, Epstein FJ, Pinto RS, et al. The tethered spine cord: diagnosis by high-resolution real-time ultrasound. Radiology 1983; 149(1):123–128.
43. Cohen AR. The mermaid malformation: cloacal exstrophy and occult spinal dysraphism. Neurosurgery 1991; 28(6):834–843.
44. Carson JA, Barnes PD, Tunell WP, et al. Imperforate anus: the neurologic implication of sacral abnormalities. J Pediatr Surg 1984; 19(6):838–842.
45. Dick EA, Patel K, Owens CM, et al. Spinal ultrasound in cloacal exstrophy. Clin Radiol 2001; 56:289–294.
46. Karrer FM, Flannery AM, Nelson MD Jr, et al. Anorectal malformations: evaluation of associated spinal dysraphic syndromes. J Pediatr Surg 1988; 23 (1 Pt 2):45–48.
47. Korsvik HE, Keller MS. Sonography of occult dysraphism in neonates and infants with MR imaging correlation. Radiographics 1992; 12(2):297–306.
48. Kriss VM, Kriss TC, Desai NS, et al. Occult spinal dysraphism in the infant. Clin Paediatr 1995; 34(12):650–654.
49. McLone DG, Naidich TP. The tethered spinal cord. In: McLayrin RL, Schut L, Venes JL, Epstein F, eds. Surgery of the developing nervous system. Philadelphia: WB Saunders; 1989:71–96.
50. Nelson MI, Segall HD, Gwinn JL. Sonography in newborns with cutaneous manifestations of spinal abnormalities. Am Fam Physician 1989; 40:198–203.
51. Robinson AJ. An audit of the value of ultrasonic examination of the lumbar spine in infants with specific reference to cutaneous markers of spinal malformation. Br Med Ultrasound Soc 2000; 77.
52. Filippigh P, Clapuyt P, Debauche C, et al. Sonographic evaluation of traumatic spinal cord lesions in the newborn infant. Pediatr Radiol 1994; 24(4):245–247.
53. Fotter R, Sorantin E, Schneider U, et al. Ultrasound diagnosis of birth-related spinal cord trauma: neonatal diagnosis and follow-up and correlation with MRI. Pediatr Radiol 1994; 24(4):241–244.

Chapter 10

The musculoskeletal system

CHAPTER CONTENTS

Technique of scanning muscles and soft
    tissues   301
Developmental dysplasia of the hip   302
Technique of hip scanning   304
    The Graf technique   304
    Dynamic sonography   306
    Terjesen femoral head coverage   308
    General principles   309
    Follow-up   310
Osteomyelitis   311
Transient synovitis (irritable hip)   312
    Ultrasound technique   313
    Aspiration technique   315
Other causes of a painful hip   315
Limb-lengthening procedures   317
Abnormalities of the tendons   317
Soft tissue masses   317

Ultrasound is now well established in the diagnosis and initial assessment of pediatric musculoskeletal disorders. The appearance of the infant skeleton and pathology encountered in children is different to that in the adult population, but the same broad principles apply. Ultrasound is particularly well suited to the pediatric population, as an exquisite view of the pediatric joints and cartilaginous bone can be obtained. Its prime importance in children is in the examination of the hip, both for the irritable hip and for developmental dysplasia of the hip. It is also particularly well suited to examining soft tissues, lumps, bumps and masses as a preliminary test before further more expensive imaging is undertaken.

TECHNIQUE OF SCANNING MUSCLES AND SOFT TISSUES

The highest frequency 15L8 linear transducers are generally the best to use for superficial musculoskeletal ultrasound in children. Older children may require a lower frequency linear transducer 8L5 to visualize deeper structures and joints. All soft tissue examinations need Doppler, as soft tissue hemangiomas and vascular malformations are common in children. Low flow settings on the equipment should be standard and applied, as sometimes the blood flow in these lesions is slow and difficult to detect.

Extended field of view capability is very useful when trying to demonstrate large soft tissue masses and their anatomical relationship to other structures, and this is best performed using a linear transducer with immediate view on the monitor. Any delay for reconstruction of the image is of no value in pediatric work as it prolongs the examination, which will often be on an uncooperative and restless child. Curvilinear or sector scanners are generally not as useful when using this technique. With good modern, high frequency transducers a gel stand-off is rarely required. It is extremely useful to image the contralateral unaffected limb for comparison with the abnormal side.

The measuring package for hip angles in developmental dysplasia of the hip is advantageous if a screening service is offered for these patients.

DEVELOPMENTAL DYSPLASIA OF THE HIP

The term developmental dysplasia of the hip (DDH), previously known as congenital dislocation of the hip, refers to a broad spectrum of disorders of hip development. It is now the preferred term to describe the abnormal relationship of the femoral head to the acetabulum, and it includes the varied appearance of the inadequately formed acetabulum together with complete dislocation of the femoral head as well as partial dislocation or subluxation.

The reliance on physical examination and newborn screening programs for the diagnosis has been disappointing, as dislocated hips are still diagnosed in later infancy and childhood. Late diagnosis of dislocation refers to the diagnosis being made after 3 months of age and implies a failure of neonatal detection.

Since the early description in the late 1970s of the use of ultrasound in the diagnosis of hip abnormalities, ultrasound has increasingly been used as a tool to try and improve patient outcome and to improve diagnosis of this late presentation. The ability to see the cartilaginous acetabulum and femoral head on ultrasound has made it an exceedingly attractive choice of modality for examining the infant hip. Radiography at this early age is not useful for this condition, as the femoral head and a large component of the acetabular roof has not ossified. The unossified head and labrum can be clearly seen on sonography, and in addition a dynamic assessment can be made where the head is manipulated in the acetabulum while the sonographer watches. Also the hip can be examined in a number of scan planes, which aids in the diagnosis. Arthrography was previously used to demonstrate abnormalities such as an inverted labrum and is occasionally still used.[1-3]

Currently there is no one universally accepted technique of performing an ultrasound examination of the infant hip, in addition to which there are two widely differing viewpoints in approaches to hip ultrasound. The European approach is based on the work of Graf, an Austrian orthopedic surgeon. His technique is based on a coronal scan plane and on the cartilaginous component of the acetabular roof. The primary American approach is related to the femoral head movement and displacement from the acetabulum. There is no universal policy for whole population screening for developmental dysplasia, and very few centers are sufficiently resourced to do so. National screening programs are present in Austria, Switzerland and Germany, where Graf established his technique. Infant screening including the use of ultrasound has still not been able to identify all children who are at risk of developmental dysplasia of the hip.

The results of ultrasound screening have consistently shown that the non-surgical treatment rate has increased. In a Norwegian study this treatment rate was almost double in the ultrasound-screened group (34 versus 18 per 1000 infants screened), and it is assumed that many children in the ultrasound group who subsequently received treatment actually had false-positive ultrasound tests. Some would argue that this is a bad thing, as there is a risk of developing avascular necrosis of the femoral head from treatment alone.

On the other hand the surgical treatment rate did not decrease significantly in newborns screened with ultrasonography compared with those screened by physical examination alone.[4]

Clinical tests

There are two clinical tests which help to identify unstable hips in newborn infants (Fig. 10.1):

- The Barlow test determines if a hip can be dislocated. The hip is flexed and the thigh adducted. With a gentle posterior pressure the femoral head can be made to move posteriorly out of the acetabulum if the hip is dislocatable.

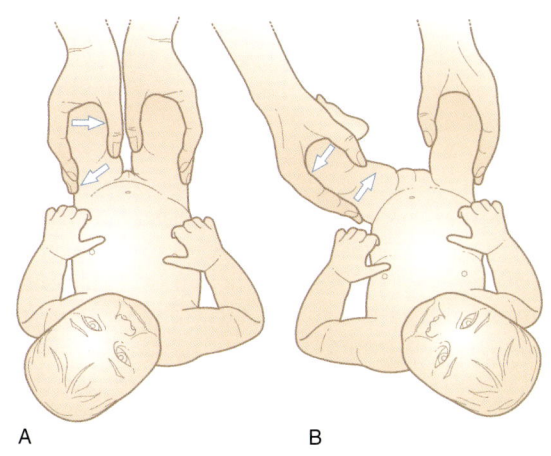

Figure 10.1 Clinical examination for developmental dysplasia of the hip. (A) The Barlow maneuver, which is gentle adduction and a push on the knee. The hip dislocates posteriorly out of the acetabulum. (B) The Ortolani maneuver. This is the reverse so that the abducted hip is gently relocated back into the acetabulum. It typically produces a click.

- The Ortolani test is the reverse of this maneuver and relocates the head within the acetabulum. The hip is flexed and abducted and gently pulled anteriorly so that on examination a 'click', or the examiner feeling the dislocated femoral head moving over the acetabulum posteriorly and returning to the acetabulum, is felt. This identifies a dislocated hip and should demonstrate whether the hip is reducible.

These examinations should be performed by an appropriately trained health professional. There is evidence that those who specialize in hip abnormalities have a better outcome with fewer late presenters. However there are those who argue that some infants are normal at birth (and therefore screening) and then go on to develop dislocation.

There are a number of risk factors associated with developmental dysplasia of the hip:

- family history of congenital dislocation of the hip—this is the most important risk factor. In some series of DDH up to 20% of infants treated had a family history
- female firstborn and pregnancies with oligohydramnios
- breech presentation
- a foot deformity that requires further treatment
- neonatal torticollis
- a clicky hip as discovered on the Barlow or Ortolani test
- where there is any doubt.

All those infants with displaced or unstable hips identified at screening and with a positive screening test should be seen by an orthopedic surgeon experienced in the field. It is very important to identify unstable hips as soon as possible, as the tissues are still supple and the chance of successful treatment is better at an earlier age.

Ideally the orthopedic surgeon will perform a joint clinic with the sonographer or have access to a hip ultrasound service. This combined approach is undoubtedly the most successful and rewarding for the sonographer and will ultimately yield the best results. Also in this milieu of increasing litigation the security of operating as a team is beneficial to all, including the patient.

Infants with displaced or unstable hips should be examined by 2 weeks of age, and for those at risk the examination is best performed when an infant is 4–6 weeks old. By this time, most immature hips have stabilized.

It is very important that the parents are kept informed and made aware that any screening program may not identify all affected children.

There are other classical signs of congenital hip displacement which may be present at birth and which become increasingly apparent after the first 6 weeks as the legs extend and the head of the femur displaces upwards, that parents should be made aware of:

- limb shortening—this is most apparent when the hips are flexed and the levels of the knees are compared
- leg posture—the thigh on the affected side tends to be held in partial lateral rotation, flexion and abduction
- thigh asymmetry—skin creases on the inside of the thigh may differ between the affected side and unaffected side
- limited abduction—in a supine position with the hips flexed, abduction may be limited as the femoral head remains dislocated.

Once the child is walking, other suspicious features are a limp or anxieties about the child's

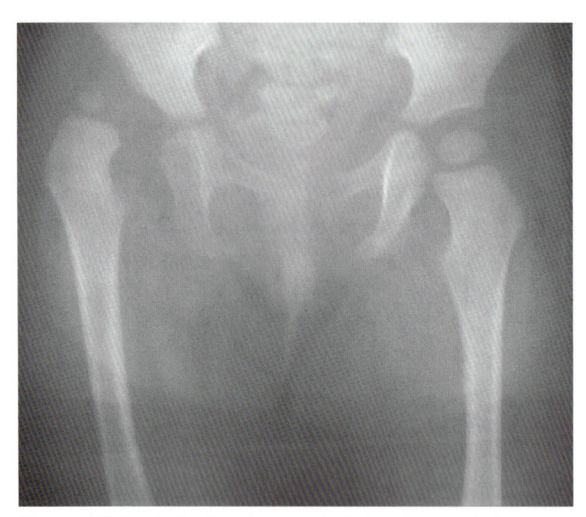

Figure 10.2 Late development of developmental dysplasia of the hip (DDH). This radiograph demonstrates the appearances of the late presentation of a dislocated hip. The acetabulum is steep and shallow and the femoral head is dislocated superiorly and posteriorly. The femoral capital epiphysis is also smaller than that on the left. The dislocated hip demonstrates how these children may present with apparent shortening of the leg on the affected side.

walk, discrepancy in leg length, and abnormalities of lower limb posture (Fig. 10.2).

TECHNIQUE OF HIP SCANNING

There is no universally accepted standard technique for ultrasound examination of the infant hip in the world today, and there are at least three methods in use:

- Graf has devised a complex classification based on the acetabular structure and position of the femoral head. Several lines and angles are measured and a single coronal image is produced. There is no dynamic (i.e. scanning and watching the femoral head movement while under stress) component to his technique. A simplified version of his technique is probably the most widely practiced method in Europe.
- Dynamic sonography of the infant hip as described by Harcke is a dynamic examination which stresses positional relationships and stability.
- The third technique is simply to use a line drawn down from the baseline to assess what percentage of the femoral head is lying within the acetabulum.

Undoubtedly the best results are obtained where the sonographer works in close collaboration with an orthopedic surgeon experienced in developmental dysplasia of the hip, so that consistent, reliable results are produced and terminology is understood by all, with improved outcomes for the infant.

The infant must be relaxed for the examination so that adequate assessment of the hip can be made and so that stress maneuvers are accurate. A screaming, kicking infant cannot be examined, and it is essential that they are given time to feed and calm down.

Commercially available supports are not essential but certainly do make the examination easier in a restless infant.

Curvilinear probes can be used, but it is now widely accepted that high frequency linear probes are undoubtedly the best and do not distort the image for angle measurements if these are to be taken. For a young infant a 15L8 can be used; a lower frequency will be needed in an older infant. Once the femoral head starts ossifying and produces a densely acoustic shadow then sonography is less reliable, but this is generally after 3–6 months. When the ossific nucleus enlarges, the acetabular floor is obscured by its acoustic shadow, but by this time plain radiographs are reliable.

The Graf technique

The Graf technique requires the sonographer to be able to identify important landmarks in the coronal plane and from these landmarks to measure the alfa and beta angles (see below). This technique requires some training and practice, and sonographers should ensure that they are adequately trained by an experienced practitioner in this method if it is to be used.[5]

It is recommended that a positioning device is used to immobilize the patient. The infant is placed on its side and the transducer is placed over the greater trochanter (Fig. 10.3). The hip should be in slight flexion. When the trochanter, femoral neck

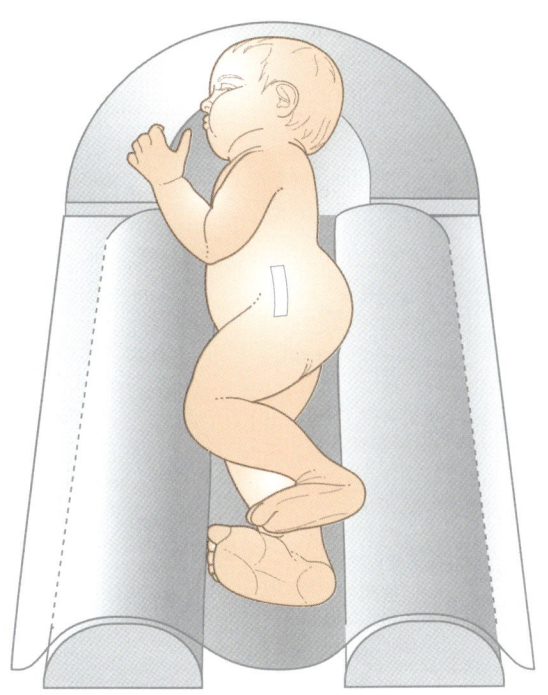

THE MUSCULOSKELETAL SYSTEM   305

Figure 10.3 The Graf cradle. The infant is positioned on its side with hip in slight flexion for the Graf method of examining the hip.

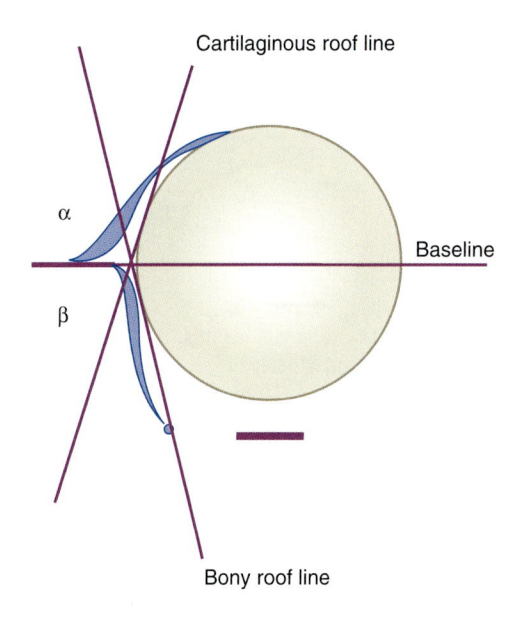

α = Bony roof angle
β = Cartliage roof angle

Figure 10.4 Graf reference lines. The diagram demonstrates how the standard reference lines are drawn and the hip angles obtained.

and acetabulum lie in the same plane, this is optimal. The transducer is positioned so that it lies exactly in the frontal plane parallel to the body's long axis and should not be tilted. The standard sonographic plane should be easily achieved in this position.

The following main reference points need to be identified:

- the acetabular labrum
- the cartilaginous portion of the acetabular roof
- the bony promontory of the superior bony acetabular rim
- the lower margin of the ilium.

Once this standard plane has been achieved then the reference lines are drawn (Fig. 10.4):

- baseline
- cartilaginous roofline
- bony roofline.

The alfa angle is described as the bony roof angle and is the most important to measure. The beta angle is the cartilaginous roof angle and is not universally used.

Table 10.1 is an adaptation of Graf's classification of hip types. Type III (subluxation) and Type IV (dislocation) are probably the easiest to identify. Graf Type III involves persistent lateral displacement of the femoral head from the acetabular floor with deviation of the labrum. Type IV hips are complete dislocations, usually posterior and towards the head, with the femoral metaphysis obscuring the acetabular floor (Fig. 10.5).

From a sonographer's point of view the standard image plane cannot be achieved when the head is dislocated, neither can accurate angles be measured. Types III and IV are very rarely detected outside specialist centers.

- Type I are the mature hips with a deep acetabulum and angles over 60°.
- Type IIa are those under three months of age with a shallow acetabulum and alfa angles of 50–59°. These are considered to be physiologically immature hips but stable.
- Type IIb are the infants of over 3 months who have shallow acetabulae with alfa angles of 50–59° who are also considered by Graf to be inherently stable.

Table 10.1 Graf classification of hip dysplasia

Graf sonographic hip type		Bony roof	Ossific rim	Cartilage roof	Alfa angle (°)
Ia	Mature	Good	Sharp	Long and narrow, extends far over femoral head	> 60
Ib	Mature	Good	Usually blunt	Short and broad but covers femoral head	> 60
IIa	Physiological delay in ossification < 3 months	Deficient	Rounded	Covers femoral head	50–59
IIb	Physiological delay in ossification > 3 months	Deficient	Rounded	Covers femoral head	50–59
IIc		Deficient	Rounded/flat	Covers femoral head	43–49
D	On point of dislocation	Severely deficient	Rounded/flat	Compressed	43–49
IIIa	Dislocated	Poor	Flat	Displaced upward and echo-poor	< 43
IIIb	Dislocated	Poor	Flat	Displaced upward and more reflective than femoral head	< 43
IV	Dislocated	Poor	Flat	Interposed	< 43

- The most important group for the sonographer to identify is the unstable Type IIc with shallow acetabulae and angles of 43–49°. These are considered to be unstable and require immediate treatment (Fig. 10.6).

The Graf classification is complex, and training is needed in order to be competent in the technique.

It is probably prudent in this age of litigation to include at least the alfa angle on any hip examination in a neonate, particularly if you are a European sonographer practicing in isolation. One major criticism of the technique has been that it produces a very high false positive rate of detection, with an excessive number of patients treated, as evidenced by the German screening program. Splinting for neonatal hip instability is not without risk, and one of the most serious complications is avascular necrosis of the femoral head.

Dynamic sonography

This technique, as described by Harcke and colleagues, is based on dynamic sonography which parallels the clinical maneuvers of Barlow and Ortolani used in the physical examination of the

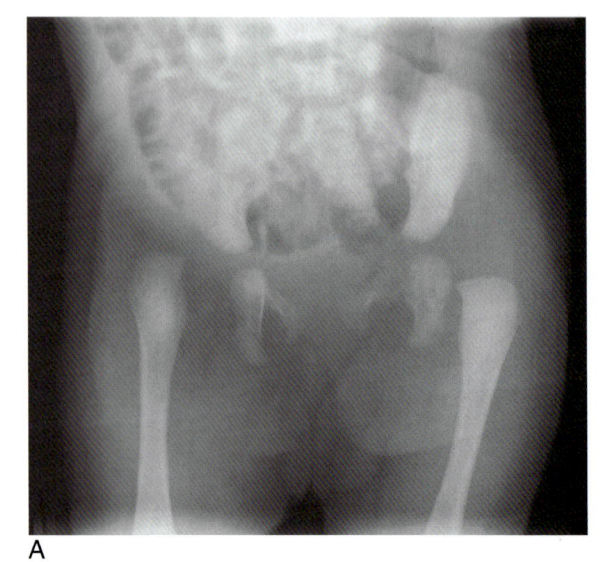

Figure 10.5 Dislocated hip. (A) This plain radiograph demonstrates the abnormalities to be detected on ultrasound. The right hip is completely dislocated. The acetabulum is steep and short and there is insufficient cup to keep the femoral head within the socket. On the left the acetabulum is abnormally short and steep, although the head is not as severely dislocated as on the right side.

THE MUSCULOSKELETAL SYSTEM 307

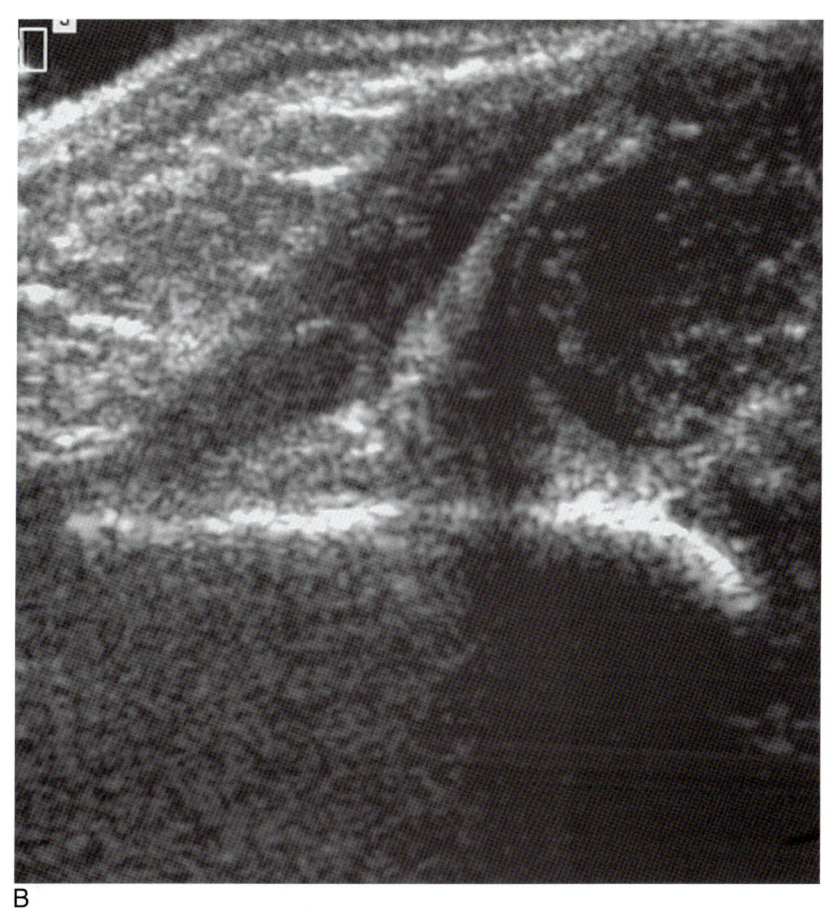

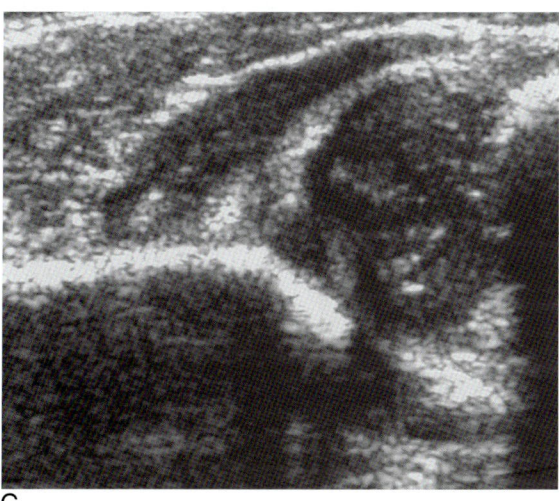

Figure 10.5, cont'd (B) Ultrasound examination of the right hip shows how the head is completely dislocated posteriorly. The normal coronal plane cannot be produced. (C) Coronal sonogram of the left hip. The left hip is decentered, also lying predominantly out of the acetabulum.

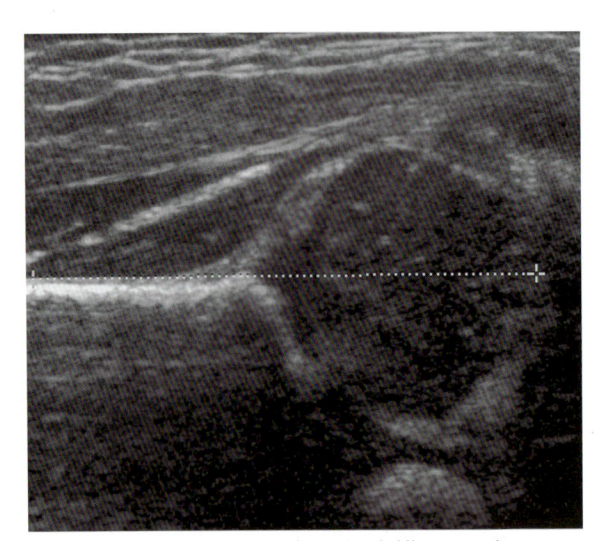

Figure 10.6 Normal hip ultrasound. Ultrasound examination in the standard plane. The iliac bone must always be parallel to the probe, otherwise errors will be made in the measurements.

hip. This technique attempts to detect subtle instability which eludes the manual examination. The baby is therefore in the supine position and the hip scanned in the coronal and transverse planes in the neutral position and in flexion.[6,7]

The objectives are to:

- note the position of the femoral head at rest in the neutral position
- assess the stability of the hip with motion and stress using maneuvers similar to those of the Barlow and Ortolani clinical examinations
- assess the development of the hip components such as the depth and configuration of the bony and cartilaginous portion of the acetabulum. No angles are measured.

The Harcke dynamic technique has four steps:

coronal neutral. This view is similar to Graf's standard plane but with no angle measurement.

coronal flexion. The same as step 1 but with the hip in 90° flexion. The triradiate cartilage is identified and then the transducer is moved posteriorly and anteriorly. When the transducer is posterior to the triradiate cartilage the femoral head should not normally be visible, and if seen it indicates that the head is abnormally sited. Then by gently pushing and pulling the knee as in the Barlow maneuver, any instability of the hip will be detected by visualizing the head move over the posterior lip of the triradiate cartilage.

transverse flexion. The infant is placed in an oblique position with the hip in 90° flexion. The hip is scanned transversely. This produces a 'U' configuration with the femoral capital epiphysis central to the femoral metaphysis and the ischium. When displaced the head cannot be seen within the 'U'. On dynamic scanning with gentle posterior pressure on the knee, if the hip is unstable then the gap between the head and the acetabulum increases. Conversely with the hip in abduction and gently pulling on the knee, the dislocated head can be relocated within the acetabulum.

transverse neutral. The hip is in the neutral position and the hip scanned transversely. The image obtained is the acetabulum centered at the level of the triradiate cartilage. The normal femoral head is located within the acetabulum, with the center of the head at this level. When dislocated the triradiate cartilage cannot be seen in this plane (Fig. 10.7).

No study of the reliability of dynamic ultrasound examination has yet been reported, and it is much more operator dependent than the static technique. It relies on the sonographer's skill in performing the dynamic maneuvers and interpreting the images.

Terjesen femoral head coverage

This technique, as described by Terjesen, positions the child supine with the hip slightly flexed and in the neutral position, which helps stabilize the child for the dynamic examination. Longitudinal and transverse scanning is performed from the lateral aspect. Subjective dynamic evaluation of hip stability and measurement of the femoral head coverage is made.

Like the other techniques, a linear transducer is used with the coronal image as standard and a line drawn perpendicular to the baseline of the image (the same as the Graf baseline).

The femoral head coverage (FHC) is equal to $a/b \times 100$, where a is equal to the distance from

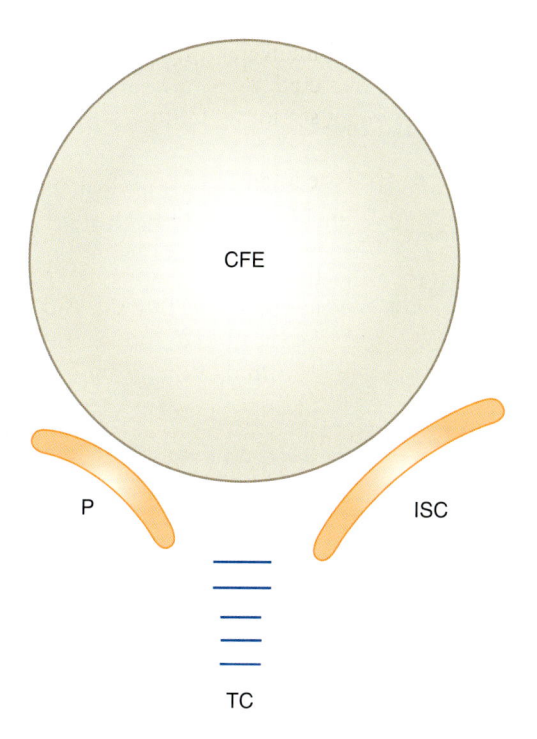

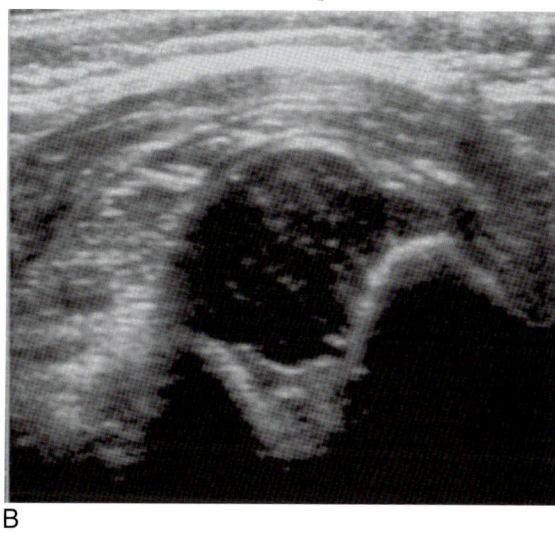

Figure 10.7 Harcke technique of hip examination. (A) Diagram showing the position of the capital femoral epiphysis (CPE) in a transverse neutral view. When the femoral epiphysis dislocates, it moves over the ischium (ISC) lateral to the pelvis (P). The triradiate cartilage (TC) lies centrally below the epiphysis. (B) Transverse neutral ultrasound of the hip showing the relationship of the femoral head to the ischium in a normal infant.

the medial wall of the acetabulum to the level of the lateral bony rim and *b* is the distance from the medial wall of the acetabulum to the lateral joint capsule (Fig. 10.8). If subluxation is present the measurements are taken from the medial tangent of the cartilaginous head instead of the acetabular floor. The hip is considered to be potentially abnormal if the femoral head cover is < 50% and/or the joint seemed unstable during manipulation (Box 10.1).

The shape of the lateral bony rim of the acetabular roof is noted. The normal bony rim is only slightly rounded, whereas the dysplastic rim is flat.

When the ossification center of the femoral head has appeared, the distance is measured from the lateral tangent of the ossification center to the lateral bony acetabular rim to define the lateral head distance (LHD). This expresses the degree of uncovering of the femoral head. When the whole ossification center is medial to the lateral acetabular rim the LHD has a minus value (Box 10.2).

The three techniques described are compared in Table 10.2.

General principles

The hip joint is a ball and socket joint and dislocation is posterior and lateral. It is generally considered that at the very minimum the ultrasound examination should consist of both a dynamic and a static component. The dynamic assessment should include the relationship of the femoral head to the acetabulum and an assessment of the movement of the femoral head within the acetabulum, whereas the static component is an evaluation of the depth and shape of the acetabulum. An image should be recorded in the standard coronal plane such that the iliac bone is in a parallel relationship to the transducer, with the triradiate cartilage on the same view (Fig. 10.9).

All infants in whom acetabular dysplasia, displacement or instability are diagnosed should be

310 PEDIATRIC ULTRASOUND

Figure 10.8 Terjesen femoral head coverage. Diagram showing how the femoral head coverage is assessed. At least 50% of the femoral head should be covered by bone in a normal hip joint.

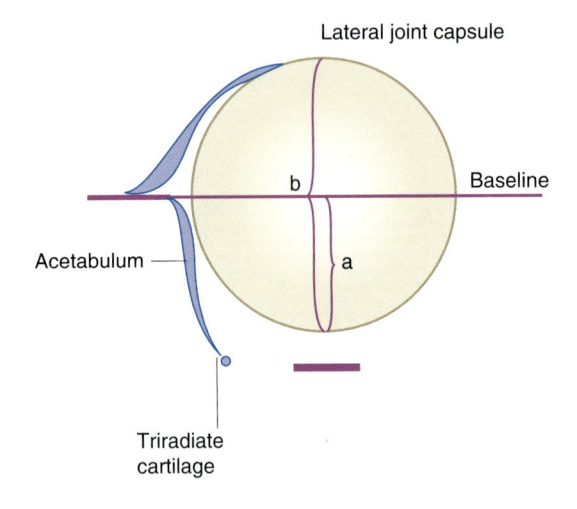

a = Bony roof angle
b = Cartliage roof angle

Box 10.1 Terjesen femoral head coverage

Femoral head coverage:
> 50%	Normal
49–40%	Possible dysplasia in newborns
49–40%	Dysplasia in infants greater than 4 months
39–10%	Subluxation
< 10%	Dislocation

Box 10.2 Lateral head distance of Terjesen

Lateral head distance:
−ve	Ossification center is medial to the lateral bony acetabular rim
+ve	Ossification center is lateral to the lateral bony acetabular rim

referred to an appropriate orthopedic surgeon. If there is no evidence of instability or dysplasia in an infant in whom the acetabular depth is considered to be normal, the patient can be discharged.

Sonographers who provide an ultrasound service for DDH should be familiar with and be able to use all techniques. In particular, they should know and understand the Barlow and Ortolani hip tests and, if possible, be trained in the examination technique.

Box 10.3 summarizes elements of best practice for hip sonography in infants.

Follow-up

Ultrasound can be used to monitor infants during treatment in a Pavlik harness. The harness is used to keep the hip in abduction, allowing the hip joint to develop normally (Fig. 10.10). The aim of the ultrasound examination is to assess the position of the head in the acetabulum. If the head is dislocated, a period of 3 weeks is usually given for the head to relocate. The role of ultrasound is to:

Table 10.2 Comparison of different techniques used in the assessment of developmental dysplasia of the hip

	Graf	Harcke	Terjesen (FHC)
Training in technique needed	+++	+++	+
Uses dynamic assessment	+	+++	++
Relies on accurate measurement	+++		+
Assessment of acetabular dysplasia	+++	+	++
Ease of understanding ultrasound image	+++	+	+++
Ease of examination related to infant position	+	+	++
Variability of interobserver assessment	+	+++	+

+++, high; +, low.
FHC, femoral head coverage.

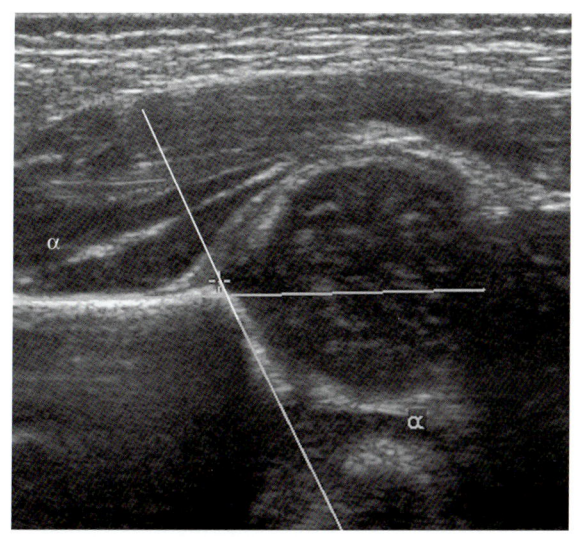

Figure 10.9 Sonographic anatomy of a normal neonatal hip. The femoral head has a speckled ultrasound appearance and is round. The socket is formed by the ilium, and lateral to the femoral head are the gluteal muscles.

- monitor the position of the femoral head so as to determine the period of treatment
- assess stability so that the harness can be adjusted.

If the femoral head cannot be maintained in the acetabulum with a Pavlik harness, then an alternative treatment strategy is undertaken.

OSTEOMYELITIS

Osteomyelitis is usually a bloodborne infection, although rarely it may be due to direct extension from an infected wound. The pyogenic organisms settle in cancellous bone. Most common is *Staphylococcus aureus*, but other organisms include streptococci and *Haemophilus influenzae*. In sickle cell anemia there is an increased risk of staphylococcus and salmonella osteomyelitis. The commonest sites are the distal femur and proximal tibia, but any bone may be affected. Where the joint capsule is inserted distal to the epiphyseal plate, osteomyelitis may spread to involve the joint, causing a septic arthritis as in the hip, shoulder or elbow. Serious and chronic complications may follow, and establishing an early diagnosis is important. Early diagnosis of osteomyelitis is often difficult, especially in the early stages of the disease, as plain radiography may be normal. Ultrasound can be very useful in the early stages, in particular to help differentiate other conditions such as soft tissue abscesses, cellulitis or even normality. Ultrasound is very useful in screening all patients who are clinically suspected of having osteomyelitis.

Clinically the child presents with a markedly painful immobile limb and an acute febrile illness. Directly over the site there is a hot erythematous swelling with exquisite tenderness. Movement causes pain. Occasionally multiple foci may be present with disseminated infection, usually staphylococcal.

The main sonographic criterion for diagnosing osteomyelitis is an abnormal collection of fluid adjacent to the bone without intervening soft tissues. Subperiosteal fluid collections appear hypoechoic or hyperechoic.[8]

Box 10.3 Tips for hip sonography in infants

- Use a high frequency linear transducer with good quality equipment
- Ensure the baby is relaxed and not struggling
- Learn to identify and produce an image of the important bony and cartilaginous landmarks for the neutral coronal image
- Whatever technique used, training and experience are important
- Optimal service is provided when there is close collaboration with experienced orthopedic colleagues
- The maximum potential for effective treatment is in the first 3 months after birth, so diagnosis and treatment are best started within this period
- Many early 'abnormal' immature hips will resolve spontaneously without treatment
- Clinically unstable hips are best examined earlier, at 2 weeks, so that treatment regimens can begin early
- Clinically normal hips in infants 'at risk' are best examined at 6 weeks, when they will have stabilized
- Static combined with dynamic examination is the most widely accepted best practice

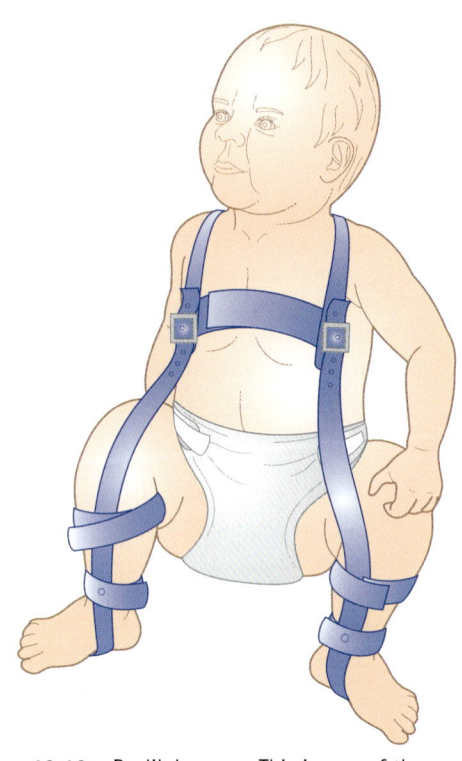

Ultrasound is also useful in differentiating osteomyelitis from other soft tissue abscesses and for localization of lesions before aspiration or surgical management. It can detect recurrence of osteomyelitis in patients with chronic osteomyelitis and a localized bone abscess which has been inadequately treated; in these the detection of sequestrated bone fragment is the aim.

The cardinal features to look for in osteomyelitis are:

- fluid collection adjacent to the bone
- joint effusion
- the ability to see internally in the bone due to bone destruction and marrow edema (Fig. 10.11).

The other main diagnostic investigations for osteomyelitis are plain radiography, radioisotope gallium scanning and, more recently, MRI.

TRANSIENT SYNOVITIS (IRRITABLE HIP)

Irritable hip is a common disorder of childhood characterized by the acute onset of pain in the hip or by a limp which gradually resolves. There is no pain at rest but a decreased range of movements, particularly external rotation. The etiology of an irritable hip remains unknown, but the commonest cause is transient synovitis. The diagnosis is generally made by exclusion. Transient synovitis occurs

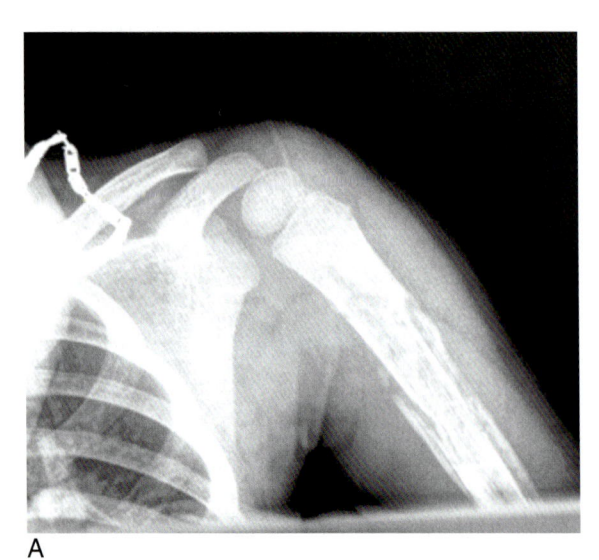

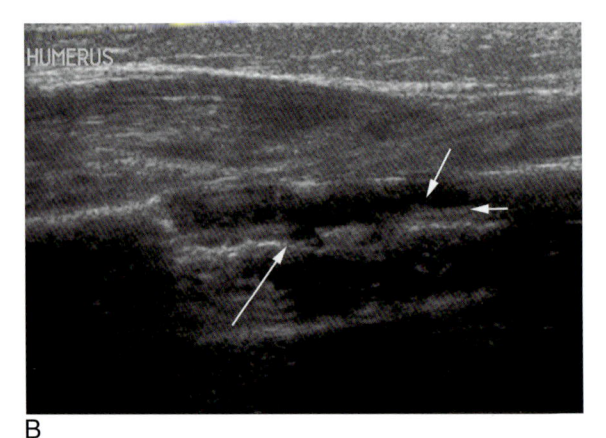

Figure 10.10 Pavlik harness. This is one of the treatment methods for developmental dysplasia of the hip. The harness holds the legs in abduction so that the femoral heads are held in the acetabulae.

Figure 10.11 Osteomyelitis. (A) Radiograph of the left shoulder and upper humerus showing the extensive osteomyelitis and bone destruction affecting predominantly the humerus. (B) Longitudinal sonogram along the shaft of the humerus showing the irregular margin of the bone (long arrow) with a periosteal reaction (short arrow) and a collection of fluid next to the bone (medium arrow).

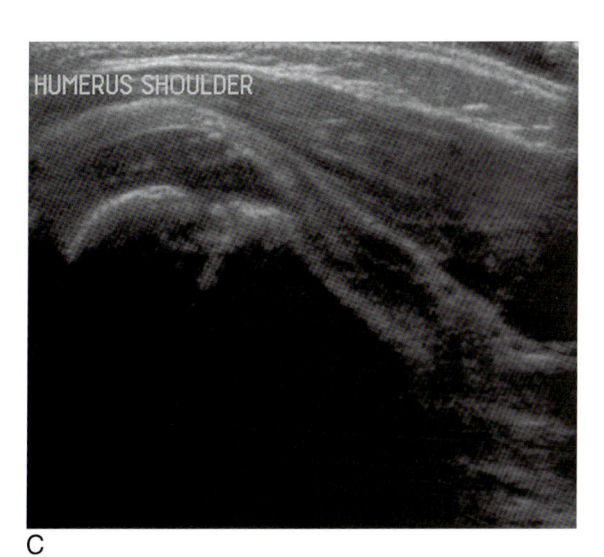

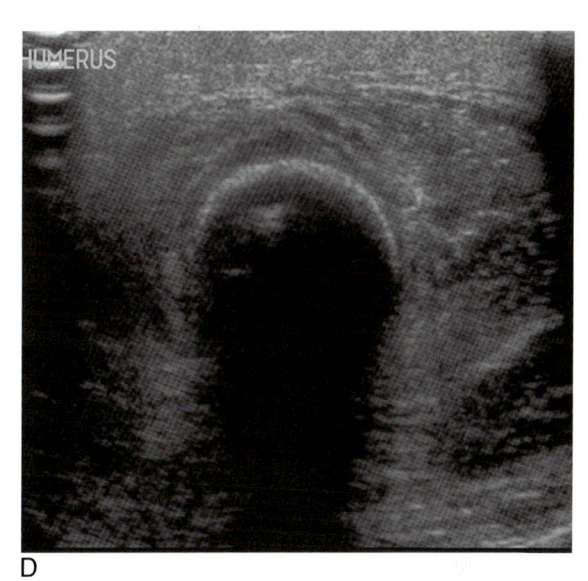

Figure 10.11, cont'd (C) Longitudinal sonogram of the left shoulder and upper humerus showing the extensive collection of fluid next to the bone extending right up to the joint capsule. This had broken through the capsule and in addition there was an infection in the joint. (D) Transverse sonogram of the contralateral (normal) upper humerus showing that the muscle is closely applied to the bone with no collections intervening.

in children from 2–12 years old and is often accompanied or follows a viral infection. The child is afebrile or has a mild fever and does not appear ill. However, patients are frequently admitted to hospital because of concerns that there may be a more serious underlying diagnosis, particularly a septic hip. In septic arthritis the child has a high fever and there is pain at rest with minimal or no movement of the hip. In some the symptoms and signs of hip sepsis and a sterile irritable hip may be identical. Sepsis requires immediate treatment, whereas irritable hip settles down within a few days of bed rest and skin traction. Clinical and laboratory tests such as irritability, fever, white cell count and ESR do not reliably predict hip sepsis. Some authors have found that 70% of children presenting with acute hip pain had an effusion on ultrasound examination. Ultrasound is an excellent technique for demonstrating fluid in the hip joint, whereas plain radiography, in particular with small hip effusions, is not as reliable.

There are other important causes of acute hip pain that may have a similar presentation to transient synovitis, including Perthes disease, slipped capital femoral epiphysis, osteomyelitis, septic arthritis, rheumatoid arthritis and bone tumors; these are discussed further below. Radiography may, at times, be normal in these conditions.[9–11]

One theoretical pitfall in using ultrasound solely for the irritable hip is the risk of missing a slipped femoral epiphysis. This condition, however, is usually seen in older children. For this reason it is recommended that radiography is still used in the older child. In addition, persisting effusions may pre-date any radiographic changes in Perthes disease.

Ultrasound technique

Fluid accumulates anteriorly in the hip joint, and so the examination is undertaken from the front (Fig. 10.12). The patient is examined in the supine position with legs in a neutral position. The hip is examined using an anterior approach with the probe parallel to the femur. When the leg is extended and externally rotated, the capsule is tightened, displacing synovial fluid posteriorly. Small effusions will be more easily demonstrated if there is slight flexion and internal rotation of the hip.

Longitudinal images of the joint capsule and psoas bursa anterior to the femoral head and neck

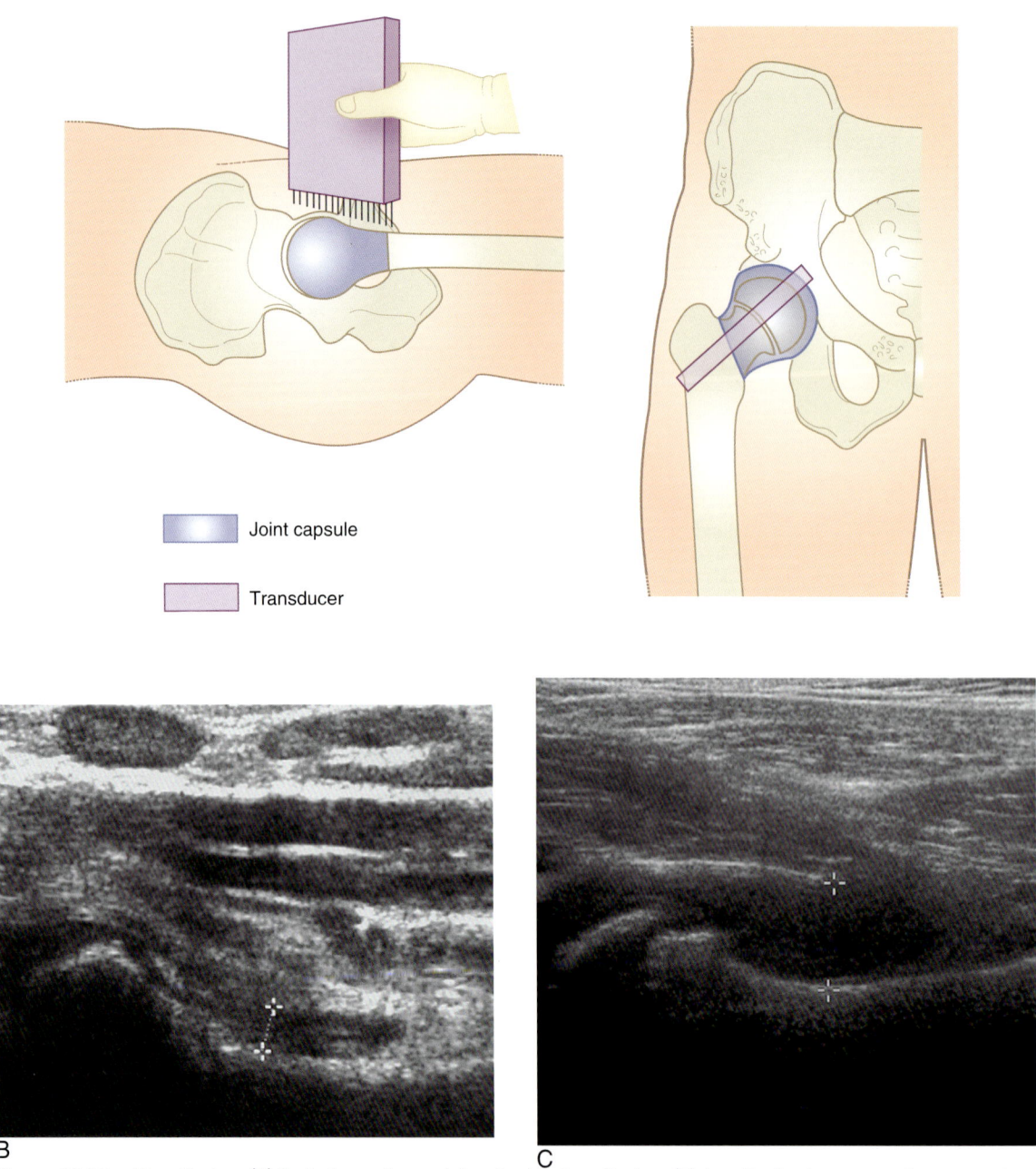

Figure 10.12 Hip effusion. (A) Technique of examining the hip for effusion. (B) Longitudinal sonogram in a normal hip. (C) This child had a large effusion in the right hip joint (between calipers).

should be obtained. The landmark to identify is the upper femur metaphysis and epiphysis. The normal joint capsule can be seen extending anterior to the femoral neck. The iliopsoas muscle can be seen just anterior to the capsule. Both right and left hips should be examined from this approach. It is important to compare the symptomatic hip with the normal hip, as there may be capsular thickening due to an inflammatory process which may otherwise be overlooked. Some hip effusions are echogenic, which may be difficult to distinguish from the adjacent capsule. The difference may be best appreciated when comparing both sides. Psoas infection or inflammation can also present with hip pain which may be indistinguishable from that of an irritable hip. The psoas muscle must always be carefully examined and pathology in the muscle excluded.

Fluid in the joint will elevate the capsule and usually appears hypoechoic. If the fluid is infected, containing cellular debris, this may cause difficulties in assessing the effusion.

Both hips must be carefully examined; a difference of 2 mm is considered abnormal. The normal capsular distention changes with age, so that the normal distance is given as 5 mm under 4 years and 7 mm over 8 years.[12]

In younger children there is a large hypoechoic zone between the ossific nucleus of the femoral head and the joint capsule. This is unossified hyaline cartilage. If the technique is not meticulous and equipment settings faulty, this may be mistaken for a hip effusion.

Also the contour of the femoral head should always be included in any hip examination so as not to miss the fragmentation and irregularity seen in Perthes disease.

Synovial thickening and pannus formation may be seen in children with rheumatoid arthritis.

Hip sepsis is an orthopedic emergency that can result in rapid permanent joint destruction, and speed of diagnosis with early treatment is essential. A delay of more than 4 days is associated with a poor outcome, with bone destruction and permanent damage to the bone and joint. The only means of confirming the diagnosis of septic arthritis is culture of synovial fluid, and hence some authors recommend immediate aspiration of the effusion and microscopy and Gram staining of the aspirate.[10]

Aspiration technique

Topical anesthetic cream is applied in the region of the anterior skin crease. It is essential to ensure absolute sterility so that organisms are not introduced into the joint. This can only be achieved by accurately marking the skin and then puncturing the joint 'blind'. Direct visualization of the needle tip is difficult to perform with dynamic scanning while keeping the whole area sterile. The key to this particular technique in maintaining sterility is accurate skin marking. Sterile gloves, gown and mask are generally recommended. Local anesthesia and infiltration together with the anesthetic cream provide a well-anesthetized area.

A 21-gauge needle or spinal needle is used and is inserted perpendicularly into the effusion. The needle is withdrawn a fraction and a few milliliters of fluid withdrawn. The original hip pain may be relieved by aspiration of the effusion.

OTHER CAUSES OF A PAINFUL HIP

Perthes disease (Legg–Calve–Perthes disease)

This is a condition of ischemia resulting in avascular necrosis of the femoral epiphysis, with irregularity and fragmentation in the early phase and revascularization and reossification in the healing phase. The femoral epiphysis ultimately appears flattened and deformed with increased density because of the collapse and new bone formation. This whole process occurs over a period of 18–36 months. It occurs in children of 5–10 years of age, is bilateral in 15% and is more common in males, with a male to female ratio of 5:1.

The clinical presentation is insidious with a limp or hip pain, and the condition is frequently misdiagnosed as transient synovitis.

One of the earliest findings in Perthes disease is a joint effusion in the hip, with a picture similar to irritable hip and transient synovitis. One difference on ultrasound is that the synovium may appear thicker. The femoral head must be visualized on all hip examinations, and any effusion that persists for longer than 2 weeks must be fully investigated.

Even if the initial X-ray is normal a repeat may be required if the clinical symptoms persist.

Slipped upper femoral epiphysis

This is a condition where the femoral epiphysis slips postero-inferiorly. It occurs in the 10–15 year age range during the adolescent growth spurt. Twenty percent are bilateral, and the condition is found particularly in obese boys. Presentation is with hip pain or a limp, and there will be restriction in abduction and internal rotation of movement. The diagnosis is made with plain radiography sometimes complemented with the frog leg view, and treatment is by pinning the epiphysis in position. It is possible to detect the slipped epiphysis with ultrasound, although it is not the first line of investigation (Box 10.4).

Juvenile idiopathic arthritis

Juvenile idiopathic arthritis (JIA) is a group of conditions in which there is chronic arthritis lasting more than 6 weeks and presenting before the age of 16 years. It was previously called juvenile chronic arthritis but the whole group of conditions has recently been reclassified according to its onset, such as: systemic, polyarticular (more than four joints) and oligoarticular (up to and including four joints) (Box 10.5). It is then further classified according to the presence of antinuclear antibodies, HLA-B27 and rheumatoid factor.

Systemic arthritis This was previously known as Still's disease and usually affects young children. Clinically they may present with an acute illness: with a high spiking fever, anorexia and weight loss. At the height of the fever there may be a pink rash. There may be aches and pains in the joints and muscles, but often at clinical presentation there is no arthritis. Children may have lymphadenopathy, hepatosplenomegaly and anemia.

Polyarticular arthritis The role of ultrasound in this whole group of children with the arthritides is twofold. First, the ultrasound examination may be requested in order to demonstrate hepatosplenomegaly or lymphadenopathy. Second, ultrasound examination of the joints is frequently requested, in particular to demonstrate joint effusions. Some may have inflammation of tendons into bone, such as the Achilles tendon, particularly in the B27-associated arthritides.

Systemic corticosteroids may be required for severe uveitis or pericarditis, and in those with severe systemic disease an ultrasound examination

---

Box 10.4 Causes of a painful hip

Age 1–3 years
- Septic arthritis (osteomyelitis)
- Transient synovitis
- Trauma

3–10 years
- Transient synovitis
- Septic arthritis (Osteomyelitis)
- Perthes
- Juvenile idiopathic arthritis
- Trauma
- Malignancy, e.g. leukemia, bone tumors

11–16 years
- Slipped upper femoral epiphysis
- Juvenile idiopathic arthritis
- Trauma
- Septic arthritis (osteomyelitis)
- Malignancy, e.g. leukemia, bone tumors

Box 10.5 Revised classification of juvenile idiopathic arthritis

Systemic 9%
Oligoarthritis
—Persistent 49%
—Extended 8%
Polyarthritis RF negative 16%
Polyarthritis RF positive 3%
Psoriatic 7%
Enthesitis-related arthritis 7%
Other arthritis 1%

RF, rheumatoid factor

may be able to detect the effects of this treatment: such as fatty infiltration of the pancreas in long term steroid therapy, and renal calculi. Amyloid is a rare but serious complication causing proteinuria and renal failure.

These children often experience considerable problems from flexion contractures and growth failure, although there have been recent improvements in the physical and pharmacological management of JIA.

LIMB-LENGTHENING PROCEDURES

Patients now increasingly present to orthopedic surgeons with short stature or unequal leg lengths in the hope of benefiting from limb-lengthening procedures. The Ilizarov distraction technique which was pioneered in Russia has become more popular, with improvements in its success rate. The technique involves fracture of the bone and the application of an external ring and bar support frame with circumferential screw threads and nuts which allows systematic distraction of bone segments. Plain radiographs are limited in detecting the small amounts of new bone formation that occur at the distraction site in the early stages of healing. Distraction of the bone is usually at the rate of 1 mm per day, and this is continued until the required length is achieved. Then there is a period of consolidation which allows the new bone to strengthen. The rate of distraction depends on the successful production of new bone at the distraction site. Early evaluation is required to monitor this process of distraction. Traditionally, radiographs have been used to monitor this distraction, but callus formation in the bone gap is not seen within the first month after the procedure. Ultrasound has been used successfully to evaluate the developing quality of the new bone at the distraction site.

The ultrasound appearance of new bone consists of echogenic foci within the distraction site which then become aligned in the longitudinal plane and which increase in number and size until they coalesce as echodense bone. Ultrasound may show the development of cysts in the developing new bone, which can be aspirated. Ultrasound has been used to monitor the rate of distraction. If the rate is too slow in proportion to the amount of new bone formation, premature fusion at the distraction site will occur, whereas, if it is too fast, insufficient new bone formation will occur to allow healing at the distraction site.

Ultrasound is a complementary technique to plain film radiography in the follow-up of patients undergoing limb-lengthening procedures. It can be useful in the early monitoring and reduces the radiation burden.[13]

ABNORMALITIES OF THE TENDONS

Abnormalities of the tendons are not very common in children, so the use of sonography to examine the tendons is limited.

The major tendinous abnormalities in children are usually seen around the ankle and include Achilles tendon tears with thinning and complete rupture of the tendon. Other abnormalities of the tendon may include tendonitis where the tendon is inflamed, with focal areas of thickening. All of these abnormalities may be associated with effusions into the ankle joint.

Ultrasound examination of all tendon abnormalities should include a full longitudinal and transverse examination. The patient should be placed in a comfortable position which is accessible for the sonographer. All tendons are characterized by polar linear echoes with well-defined margins.

SOFT TISSUE MASSES

Soft tissue masses are commonly encountered in children, and ultrasound is an excellent modality to use in the first instance to help characterize, locate and determine the anatomical relationship to other adjacent structures. While it is not always possible on ultrasound to exactly determine the diagnosis, it can guide further imaging and localize the mass for biopsy or drainage. In addition, with the use of Doppler, the vascular characteristics of the mass can be determined, which is important in children because hemangiomas are common.[14]

Box 10.6 lists considerations to be borne in mind when examining soft tissue masses.

Box 10.6 Ultrasound of soft tissue masses

- Always compare with the unaffected side
- Is the mass solid or cystic?
- Observe the margins of the mass. Well-defined masses are more likely to be benign
- Observe the surrounding tissues. Is the mass ill-defined and infiltrating the surrounding muscle planes? This is found in infection, hematomas, malignant and some benign masses
- Identify the structure from which the mass is arising, such as tendon nerve sheath or muscle
- Inflammation and infection of the muscle will cause swelling of the muscle initially with an increase in echogenicity and loss of the normal muscle architecture
- Cellulitis is inflammation in the subcutaneous tissue
- Abscesses are ill defined and predominantly hypoechoic. They may contain gas if the organism produces gas. Doppler signals will be enhanced around the periphery of the abscess
- Hemangiomas are common and may be hypo-, hyper- or of mixed echogenicity. Vessels may be identified supplying the mass on Doppler
- Aneurysms, pseudoaneurysms (Fig. 10.13) and arteriovenous fistulae may be pulsatile and are sometimes seen after femoral artery catheterization. Doppler is essential to characterize the different vascular masses
- Lipomas are echogenic and well defined (Fig. 10.14)
- Hematomas are echogenic when fresh and, when resolving with central liquefaction, become anechoic
- Myositis ossificans can occur as a result of trauma and appears as echogenic foci and acoustic shadowing in the muscle

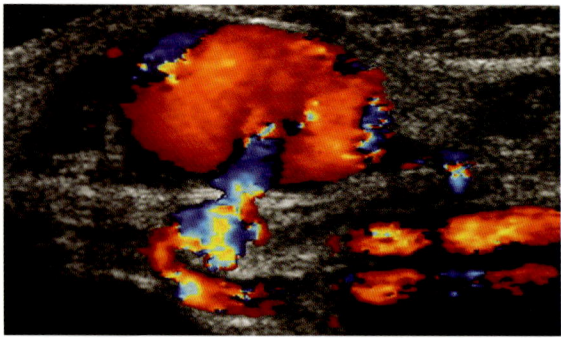

Figure 10.13 Pseudoaneurysm. This child presented with a lump in the groin after having had a femoral cardiac catheterization. Clinically the child had a large bruise. The ultrasound examination shows that there is a large pseudoaneurysm related to the femoral artery. This is clearly demonstrated on Doppler examination, which can differentiate hematomas, aneurysms and arteriovenous fistulas.

A

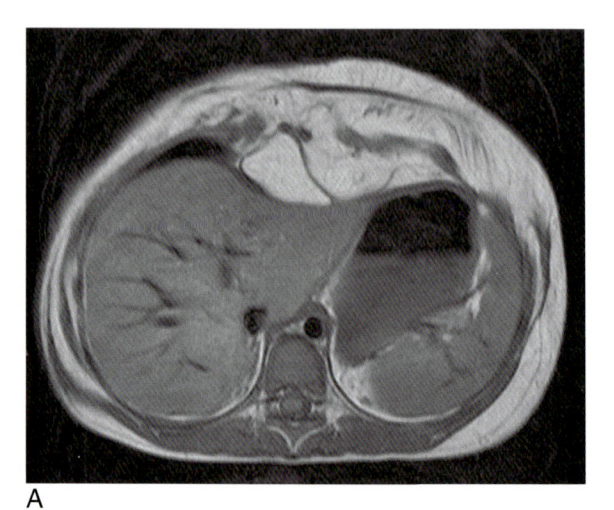

Figure 10.14 Soft issue lipoma. (A) MRI examination in the coronal view showing the large subcutaneous lipoma beneath the anterior abdominal wall.

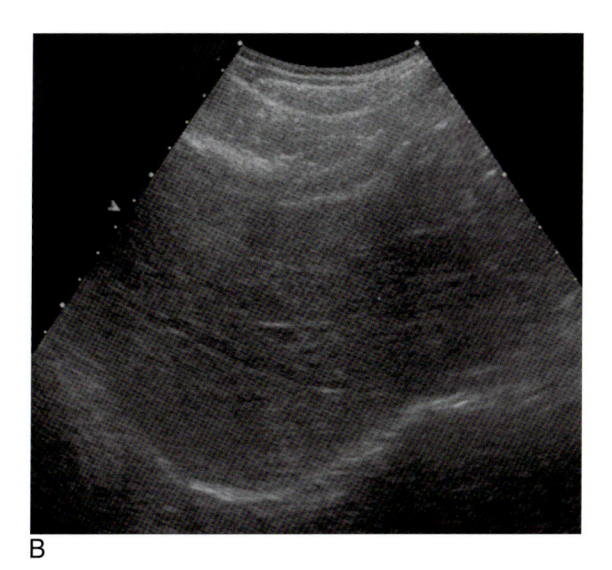

Figure 10.14, cont'd (B) Transverse sonogram in the same position showing the echogenic soft tissue lipoma just anterior to the liver.

References

1. Poul J, Bajerova J, Skotakova J, et al. Selective treatment program for developmental dysplasia of the hip in an epidemiologic prospective study. J Pediatr Orthop B 1998; 7(2):135–137.
2. Rosendahl K, Aslaksen A, Lie RT, et al. Reliability of ultrasound in the early diagnosis of developmental dysplasia of the hip. Pediatr Radiol 1995: 25(3):219–224.
3. Rosendahl K, Markestad T, Lie RT. Developmental dysplasia of the hip: prevalence based on ultrasound diagnosis. Pediatr Radiol 1996; 26(9):635–639.
4. Rosendahl K, Markestad T, Lie RT. Ultrasound screening for developmental dysplasia of the hip in the neonate: the effect on treatment rate and prevalence of late cases. Pediatrics 1994; 94:47–52.
5. Graf R, Schuler P. Sonography of the infant hip: an atlas. Germany: VCH; 1986.
6. Harcke HT, Grissom LE. Performing dynamic sonography of the infant hip. AJR Am J Roentgenol 1990; 155:837–844.
7. Harcke HT. Screening newborns for developmental dysplasia of the hip: the role of sonography. AJR Am J Roentgenol 1994; 162:395–397.
8. Abiri MM, Kirpekar M, Ablow RS. Osteomyelitis: detection with US. Radiology 1989; 172:509–511.
9. Zawin ZK, Hoffer FA, Rand FF, et al. Joint effusion in children with an irritable hip: US diagnosis and aspiration. Radiology 1993; 187:459–463.
10. Berman L, Fink AM, Wilson D, et al. Technical note: Identifying and aspirating hip effusions. Br J Radiol 1995; 68:306–310.
11. Fink AM, Berman L, Edwards D, et al. The irritable hip: immediate ultrasound guided aspiration and prevention of hospital admission. Arch Dis Child 1995; 72:110–114.
12. Marchal GJ, Van Holsbeeck MT, Raes M, et al. Transient sinovitis of the hip in children: role of ultrasound screening. Radiology 1987; 162:825–828.
13. Young JWR, Kostrubiak IS, Resnik C, et al. Sonographic evaluation of bone production at the distraction site in Ilizarov limb-lengthening procedures. AJR Am J Roentgenol 1990: 154:125–128.
14. Fornage BD, Tassin G. Sonographic appearances of superficial soft-tissue lipomas. J Clin Ultrasound 1991; 19:215–220.

Chapter 11

Pediatric interventional ultrasound

Derek J. Roebuck

CHAPTER CONTENTS

Anesthesia   321
Venous access   322
   Technique   323
   Venous access sites   324
   Complications   329
Biopsy   330
   Renal biopsy   330
   Liver biopsy   332
   Biopsy of other organs   334
Aspiration and drainage of fluid
   collections   335
Sclerotherapy of vascular malformations   336
Urological intervention   337
Other ultrasound-guided intervention   338

Pediatric interventional radiology is a rapidly growing subspecialty, and many procedures formerly the responsibility of pediatricians and pediatric surgeons are now performed by radiologists.[1,2] Ultrasound guidance is ideal for interventional radiology in children (Box 11.1). It is the only imaging required for some procedures and is the starting point for many others (Box 11.2).

ANESTHESIA

There are widely differing ideas about the appropriate form of anesthesia for pediatric interventional radiology. Some centers use mainly intravenous sedation (using various drugs), with good results.[2] At our institution, we prefer general anesthesia (GA) on the grounds that it is less unpleasant for the child and may make the procedure safer.

General anesthesia is required for particularly painful or prolonged procedures, and also for insertion of tunneled central venous catheters, where air embolism may occur in procedures on uncooperative children.

If GA is not used, topical anesthetic cream is applied to the appropriate area before the procedure. Buffered lidocaine is then injected through this anesthetized area. If the procedure is performed under GA, we use bupivacaine, a longer-acting local anesthetic, for postoperative pain control.

For brief procedures, the child can breathe an equimolar mixture of oxygen and nitrous oxide (Entonox). In combination with topical and local anesthetic this is particularly effective for brief but

> **Box 11.1 Advantages of ultrasound for image-guided intervention in children**
>
> Excellent resolution
> Real time imaging
> Speed
> Portability
> Low cost
> Safety
> —better image quality
> —no ionizing radiation

painful procedures such as renal biopsy or pleural aspiration.

VENOUS ACCESS

Central venous access procedures form a large part of the workload in pediatric interventional radiology, comprising nearly 50% of the cases in our practice.[1] The ability to provide routine venous access both for the administration of medication and for diagnostic blood sampling has become a basic requirement in the acute medical care of the child. The major indications for central venous access in children include total parenteral nutrition, prolonged intravenous therapy, use of toxic chemotherapies, difficult access, frequent blood transfusions or sampling and hemodialysis.

The following types of device are used:

- *PICC: peripherally inserted central venous catheters* are often used for toxic therapies, long term antibiotics and total parenteral nutrition. They are unsuitable if high infusion rates are necessary.
- *Tunneled catheters* (e.g. Hickman or Broviac catheters) pass through a subcutaneous tunnel before entering a central vein. They can have more than one lumen, and are intended for long term use.
- *Ports* (e.g. Port-a-Cath) are subcutaneously implanted reservoirs attached to central venous catheters. They are intended for long-term intermittent use.

We check full blood count and coagulation profiles in all children with chronic systemic or severe acute disease before the procedure. Uncorrected coagulopathy and more than moderate thrombocytopenia (platelet count <50 µL^{-1}) are relative contraindications to central line insertion.

It is sometimes necessary to insert a central venous access device in a child with positive blood cultures, but this should be avoided where possible.

The selection of catheter to be inserted depends on several factors:

- intended duration of use
- type of infusion and frequency with which it will be infused
- venous anatomy and access sites
- previous intervention at the intended site for access and future needs for access
- clinical history and coagulation status
- preference of the physician or patient
- ability of the patient or carers to maintain the device.

The use of ultrasound guidance makes central venous access easy, quick and safe in all but the most difficult cases. Potential advantages over surgical placement of central lines include a very high

> **Box 11.2 Ultrasound-guided interventional techniques**
>
> Venous access (see Table 11.1)
> —central venous catheterization
> —venous intervention
> Biopsy
> —renal biopsy
> —liver biopsy
> —tumor biopsy
> Aspiration and drainage of fluid collections
> Sclerotherapy of vascular malformations
> —venous malformations
> —cystic lymphatic malformations
> Urological intervention
> —nephrostomy
> —other intervention
> Other intervention
> —biliary intervention
> —joint aspiration and injection
> —arterial access

success rate at the first site attempted, a good cosmetic result because of the short puncture site incision, a short procedure time and no need for preoperative imaging in children who have had multiple central veins accessed in the past.[1] Table 11.1 lists, for various veins, indications for access.

Technique

A high frequency linear array probe is used for most procedures. The puncture can be performed with the needle either parallel to or perpendicular to the long axis of the probe. A 21-gauge needle (which accepts a 0.018-inch guidewire) is usually used in small children. In older children it is possible to use 19- and 18-gauge needles (which accept 0.035- and 0.038-inch guidewires, respectively). Non-tunneled catheters can be inserted over the guidewire following dilation of the tract with a vascular dilator. The insertion of tunneled catheters requires the use of a peel-away sheath (Fig. 11.1).

The standard method for central venous catheter insertion can be seen from the procedure for insertion of an internal jugular Hickman catheter. The patient's skin is prepared and draped in a standard fashion. The puncture and exit sites are identified, and bupivacaine 0.25% is injected at and between these sites. Stab incisions are made, and the catheter is tunneled through the subcutaneous tissue between them using a tunneling probe. The puncture needle is inserted through the puncture site incision, taking care not to damage the catheter. It is important to puncture the vein with a sharp, stabbing motion to ensure that the tip of the needle enters the lumen of the vein. The needle should be seen to move freely in the lumen, without a 'tent' of intima over the tip. It is easy to advance the guidewire along a subintimal plane if care is not taken at this stage. Inadvertent puncture of the opposite wall of the vein is usually not a problem. The guidewire is then advanced into the vein in a central direction, and its position confirmed by fluoroscopy. If it is easy to pass the guidewire through the right atrium and down the inferior vena cava, this should be done, as it makes insertion of the peel-away sheath easier. Following removal of the needle, the peel-away sheath is advanced over the guidewire. It is crucial to fix the guidewire (relative to the patient) at this stage. If this is not done, the dilator of the peel-away sheath may cause serious damage to the superior vena cava or heart. I suspect that the occasional reports of cardiac tamponade following Hickman insertion are due to injury occurring at this stage. The next step is to cut the catheter to the desired length. In many centers, the catheter tip is left in the superior vena cava, although this appears to be associated with an increased risk of superior vena cava

Table 11.1 Ultrasound-guided venous access

Access	Common indications	Other indications
Internal jugular veins	Central venous catheterization	Transjugular liver biopsy TIPS IVC filter insertion Other venous intervention
Subclavian veins	Central venous catheterization	Pacemaker insertion
Femoral veins	Central venous catheterization	Venous sampling Transvenous biopsy IVC filter insertion Other venous intervention
Upper limb veins	PICC insertion	Other venous intervention
Hepatic veins	Cardiac intervention	Central venous catheterization
Portal venous system	Pancreatic venous sampling	Islet cell infusion Portal vein embolization

IVC, inferior vena cava; PICC, peripherally inserted central venous catheter; TIPS, transjugular intrahepatic portosystemic shunt.

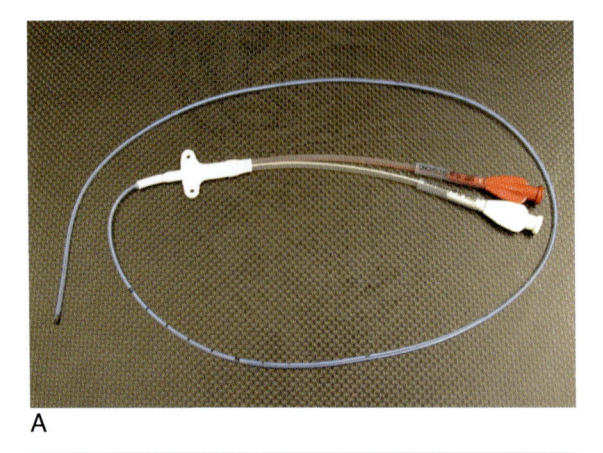

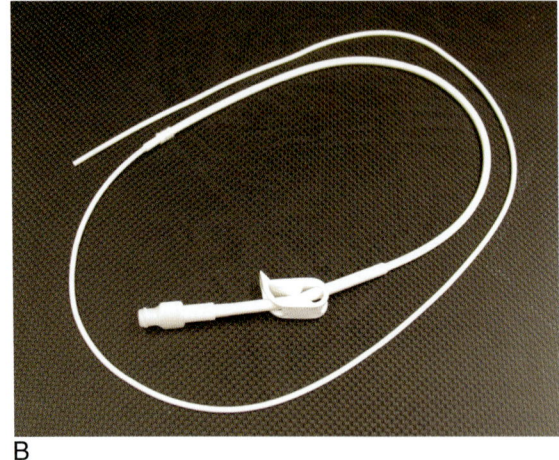

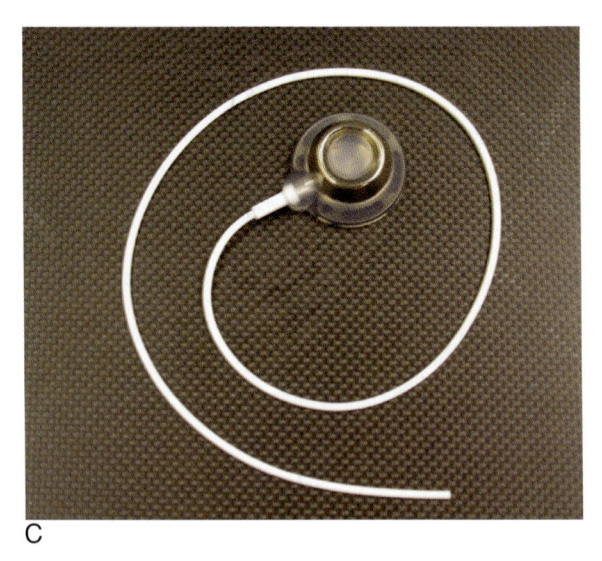

Figure 11.1 Catheters used for central venous access. (A) Dual lumen PICC line. (B) Single lumen Hickman line. (C) Port device.

thrombosis. We prefer to leave the tip in the right atrium. Fluoroscopy can be performed with the catheter on the anterior chest wall, projected over the peel-away sheath. If the catheter is then cut at the T7 level, its tip will lie in the upper right atrium. The guidewire and the dilator of the peel-away sheath are removed, and the catheter advanced through the sheath. The sheath is then split and removed. The position of the catheter tip is confirmed with fluoroscopy. The catheter is flushed with heparin (10 unit/ml) and sutured to the skin at the exit site. The puncture site can be closed with a subcuticular suture, tissue glue or adhesive tape.

Venous access sites

The most frequently used central veins are the internal jugulars, subclavians and femorals. The right internal jugular vein (Fig. 11.2) is usually the preferred site for insertion of temporary and tunneled central venous catheters and venous port devices. When this vein cannot be used, the left internal jugular vein is preferred to the subclavian veins. This advice is not evidence-based but relies on the assumption that the risks of pneumothorax and inadvertent arterial puncture are less with ultrasound-guided jugular puncture.

The subclavian veins can be punctured, with ultrasound guidance, from either a supraclavicular or infraclavicular approach. In patients with chronic renal failure the subclavian veins are not used, because the large catheters used for hemodialysis often cause subclavian vein stenosis, which may prevent the use of the ipsilateral upper limb for creation of a dialysis fistula (Fig. 11.3).

Although femoral puncture is easy (Fig. 11.4) femoral catheters have several disadvantages, partic-

PEDIATRIC INTERVENTIONAL ULTRASOUND

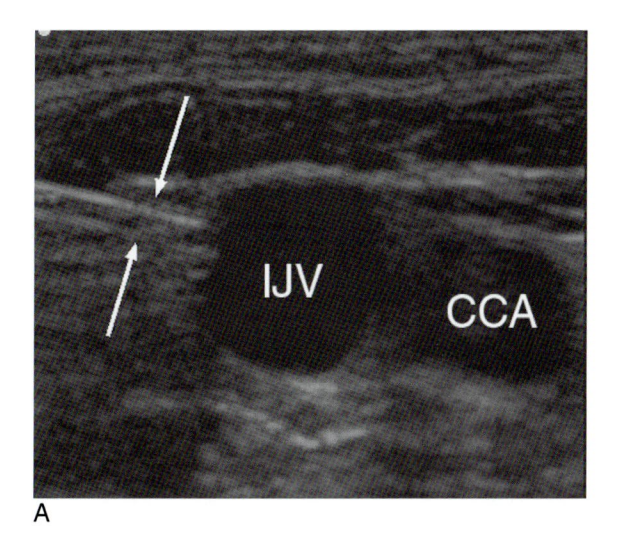

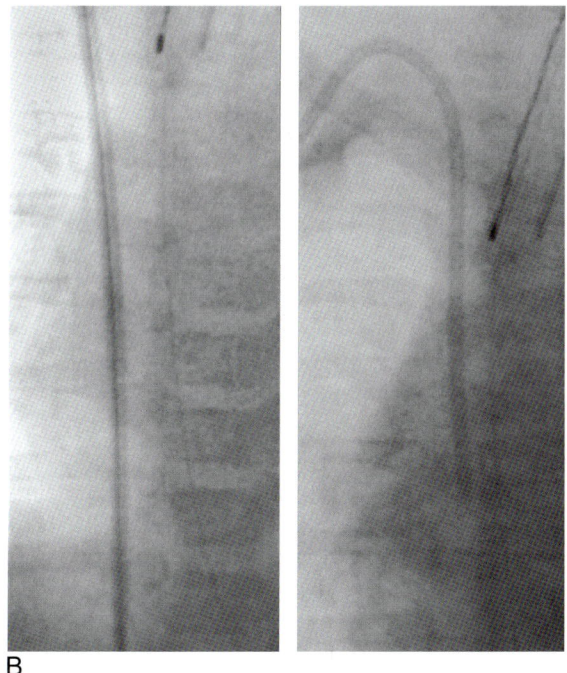

Figure 11.2 Jugular puncture. (A) Transverse image of the right side of the anterior neck. The needle has been advanced through the sternocleidomastoid muscle and is about to enter the internal jugular vein (IJV). The common carotid artery (CCA) lies medially.
(B) A guidewire has been inserted, followed by a peel-away sheath (left panel). A Hickman catheter has been inserted through the peel-away sheath, which has been split and removed (right panel).

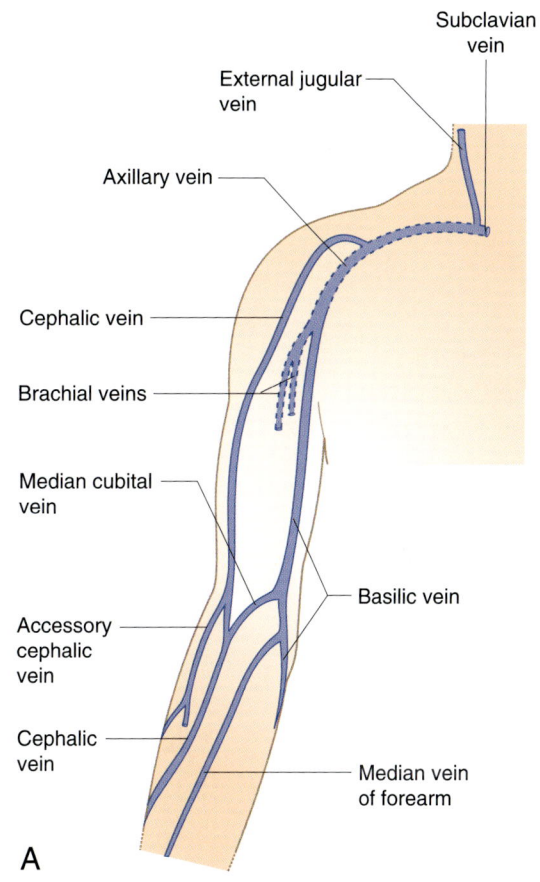

Figure 11.3 Venous access sites in upper body for insertion of lines.

ularly in infants. The risk of infection appears to be higher than at other sites. Femoral catheters may cause impairment of venous return from the ipsilateral lower limb in neonates and infants. Short (non-tunneled) femoral venous catheters frequently cause iliac vein occlusion in very small babies. They should also be avoided in children with renal failure who may become candidates for renal transplantation, as iliac venous occlusion may make this operation much more difficult (Fig. 11.5).

Children with chronic disease and multiple previous central venous access procedures may have venous occlusions, rendering all of the usual sites of access unusable with standard techniques. There are three solutions to this problem. First, occluded veins can often be recanalized with a dilator and guidewire following puncture of a vein peripheral to the occlusion. Longstanding occlusions are

326 PEDIATRIC ULTRASOUND

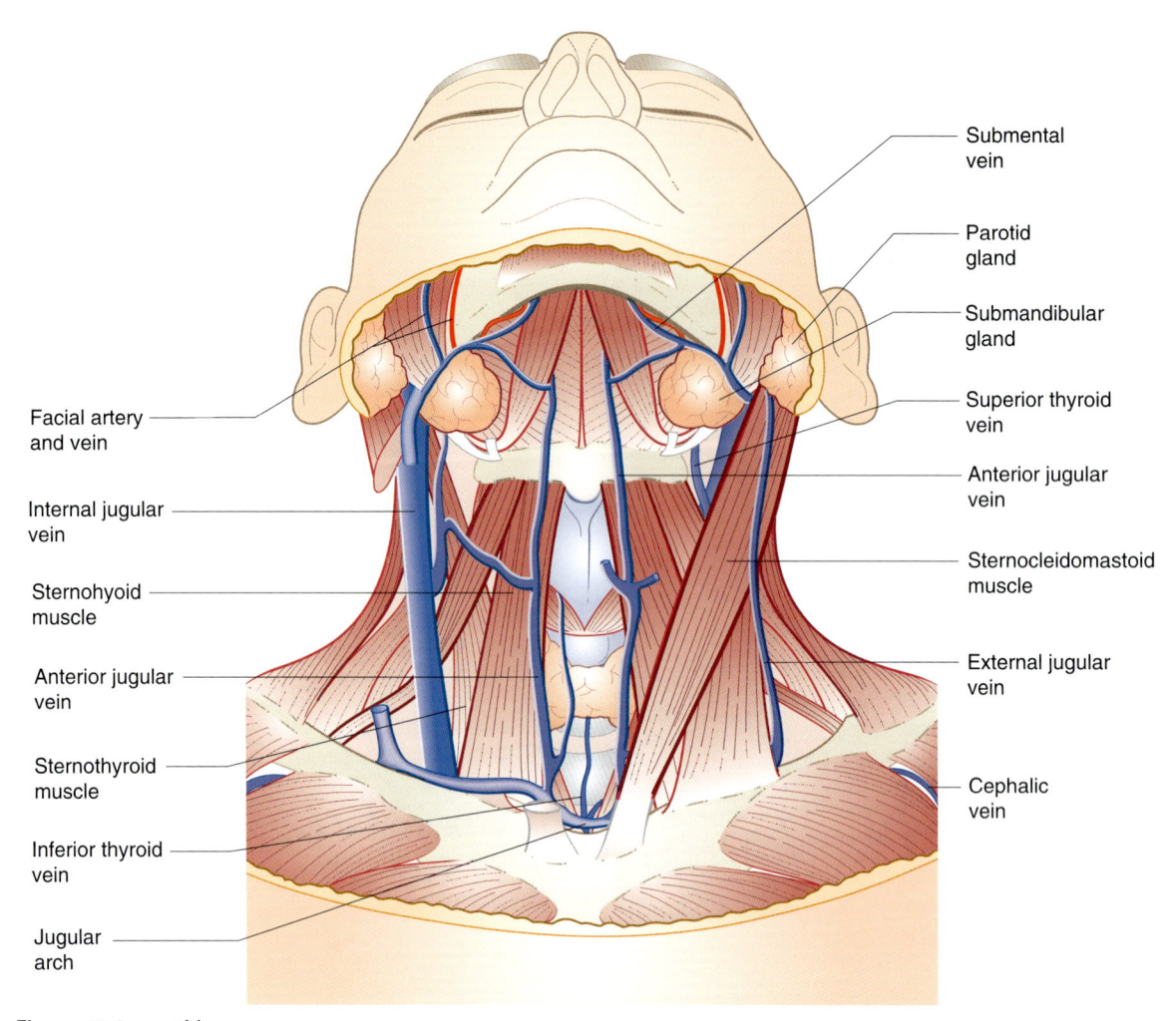

Figure 11.3, cont'd

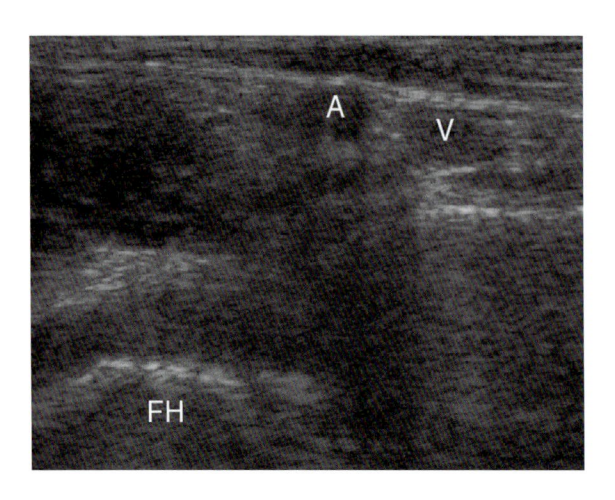

Figure 11.4 Femoral puncture. Oblique transverse image of the right groin. The common femoral artery (A) and vein (V) can be punctured at the level of the femoral head (FH).

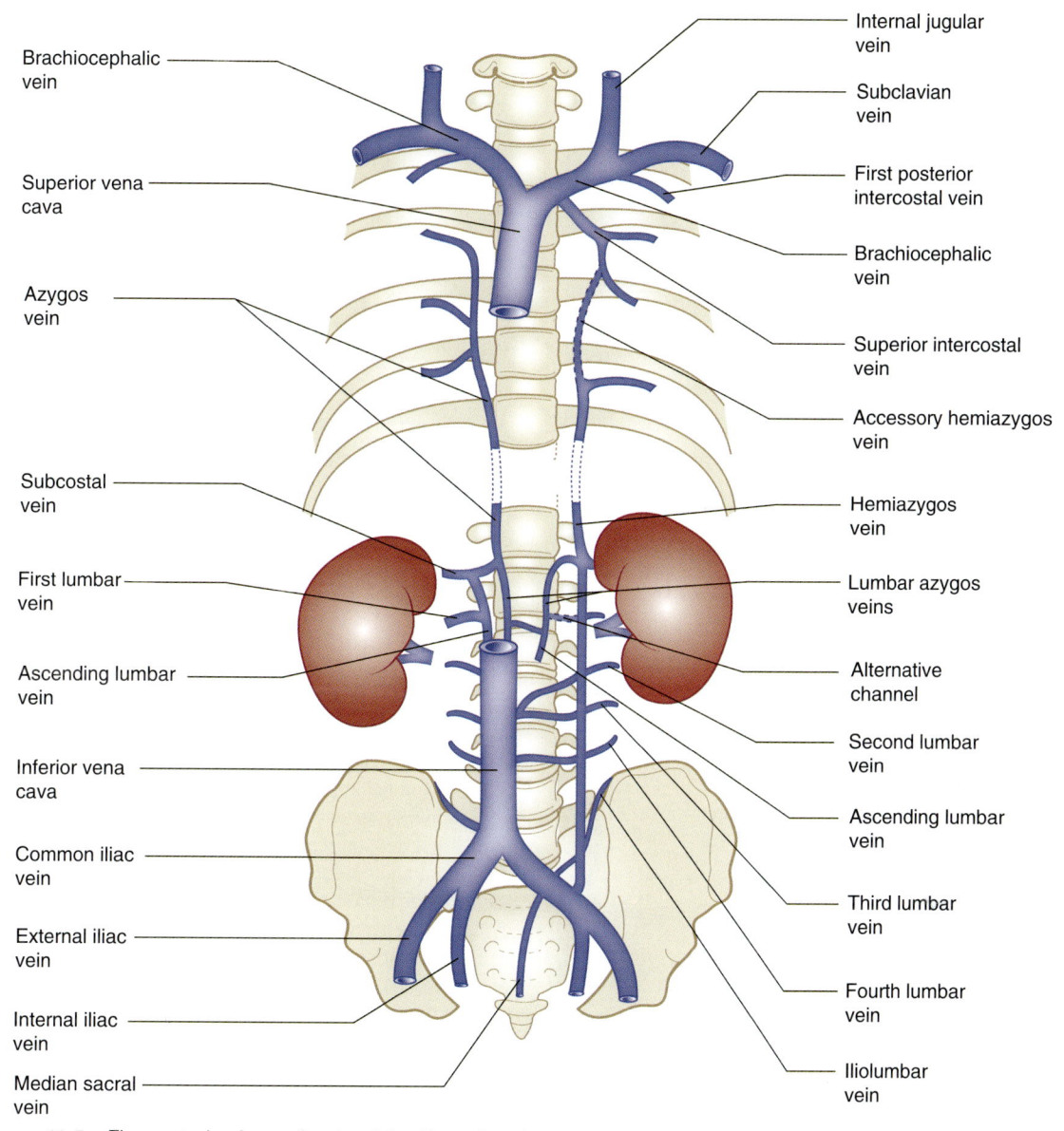

Figure 11.5 The central veins and potential collateral pathways.

difficult to treat in this way, but are always associated with the development of collateral veins. These small veins can sometimes be used for central venous access (Fig. 11.6).

Finally, the use of unconventional puncture sites can be considered. The best of these in small children are the brachiocephalic veins (Fig. 11.7), which may remain patent even in the presence of ipsilateral jugular and subclavian occlusion. In older children it may be difficult to see the brachiocephalic vein with ultrasound, in which case a catheter can be advanced from a femoral vein into the superior vena cava, and a stiff guidewire pushed under fluoroscopic guidance through the wall of the vein and into the soft tissues of the neck. This can be seen with ultrasound, and retrieved via a

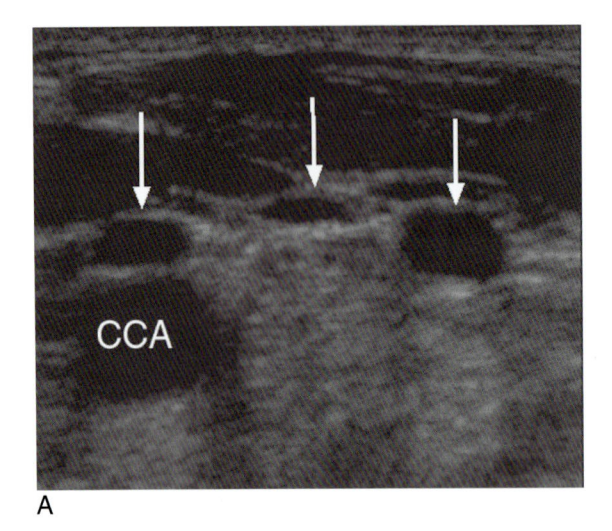

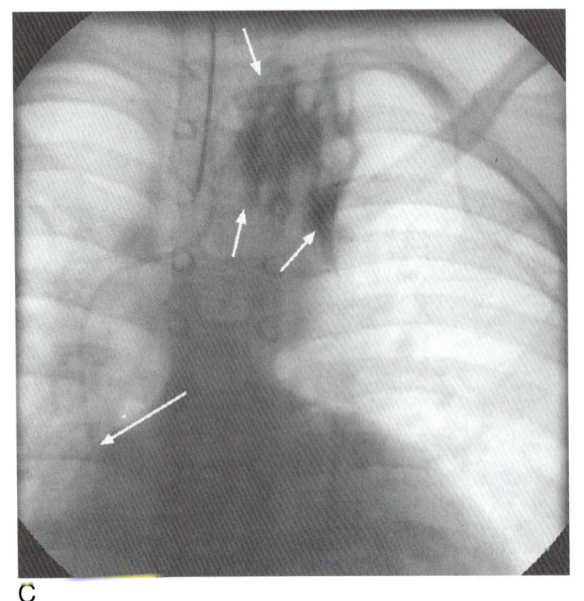

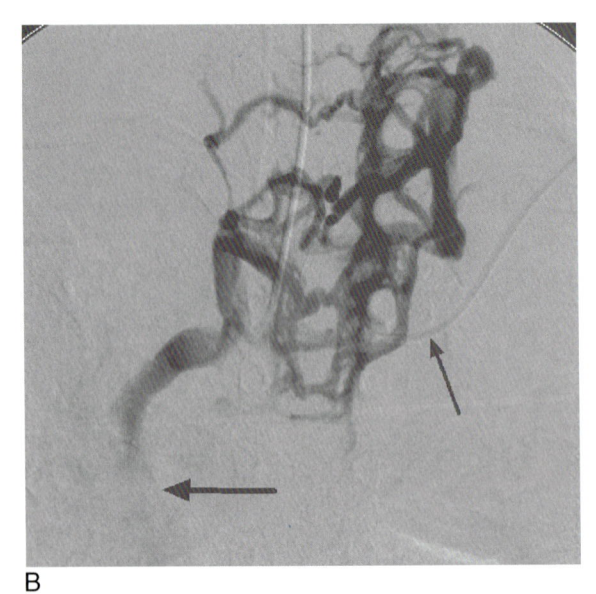

Figure 11.6 Collateral venous access. (A) Transverse image of the left side of the neck. The common carotid artery (CCA) is present, but there is no internal jugular vein. Several collateral veins are present (arrows). (B) One of the collaterals was punctured, and a dilator (small arrow) inserted. Injected contrast flows through paraspinal and epidural collaterals, eventually reaching the superior vena cava (large arrow). (C) A Hickman catheter has been inserted through a collateral pathway. Its tip (long arrow) lies at the junction of the superior vena cava and right atrium. Extravasated contrast (short arrows) is present from a previous unsuccessful attempt to negotiate the collaterals.

small cutdown. This access can then be used to insert a catheter. Ultrasound-guided transhepatic central venous access is occasionally useful, especially for cardiac intervention, but also sometimes for insertion of central venous catheters.[3,4] This form of access may be very effective in older children. However, in very young children (less than 2 years old) the catheter may back out of the venous system and migrate into the peritoneal cavity. A final alternative is the translumbar approach to the inferior vena cava.[3,5] This is performed with fluoroscopic rather than ultrasound guidance.

The type of central venous access device used will depend on the precise indication for intravenous therapy (Table 11.2). I have a strong preference for inserting central venous port devices rather than Hickman catheters, except for certain indications such as total parenteral nutrition and bone marrow transplantation. Ports have a lower infection rate, cannot be inadvertently removed, and are less conspicuous and limiting of patient activities. They are not suitable for children who cannot tolerate regular needle access (Fig. 11.8).

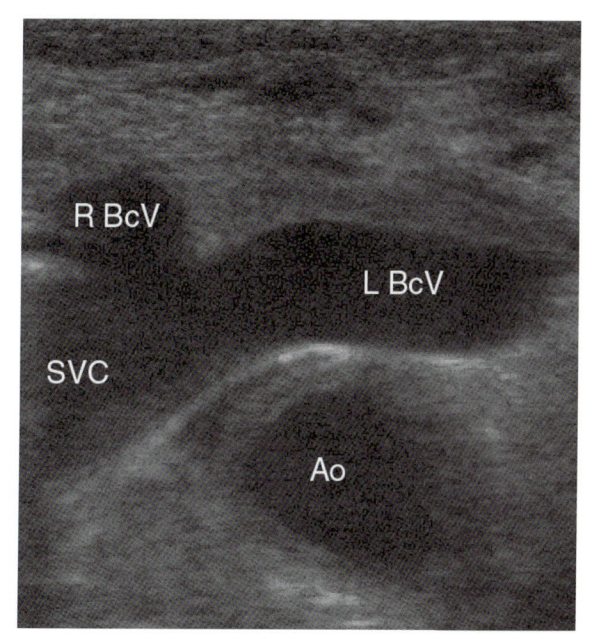

Figure 11.7 Brachiocephalic (innominate) venous access. Angled transverse suprasternal image of the anterior mediastinum. SVC = superior vena cava, Ao = aorta. The right (R BcV) and left (L BcV) brachiocephalic veins can be used for central venous access when they can be visualized with ultrasound. A thin strip of thymus lies anterior to the left brachiocephalic vein.

Upper limb veins are used for most peripherally inserted central venous catheters (PICCs). Ultrasound guidance allows puncture of the venae comitantes of the brachial artery (Fig. 11.9).[6] The use of superficial (cephalic and basilic) veins does not require image guidance and is easier in older children.

Because central venous access in children comprises mostly high volume, low complexity work, it is ideal for role extension for nurses and radiographers (radiologic technicians). Nurses now perform most PICC insertion procedures in many centers.

Venous interventions such as venous sampling, recanalization and stenting, vena cava filter insertion and transvenous biopsy (Fig. 11.10) are usually performed through jugular or femoral venous access. Transhepatic access to the portal venous system (Fig. 11.11) is necessary for pancreatic venous sampling, portal vein embolization or islet cell infusion.

Education of the patients and their carers in the maintenance of the catheters is essential in order to maintain good function and avoid complications such as infection or catheter thrombosis.

Complications

Complications associated with central venous access are twofold: procedural and delayed.

Procedural complications

Procedural complications are very unusual, but include:

- *pneumothorax* (due to puncture of the lung) probably occurs in less than 0.1% of jugular punctures and can generally be managed expectantly
- *arterial puncture* does not usually cause symptomatic complications if a small needle (e.g. 21-gauge) is used
- *air embolism* can be avoided by maintaining positive airway pressure at the time of inserting the catheter into the peel-away sheath
- *arrhythmias* are usually self-limiting
- *catheter malposition*.

Delayed complications

Delayed complications are not uncommon, and include:

- Infection is the most common complication, especially in immunocompromised children, and may be caused by skin organisms (such as *Staphylococcus epidermidis*), gut organisms or fungi. Systemic and local (tunnel or exit site) infections can be treated with antibiotics, but often it is necessary to remove the affected catheter or port. Catheters with more than one lumen may be more likely to become infected.
- Catheter tip thrombosis and fibrin sheath formation show an association with infection.
- Accidental removal of central venous catheters is not unusual, especially in small children.
- Embolism of a fragment of catheter (usually to a pulmonary artery) is rare. Percutaneous snaring and extraction with a transvenous approach is usually straightforward.

Table 11.2 Types of central venous access device

Device	Characteristics	Advantages	Disadvantages	Typical indications
Non-tunneled central venous catheter	Short, relatively stiff, usually multiple-lumen catheter	Ease of insertion	High infection rate	Short term intravenous therapy or pressure monitoring
Single lumen Hickman catheter	Relatively soft catheter	Relatively low infection rate	No possibility of coadministration of incompatible infusions	Total parenteral nutrition Low intensity chemotherapy (e.g. Wilms)
Multiple lumen Hickman catheter	Relatively soft catheter with two or three lumens	Coadministration of blood products, parenteral nutrition and drugs	Higher infection rate	Intensive chemotherapy protocols Bone marrow transplantation
Non-tunneled hemodialysis catheter	Large diameter catheter with offset lumens	Ease of insertion	Short life span Higher infection rate	Short term hemodialysis Plasmapheresis Stem cell harvest
Tunneled (permanent) hemodialysis catheter	Large diameter catheter with offset lumens	Long life span Low infection rate	Higher incidence of damage to vein	Long term hemodialysis
Central venous port device	Subcutaneous port with attached venous catheter	Even lower infection rate than Hickman catheter	Requires needle access Longer scar than Hickman catheter	Chemotherapy Conditions requiring regular transfusions of blood products (e.g. hemophilia) or antibiotics (e.g. cystic fibrosis)
Peripherally inserted central venous catheter	Small caliber soft catheter with one or two lumens	Safe insertion without general anesthetic	Higher catheter occlusion rate	Short to medium term access (e.g. for antibiotic therapy)

- Catheter migration into a non-central vein (such as the azygos vein) may cause malfunction or thrombophlebitis.

Recent advances in imaging and, in particular the growth of interventional radiology as a specialty, mean that central venous access and catheters are now a routine part of the interventionalist's workload. The success rate is probably highest and complication rate lowest when imaging guidance is used for central venous access.

BIOPSY

Percutaneous biopsy in children is usually performed with semi-automatic core needles. These needles have a cutting tip that can be advanced to expose a slot into which tissue can be trapped by an outer cutting sleeve that advances when the needle is fired. Fine needle aspiration cytology is sometimes used in the diagnosis of pediatric tumors[7] but requires specialized cytology expertise and may not provide a sufficient quantity of tumor cells for necessary biological tests.

Renal biopsy

Renal biopsy can be performed under GA or with sedation or Entonox. Either kidney can be biopsied. Although the prone position is often used, it is usually easier to place the patient in a lateral position. This

PEDIATRIC INTERVENTIONAL ULTRASOUND 331

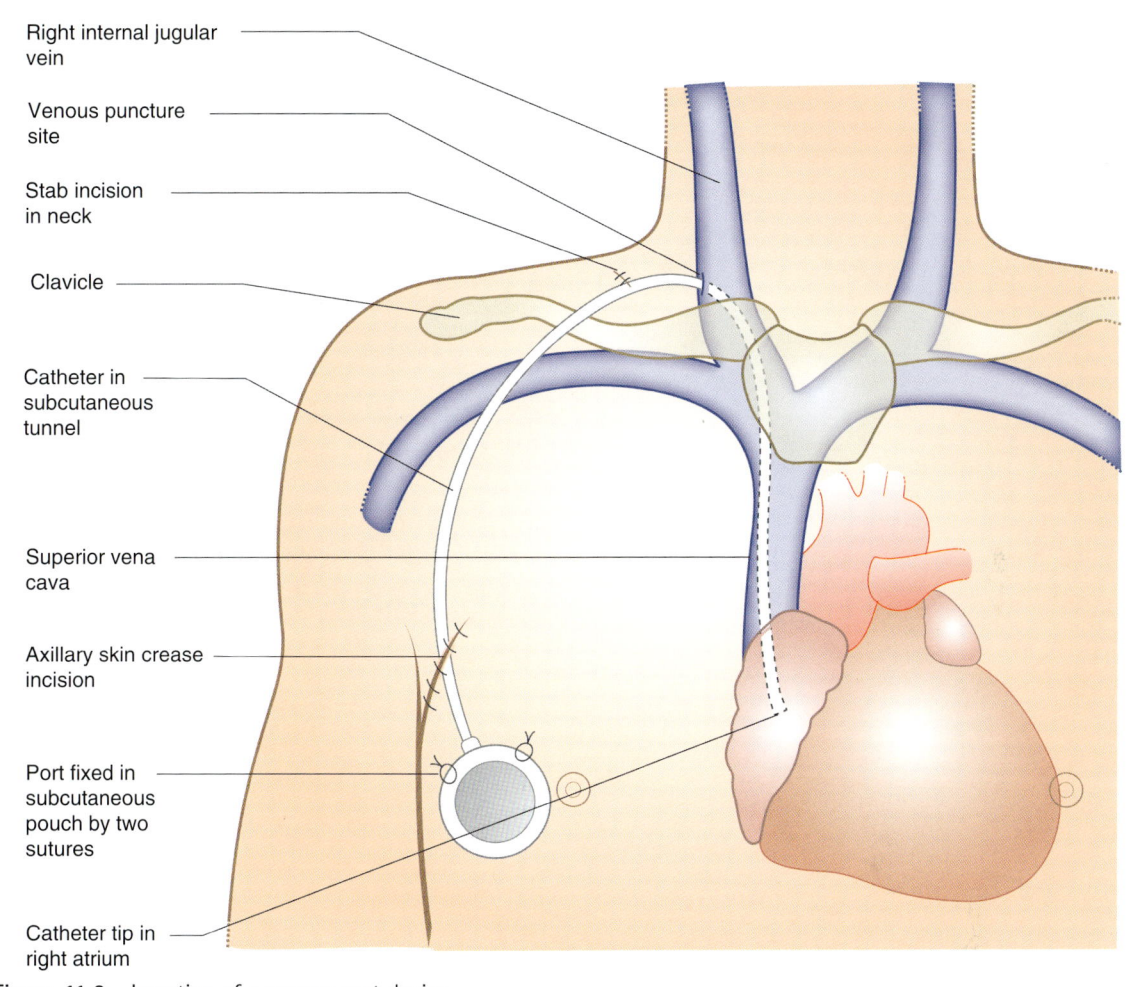

Figure 11.8 Insertion of a venous port device.

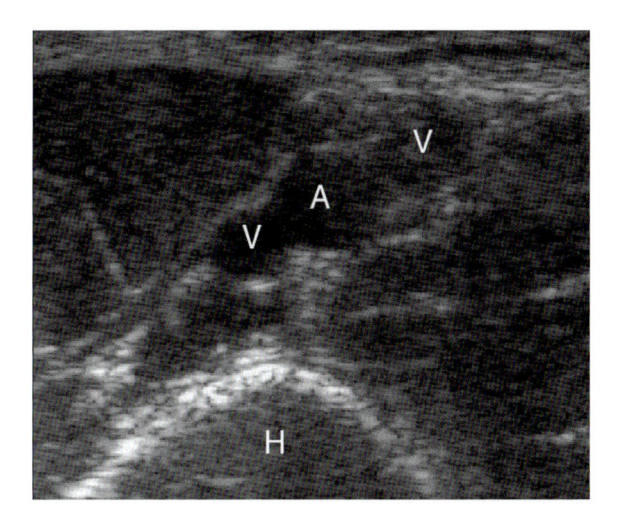

Figure 11.9 Catheterization of venae comitantes. Transverse image of the anterior upper arm. The brachial artery (A) is flanked by its venae comitantes (V), which are useful for peripherally inserted central venous catheters. The humeral shaft (H) lies posteriorly.

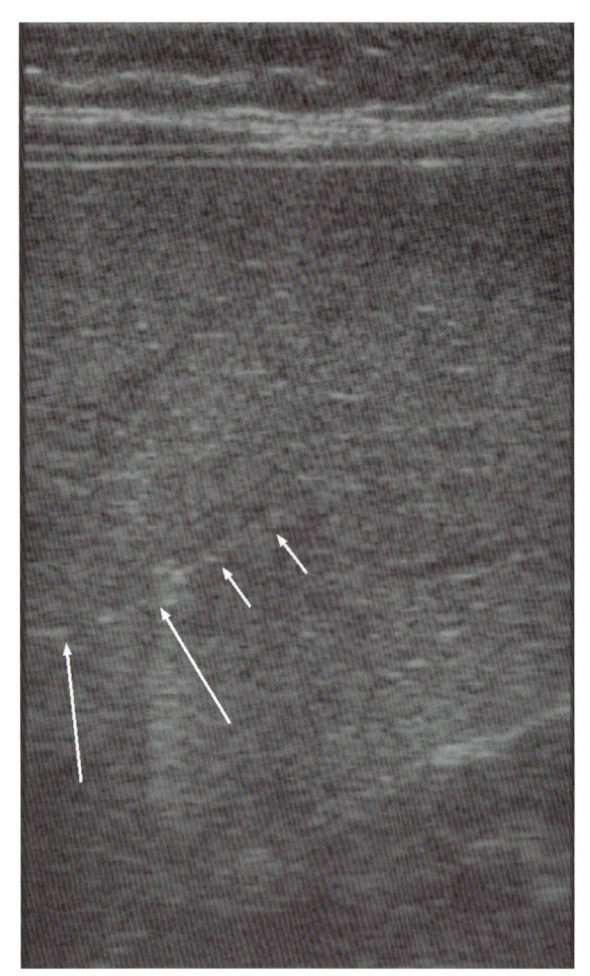

Figure 11.10 Transhepatic biopsy. Oblique sagittal image of the liver. Transjugular biopsy of the liver is achieved by advancing a core biopsy needle (short arrows) into the liver parenchyma through a curved vascular sheath (long arrows).

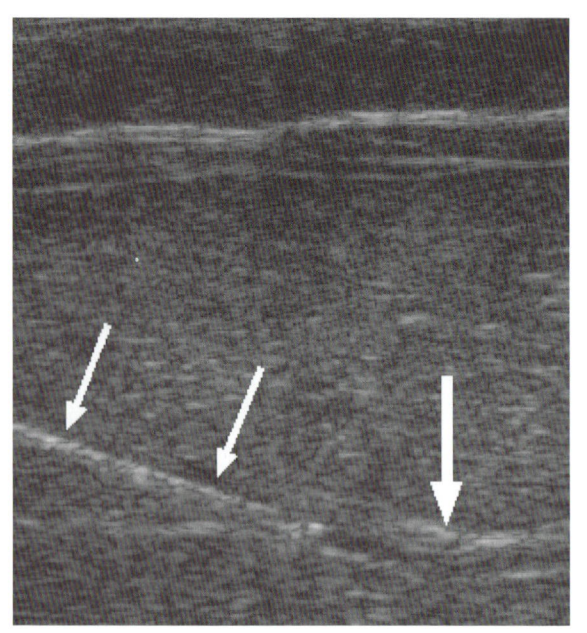

Figure 11.11 Transhepatic access to portal vein. Oblique transverse image of the right lobe of the liver. Transhepatic access to the portal venous system is achieved by puncturing the right portal vein (large arrow) with a 21-gauge needle (small arrows).

makes the use of Entonox simpler or, if GA is preferred, means that endotracheal intubation will not be required. It is necessary to place a large pad under the patient's abdomen to make the side to be biopsied convex. Renal transplant biopsy is performed in the supine position, and does not usually require GA.

The intended biopsy tract is infiltrated with local anesthetic down to the level of the renal capsule. In our center we use 16-gauge semi-automatic core biopsy needles. The needle is inserted through a stab incision. If able to cooperate, the child is asked to hold his or her breath as the needle is inserted into the kidney and the biopsy taken (Fig. 11.12).

Suspension of breathing is not necessary for safe renal biopsy, however, and the anesthesiologist may prefer to allow the patient to breathe spontaneously.

We ask a pathology technician to examine the core to confirm that sufficient glomeruli are present. If not, another core is taken. This technique should be sufficient to ensure that 99% of biopsies have a definitive histological report.[8] The complication rate is very low. Significant complications, such as hematuria requiring transfusion and injury to other organs, should occur in < 1% of biopsies.[8]

Liver biopsy

Percutaneous liver biopsy can be performed by several techniques. The old method of blind biopsy is obsolescent, and it would now be difficult to justify a randomized trial comparing liver biopsy performed with and without ultrasound guidance. In any case, imaging guidance is necessary for biopsy of small focal lesions. It is extremely unusual (< 1% of cases) for ultrasound to be inadequate for biopsy of focal liver lesions in children (Fig. 11.13).

PEDIATRIC INTERVENTIONAL ULTRASOUND   333

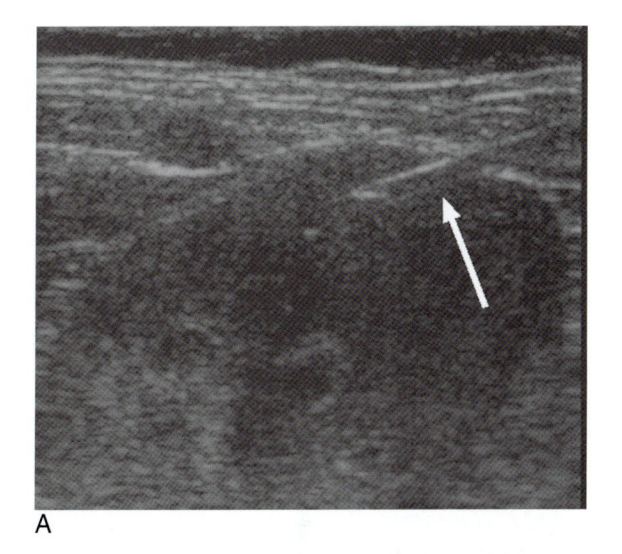

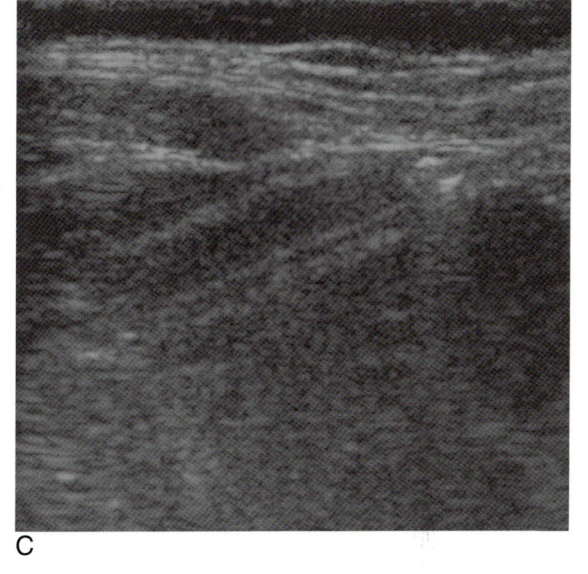

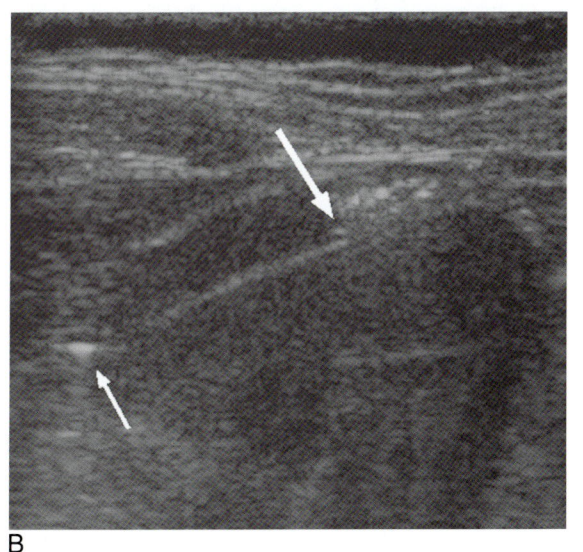

Figure 11.12 Renal biopsy. (A) The core biopsy needle is seen entering the lower pole of the kidney, angled to sample predominantly cortex. (B) The tip (small arrow) is advanced, exposing a slot between it and the tip of the outer cutting sleeve (large arrow). (C) The needle is fired, and the cutting sleeve advances rapidly, trapping a core of tissue in the slot.

We use a coaxial technique with a 17-gauge outer needle and 18-gauge biopsy needle. A safe biopsy tract is selected, and the outer needle is advanced into the liver. A subcostal approach is preferred where possible to reduce the risks of pneumothorax or hemothorax.[9] The trocar is then removed and replaced with the biopsy needle, which is used to take several biopsy cores. When sufficient tissue has been obtained, gelatine foam plugs are injected to prevent bleeding from the liver. A slurry of collagen is an alternative to gelatine foam.[9]

The main potential complication is intraperitoneal bleeding. Bleeding of sufficient severity to require blood transfusion, embolization or emergency surgery should occur in less than 1% of children with normal coagulation parameters.[9,10] It is more common in children with coagulopathy or thrombocytopenia, or who have undergone bone marrow transplantation.[10,11] Transjugular biopsy has been adopted in these patients to try to reduce the risk of postbiopsy bleeding.[9] It should be noted, however, that delayed intraperitoneal

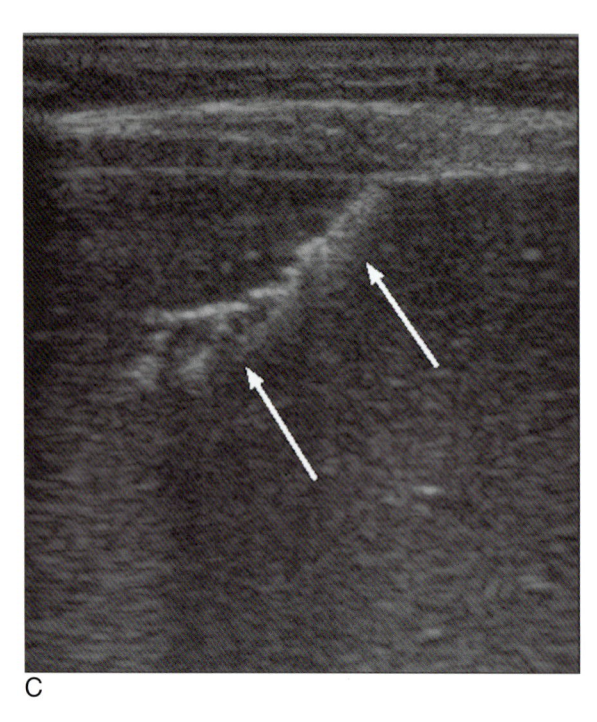

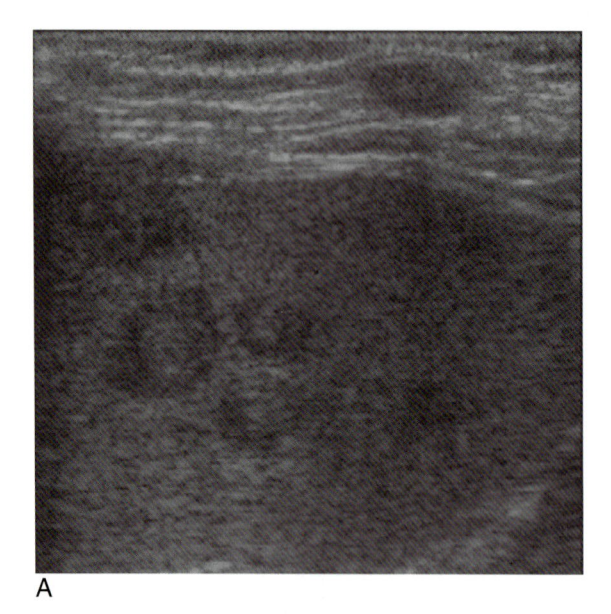

Figure 11.13 Liver biopsy. (A) Oblique image in a child with acute lymphoblastic leukemia and disseminated fungal infection shows multiple liver lesions. (B) The biopsy needle has been inserted through the outer coaxial needle (arrowhead) and through one of the lesions (arrows). (C) The biopsy tract (arrows) has been plugged with gelatine foam plugs.

hemorrhage has been reported following transjugular liver biopsy. Overall mortality for percutaneous liver biopsy is less than 1%.[9,12]

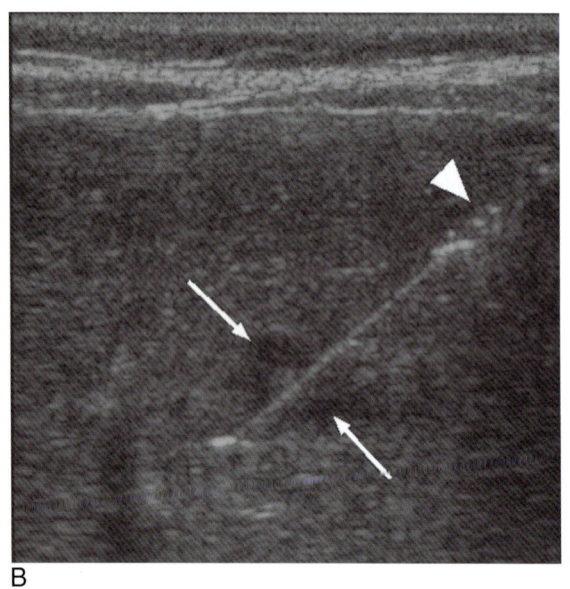

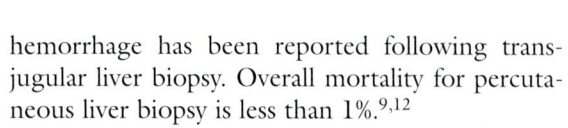

Biopsy of other organs

It is possible to biopsy most other organs and tissues with ultrasound guidance. In our practice, the most common are lymph node, bone, soft tissue and spleen.[13] Peripheral lung lesions may also be biopsied using ultrasound guidance.

Tumor biopsy

At our center, almost all tumors outside the central nervous system are diagnosed by ultrasound-guided needle biopsy (Box 11.3). In addition to the more familiar abdominal biopsies, we biopsy tumors in the thorax, head, neck and limbs. This approach has several advantages over open biopsy. It is less invasive than and, perhaps surprisingly, apparently equally accurate to open (surgical) biopsy. The period of convalescence is shorter, and

> **Box 11.3 Ultrasound-guided tumor biopsy in children**
>
> Neuroblastoma
> Renal tumors
> —Wilms tumor
> —other renal tumors
> Lymphoma
> —non-Hodgkin lymphoma
> —Hodgkin lymphoma
> Soft tissue tumors
> —rhabdomyosarcoma
> —peripheral primitive neuroectodermal tumor
> —other soft tissue tumors
> Liver tumors
> Germ cell tumors
> Other abdominal and thoracic tumors

this may allow earlier commencement of chemotherapy. In most patients at our hospital, ultrasound-guided tumor biopsy is performed at the same GA as insertion of a central venous access device and, where appropriate, bone marrow aspiration and trephines.

Although the technique is very accurate in the diagnosis of most tumor types, there may be problems making the diagnosis of Hodgkin lymphoma on needle biopsies alone. Needle biopsy of pediatric tumors is less often performed in North America, where protocols for most common tumors require a surgical approach at diagnosis.

Tumor biopsy can also be performed with a coaxial technique. This means that numerous cores of tissue can be obtained, but the tumor capsule is only punctured once. Plugging the tumor biopsy tract may have the added advantage of preventing seeding of malignant cells.

ASPIRATION AND DRAINAGE OF FLUID COLLECTIONS

Most radiological aspiration and drainage is required for abdominal and pelvic abscesses (Fig. 11.14), pleural effusion (Fig. 11.15) and empyema and pericardial effusions.[14] In children, most aspirations can be performed with ultrasound guidance. Pelvic

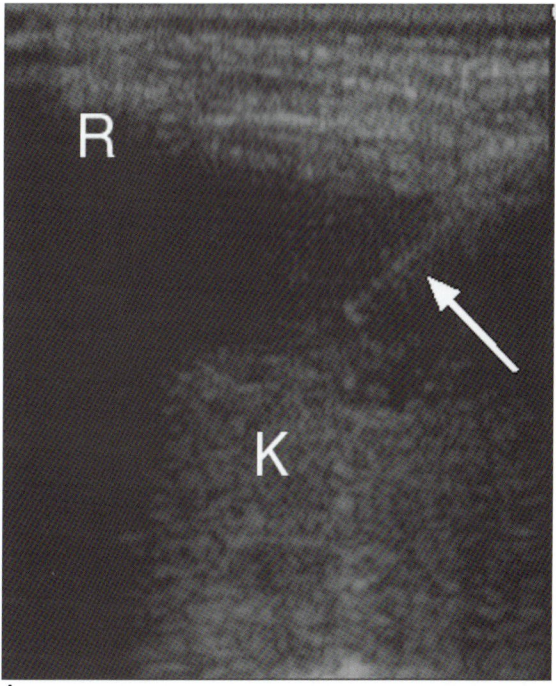

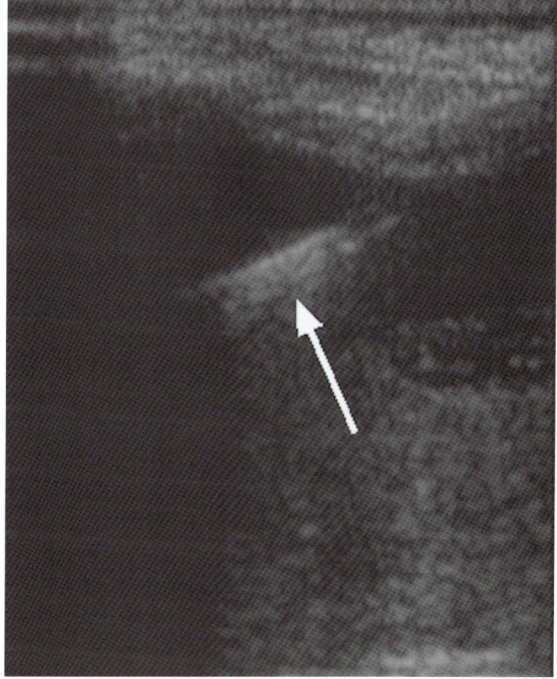

Figure 11.14 Perirenal collection. (A) A needle (arrow) has been inserted into a perinephric abscess surrounding the right kidney (K). Note the acoustic shadowing from the 12th rib (R). (B) A guidewire (arrow) has been inserted through the needle.
Continued

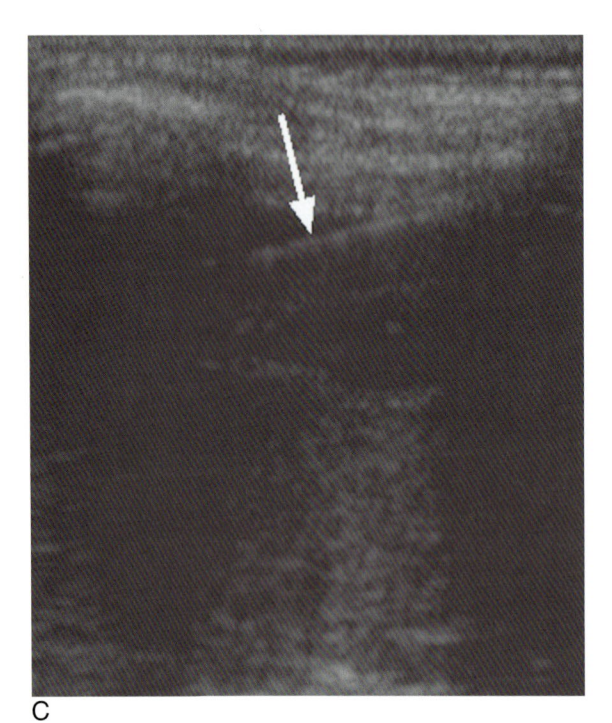

Figure 11.14, cont'd (C) Following dilation of the tract, a 12-French pigtail drainage catheter (arrow) has been advanced into the collection over the guidewire.

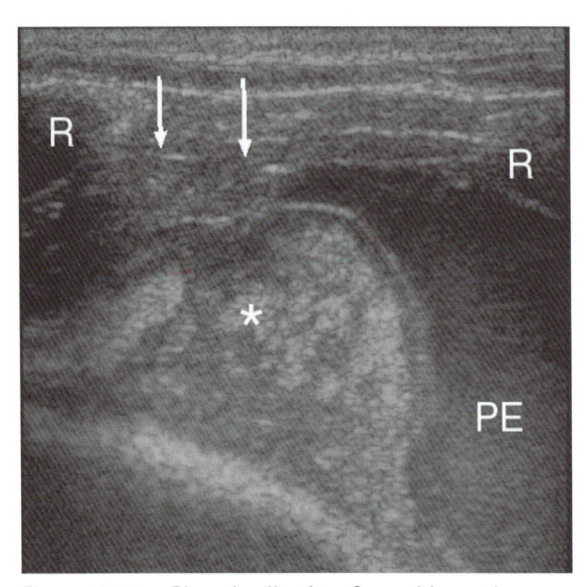

Figure 11.15 Pleural collection. Coronal image in a child with lymphoblastic lymphoma shows a malignant pleural effusion (PE), with a small mass on the parietal pleura (arrows) and a large mass on the mediastinal pleura (*). The effusion was drained following intercostal puncture and biopsy of the parietal pleural mass.

collections can be approached through the anterior abdominal wall, vagina or rectum, or from the buttock. In principle, ultrasound guidance can be used to aspirate fluid collections almost anywhere in the body. In infants, intracranial abscesses can be aspirated through the anterior fontanelle.

Drainage procedures usually require ultrasound-guided puncture of the fluid collection, followed by guidewire insertion and positioning of a drainage catheter. The latter stages can be performed with ultrasound or fluoroscopic guidance as appropriate. The use of ultrasound throughout has the advantage that the procedure can be carried out at the bedside or in the intensive care unit.

SCLEROTHERAPY OF VASCULAR MALFORMATIONS

Vascular anomalies may be classified as vascular tumors (such as hemangioma) or vascular malformations. The most common vascular malformations seen in children are venous and lymphatic.

Venous malformations

Venous malformations contain spongy spaces of varying size, filled with stagnant blood. They are most frequently seen in the lower limbs, face and upper limbs. In the lower limb these malformations may bleed into the knee joint and cause premature arthritis. Venous malformations are suitable for sclerotherapy with agents such as sodium tetradecyl sulfate[15] or ethanol.[16] The purpose of sclerotherapy is to reduce the size of the malformation in order to give symptomatic relief. There may also be some cosmetic improvement following treatment.

Following ultrasound-guided placement of one or two needles in the lesion, radiographic contrast can be injected to confirm the nature of the malformation and identify its pattern of venous drainage. During injection, connections with normal deep veins may be temporarily occluded by external pressure.

Cystic lymphatic malformations

Cystic lymphatic malformations ('cystic hygromas') appear to be the result of abnormal develop-

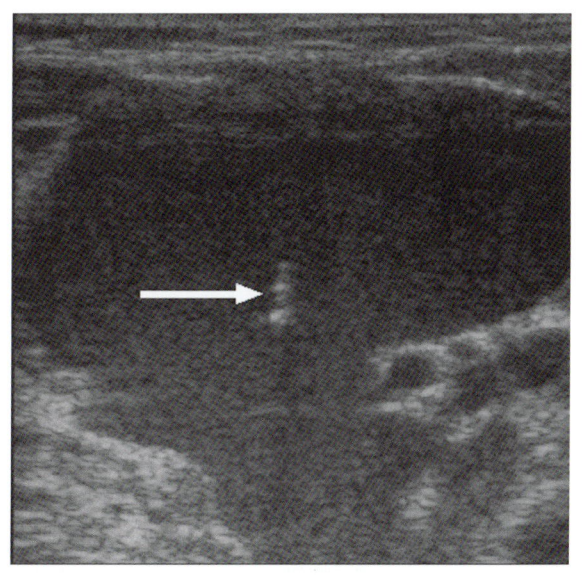

Figure 11.16 Sclerotherapy of a cystic lymphatic malformation of the neck. Transverse image shows a large cystic lesion containing dependent low-level echoes. This is common, and corresponds to intracystic hemorrhage. A needle tip (arrow) is seen within the cyst.

laxis is usually given.[19] The nephrostomy tract can be used for other interventions such as antegrade ureteric stenting or percutaneous stone removal.

The most common indications for nephrostomy in children are congenital and postoperative obstruction.[20] Local anesthetic is infiltrated as for renal biopsy. When the collecting system is dilated it can usually be punctured easily with a single pass of a needle (Fig. 11.17). Various needle systems are available for nephrostomy. I prefer to use a trocar needle (18- or 20-gauge) because when the trocar is removed the outer part of the needle has a blunt tip, which is unlikely to damage the collecting system. Following aspiration of urine for culture, contrast may be injected to assess the level and degree of obstruction. A guidewire is then inserted and its tip coiled in the renal pelvis. A locking pigtail catheter can

ment of the lymphatic system. Various agents have been used to sclerose these lesions, either as definitive treatment or to reduce their size before surgical excision. The most popular are currently bleomycin, picibanil (OK432)[17] and ethanol, or preparations including ethanol, such as Ethibloc.[18] Most of these lesions are located in the face and neck (Fig. 11.16). Even when the lesion is palpable, ultrasound guidance is useful to ensure that the sclerosant is injected entirely into the lesion and to treat separate locules, which are not uncommon.

UROLOGICAL INTERVENTION

Urological interventions are based on nephrostomy (Fig. 11.17), which is usually a simple procedure in children. The patient can be placed in the lateral position, as for renal biopsy (see above), although for bilateral nephrostomy it is probably better to perform the procedure with the patient prone, under GA with endotracheal intubation. Intravenous antibiotic prophy-

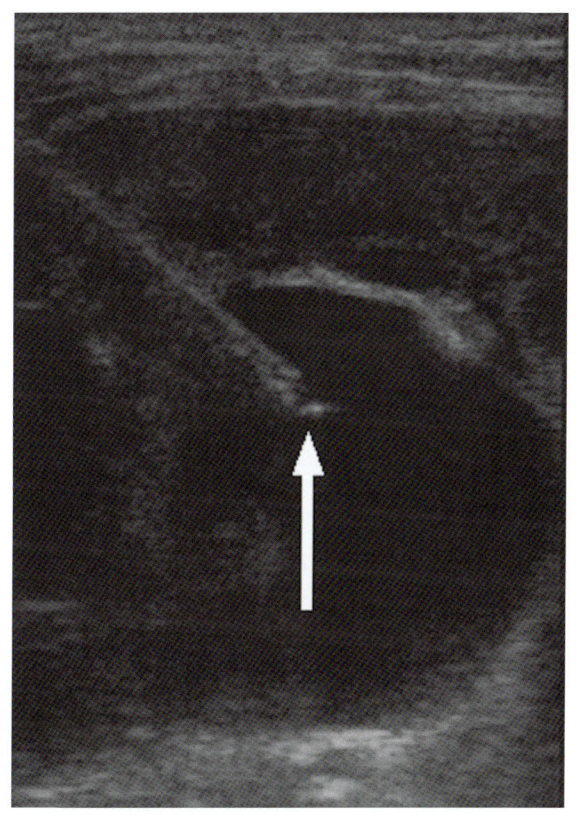

Figure 11.17 Nephrostomy. The dilated pelvicaliceal system has been punctured with an 18-gauge trocar needle (arrow).

then be inserted over a stiffener. When the collecting system is not dilated, a coaxial access set may be used. This allows puncture to be performed with a 21-gauge needle. A 0.018-inch guidewire is inserted, and then exchanged for a 0.035-inch wire after insertion of a two part coaxial dilator.

OTHER ULTRASOUND-GUIDED INTERVENTION

Arterial access

Arterial access in small children is not always straightforward. I now use ultrasound guidance for

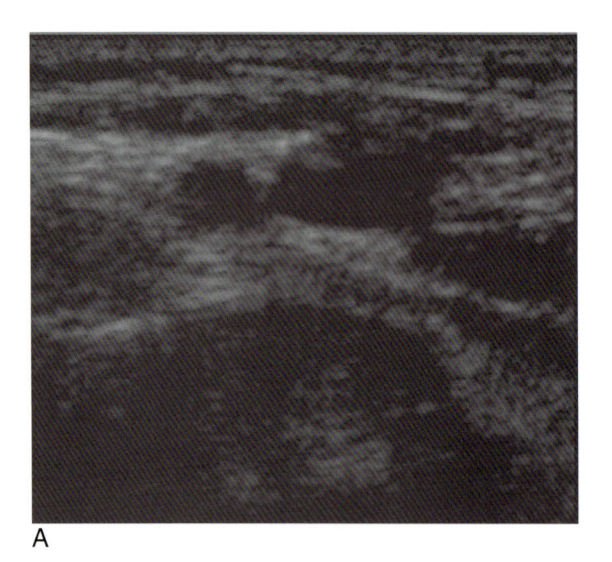

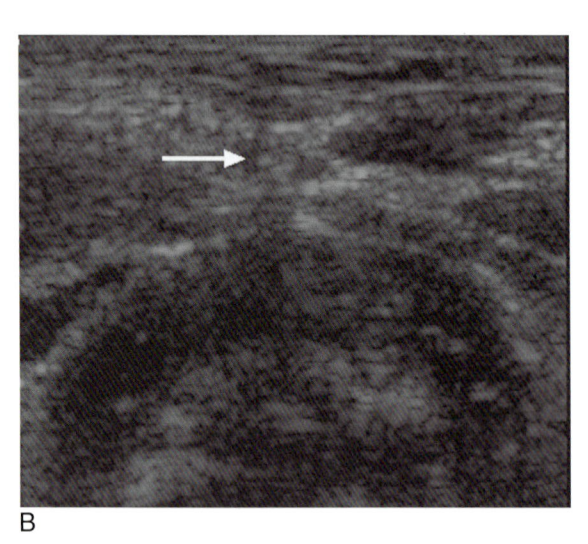

Figure 11.18 Arterial puncture in a 6-month-old child. (A) The femoral artery and vein are shown in a slightly oblique transverse section. (B) The needle tip (arrow) is compressing the common femoral artery. The needle is then advanced abruptly to puncture the artery. The femoral head is seen posteriorly, and this confirms that the puncture is being made in the correct position.

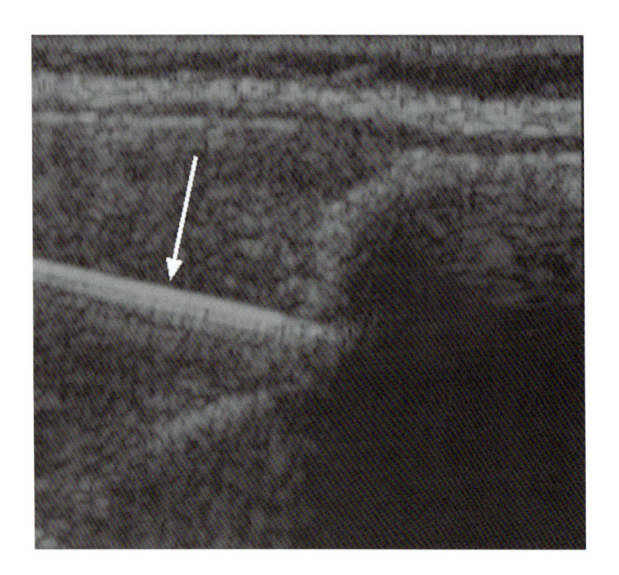

Figure 11.19 Transhepatic puncture of the gallbladder. A 22-gauge needle (arrow) has been advanced through the liver and is about to puncture the gallbladder.

all arterial punctures. This technique makes femoral arterial punctures much easier (Fig. 11.18) and can be adapted for puncture at other sites (e.g. the axillary artery).

Biliary intervention

Diagnostic percutaneous transhepatic cholangiography (PTC) is rarely required in children. One indication is sclerosing cholangitis (seen most often in children with Langerhans cell histiocytosis at our center), when PTC can be performed at the same time as liver biopsy. When the intrahepatic bile ducts are not dilated, the simplest method is to puncture the gallbladder under ultrasound guidance (Fig. 11.19).

PTC with or without biliary drainage or balloon dilation of biliary strictures may also be required following liver transplantation.[21,22] Although malignant obstructive jaundice is unusual in children, it may also require biliary drainage.[23] In these circumstances, ultrasound-guided puncture of a dilated intrahepatic duct is usually easy.

References

1. Roebuck DJ. Interventional radiology in children. Imaging 2001; 13:302–320.
2. Kaye RD, Sane SS, Towbin RB. Pediatric intervention: an update—part I. J Vasc Interv Radiol 2000; 11:683–697.
3. Azizkhan RG, Taylor LA, Jaques PF, et al. Percutaneous translumbar and transhepatic inferior vena caval catheters for prolonged vascular access in children. J Pediatr Surg 1992; 27:165–169.
4. Bergey EA, Kaye RD, Reyes J, et al. Transhepatic insertion of vascular dialysis catheters in children: a safe, life-prolonging procedure. Pediatr Radiol 1999; 29:42–45.
5. Robertson LJ, Jaques PF, Mauro MA, et al. Percutaneous inferior vena cava placement of tunneled silastic catheters for prolonged vascular access in infants. J Pediatr Surg 1990; 25:596–598.
6. Donaldson JS, Morello FP, Junewick JJ, et al. Peripherally inserted central venous catheters: US-guided vascular access in pediatric patients. Radiology 1995; 197:542–544.
7. Hugosson CO, Nyman RS, Cappelen-Smith JM, et al. Ultrasound-guided biopsy of abdominal and pelvic lesions in children: a comparison between fine-needle aspiration and 1.2 mm-needle core biopsy. Pediatr Radiol 1999; 29:31–36.
8. Webb NJ, Pereira JK, Chait PG, et al. Renal biopsy in children: comparison of two techniques. Pediatr Nephrol 1994; 8:486–488.
9. Hoffer FA. Liver biopsy methods for pediatric oncology patients. Pediatr Radiol 2000; 30:481–488.
10. Lachaux A, Le Gall C, Chambon M, et al. Complications of percutaneous liver biopsy in infants and children. Eur J Pediatr 1995; 154:621–623.
11. Cohen MB, A-Kader HH, Lambers D, et al. Complications of percutaneous liver biopsy in children. Gastroenterology 1992; 102:629–632.
12. Scheimann AO, Barrios JM, Al-Tawil YS, et al. Percutaneous liver biopsy in children: impact of ultrasonography and spring-loaded biopsy needles. J Pediatr Gastroenterol Nutr 2000; 31:536–539.
13. Muraca S, Chait PG, Connolly BL, et al. US-guided core biopsy of the spleen in children. Radiology 2001; 218:200–206.
14. Towbin RB, Strife JL. Percutaneous aspiration, drainage, and biopsies in children. Radiology 1985; 157:81–85.
15. O'Donovan JC, Donaldson JS, Morello FP, et al. Symptomatic hemangiomas and venous malformations in infants, children, and young adults: treatment with percutaneous injection of sodium tetradecyl sulfate. AJR Am J Roentgenol 1997; 169: 723–729.
16. Yakes WF. Extremity venous malformations: diagnosis and management. Semin Interv Radiol 1994; 11:332–339.
17. Ogita S, Tsuto T, Deguchi E, et al. OK–432 therapy for unresectable lymphangiomas in children. J Pediatr Surg 1991; 26:263–270.
18. Dubois J, Garel L, Abela A, et al. Lymphangiomas in children: percutaneous sclerotherapy with an alcoholic solution of zein. Radiology 1997; 204:651–654.
19. Hogan MJ, Coley BD, Jayanthi VR, et al. Percutaneous nephrostomy in children and adolescents: outpatient management. Radiology 2001; 218:207–210.
20. Laurin S, Sandström S, Ivarsson H. Percutaneous nephrostomy in infants and children. Acad Radiol 2000; 7:526–529.
21. Lorenz JM, Funaki B, Leef JA, et al. Percutaneous transhepatic cholangiography and biliary drainage in pediatric liver transplant patients. AJR Am J Roentgenol 2001; 176:761–765.

22. Khong PL, Sreeram N, John PR. Metallic stenting of the biliary tree following liver transplant hepatic artery thrombosis in an infant. Pediatr Radiol 1997; 27:79–81.

23. Roebuck DJ, Stanley P. External and internal-external biliary drainage in children with malignant obstructive jaundice. Pediatr Radiol 2000; 30:659–664.

Chapter 12

The chest

CHAPTER CONTENTS

Technique of ultrasound examination   341
Juxtadiaphragmatic lesions   342
   Masses arising in the chest   343
   Diaphragmatic hernias   345
   Masses arising from the diaphragm   347
The mediastinum   347
   The thymus   347
   Lymphadenopathy   348
The opaque hemithorax   348
   Lung abnormalities   348
   Pleural fluid   349
Congenital cysts   350

Ultrasound of the pediatric chest is an area often neglected because of the presence of air in the lungs and the difficulty which the bony rib cage poses to access. However, as a result of the smaller footprint and higher resolution of modern equipment, there are a number of chest conditions where ultrasound can be usefully used in children. While CT and MRI are still considered the techniques for evaluating the chest, ultrasound has a definite and useful role in certain circumstances. In particular, ultrasound is most useful in the remote intensive care situation where children are often too ill and unstable to be moved to a scanner.[1]

TECHNIQUE OF ULTRASOUND EXAMINATION

All patients should be examined in the knowledge of what the chest radiograph shows and the exact clinical question to be answered. Always look at the chest radiograph before starting the ultrasound examination.

Depending on the location of the abnormality, different approaches can be used (Fig. 12.1).

Patients with superior mediastinal abnormalities can be examined from the supraclavicular or suprasternal notch. This can be achieved by positioning the patient's shoulders on a pillow to help extend the neck for better access.

For juxtadiaphragmatic lesions the abdominal approach is best, with particular views of the diaphragm using the transdiaphragmatic and subxiphisternum views. Use a curvilinear transducer

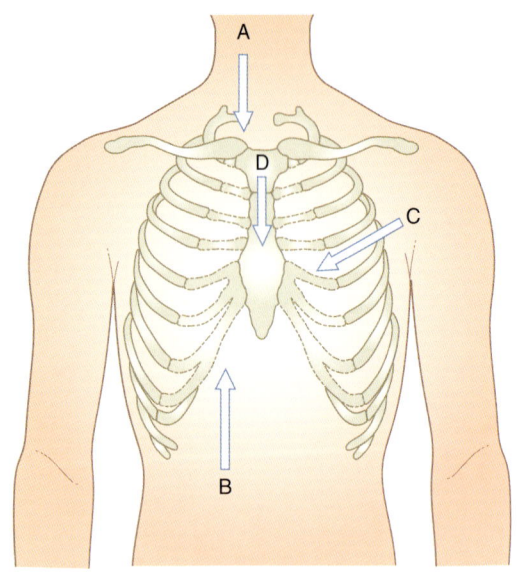

Figure 12.1 Windows of access to the chest and thoracic cavity. The chest can be examined superiorly from the suprasternal notch, the supraclavicular approach (A). It can be examined inferiorly by the subcostal or sub-xiphisternum approach (B). For masses within the thoracic cage it can be examined by an intercostal approach (C). Mediastinal masses can be examined by a sternal or parasternal approach (D).

Doppler and color flow imaging must be used in all lesions next to the diaphragm. In particular when assessing for suspected pulmonary sequestration, anomalous feeding vessels may be demonstrated arising from the aorta in the abdomen.

Mass lesions in the chest are usually described according to their location either in the anterior, middle or posterior mediastinum[3] (Fig. 12.2). Box 12.1 gives a differential diagnosis of the more common masses seen in children and where they lie in the mediastinum.

JUXTADIAPHRAGMATIC LESIONS

Lesions next to the diaphragm, whether they be anterior or posterior, should be scanned with a sub-xiphoid or transdiaphragmatic approach.

Lesions will fall into three broad groups:

- those arising in the chest
- those arising in the abdomen and herniating into the chest
- those arising from the diaphragm.

with the liver or spleen as an acoustic window. When examining any juxtadiaphragmatic mass the upper abdomen must be carefully examined as well, in particular the liver, spleen and kidneys in case of herniation. Pathology in the liver parenchyma, such as an abscess, may cause a sympathetic effusion in the chest.

Intrathoracic pathology is best examined using the intercostal and parasternal approaches. The posterior chest must always be examined in suspected pleural effusions, as fluid tends to accumulate posteriorly as the patient lies supine in bed.[2]

High frequency linear and curvilinear probes are generally the best as fluid collections are superficial and will not be appreciated if a small footprint vector scanner is used. A small footprint vector transducer can be useful for access but causes distortion of the near field image. Generally speaking the choice of frequency and transducer will depend on the position of the lesion and the age of the patient.

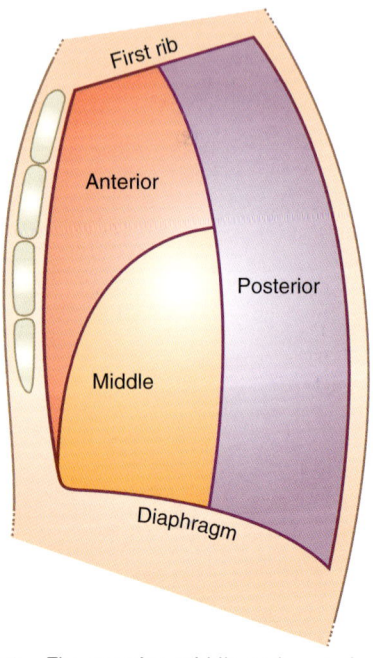

Figure 12.2 The anterior, middle and posterior mediastinum. Box 12.1 gives a differential diagnosis of masses in these three regions.

Box 12.1 Causes of mediastinal masses

Anterior
- Thymus, e.g. normal, cysts, hemorrhage
- Teratoma, teratodermoid
- Lymphadenopathy, e.g. lymphoma
- Cysts, e.g. cystic hygroma
- Thyroid, e.g. ectopic
- Vascular, e.g. aorta or SVC

Middle
- Diaphragmatic hernias, e.g. Morgagni
- Bronchogenic cysts
- Lymphadenopathy, e.g. TB
- Neurenteric cyst
- Duplication cyst of the esophagus
- Extralobar sequestration

Posterior
- Neurogenic tumors: neuroblastoma, ganglioneuroma
- Neurenteric cysts
- Lateral meningocele
- Bochdalek hernias
- Herniation of kidney
- Extralobar sequestration

SVC, superior vena cava.

Masses arising in the chest

The clue to the potential diagnosis will usually lie on the appearances on the chest radiograph and the clinical presentation. The contour of the mass and whether it is lying anterior or posterior in the chest is important in the differential diagnosis.[4]

Neurogenic tumors

These arise posteriorly along the sympathetic chain, are often incidental findings and are usually ganglioneuromas. They are usually well defined, clearly posterior and hyperechoic, often containing small granular calcification. There may be associated rib erosions on the chest radiograph. Posterior mediastinal masses are almost always neurogenic in origin, and if the patient is young can be turned prone and a spinal examination undertaken to look for spinal extension. Neuroblastoma is the malignant form of neurogenic tumor, and intraspinal extension must be sought.

Ultrasound is particularly useful to help differentiate lateral intrathoracic meningoceles from solid masses.

Neurenteric cysts

Neurenteric cysts are essentially cysts of bowel that have failed to separate from the neural canal during development. On the chest radiograph there may be a spinal abnormality, and usually this is higher than the lesion (Fig. 12.3). On ultrasound the neurenteric cyst has a well-defined border with a thin wall similar to a duplication cyst of the bowel. It may be completely hypoechoic or, if infection or hemorrhage has occurred, the cyst may contain cellular debris due to blood, mucus or white cells.

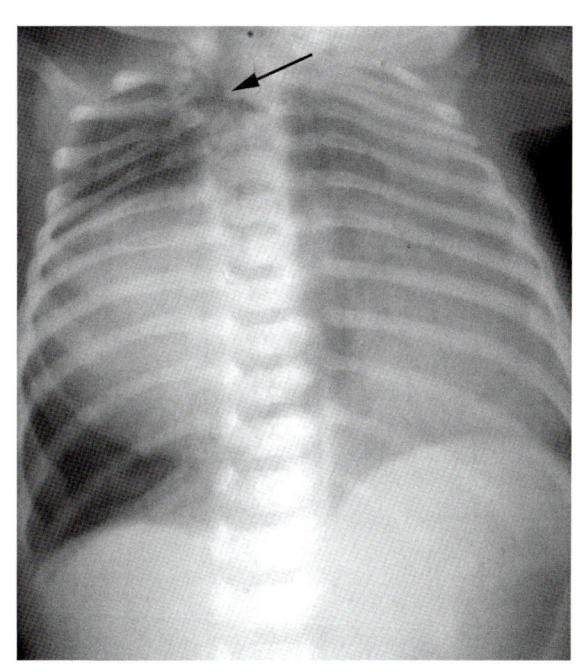

Figure 12.3 Neurenteric cyst. Chest radiograph on a child with a mass in the right chest. There is a well-defined oval mass in the right chest with displacement of the heart to the left. There are multiple abnormal ribs and a spinal abnormality higher than the mass. These are the typical appearances of a neurenteric cyst with a spinal deformity higher than the mass (arrow).

Pulmonary sequestration

Also called a bronchopulmonary foregut malformation, pulmonary sequestration refers to a segment of lung which does not function, has an anomalous arterial blood supply from the systemic circulation and has no communication with the tracheobronchial tree. It is due to a developmental abnormality in which there is an accessory tracheobronchial foregut bud.[5]

The majority are diagnosed in children with a typical clinical presentation of a lower lobe consolidation that never clears completely. If infected and communication with the bronchial tree occurs, there may be multiple fluid levels on the chest radiograph. There are two types of sequestration: the intralobar form and the extralobar form which is more common in infants and children.

Extralobar sequestration This type of sequestration occurs more commonly in neonatal males and is four times more common on the left. In over 60% there are associated anomalies, the most common of which is a defect in the diaphragm and cystic adenomatoid malformation of the lungs. Many are asymptomatic in the neonatal period and often only diagnosed by antenatal detection. Some may be found below the left hemidiaphragm, and the differential diagnosis is an antenatal neuroblastoma as both may appear solid and highly echogenic. The main difference on ultrasound is that in extralobar sequestration the left adrenal can be seen separately and an abnormal arterial vascular supply may be detected from the aorta.

Intralobar sequestration This is different to extralobar sequestration in that the abnormal lung is enclosed in the visceral pleura of the affected lobe. These usually present in the older age group, often young adults.

Ultrasound appearances A diagnosis will generally be suspected on a chest radiograph, and the role of ultrasound is to demonstrate the anomalous blood supply which will confirm the diagnosis (Fig. 12.4). The upper abdomen must be carefully examined, with particular attention paid to the upper aorta and IVC and any abnormal vasculature

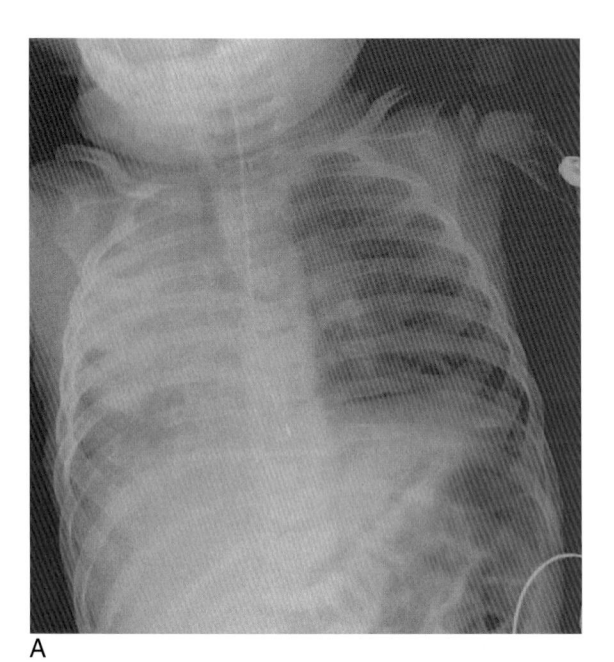

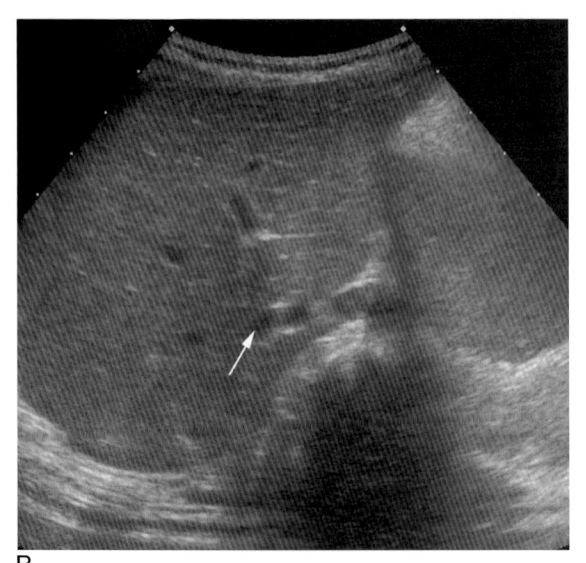

Figure 12.4 Sequestration. (A) This radiograph on a young child shows the mediastinum and heart shadow displaced to the right. The right hemithorax appears opaque with some aeration at the right base. The clinical question was whether this appearance was due to a hypoplastic lung on the right with a sequestrated segment. (B) Ultrasound examination was performed to look for an anomalous blood vessel supplying the sequestrated segment. This is a transverse sonogram of the upper abdomen showing a second vessel next to the inferior vena cava (arrow).

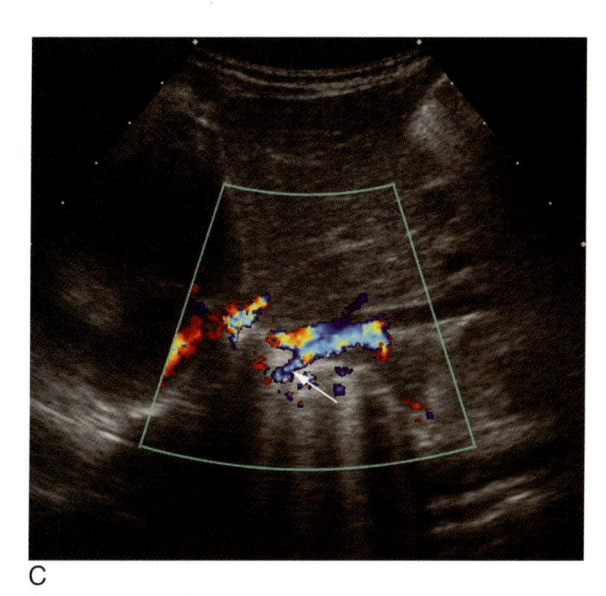

Figure 12.4, cont'd (C) Longitudinal sonogram with Doppler showing the IVC and a second anomalous vessel which was leading up to the sequestrated segment at the right base of the lung. Ultrasound is an excellent modality for detecting these anomalous vessels.

on Doppler examination. The systemic or arterial supply is usually from the distal thoracic or upper abdominal aorta. The abnormal venous drainage is via the pulmonary veins. The lung on that side may be hypoplastic with a small hemithorax and shift of the mediastinum.

The appearance of sequestrated segments is variable depending on their communication with the bronchial tree and whether infection and abscess formation has occurred. If there is no communication with the bronchial tree, sequestrated segments will appear solid and are usually close to the hemidiaphragm. They rarely occur in the upper lobe and are usually in the posterior basal segment of the lower lobe. Further investigation will include MRI and angiography in order to embolize the sequestrated segment.

Cystic adenomatoid malformation

Cystic adenomatoid malformations (CAM) of the lung are commonly diagnosed prenatally (see Ch. 2) or in the early neonatal period on the basis of respiratory distress. They are congenital hamartomatous lesions of the lung resulting in a mass of disorganized lung tissue. They normally communicate with the bronchial tree and on chest radiograph appear as multiple cysts.

Ultrasound plays little role in these lesions except when there is a suspected sequestrated segment in association with the CAM.

Diaphragmatic hernias

The diaphragm is a thin muscle that separates the thoracic cavity from the abdominal cavity. There may be a defect in the diaphragm, in which case there may be herniation of abdominal contents into the chest. Diaphragmatic hernias in infants are generally congenital but in older children may also be acquired as a result of trauma. They are the commonest intrathoracic anomaly seen in the fetus. There is also a known association between streptococcus B chest infection and the delayed appearance of a hernia.

There are two types of congenital diaphragmatic hernias: those occurring at the front, which are called Morgagni hernias, and those occurring at the back, which are known as Bochdalek hernias. Congenital hernias result from failure of closure of the pleuroperitoneal fold during intrauterine life.

Diaphragmatic hernias are more common on the left in all types, and this is thought to be due to the protective effect of the liver or else the plugging of the defect by the liver.

Bochdalek hernias are more common than Morgagni hernias, and there may be herniation of the liver, spleen, stomach and small bowel. Kidneys may herniate through posterior defects in the diaphragm, and ultrasound will very clearly show the herniated kidney.

Morgagni hernias occur anteriorly and are best seen on a radiograph lying in the right cardiophrenic angle. Transverse colon and liver may herniate (Fig. 12.5).

There are a number of abnormalities associated with diaphragmatic hernias: in particular, neural tube defects, malrotation of the bowel, cardiac and genitourinary tract anomalies.

Eventration of the diaphragm refers to a localized weakness of the diaphragmatic muscle where this is due to a fibrous band. Ultrasonically it is not possible to differentiate an eventration from a diaphragmatic hernia.

346 PEDIATRIC ULTRASOUND

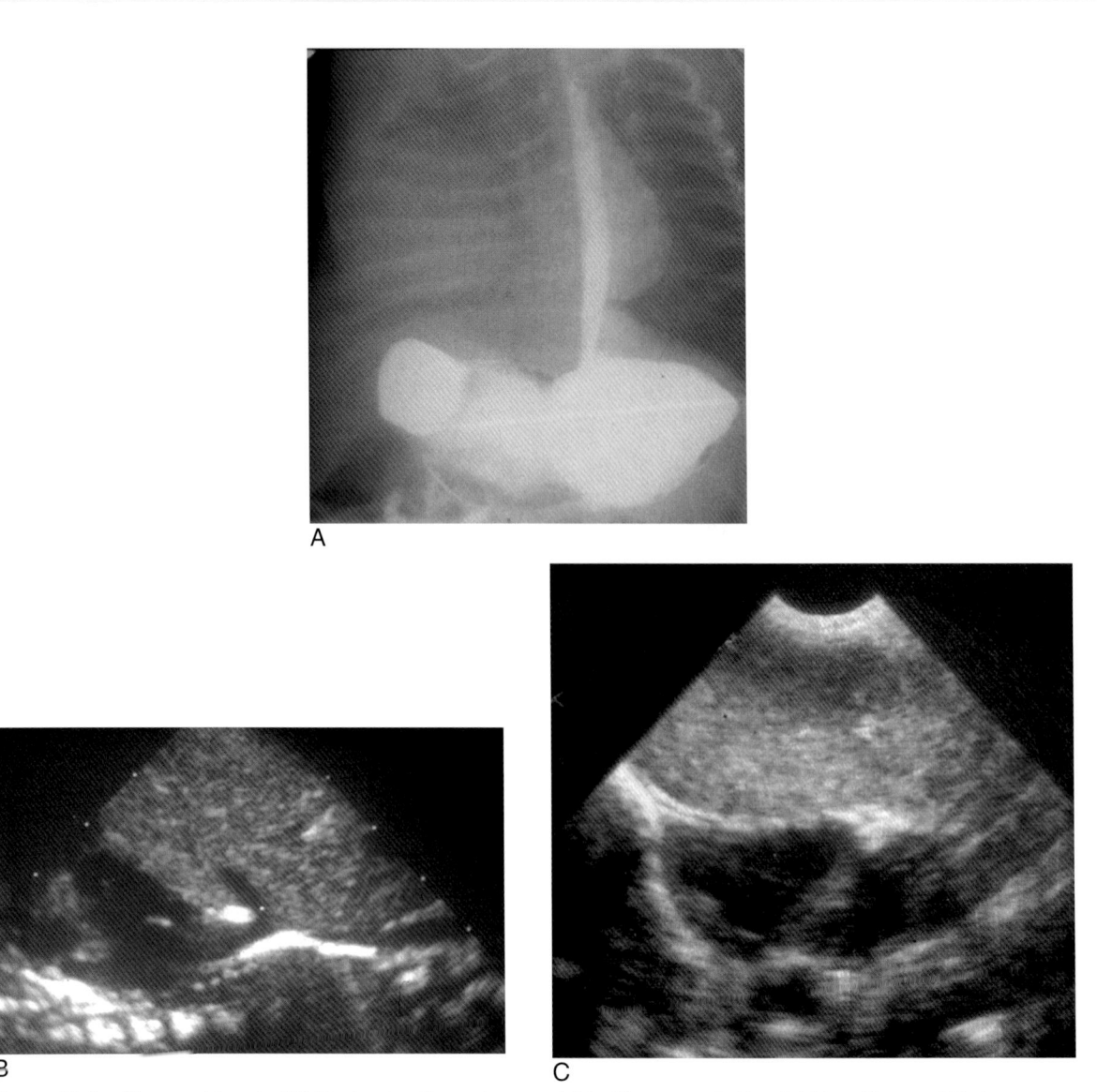

Figure 12.5 Morgagni hernia. (A) PA chest radiograph on a child with a mass in the right hemithorax. This is a barium examination showing the stomach and antrum lying high and apparently close to the hemidiaphragm. (B) Longitudinal sonogram of the liver showing anterior herniation of the liver into the chest. The hepatic veins are entering the IVC in the opposite direction, i.e. craniocaudally, to normal. (C) Transverse sonogram of the lower chest showing the liver lying anterior to the heart.

Diaphragmatic movement

The diaphragm normally moves down on inspiration and up on expiration. With paralysis of the diaphragm it will either remain high and fixed or may exhibit paradoxical movement so that on inspiration it moves upwards. This movement of the diaphragm has traditionally been examined by fluoroscopic screening, but careful ultrasound examination of both hemidiaphragms will give excellent information regarding the diaphragmatic movement.

The ultrasound examination must be performed with the child in quiet respiration and both diaphragms scanned in both longitudinal and transverse planes. High transverse scans must be undertaken with both diaphragms in view for comparison of movement. Difficulties arise for the sonographer when the child is on a ventilator. It is best to assess the diaphragms while attached to the ventilator and also for a short period when removed. The ventilator fills the lungs with air which will cause the diaphragms to move down with inspiration even when paralyzed.

Paralysis of the diaphragm is associated with damage to the phrenic nerve and may occur after thoracic surgery. Ultrasound will help differentiate other causes of an apparently high hemidiaphragm, such as subpulmonary fluid or diaphragmatic defects or eventration.

Masses arising from the diaphragm

Malignant rhabdomyosarcomas are rare tumors that may arise from the muscle of the diaphragm. Children will present with an opaque hemithorax, and ultrasound will detect a solid mass in the hemithorax.

THE MEDIASTINUM

The superior mediastinum is an area easily accessible with ultrasound in children, especially very young children, using the suprasternal notch as the window. This area contains the thymus, the origins of the major vessels of the heart, the aortic arch, esophagus and lymph nodes most notably. Ultrasound is most useful in the evaluation of the superior mediastinum for masses thought to be related to the thymus and is generally used before other cross sectional imaging. It is particularly useful for ill children in intensive care. In very young children the bones are not yet well ossified, making ultrasound access more feasible.

The thymus

The thymic gland is largest in the first 2 years of life, and the normal thymus is readily visible on ultrasound using the suprasternal approach. The size and shape of the normal thymus are very variable, and the gland may extend from the neck as far down as the diaphragm (Fig. 12.6).[6]

On ultrasound the normal thymus has a homogeneous echo texture and is slightly less echogenic than the liver. It is hypovascular on Doppler imaging and has a well-defined margin, as it is surrounded by capsule.

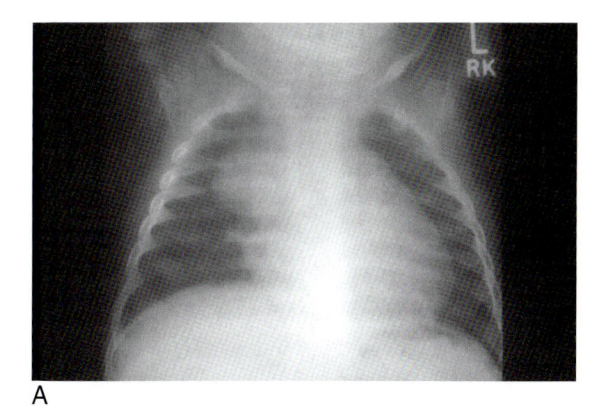

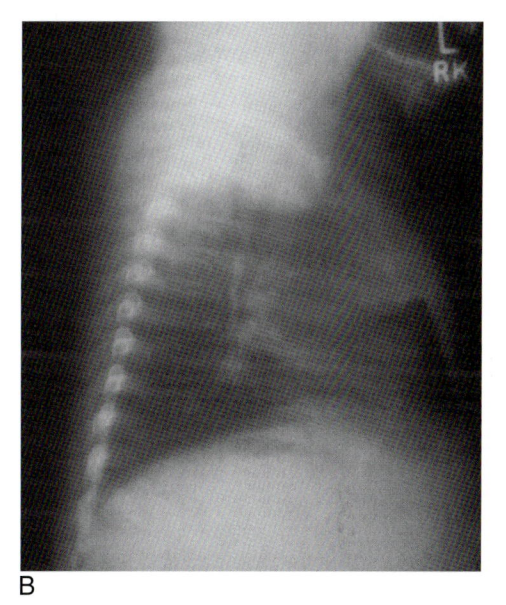

Figure 12.6 Normal thymus. (A) Chest radiograph showing the normal thymus. The thymus is lying in the superior mediastinum to the right of the heart and major vessels. It appears as a well-defined mass sometimes taking a sail shape. (B) Lateral chest radiograph of a normal thymus showing the anterior position of the thymic shadow.

The normal thymus has many variations in appearance and may sometimes be mistaken for a mass lesion in the chest. A normal thymus should never compress the trachea. It is in this scenario where ultrasound is most useful in differentiating the normal thymus from a mediastinal mass or upper lobe consolidation and collapse (see Fig. 9.31).

Abnormalities of the thymus

The thymus is abnormal when enlarged. Benign enlargement may occur in intrathymic hemorrhage, thymic cysts and lymphangiomatous malformations. Hemorrhage and later liquefaction of the hematoma are very well evaluated using ultrasound.

Malignancy Malignant thymomas are rarely encountered in childhood.

Infiltration by lymphoma or leukemia is one of the most common tumors involving the superior mediastinum. The thymus may have a lobulated outline and have a generally more hypoechoic appearance. In addition there may be nodal masses in the neck and symptoms of superior vena cava obstruction.

Langerhans cell histiocytosis may also infiltrate the thymus.

Lymphadenopathy

Lymphadenopathy is generally in the middle mediastinum but if sufficiently large may extend into the anterior mediastinum. Lymphadenopathy is found in older children. Causes include infections such as tuberculosis (TB) and, rarely, fungal infections. Lymphoma may cause massive mediastinal lymphadenopathy, even obstruction of the superior vena cava. Large pleural effusions are commonly associated with lymphoma.

THE OPAQUE HEMITHORAX

Ultrasound is particularly useful in evaluation of the chest in complete opacification of a hemithorax, and will help differentiate consolidated lung, large pleural effusion and solid mass arising from a rib or the diaphragm. The chest radiograph must always be carefully evaluated in particular for any rib destruction[7] (Fig. 12.7).

Lung abnormalities

The normal lung on ultrasound appears as air, and no internal architecture can be demonstrated.

Consolidation

Consolidation of the lung occurs in infection when the lung is filled with mucus and inflammatory exudates. Lung volume is increased, as the lung is filled with fluid, but the bronchi still contain air and produce the typical air bronchogram on a plain radiograph. These appearances may be seen on ultrasound.

Small echogenic areas of air trapped within alveoli may also be visible. The lungs may become consolidated as a result of mucoid impaction as seen in asthmatics. Ultrasound will then demonstrate tubular cystic areas within the consolidated lung. There may be complete consolidation of the lung with absence of air or fluid

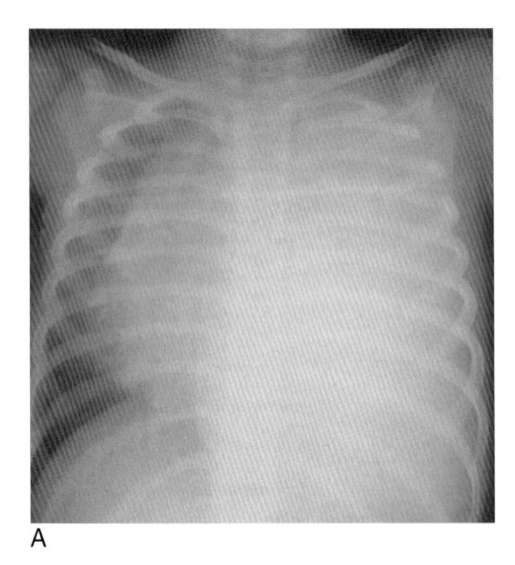

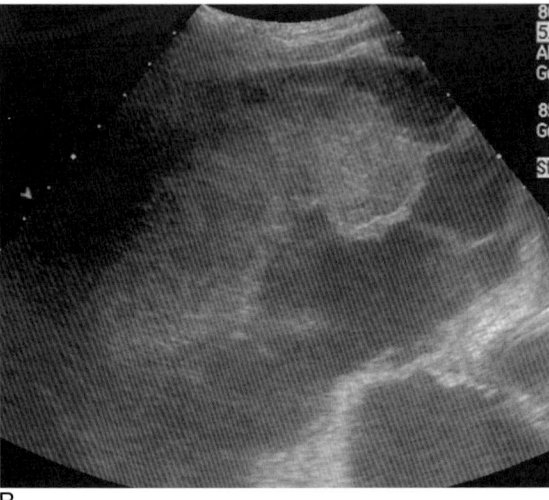

Figure 12.7 Opaque hemithorax. (A) Chest radiograph of a child presenting with breathlessness. The left hemithorax is completely opaque and the heart is shifted to the right. These radiographic appearances suggest that there is a space-occupying mass in the left hemithorax displacing the heart, such as a large pleural effusion or a mass. Ultrasound examination can readily differentiate the two. This is a common clinical request. (B) Upper chest longitudinal sonogram of the left chest in the same child.

C

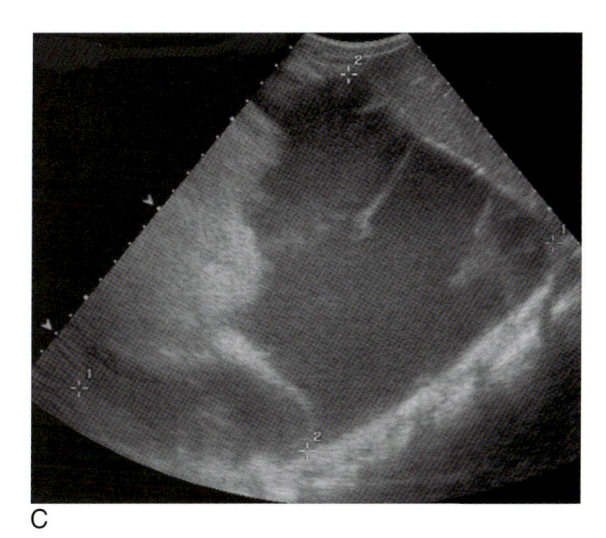

Figure 12.7, cont'd (C) Lower chest longitudinal sonogram of the left chest in the same child. The lung is solid and completely collapsed. There is a large amount of fluid displaying multiple echoes and septations surrounding the collapsed lung. In (C) the diaphragm and spleen can be seen. This child had an empyema.

in the bronchial tree. Doppler evaluation of the pulmonary vasculature may then prove useful and demonstrate a radiating pattern which will help distinguish consolidated lung from an intrathoracic mass. In addition the use of Doppler will help differentiate fluid in the bronchi from vascular structures.[8]

In atelectasis, or collapsed lung, volume is decreased. The ultrasound differentiation lies between a lung mass and consolidated lung, and it is important for the sonographer to be able to differentiate these two.

Tumors

Primary lung tumors are extremely rare and include blastoma, bronchogenic carcinoma, hemangiopericytoma and leiomyosarcoma. Ewing's tumor of the rib may present as a large intrathoracic mass and pleural effusion. Ultrasound is helpful in distinguishing these large solid masses from a massive pleural effusion.

Pleural fluid

Ultrasound is the ideal modality for the detection of pleural fluid (Fig. 12.8). The role of ultrasound lies in:

- establishing the diagnosis of a pleural effusion
- establishing the extent and position of the fluid
- assessing the position for aspiration or drainage
- determining whether the collection looks simple, i.e. clear fluid, or complex.

A

B

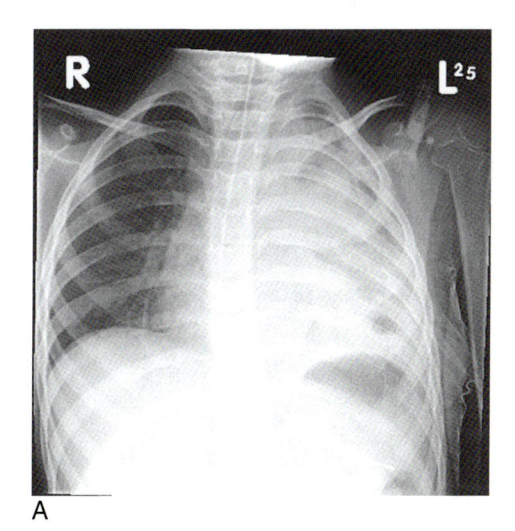

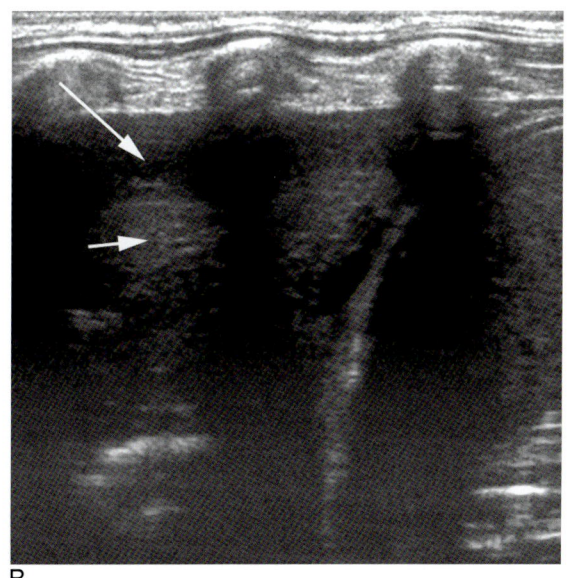

Figure 12.8 Pleural effusion. (A) Chest radiograph on a girl presenting with a high fever and a pleural effusion on the left. An intercostal drain was in position but was not draining. (B) Longitudinal sonogram of the left lower chest showing the spleen and diaphragm. There is consolidated lung at the left base (short arrow) with a pleural effusion (long arrow) lying around the lung.

Continued

350 PEDIATRIC ULTRASOUND

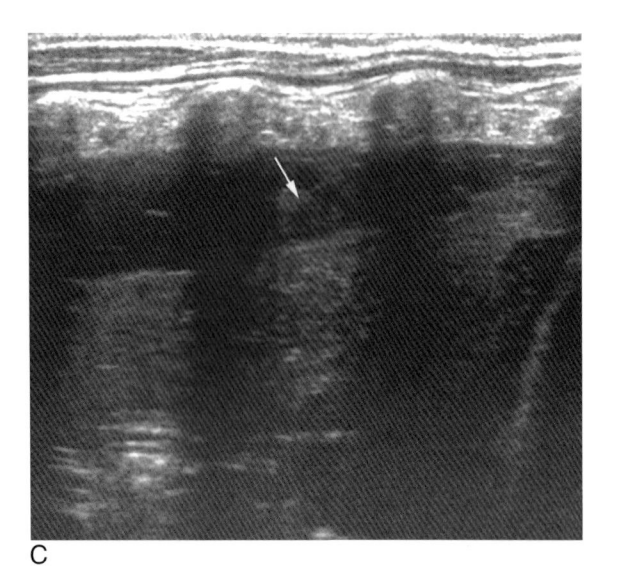

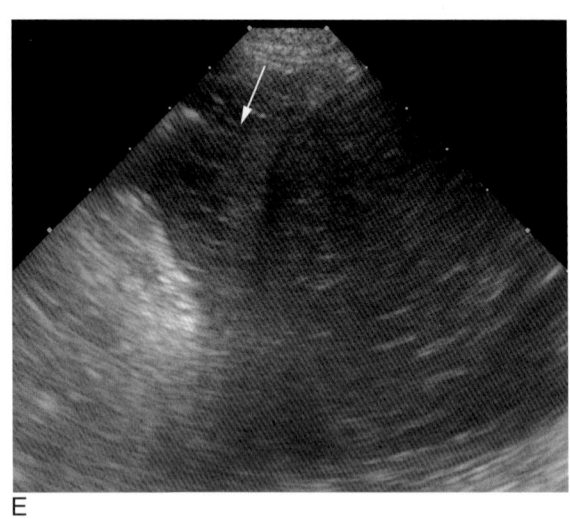

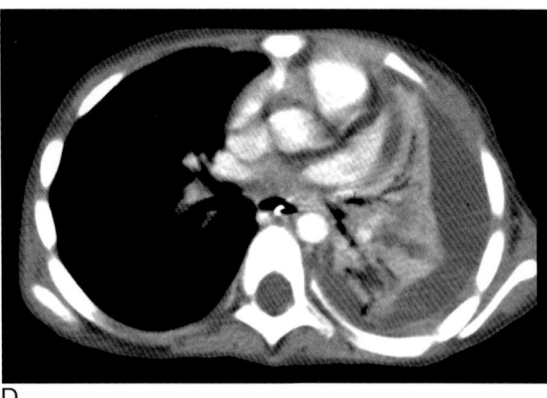

Figure 12.8, cont'd (C) Longitudinal sonogram showing the consolidated lung. The pleural effusion (arrow) contains multiple echoes with septations. (D) CT examination of the chest in the same girl showing the pleural effusion lying around the lung with consolidated collapsed lung medially. (E) This is another child who also presented with a pleural effusion. Ultrasound examination revealed very echogenic fluid (arrow) above the spleen and just beneath the aerated lung. Potentially this fluid will be much more difficult to drain, as it contains cellular debris and will be thick.

The abdomen must always be carefully examined in these children in order to detect intra-abdominal pathology causing a reactive pleural effusion (Fig. 12.9). Other features to look for are change in shape or fluid shifts when the patient's position is changed.

Different types of pleural effusion reflect the nature of the fluid content. Chylothorax is a pleural effusion containing chyle, hemothorax contains blood, and empyemas are infected and contain pus.[9]

A simple effusion appears as a clear fluid collection. A complex effusion has multiple internal echoes with dense septations, multiple loculations and thickened echogenic pleura.

Once fluid collections become organized, such as in empyemas, they produce dense septae which make both drainage and thoracentesis extremely difficult. These appearances on ultrasound are not always visible on CT, which makes ultrasound a very useful mode of investigation.

The use of ultrasound for characterization is extremely helpful in guiding further management and treatment.

CONGENITAL CYSTS

Congenital cysts occur in the chest in a number of positions, usually related to the superior mediastinum.[10]

CT is still the examination of choice when intrathoracic masses are suspected.

Bronchogenic cysts

Bronchogenic cysts are the commonest intrathoracic cysts and are found around the carina such

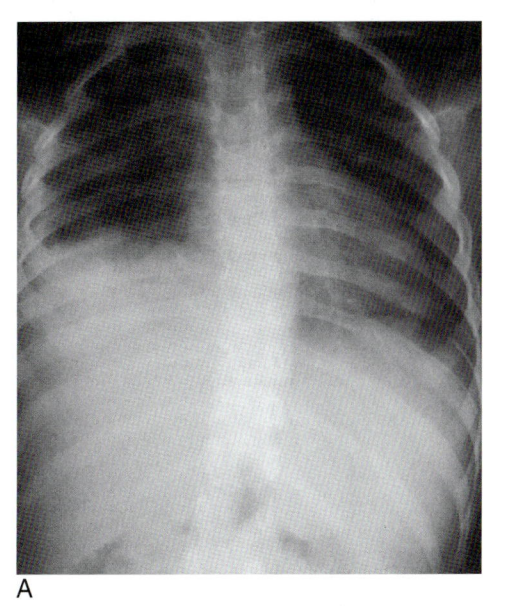

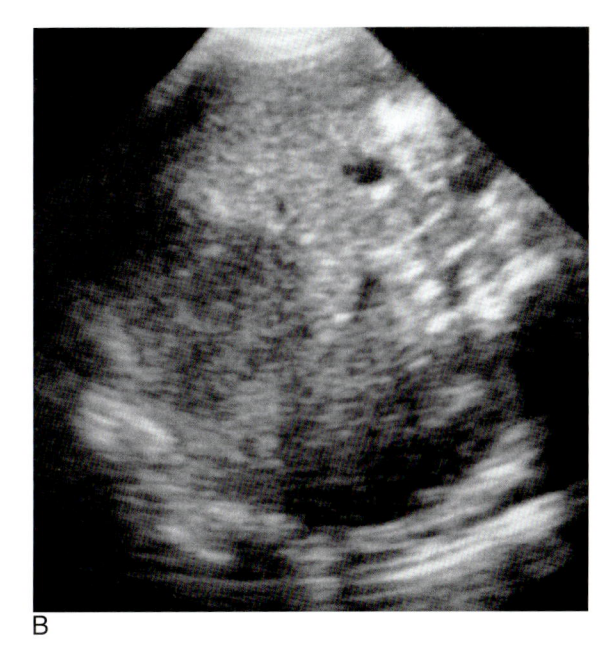

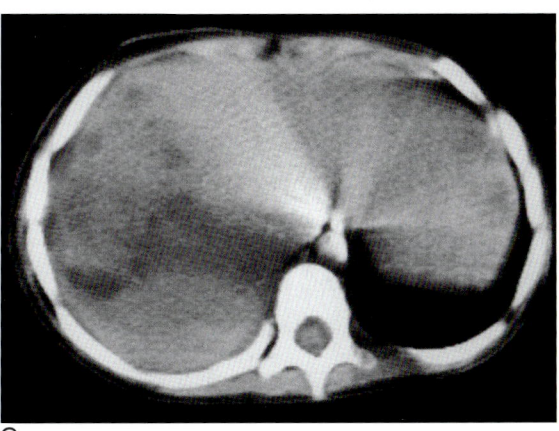

Figure 12.9 Liver abscess and effusion. (A) Chest radiograph on a child with a fever and cough. The right hemidiaphragm appears to be high and there is a small right basal pleural effusion. (B) Longitudinal sonogram of the liver showing that the liver has an abnormal texture. (C) CT examination on the same child showing that the apparent elevation of the hemidiaphragm was caused by a liver abscess with a small reactive effusion in the chest.

as the subcarina or subparatracheal regions. They may also be found in the paratracheal region. They arise from abnormal budding of the tracheobronchial tree and may communicate with the trachea or compress it, resulting in collapse of a lobe.

Gut duplication cysts from the esophagus

These duplication cysts occur next to the esophagus and may extend down into the abdomen. They typically have a bowel wall and may be clear or contain cellular debris on ultrasound.

SUMMARY

Ultrasound is a useful technique in the chest, and its main role is to answer specific clinical questions, in particular relating to pleural effusions, juxtadiaphragmatic masses and aberrant vessels. Chest radiography and cross sectional imaging are still the primary imaging modalities.

References

1. Rosenberg HK. The complementary roles of ultrasound and plain film radiography in differentiating pediatric chest abnormalities. RadioGraphics 1986; 6:427–445.
2. Ben-Ami TE, O'Donovan JC, Yousefzadeh DK. Sonography of the chest in children. Radiol Clin North Am 1993; 31:517–531.
3. Tecce PM, Fishman EK, Kuhlman JE. CT evaluation of the anterior mediastinum: spectrum of disease. RadioGraphics 1994; 14:973–990.
4. Merten DF. Diagnostic imaging of mediastinal masses in children. AJR Am J Roentgenol 1992; 158:825–832.
5. Schlesinger AE, DiPietro MA, Statter MB, et al. Utility of sonography in the diagnosis of bronchopulmonary sequestration. J Pediatr Surg 1994; 29:52–55.
6. Adam EJ, Ignotus PI. Sonography of the thymus in healthy children: frequency of visualization, size, and appearance. AJR Am J Roentgenol 1993; 161:153–155.
7. Acunas B, Celik L, Acunas A. Chest sonography: differentiation of pulmonary consolidation from pleural disease. Acta Radiol 1989; 30:273–275.
8. Targhetta R, Chavagneux R, Bourgeois JM, et al. Sonographic approach to diagnosing pulmonary consolidation. J Ultrasound Med 1992; 11:667–672.
9. Lomas DG, Padley SG, Flower CD. The sonographic appearances of pleural fluid. Br J Radiol 1993; 66:619–624.
10. Hernanz-Schulman M. Cysts and cystlike lesions of the lung. Radiol Clin North Am 1993; 31:631–649.

Recommended reading

Carty H, Brunelle F, Shaw D, Kendall B. Imaging children. Edinburgh: Churchill Livingstone; 1994.

Dewbury K, Meire H, Cosgrove D, et al. Clinical ultrasound: a comprehensive text. 2nd edn. Churchill Livingstone; 2001.

Petterson H, Ringertz H. Measurements in pediatric radiology. London: Springer-Verlag; 1991.

Rennie J. Neonatal cerebral ultrasound. Cambridge: Cambridge University Press; 1997.

Sadler TW. Langman's medical embryology. 8th edn. Baltimore: Lippincott Williams & Wilkins; 2000.

Taybe H, Lachman R. Radiology of syndromes, metabolic disorders, and skeletal dysplasias. 4th edn. St Louis: Mosby; 1996.

Te Haar G, Duck FA. The safe use of ultrasound in medical diagnosis. London: British Medical Ultrasound Society; 2000.

Glossary

Acetabular dysplasia: Defective development of the acetabulum.

Acetabulum: Hip socket.

Achondrogenesis: Severe lethal form of dwarfism. Antenatal diagnosis can be made.

Acoustic shadow: The dark area that occurs behind a highly attenuating structure. For example, the dark area that occurs behind a calculus in the kidney.

Acoustic window: A structure such as the bladder that has little or no acoustic impedance and as a result allows the passage of sound so that deeper structures (e.g. the uterus and ovaries) can be seen.

Alagilles syndrome (arteriohepatic dysplasia): In this autosomal dominant condition infants have characteristic triangular facies, skeletal abnormalities, peripheral pulmonary stenosis, renal tubular disorders, defects in the eye and intrahepatic biliary hypoplasia with severe itching and failure to thrive.

Alfa-fetoprotein: A protein produced by the yolk sac or fetal liver. High blood levels are found in liver tumors such as hepatoblastoma or maternal blood and neural tube defects in the fetus.

Alport syndrome: Nephropathy (hematuria, proteinuria, progressive renal failure), sensorineural deafness, ocular abnormalities, inguinal hernia, anomalies of fingers, cryptorchidism, CNS tumors, myasthenia.

Aneuploidy: Any deviation from an exact multiple of the haploid number of chromosomes, whether fewer or more.

Aniridia: Chromosomal abnormality (deletion 11p 12–14.1) resulting in absent iris and association with Wilms tumors, mental retardation, skull or craniofacial dysmorphism, various skeletal defects, deformities of pinna, genitourinary anomalies.

Aperts syndrome: Many abnormalities. Main features to look for on ultrasound include deformed head with flat forehead and intracranial abnormalities, mitten hand and sock foot.

Ascites: Free fluid in the abdominal cavity.

Asplenia: Absence of spleen

Atresia: Congenital absence or closure of a normal body opening or tubular structure.

Autosomal recessive: A mode of inheritance which gives the offspring a 1 in 4 chance of having the disease.

Bartter syndrome: Nephromegaly and nephrocalcinosis. Growth retardation, mental retardation; craniofacial features: large head, prominent forehead, triangular facies, large eyes, drooping mouth, large pinnae; muscle weakness, tetany, vomiting, polydipsia, polyuria,

Beckwith–Wiedemann syndrome: Sometimes referred to as EMG (exomphalos-macroglossia, gigantism): omphalocele, visceromegaly, umbilical hernia. Association with neoplasms, nephroblastoma, neuroblastoma and hepatoblastoma.

Branchial cleft: Part of the development of the head and neck in embryogenesis.

Budd–Chiari syndrome: Obstruction of major hepatic veins or obstruction in intrahepatic portion of inferior vena cava or ostium of a hepatic vein.

Campomelic dysplasia: Dwarfism characterized by bowing of lower limbs, detectable antenatally. Peculiar small facies. Cleft palate. Poor or absent pelvic ossification. Death in infancy.

Caroli syndrome: Segmental saccular dilation of intrahepatic bile ducts with extension to hepatic periphery, absence of liver cirrhosis or portal hypertension in pure form of disease, cholangitis, liver abscess, hepatic fibrosis, renal tubular ectasia, or other renal cystic lesions.

Caudal regression: Also called caudal dysplasia syndrome. Vertebral agenesis, from partial sacral agenesis to total absence below the lumbar vertebrae. Associated with maternal diabetes.

Cavum septum pellucidum: A space between the membranes that separate the anterior horns of the lateral cerebral ventricles.

CHARGE association: Coloboma, heart disease, choanal atresia, retarded growth/development and/or CNS anomalies, genital hypoplasia, ear anomalies and/or deafness.

Chronic granulomatous disease: Neutrophil dysfunction syndrome. The white cells are unable to kill certain bacteria. Chronic and recurrent severe suppurative infections in lung, lymph nodes, bones, spleen, liver caused by particularly staphylococci, *Klebsiella*, *Pseudomonas*, *E. coli* and salmonella infections.

Cloaca: A common passage for fecal, urinary and reproductive discharge in most lower vertebrates such as frogs.

CMV: Cytomegalovirus.

Cornelia de Lange syndrome: Anomalies of limbs and digits, delayed skeletal maturation, microbrachycephaly.

'Dancing eyes' syndrome: Jerking eye movements in patients with neuroblastoma.

Dandy–Walker malformation: Hydrocephalus associated with congenital anomaly of fourth ventricle and cerebellum with atresia of foramen of Magendie and atresia of one or both foramina of Luschka; absence of cerebellar vermis (partial or complete).

Denys–Drash syndrome: Male pseudohermaphroditism, progressive nephritis, Wilms tumor.

Developmental dysplasia of the hip (DDH): This term is used to refer to a spectrum of disorders which includes unstable hips and acetabular dysplasia.

DiGeorge syndrome: Also known as third and fourth pharyngeal pouch syndrome. Complete DiGeorge syndrome: absent parathyroid, no T cell function. Partial DiGeorge syndrome: some T cell function. Abnormalities of the third and fourth pharyngeal pouches, malformation and hypoplasia or maldescent of thymus or parathyroid glands.

Displaced hips: Synonyms are dislocated or subluxated. There are two types: reducibly displaced (detectable by the Ortolani test) and irreducibly dislocated (not detectable by the Ortolani test, but may manifest as limited abduction). They may also be detected by ultrasound examination or (in older infants) by X-ray.

Down syndrome: See Trisomy 21.

Ductus venosus: A fetal vessel that runs through the liver and joins the umbilical vein to the vena cava.

Eagle–Barrett syndrome (Prune Belly syndrome): Most reported cases in males; partial or complete absence of abdominal musculature; dysplasia of urinary tract, large irregularly shaped bladder, patent urachus and dilated posterior urethra. Undescended testes. Other reported anomalies include malrotation of the bowel, hip dislocation, foot and leg deformities, polydactyly, congenital heart disease.

ECMO (extracorporeal membrane oxygenation): Treatment for some severe lung conditions usually in neonates. Lungs are effectively 'bypassed'.

Epstein–Barr virus: A herpes-like virus that causes infectious mononucleosis and is associated with Burkitt lymphoma and nasopharyngeal carcinoma.

ESWL (extracorporeal shock wave lithotripsy): A treatment used for fragmenting renal stones using ultrasound shock waves.

Exstrophy of the bladder: A ventral body wall defect in which the bladder mucosa is exposed onto the anterior abdominal wall.

Femoral head: That part of the top of the femur which fits into the acetabulum.

Fistula: An abnormal passage or communication, usually between two internal organs or leading from an internal organ to the body surface.

Fryn syndrome: Nuchal edema, cataracts, contractures, micrognathia, CNS abnormalities, intrauterine growth retardation (IUGR).

Genotype: The entire genetic constitution of an individual; also the alleles present at one or more specific loci.

Glycogen storage disease type I: Von Gierke disease: Onset of symptoms in infancy include failure to thrive; massive hepatomegaly; repeated episodes of hypoglycemia and acidosis; progressive enlargement of the kidneys; pathologic fracture; retarded bone maturation, renal calculi; liver masses (adenoma, carcinoma). There are three other types of glycogen storage disease with different clinical manifestations.

Goodpasture syndrome: Weakness, cough, pallor, low grade fever, tachycardia; pulmonary hemorrhage, hemoptysis; renal disease, hematuria, albuminuria, uremia; microcytic anemia.

Haploid: Having half the number of chromosomes characteristically found in the somatic (diploid) cells of an organism. In a human, diploid is 46 chromosomes and haploid is 23 chromosomes, the latter being typically found in the sperm or ovum.

Henoch–Schönlein syndrome: Allergic arteritis with submucosal hemorrhage affecting bowel and urinary tract. Insidious or sudden onset of pain in abdomen, vomiting, painful joints, cutaneous purpura, gastrointestinal hemorrhage, nephritis.

Hepatoblastoma: A malignant intrahepatic tumor consisting chiefly of embryonic tissue, occurring in infants and young children.

Holoprosencephaly: Failure of cleavage of the prosencephalon (early forebrain) associated with defects in midline facial structures or cyclops. Single cerebral structure with a common ventricle and typical facial anomaly.

Holt–Oram syndrome (heart–hand syndrome): Absent thumb and congenital heart disease (atrial septal defect/ventricular septal defect) and shoulder anomalies.

Hypoxia: A shortage of oxygen.

Jeune syndrome: Respiratory distress, short ribs, small narrow thoracic cage, cone shaped epiphyses of hands, trident acetabulum, medullary cystic renal disease in adolescence, hepatic fibrosis.

Joubert syndrome: Autosomal recessive. Aplasia of cerebellar vermis, occipital meningocele, microcephaly and polydactyly.

Kasabach–Meritt syndrome: Hemangiomas in any location causing platelet trapping which results in severe, often life-threatening thrombocytopenia.

Klinefelter syndrome: Males with poorly developed penis and testicular atrophy. Eunuch appearance. It is associated typically with an XXY chromosome complement or other various mosaic patterns.

Klippel–Feil syndrome: Shortness of the neck due to reduction in the number of cervical vertebrae or the fusion of multiple hemivertebrae into one osseous mass with limitation of neck motion and low hairline.

Laurence–Moon–Biedl syndrome: A hereditary syndrome transmitted as an autosomal recessive trait characterized by mental retardation, obesity, retinitis pigmentosa, polydactyly, hypogonadism and renal dysplasia.

Lesch–Nyhan syndrome: A hereditary disorder of purine metabolism with physical and mental retardation, compulsive self-mutilation of fingers and lips by biting, choreoathetosis, spastic cerebral palsy, impaired renal function and by extremely excessive purine synthesis and consequently hyperuricemia and excessive urinary secretion of uric acid. It is transmitted as a sex-linked recessive trait.

Li–Fraumeni syndrome: Also known as the SBLA: sarcoma, breast and brain tumors, leukemia, laryngeal carcinoma and lung cancer and adrenocortical carcinoma.

Meckel–Gruber syndrome (Meckel syndrome): Autosomal recessive; occipital encephalocele, cleft lip and palate, polydactyly, polycystic kidneys.

Megahertz (MHz): Million(s) of cycles per second.

Metaphysis: The wider part at the end of the shaft of the long bone.

Micrognathia: Small jaw.

Mitrofanoff procedure: Drainage procedure used in augmented bladders. Patients catheterize a track fashioned from either ureter or appendix.

Müllerian ducts: Also known as paramesonephric ducts. They go on to form the uterus, fallopian tubes and upper vagina in adult females.

Multiple endocrine neoplasia (types IIa and IIb): Multiple tumors or hyperplasia of several endocrine glands such as parathyroid, pituitary, adrenal, thyroid and pancreas.

Nager acrofacial dysostosis: Micrognathia, microcephaly, intrauterine growth retardation and upper limb anomalies.

Neonatal hip instability: Describes displaced or unstable hips identified through clinical screening examination in newborn or young infants.

Neoplasm: A tumor. May be benign or malignant.

Nephroblastoma: Kidney tumor otherwise known as a Wilms tumor.

Nesidioblastosis: Beta cell hyperplasia of the pancreas frequently seen in neonates with hypoglycemia.

Nephrocalcinosis: The deposition of calcium in the kidneys.

Neuroblastoma: Tumor from the sympathetic chain most commonly arising in the adrenal gland.

Noonan syndrome: The male phenotype of Turner syndrome.

Osteogenesis imperfecta: Otherwise known as brittle bone disease. There are four types with varying severity.

Pallister–Killian (tetrosomy 12p): Nuchal edema, intrauterine growth retardation, rocker-bottom feet, polydactyly.

Parvus–tardus phenomenon: Flattening of the Doppler spectral waveform downstream to a renal artery stenosis.

Perlman syndrome: Gigantism, visceromegaly, hypotonia, facial dysmorphism.

Phenotype: The entire physical, biochemical and physiological make-up of an individual as determined both genetically and environmentally.

Pleural effusion: A collection of fluid between the lung and the chest wall.

Polydactyly: More than five digits.

Polysplenia: Refers to a transverse liver, multiple aberrant nodules of spleen on the right side of the abdomen and an interrupted inferior vena cava.

Prader–Willi syndrome: Short stature, hypogonadism, undescended testes, mental retardation.

Proteinuria: More than 300 mg/l of protein in the urine.

Prune belly syndrome: See Eagle–Barrett syndrome.

Recessive: Refers to a hereditary condition which cannot be expressed unless carried by both parents with homologous chromosomes. The child has a 1:4 chance of inheriting the condition.

Shwachman syndrome: An autosomal recessive condition characterized by the impairment of neutrophil function. Other features seen in the syndrome include metaphyseal chondrodysplasia, metaphyseal widening and a 'cup' deformity of the ribs, together with bone marrow hypoplasia and exocrine pancreatic insufficiency leading to malabsorption.

Simpson–Golabi–Behmel: Polydactyly, developmental dysplasia, cardiac abnormalities, genital and vertebral anomalies.

Situs inversus: The abdominal contents appear normal but are on the opposite side from that usually expected, so that the spleen is on the right and the liver is on the left.

Smith–Lemli–Opitz syndrome: Autosomal recessive; cardiac anomalies, short limbs, microcephaly and polydactyly.

Sonolucent: Producing few echoes.

Sturge–Weber syndrome: A congenital syndrome of angiomatous lesions of the face and angiomas of the meninges and choroid. Frequently associated with intracranial calcification, epilepsy and mental retardation.

Syndactyly: Webbed fingers or toes.

Tamm–Horsfall proteinuria: Term used to describe a specific echogenic appearance of medullae in neonates which resolves without treatment.

Thanatophoric dysplasia: A lethal form of dwarfism. Thanatos is the Greek word for death.

Thrombocytopenia absent radius (TAR syndrome): Congenital deformity of forearm and hand, with hand at right angles to forearm. Normal thumbs, cardiac abnormalities and bowed limbs.

TORCH: A group of congenital disorders which are made up of toxoplasmosis, rubella, cytomegalovirus, herpes virus. These are the common infections that affect multiple systems in the fetus.

Total parenteral nutrition (TPN): Long term intravenous feeding therapy.

Transducer: A device (and its housing) composed of one or more piezoelectric crystals that will convert voltages to ultrasound energy and ultrasound to voltages.

Transonic: Allowing sound to pass through it, i.e. a poor attenuator.

Trisomy 13 (Patau syndrome): Microcephaly, holoprosencephaly, hand and foot deformities.

Trisomy 18 (Edward syndrome): Abnormal craniofacial appearance, congenital heart disease, deformed fingers and rocker-bottom feet.

Trisomy 21 (Down syndrome): Mongolism: typical craniofacial anomalies; congenital heart disease; gastrointestinal abnormalities such as duodenal atresia or anorectal anomalies; excess skin on back of neck.

Turner syndrome (chromosome XO syndrome): Short web-shaped necks; urinary tract anomalies such as horseshoe kidneys, malrotation and duplication; ovarian dysgenesis with primary amenorrhea; coarctation of the aorta; bony abnormalities of the wrist.

Tyrosinemia: Chronic hereditary tyrosinemia: hepatic cirrhosis, generalized renal reabsorption defects developing nephrocalcinosis and rickets. Associated with mental retardation. High incidence of hepatomas developing.

Ultrasound examination: Sound with frequencies above the range of human hearing (more than 20 KHz). Diagnostically usable ultrasound is usually in the range of 2–10 MHz. Synonyms are ultrasonography and sonography. There are two types: static and dynamic.

Unstable hips: Synonyms are subluxatable or dislocatable. These are characterized by partial or complete displacement of the femoral head from the acetabulum on stress but not at rest. They are identified by the Barlow test or dynamic ultrasound examination with stress.

Urachus: A fetal canal connecting the bladder with the allantois via the umbilicus.

Ureteric bud: Outpouching of mesonephric duct near cloaca, which goes on to form the collecting system of the kidney.

Ureterocele: Outpouching of mucosa in bladder, most commonly associated with duplex kidneys in children.

Urolithiasis: Stones in the renal tract.

VA(C)TER(L) association: Association of some or all of the following anomalies: vertebral anomalies, vascular anomalies, anal anomalies, tracheo-esophageal fistula, esophageal atresia, renal anomalies, radial defects, rib anomalies, cardiovascular anomalies, limb anomalies. If there are three or more anomalies in the same patient it is termed the VATER (or VACTERL) association.

Wagr syndrome: Aniridia, hemihypertrophy and Wilms tumor.

Wegener granulomatosis: Granulomatous reaction usually starting in the respiratory tract, particularly affecting the nasal passages, trachea and lungs. Also affects heart and kidneys with a panarteritis.

Williams syndrome: Elfin facies associated with supravalvular aortic stenosis and hypercalcemia.

Wilson disease: Otherwise known as hepatolenticular degeneration. An abnormality of copper metabolism. Onset in childhood. Profound neurological symptoms, liver cirrhosis and renal dysfunction.

Wolffian ducts: Otherwise known as mesonephric ducts, these are the ducts of the interim embryological kidneys or mesonephroi. They disappear in the female but have some adult male derivatives.

Zellweger syndrome (cerebrohepatorenal syndrome): Soft tissue calcification, limb anomalies, renal cysts, brain dysgenesis, liver fibrosis.

Index

Note: page numbers in *italics* refer to figures, tables and boxes.

A

abdomen
 abscess 335
 cystic masses 198–9, 200, *201*
  ovarian cysts 219–20
 developmental abnormalities 183–4
 embryology 181–3
 fetal ultrasound 18, *21*
 herniation of viscera 183
 perihepatic spaces 200, *201*
 ultrasound technique 184
  probes 5
 wall defects 237
abscess
 abdomen 335
 adrenal glands 116
 appendix 195, *197*
 kidneys 65, 66
  perinephric *335, 336*
 liver *151, 155, 351*
 neck *286*
 pelvis 335
 peritoneum 202
 psoas *204*
 soft tissue *318*
 spleen 167–8
 testes 248
acetabulum 302, 303, 308
 dysplasia 309
Achilles tendon 317
achondrogenesis 25
adolescence, menstrual dysfunction 225, 227–8

adrenal glands
 abnormalities 115–17
 abscess 116
 congenital hyperplasia 115, 222, 227
 cystic lesions 116–17
 diameters *114*
 ectopic rests in testes 248
 haemorrhage 115–16
 normal appearance 113, *114*
 size 114
 tumors 117–18, *119–20,* 121–7, *128*
 ultrasound technique 114–15
adrenarche
 isolated premature 223–4
 polycystic ovarian syndrome 227
adrenocortical tumors 124–5, *126, 127*
Alagille syndrome 143
alfa-fetoprotein
 hepatoblastoma 157
 hepatocellular carcinoma 158
 ovarian teratoma 228
amenorrhea 225
amoebic liver abscess 155
amyloid 317
andrenoblastoma 228
androgenital syndrome 219
androgens
 excess 219, 227
 testicular descent 236, 237
anencephaly 22, 291, *292*
anesthesia 321–2
 general 321, 330, 334
anesthetic cream, topical 321
aneuploidy
 fetal ultrasound markers 19, *23*
 renal anomalies 33

aneurysm *318*
 vein of Galen 275–6
angiomyolipoma, renal echogenic 76, *77*
anorectal anomalies 182–3, 197–8
 agenesis 298
 atresia 183, 198
anorexia nervosa 225
antinuclear antibody 316
aorta
 coarctation 91
 Doppler velocimetry 21
appendicitis 194–5, *196,* 197
 mesentery echogenicity 203
appendicoliths 195, *196*
appendix
 abscess 195, *197*
 development 182, *183*
 mucocele 197
 normal 194
 solid masses 197
 ultrasound technique 195
appendix testis 238, 240
 torsion 246
appointment letter 1–2
aqueduct of Sylvius 255
arachnoid cysts 23, *24,* 272
Arnold–Chiari II malformation 272
arterial access, ultrasound-guided 338
arteriovenous fistula, renal 102
arteriovenous malformations, cranial 275–6
arthritis
 juvenile idiopathic 316–17
 polyarticular 316–17
 septic 313
 systemic 316
 venous malformations 336
 see also rheumatoid arthritis

INDEX

ascites 135
aspergillus, splenic abscess 168
aspiration, ultrasound-guided 335–6
asplenia 134, 166
axillary artery 338
axillary hair, premature development 223–4

B

bacterial infection
  osteomyelitis 311
  parotid gland 288
  thyroiditis 279
  see also named bacteria
bacteriuria 65
barium study
  bezoars 189
  gastroesophageal reflux 184
  malrotation of bowel 190
Barlow test 302, 309
basal ganglia 255
Beckwith–Wiedemann syndrome
  adrenal cystic lesion association 117
  adrenocortical tumor association 125
  echogenic kidneys 83
  hepatoblastoma *157–8*
  neuroblastoma association 118
  pancreaticoblastoma 178
  splenic hemangioma 167
bell and clapper deformity 244
bezoars 189
bile duct
  carcinoma 148
  common 132, 173
    biliary atresia 143
    patent 142
  dilation 177
  intrahepatic 143
  rhabdomyosarcoma 162
  spontaneous perforation 144
bile plug syndrome, inspissated 143
biliary hypoplasia, intrahepatic 143
biliary system
  abnormalities 140–4
  atresia 142–3, *144*
    ultrasound findings 143
  complications in liver transplantation 163
  cystic dilation 144–8
  ultrasound-guided intervention 338–9
biliary tree
  cystic dilation 73
  Doppler examination 8

normal appearance 135–6
obstruction 177
biopsy, ultrasound-guided 330, 332–5
  needle 334–5
  percutaneous 330
  tumors 334–5
bladder
  anomalies 45–6
  calculi *87*
  diverticulae 46
  duplication 45
  exstrophy 31, 85, 356
  fistula 183
  function in renal transplantation 96
  neurogenic 85
  neuropathic 44
  outflow obstruction 30, *31*
  preparation for scan 2, 210
  thickened wall 30, *31*, 60, *61*
  wall 50, *52*
bleomycin sclerotherapy 336
blood group, fetomaternal incompatibility 22, 34
blood transfusion, intrauterine 22
blood–gonad barrier 248
bone tumors 313
bowel
  developmental abnormalities 183–4
  duplication cysts 190–1
  echogenic 28, *29*
  embryology 181–3
  herniation 202
  infiltrative disorders of wall 197
  malrotation 182, 189–90
    diaphragmatic hernia association 345
    ultrasound technique 190
  obstruction 154
  perforation 177
  ultrasound technique 184
  wall thickening 197, *198*, *199*
  mesenteric infection 203
  see also gastrointestinal tract
brachial artery, venae comitantes 328–9, *331*
brachiocephalic vein puncture 327, *329*
brain
  embryology 291
  measurement 252–3, *254*
  non-accidental injury 274
  parenchymal abnormalities 274–5
  secondary damage 275
  ventricular system 255, *260*
brain-sparing effect 21

branchial cleft anomaly 283, *284*
branchio-oto-renal dysplasia 83
breast development 211, 221
  menarche 224
  normal *225*
  precocious puberty 223
  premature 223, *227*
breech presentation 303
bronchial tree 344, 345
bronchogenic cysts 350
bronchopulmonary sequestration (foregut malformation) 27–8, 344–5
Budd–Chiari syndrome 134, 151, 152
  veno-occlusive disease 153
bulimia nervosa 225, 227
bupivacaine 321

C

caecum echogenicity 195
calcification
  hepatic hemangioma 137, 138
  testes 246, 247
Campylobacter 203
candidiasis
  liver abscess 155
  renal 69–70, 88
  splenic abscess 168
cardiac abnormalities
  diaphragmatic hernia association 345
  fetal 25–6
cardiac conditions
  complex cyanotic congenital disease 166
  congestive failure 136, *137*
Caroli syndrome i146, 73, 145, 356
catheterization, voiding urosonography 12
catheters
  fracture 329
  migration 329
  selection for venous access 322
  thrombosis 329
  tunneled 322, 323, 330
cauda equina 291, 294
caudal eminence 291
caudal regression syndrome 25, 297–8, 356
caudate nucleus 255, *259*
caudothalamic groove 255, *259*, *262*
cavum septum pellucidum 255, *266*, 356
cavum vergi 255
cellulitis *318*

central venous access 322–5, *326*, 327–30, *331*, *332*
  complications 329, 330
  devices (CVAD) 322, 328–9, *330*
  guidewire 323, *325*
  sites 324–5, *326*, 327–9
  ultrasound
    guidance 322–5, *326*, 327–30, *331*, *332*
    technique 323–4
  venous occlusion 325, 327
cerebellar vermis *259*
  herniation 297
  partial agenesis 271
cerebellum 255
  banana-shaped 24, *25*
  hemorrhage 260
cerebral artery, middle (MCA)
  flow velocity 21
  pulsatility index 21, 22
cerebral atrophy 275
cerebrospinal fluid (CSF) 275
cervical lymphadenopathy 284–5, *286*
cervix, uterine 212, *213*
  development 208
chest
  congenital cysts 350–1
  cystic adenomatoid malformation 345
  ganglioneuroma 343
  intercostal approach 342
  mass lesions 342, 343–5
  neurenteric cysts 343
  neuroblastoma 343
  neurogenic tumors 343
  parasternal approach 342
  probes 342
  pulmonary sequestration 344–5
  ultrasound examination 341–2
  see also diaphragm
Chiari II malformation 297
children, older
  echogenic kidneys 83–4
  hypertension 89–94
cholangitis 146
cholecystitis 160
choledochal cysts 141–8, 191
  ultrasound examination 147–8
choledochocele 142
cholelithiasis 160–1
chondrodysplasia
  metaphyseal 175
  punctata 25
  syndromes 145
choroid plexus 255, *258*, *263*
  cysts 22, *24*, 255, 272
  echogenic *267*
  hemorrhage 260

chromosomal anomalies 19, *23*
  echogenic kidneys 83
chylothorax 349–50
cirrhosis 149–50
  cystic fibrosis 154
cloaca 356
cloacal abnormalities 30, 46, 216
  anorectal atresia 198
  exstrophy 46
collagen slurry 333
collateral vein canalization 327, *328*
colon 200
  development 182
color Doppler
  chest 342
  fetal cardiac 26
  kidneys 94
  subarachnoid hemorrhage 263
  urinary tract 50, 52
computed tomography (CT)
  appendix 195
  inflammatory bowel disease *199*
  kidneys 94
congenital adrenal hyperplasia (CAH) 115, 222, 227
congenital anomalies
  before 24 weeks *18*
  cardiac abnormalities 25–6
  cranial 22–5
  detection before 14 weeks *17*
  gastrointestinal abnormalities 28
  prenatal diagnosis 15–36
  pulmonary abnormalities 26–8
  routine screening 16, 18–22
  skeletal abnormalities 33–4
  spectrum 16
  spine 22–5, *26*
  urinary tract abnormalities 28–33, *34*
  see also named organs and conditions
congenital cystic adenomatoid malformation of the lung (CCAML) 26–7
contrast agents 11–12
corpus callosum *259*
  agenesis 23, 272, *273*
corpus luteum 209, 211–12
corticosteroids, systemic 316
coupling gel, warming 4
cranium
  accidental injury 275
  congenital cystic abnormalities 269, 271–2
  contusions 274–5
  measurements 252–3, *254*
  normal anatomy 253–5, *256–7*
  trauma 272, 274–5

  ultrasound 249–50
  axial planes 254–5
  coronal planes 253, *256–8*
  fetal 22–5
  probes 5
  sagittal planes 254, *256–7*, *259*, *262*
  technique 252–5, *256–7*
  vascular abnormalities 275–6
  see also intracranial hemorrhage
cremasteric artery 238
cremasteric reflex 238
Crohn disease 188
cryptococcus, splenic abscess 168
cryptorchidism 237, 241
  testicular calcification 246
Cushing syndrome 125, *126*
cysteine renal stones 85, 86
cystic adenomatoid malformation of lung 345
cystic fibrosis 154
  intussusception risk 192
  pancreas 174–5
  ultrasound appearance 174–5
cystic hygroma 283–4, *285*
  sclerotherapy 336–7
cystography
  bladder catheterization 2
  nuclear medicine 49
  vesicoureteric reflux 53–4
  see also micturating cystourethrogram (MCU)
cytomegalovirus (CMV) 88, 356

D

Dandy–Walker cysts 271, 356
  agenesis of corpus callosum 272
deferential artery 238
dermal sinus, dorsal 295–6
diaphragm
  eventeration 345, 346
  masses 346–7
  movement 346
  paralysis 346
  rhabdomyosarcoma 346–7
diaphragmatic hernia, congenital 26, 345–6
  Bochdalek 345
  Morgagni 345, *346*
diastematomyelia 296, 297
^{99}Tc-diethylenetriaminepentaacetate (DTPA) *48*, 99
DiGeorge syndrome 118, 356
Digital Image Communications in Medicine (DICOM) standards 7, 10

^{99}Tc-dimercaptosuccinic acid
  (DMSA) *48*, 54, 55
  duplex kidneys 64
  hypertension 91, 93, 94
  urinary tract infection 66, 68
direct isotope cystogram (DIC) *48*,
  68
disseminated intravascular
  coagulation (DIC) 137, *140*
Doppler examination 5, 7–8
  cavernous hemangioma 140
  chest 342
  fetal 20–2
    bladder 31
  goiter 280
  hepatobiliary system 133
  hypertension 90, 92, 93, 99
  kidneys 50, 52
  lung consolidation 348
  power 5, 7
  pulmonary sequestration 345
  renal transplantation 97, *98*, 99
  safety 12
  soft tissue masses 317
  splenic focal lesions 167
  testicular torsion 245–6
  thyroiditis 278–9
  urinary tract 50, 52
  velocimetry 21–2
  see also color Doppler
Down syndrome 359
  cystic hygroma 284
ductus deferens 235
ductus venosus 132, 356
duodenum
  atresia 172, 181
  Ladd bands 202
  malrotation 172
  stenosis 181

E

Eagle–Barrett syndrome see prune
  belly syndrome
echocardiography, fetal 26
ejaculatory duct 236
empyema 335, 350
encephalocele 33
  agenesis of corpus callosum 272
endometrium 212, *213*
endoscopic retrograde
  cholangiopancreatography
  (ERCP)
  choledochal cysts 141, *148*
  pancreatitis 175
Entonox 321, 330
epidermoid cysts, spleen 167

epididymis 235, 238
  cystic lesions 248
  hyperechoic 245
epididymitis 246
epididymo-orchitis 246
equipment choice/capabilities 5, 7
Escherichia coli
  adrenal abscess 116
  xanthogranulomatous
    pyelonephritis 69
esophageal atresia 28
esophagus
  duplication cysts 351
  pH monitoring 184
ethanol sclerotherapy 336
Ewing's tumor of rib 349
examination 3–5
  protocols 4
extended field of view imaging 11
extracorporeal membrane
  oxygenation (ECMO) 269,
  270, 356
extracorporeal shockwave lithotripsy
  86, 356

F

face, fetal ultrasound 19
fallopian tubes
  development 208
  regression 219
falls 275
fasting 2
femoral artery
  pseudoaneurysm *318*
  puncture 324–5, *326*, 338
femoral epiphysis 309
  slipped capital 313, 316
femoral head 308, *309*, 356
  avascular necrosis 302, 306
  contour 315
  coverage 308–9, *310*
  lateral head distance 309, *310*
  ossification center 309
  Perthes disease 315
  puncture *326*
femoral vein puncture 324–5, *326*,
  329
fetal ultrasound 15
  abdomen 18, *21*
  aneuploidy markers 19, *23*
  cardiac abnormalities 25–6
  cranium 22–5
  detectable syndromes *35*
  face 19
  gastrointestinal abnormalities 28
  gender 19

gestational age *16*
  head 18, *20*
  limbs 19
  pulmonary abnormalities 26–8
  skeletal abnormalities 33–4
  spectrum of abnormalities *16*
  spine 18–19, *21*, 22–5, *26*
  thorax 18, *20*
  urinary tract abnormalities 28–33,
  34
fetus
  small for gestational age 20
  three-dimensional
    echocardiography 26
fibromatosis colli 284, *285*
fibromuscular hyperplasia 94
filum terminale
  fibrolipoma 296
  tight 297
fine needle aspiration cytology 330
fistula 357
  arteriovenous renal 102
  bladder 183
  tracheo-esophageal 28
  urethral/vaginal 183
fluid drainage, ultrasound-guided
  335–6
fluoroscopy 324
  brachiocephalic vein puncture
    327, *328*
  drainage procedures 336
  inferior vena cava translumbar
    approach for puncture 328
  intussusception reduction 193
follicle-stimulating hormone (FSH)
  211
  precocious puberty 223
follicles 209, 211
foot deformity 303
foramen
  of Luschka 271
  of Magendie 271
  of Munro 255, *257*
  of Winslow 200
foregut 181
fungal infections 168

G

gallbladder
  abnormalities 160–2
  biliary atresia 143
  congenital anomalies 136
  cystic fibrosis 154
  hepatitis 153
  hydrops 162
  normal appearance 135–6

puncture 338
sludge 161–2
gallstones 160–1
    carcinoma 148
    causes 162
    cystic fibrosis 154
    splenic infarct in sickle cell disease 169
ganglioneuroblastoma 117, 123
ganglioneuroma 117, 123
    chest 343
gastric mucosa thickening 188
gastric outlet obstruction 171, 190
gastroesophageal junction 184–5
gastroesophageal reflux 184–5
gastrointestinal tract
    abnormalities 184–95, *196*, 197–9
    enteric duplication 190–1
    intussusception 191–3
    neuromatosis 280
    stomach abnormalities 188–9
    see also bowel
gastroschisis 183
Gaucher disease 169
gelatine foam plugs 333
gender
    assignment 218–19
    fetal ultrasound 19
genital ducts, development 208
genital tract, female 207
    congenital abnormalities 214
    embryology 208–10
    normal 210–13, *214*
    obstruction 216–18
    ultrasound technique 210–13, *214*
genital tract, male
    congenital anomalies 241–3
    embryology 235–8
    normal anatomy 238–9, *240*
    ultrasound technique 240–1
genitalia, ambiguous 207, 218–19, *220, 221*
germ cell tumors 228–9, 246
germ cells, female 209
germinal matrix hemorrhage 259, 260, *262, 263, 264, 265*
    with periventricular leukomalacia 268
giant cell astrocytoma 75, *77*
glucocerebrosidase 169
glucose-6-phosphatase deficiency 159
glycogen storage disease 149, 357
    liver adenoma 159
    polycystic ovaries 227
goiter *278*, 279–80
gonadotropins 210, 211, 236–7
gonads, development 208

Graafian follicle 209, 211
granulomatous disease, chronic 356
    liver 156
    stomach 188
granulosa cells 209
granulosa theca cell tumors 223, 228
Graves disease 278–9
gubernaculum 236
gut, primordial 181
Guthrie test 277

H

Haemophilus influenzae 311
Hashimoto thyroiditis *278*, 279
head 251–2
    congenital anomalies 22–5, *26*
    fetal ultrasound 18, *20*
    non-accidental injury 272, 274
    tumors 288–91
    see also cranium; intracranial hemorrhage; skull
health care staff
    occupational injury avoidance 8
    safety 12
heart
    four-chamber view 26
    see also cardiac abnormalities; cardiac conditions
heart-sparing effect 21
hemangioendothelioma, hepatic 136–8, *139*, 140
hemangioma
    hepatic 136–8, *139*, 140, *141*
        calcification 137, 138
        cavernous 138, *139*
        ultrasound appearance 137–8, *139*, 140
    soft tissue 318
hematologic malignancies, peliosis 169
hemidiaphragm, high 346, *351*
hemihypertrophy 125
hemithorax, opaque 347, 348–50
hemivertebrae 24–5, *26*
hemoperitoneum 202
hemothorax 350
Henoch–Schönlein purpura 188, 357
hepatic artery 135
    liver transplantation 162
    thrombosis 163
hepatic fibrosis, congenital 72–3, 144–5
hepatic iminodiacetic acid (HIDA) scan 73–4
    choledochal cysts 148

hepatic veins 134–5
    dilation 136
    veno-occlusive disease 154
hepatitis 152–3
    carriers 153
    neonatal 143, *144*
    viral 152–3
hepatobiliary system
    normal 133–6
    ultrasound technique 133–4
hepatoblastoma 157–8, 357
    neonate 140, *141*
hepatocellular carcinoma 149, 153, 158
hepatomegaly 136, 137
hepatosplenomegaly 169
hernia
    inguinal 241, 242
    scrotum 241–2
Hickman line 322, 323, *324*, 330
    collateral pathway 328
hindgut 182–3
hip
    alfa angle 305
    angle measurement 302, 305
    developmental dysplasia 302–4, 356
        clinical tests 302–4
        follow-up 310–11
        Graf classification 305, *306*
        risk factors 303
        ultrasound technique 304–6, *307*, 308–11
    dislocation 305, *306*, 306–7
    displaced 356
    dynamic assessment 309
    dynamic sonography of Harcke 304, 306, 308, *309*, 310
    effusion 313, *314*, 315
    Graf technique 304–6, *310*
    instability 358
    irritable 312–13, *314*, 315
    painful 311–13, *314*, 315–17
    septic 313, *314*, 315
    stability assessment 306
    subluxation 305, *306*
    Terjesen femoral head coverage 308–9, *310*
    ultrasound
        principles 309–10
        technique 304–6, *307*, 308–11
    unstable 303, 359
Hirschsprung disease 118
histiocytosis, testicular metastases 248
HLA-B27 316
Hodgkin lymphoma 335
holoprosencephaly 22, 271–2, 357
    agenesis of corpus callosum 272

hydatid infections
  liver disease 155–6
  spleen 167
hydrocele 238, 241–2, 248
hydrocephalus
  detection 269
  intraventricular hemorrhage 265–7
  ultrasound examination 275
hydrocephaly 23
hydrocolpos 216
hydrometrocolpos 115, 216, *218*
hydromyelia 296, 297
hydronephrosis
  bilateral 59, 60
  differential diagnosis of prenatal 53
  genital tract obstruction 216, 217
  nephrocalcinosis coexistence 88
hydrops, fetal 27, *28*, 34, *36*
  immune 22, 34
  non-immune 34, *36*
hydroureter, bilateral 60
hymen, imperforate 216
hyperbilirubinemia
  conjugated 142
  unconjugated 141
hyperoxaluria 84–5
hyperparathyroidism 281
hypertension
  causes 90
  children 89–94
  Doppler examination 90, 92, 93, 99
  imaging 90–4
  normal kidneys 94
  pheochromocytoma 92–3, 94
  renovascular disease 90
  small kidneys 93–4
  see also portal hypertension
hypoplastic left heart syndrome 26
hypospadias 218
hypotelorism 271–2
hypothalamic–pituitary axis 210
hypothalamic–pituitary–ovarian axis 225
hypothyroidism, congenital 277

I

iliac vein occlusion 325
Ilizarov distraction technique 317
images
  analogue 9
  digital 9–10
  dynamic clips 10
  recording 8–10
  storing 8–10

immunocompromised patients 329
indirect radioisotope cystogram (IRC) 48
infants, preparation for scan 2
infection
  central venous access 329
  fungal 168
  muscles *318*
  viral 312
  see also bacterial infection
inferior vena cava
  adrenal scanning 115
  anomalies 133
  congenital web 153, 154
  development 132
  dilation 136
  Doppler velocimetry 21
  examination 134, 135
  patency for liver transplantation 162
  thrombus 243
  translumbar approach for puncture 328
infertility
  risk with cryptorchidism 241
  testicular calcification 246
inflammatory bowel disease *199*
  appendicitis differential diagnosis 195
information leaflet 1–2
infratentorial hemorrhage 268
inguinal canals 236, 237
  anatomy 238
  hydrocele 238, *239*
inguinal hernia 241, 242
inspissated bile plug syndrome 143
insulin, polycystic ovaries 227
intersex 207
intracranial hemorrhage 257–60, 261–2, 263–4
  classification 263–4, 265
  extra-corporeal membrane oxygenation (ECMO) 269, 270
  neonates 268–9
  types 259–60, *262*, 263
intrauterine growth retardation (IUGR) 20–1, 31
  Doppler velocimetry 22
intravenous urogram (IVU) 48
  caliceal renal cysts 79
  duplex kidneys 64
  hypertension 93
  medullary sponge kidney 79
  PKD
    autosomal dominant 75
    autosomal recessive 73, *74*
  renal transplantation 101
  urinary tract infection 68

intraventricular hemorrhage 265–7
intraventricular rupture 260
intussusception 191–3
  appendicitis differential diagnosis 195
  treatment 193
  ultrasound technique 192–3

J

jaundice
  malignant obstructive 339
  neonatal 140–2
    ultrasound 144
Jeune syndrome 145, 357
jugular vein puncture 324, *325*, 329
juvenile nephronophthisis/medullary cystic disease complex 76, 78
juxtadiaphragmatic lesions 341–2, 342–7

K

Kasabach–Meritt syndrome 137, 357
  splenic hemangioma 167
Kawasaki disease 162
kidneys
  abnormalities 195
  abscess 65, 66
    perinephric *335*, 336
  angiography 93, 94, 101
  angiomyolipoma 76, *77*
  anomalies 28–33, *34*, 41, *42*
  arteriovenous fistula 102
  biopsy 330, 332, *333*
  calculi 66, 84–6, 88
    infectious 85
    staghorn 85, *86*
    stents 88
  candidiasis 69–70, 88
  clear cell sarcoma 106
  cortex
    nephrocalcinosis 88–9
    thickness 66–7
  cross-fused ectopia 42, *43*, 198
  cystic 70–6, *77*, 78–9, *80*
    acquired disease 79
    caliceal 79
    genetic disease 71, 72–6, *77*, 78
    medullary disease 76, 78, 88
    multilocular nephroma 79, *80*
    non-genetic disease 72, 78–9
    simple 78, *80*
  Doppler examination 50, 52
  duplex 30, 43, 62–4, *65*
  dysplasia 31–2, 59

cystic 60, 71, *80*
echogenic 83
multicystic 57–9, 71, *80*
prenatal diagnosis 54
echogenic 32–3, *34*, 63, 65, 79–84
hypertension 91
neonates 80–3
urinary tract infection 68
ectopic 41–2, *43*
embryology 39–41
fetal 28–33, *34*
lobulation 67
glomerulocystic 78
horseshoe 42
investigations 48–50, *51*, 52
medulla
cystic disease 76, 78, 88
necrosis 82
nephrocalcinosis 88–9
medullary sponge 79
multicystic 57–9, *60*, 71
postnatal ultrasound 58–9
pelvic 217
position abnormalities 41–2, *43*
pseudoaneurysms 102
renal cell sarcoma 106
rhabdoid tumor 106
single 42, *43*, 198
size in hypertension 91, *92*
small in hypertension 93–4
tissue harmonic imaging 11
transplantation 94–7, *98*, 99–102
anatomy 95
arteriovenous fistula 102
complications 96, 99–102
donation 95
Doppler examination 97, *98*, 99
late dysfunction 101
malignancy 102
obstruction 100–1
post-transplantation 96
pre-transplantation 95–6
primary non-function 97
pseudoaneurysms 102
trauma 94
tumors 102–9, *110*
varicocele 242
see also polycystic kidney disease (PKD); renal *entries*
kyphoscoliosis 23

L

lactobezoars 189
Ladd bands 182, 190, 202
Langerhans cell histiocytosis 169, 338, 348
lateral head distance (LHD) 309, *310*
Legg–Calvé–Perthes disease *see* Perthes disease
Lesch–Nyhan syndrome 357
nephrocalcinosis 88
uric acid renal stones 85
leukemia
ovarian metastases 229
renal involvement 107–8
salivary glands 291
spleen 168, 169
testes 248
thymus infiltration 347
Li–Fraumeni syndrome 357
adrenocortical tumor association 125
ligamentum teres 132
ligamentum venosum 132
limbs
congenital abnormalities 33–4
fetal ultrasound 19
lengthening procedures 317
lipoma, soft tissue *318*, *319*
lipomyelomeningocele 296
litigation 4
liver
abnormalities
diffuse 148–54
neonatal 136–8, *139*, 140
abscess *151*, 155, *351*
adenoma 159
angiomatous lesions 156
bare area 200
biopsy 332–3, *334*
transjugular 333
bright 148–9
calcification 157
chronic disease *150*
granulomatous 156
cirrhosis 149–50
cystic fibrosis 154
cysts 155
Doppler examination 8
embryology 131–2
failure 143
fatty infiltration 148–9
fetal vascular anatomy 132–3
focal lesions 154–7
focal nodular hyperplasia 159
hemangioendothelioma 136–8, *139*, 140
hemangioma 136–8, *139*, 140
hematoma 156
hydatid disease 155–6
investigations *164*
lobe size 134–5
mesenchymal hamartoma 156–7
metastases 160
normal appearance 134
perihepatic spaces 200, *201*
segments 134–5
transplantation 162–3
complications 163
percutaneous transhepatic cholangiography 339
tumors 157–60
undifferentiated embryonal sarcoma 158–9
vasculature 134–5
see also hepatic entries
low birth-weight 241
lung
abnormalities 348–9
fetal ultrasound 26–8
atelectasis 348–9
consolidation 348–9, *350*
cystic adenomatoid malformation 345
tumors 349
see also pulmonary *entries*
luteinizing hormone (LH) 211
precocious puberty 223
lymph nodes, neck 285, *286*
lymphangioma
mesentery 202
neck 290–1
spleen 167
lymphatic malformations, cystic 336–7
lymphocele 101
lymphoma
liver metastases 160
mediastinum 348
neck 285
needle biopsy 335
ovarian metastases 229
pancreatic metastases 178
peritoneal cavity 203
renal involvement 107–8
salivary glands 291
spleen 168–9
stomach infiltration 188
testes 248
thymus infiltration 347
thyroid gland *278*, 280
lymphoproliferative disorder 102

M

magnetic resonance angiography (MRA) 101
magnetic resonance imaging (MRI)
autosomal recessive PKD 74

magnetic resonance imaging (MRI) (*Continued*)
  neuroblastoma 121
  renal transplantation 100
malabsorption 154, 174
malignancy
  extratesticular mass 249
  risk with cryptorchidism 241
  testes 247–8
  thymus 347–8
  thyroid gland 280, *281*
masculinization of female 219
massa intermedia 255
Meckel diverticulum 184, 192
Meckel–Gruber syndrome 33, 145, 357
meconium ileus 154
mediastinum 342, 347–8
  lymphadenopathy 348
  masses *343*
  superior 341
mediastinum testis 238
megacystis microcolon 30–1
megaureter 56–7, 85
  primary 43–4
menarche 210, 211–12, *224*
meningocele 297
  anterior 216, *217*
meningomyelocele 291, *292*, 298
menstrual cycle 225
menstrual dysfunction 225, 227–8
^{99}Tc-mercaptoacetyltriglycine (MAG3) scan *48*
  duplex kidneys 64
  hypertension 93
  renal transplantation 101
  urinary tract infection 68
mesenteric artery, superior 172, 182
  thrombosis 177
  ultrasound technique 190, *191*
  volvulus 189
mesenteric vein, superior 173
  thrombosis 177
  ultrasound technique 190, *191*
mesentery 199–201, 202–3, *204*
  abnormalities 202–3, *204*
  cysts 198–9, *200, 201*
  infections 203
  inflamed 195
  lymphadenitis 195
  lymphadenopathy 203, *204*
mesonephric (Wolffian) ducts 208, 219, 235–6, 359
mesonephroi 39–40
^{123}I-metaiodobenzylguanidine (^{123}I MIBG) scan 94
  neuroblastoma 121
  phaeochromocytoma 128

metanephroi 40
metaphysis, Schwachman syndrome 175
metastases
  liver 160
  neuroblastoma 118, 121
  ovarian 229
  pancreas 178
  testes 248
  Wilms tumor 203
^{99m}Tc-methylene diphosphonate scan 121
microbubbles, echogenic 12
microcephaly 23
microlithiasis, testicular 246, *247*, 248
micropenis 218
micturating cystourethrogram (MCU) *48*, 55
  posterior urethral valves 60
  renal pelvic dilation 57
  urinary tract infection 68
middle aortic arch syndrome 91, 94
midgut 181–2
Morrison's pouch 200, *201*
Müllerian ducts *see* paramesonephric (Müllerian) ducts
Müllerian inhibitory substance 208, 219
multiple endocrine neoplasia 280, 358
muscles
  inflammation/infection 318
  ultrasound technique 301–2
myelomeningocele 297
myositis ossificans *318*

N

neck
  abscess *286*
  cystic hygroma 283–4, *285*
    sclerotherapy 337
  fibromatosis colli 284, *285*
  lymph nodes 285, *286*
  lymphangioma 290–1
  lymphoma 285
  masses 281, *282*, 283–5, *286*
  neuroblastoma 291
  rhabdomyosarcoma 291
  salivary glands 287–8
  thymus 286–7
  tumors 288–91
  ultrasound technique 278
  see also thyroid gland
needle biopsy 334–5

neonates 4–5
  echogenic kidneys 80–3
  female 214, 216–20
    masculinization 219
  hepatic abnormalities 136–8, *139*, 140
  hepatoblastoma 140, *141*
  intracranial hemorrhage 268–9
  jaundice 140–2
  ovarian cysts 219–20
  traumatic spinal cord lesions 298
nephroblastoma 358
  see also Wilms tumor
nephroblastomatosis 108–9
nephrocalcinosis 84, 86–9, 358
  cortical 88
  grading 88, *89*
  iatrogenic 87, 88
  medullary 88–9
  tyrosinemia 149
nephroma
  mesoblastic 106, *108*
  multilocular cystic 79
nephronia, focal 65, 66
nephronophthisis, juvenile 76, 78
nephropathy, reflux 68
nephrostomy 337
nesidioblastosis 175
neural tube defect 23–4, *25*
  diaphragmatic hernia association 345
neurenteric cysts 343
neuroblastoma 117–23, *124*, 358
  4S 122–3, *124*, 140
  adrenal hemorrhage differential diagnosis 116
  calcification 118, 121
  chest 343
  clinical presentation 118
  imaging 118, *119–20*, 121–2
  intraspinal extension 121
  metastases 118, 121
    liver 160
    testicular 248
  neck 291
  staging 122, *123*
  Wilms tumor differential diagnosis 121, *122*
neurofibromatosis, neuroblastoma association 118
nevus, cutaneous 295
nitrous oxide 321, 330
non-accidental injury 272, 274
non-pancreatic pseudocyst 199
nuchal translucency thickness 26
nuclear medicine cystography *49*

O

occupational injury avoidance 8
ocular scanning, probes 5
oligohydramnios
    developmental dysplasia of hip risk 303
    posterior urethral valves 59
    renal agenesis 41
omental cysts 198–9, *200, 201*
omental fat, inflamed 195
omentum 199–201, 202–3, *204*
    abnormalities 202–3
omphalocele 183
oocytes 209
orchidopexy 246
orofacial digital syndrome 78
Ortolani test 303, 309
osteal stenosis 94
osteomyelitis 311–12, *313*
    transient synovitis differential diagnosis 313
ovarian cysts 191, 219–20
    appendicitis differential diagnosis 195
    polycystic 225, 227–8, *229*
    precocious puberty 222–3
    torsion 220, *223*
ovaries
    development 208–9
    endocrinology 210
    growth 209–10, 211
    masses 216
        malignant 229, *231*
    metastases 229
    multifollicular 222
    neoplasms 228–9, *230–1*, 232
        secondary 229
    polycystic 225, 227–8, *229*
        bulimia nervosa 225, 227
    streak 225, *228*
    ultrasound technique 210–11
    vascularization 209–10
    volume 211
ovulation 209
ovulatory cycles 210
oxalate stones, renal 85
oxalosis 88
oxygen and nitrous oxide (Entonox) 321, 330

P

pain control 321–2
    postoperative 321
pampiniform plexus 239, 240
    varicocele 242

pancreas
    abnormal 174–5, *176*, 177–9
    annular 171
    congenital anomalies 171–2
    cystic fibrosis 174–5
    cysts 177–8
        congenital 171
    divisum 171
    echogenicity 173, 177, *178*
    ectopic 171–2
    embryology 170–1, *172*
    focal lesions 177–9
    insufficiency 154, 174
    metastases 178
    neoplasms 178
    nesidioblastosis 175
    normal anatomy 172–4
    pseudocysts 175, *176*, 177
    Shwachman syndrome 175
    size 173
    trauma 178–9
    ultrasound technique 173–4
pancreatic duct 171
pancreaticoblastoma 178
pancreatitis 146
    acute 175, *176*, 177
    chronic 177
paracolic spaces 200, 202
paraesophageal varices 152
paramesonephric (Müllerian) ducts 208, 214, 216, 240, 358
parathyroid glands 277, 280–1
    adenoma 281
    hyperplasia 280
paravesical recesses 200–1, 202
parotid gland 287–8
    enlargement 288
    hemangioma 288–90
    infection 288
    tumors 288–90
    ultrasound technique 288
parotitis 288
patients
    examination 3–5
    information for 1–2
    positioning 5, *6*
    preparation for scan 2
    rewards 5
    safety of ultrasound 12
    waiting area 2–3
Pavlik harness 310, *312*
peliosis 169
pelvis
    abscess 335
    masses in neonates 214, 216–18
    teratoma 230
pelviureteric junction obstruction 30, 58

multicystic kidneys 59
renal transplantation 101
percutaneous transhepatic cholangiography (PTC) 338–9
pericardial effusion 335
pericarditis 316
perihepatic spaces 200, *201*
peripheral vascular studies 7
peripherally inserted central venous catheters (PICC) 322, *324, 328–9, 330, 331*
peritoneal cavity 200
    infection 202
    neoplasms 203
    trauma 202
peritoneal fluid 201–2
peritoneum 199–202, 203
    abscess 202
    development 183
peritonitis 202
periventricular hemorrhage 257–8, 260
    grading 263–4, *265*
periventricular leukomalacia 255, *261*, 264–5, 267–8
    causes 265
    grading 267, *269*
    ultrasound examination 265, 267–8, *269–70*
Perthes disease 313, 315–16
Peutz–Jaeger syndrome 192
pheochromocytoma 92–3, 94, *125, 127, 128*
    multiple endocrine neoplasia 280
phrenic nerve damage 346
phytobezoars 189
picibanil sclerotherapy 336
picture archiving and communication system (PACS) 9–10
PKD1 gene 74
placental insufficiency 21
play specialists 2
pleural effusions 335, *336*, 349–50, *351*, 358
    lymphoma 348
pleural fluid 349–50
    collections 202
pneumoperitoneum 202
polycystic kidney disease (PKD) 71
    autosomal dominant 71, 74–5, *80*
        pancreatic cysts 171
    autosomal recessive 71, 72–4, *80*
        Caroli syndrome association 145
        congenital hepatic fibrosis association 144, 145
    echogenic kidneys 82–3
    liver cysts 155

polycystic ovarian syndrome 227
polyhydramnios 27, 28
  congenital diaphragmatic hernia 26
polysplenia 134, 165, 358
porencephalic cyst 264, 271
port device 322, *324*, 328, *330*
  insertion *331*
portal cyst 143
portal hypertension 146, 149, 150–2
portal system, Doppler examination 8
portal vein 132, 134, 135, 152
  arterioportal shunts 152
  cavernous transformation 152
  congenital variations 135
  gastric varices 152
  obstruction 151
  pancreatic neck 173
  paraesophageal varices 152
  paraumbilical collaterals 152
  patency for liver transplantation 162
  splenorenal collaterals 152
  thrombosis 152, 163
  transhepatic biopsy 329, *332*
posterior fossa cysts 22, 24
postnatal investigations, urinary tract 52–64
pouch of Douglas 201, 202
Prader–Willi syndrome 237, 358
pre-eclampsia 22
precocious puberty 221–3
  causes 223
  isosexual 223, *226*
  ovarian tumors 228
pregnancy, red cell alloimmunized 22
prematurity
  intracranial hemorrhage 257
  periventricular leukomalacia *267*
  scrotal hernia association 241
prenatal diagnosis *see* congenital anomalies, prenatal diagnosis
preparation for scan 2
  urinary tract abnormalities 47
presacral mass 217–18
probes 5
processus vaginalis 236, 238
  hydrocele 241
prostate 236
Proteus infection
  renal calculi 84
  urinary tract infection 66
  xanthogranulomatous pyelonephritis 69
prune belly syndrome 46, 237, 356, 358
pseudoaneurysm *318*

Pseudomonas aeruginosa 329
pseudoprecocious puberty 222
psoas abscess *204*
puberty 210
  abnormal development 221–5, *226*
  delayed 224–5
  disorders 220–5, *226*, 227–8
  normal in girls *224*
  precocious 221–3
    ovarian tumors 228
  pseudoprecocious 222
pubic hair, premature development 223–4
pulmonary abnormalities
  fetal ultrasound 26–8
  see also lung
pulmonary emboli 329
pulmonary sequestration 27–8, 344–5
pulsatility index (PI) 97
  middle cerebral artery 21, 22
  umbilical artery 22
pyelonephritis 65
  xanthogranulomatous 69, 103
pyloric canal measurement 186, 187
pyloric muscle thickening 186, *187*
pyloric stenosis, hypertrophic 185–7
pylorospasm 187
pylorus
  double mucosal channel 187
  normal 185, *186*

R

radiation contamination/exposure 2
 radioisotope injection 2
rectovesical space 201
rectum
  atresia 183
  duplication 216–17
renal agenesis 31, 41
  see also kidneys
renal artery
  Doppler examination 99
  stenosis 93, 101
  thrombosis 97
renal caliceal dilation 56, *57*, *60*
  urinary tract infection *67, 68*
renal cell sarcoma 106
renal failure, end-stage/chronic 94–5
renal length 50
renal pelvis
  bifid 62, *64*
  diameter 56
  dilation 30

bilateral 56
  postnatal scan 53–5
  unilateral 55–6
renal size 49–50, *51*
renal tract investigations 48–50, *51*, *52*
renal tubules
  acute necrosis 82, 97, *98*
  ectasia 73
renal vein thrombosis 81–2, 97, 115, 116, *117*
  adrenal hemorrhage association 115
  tumor 243
  varicocele 242, 243
renal–hepatic–pancreatic dysplasia 83
renovascular disease in hypertension 90, 94
repetitive strain injury 8
resistive index (RI) 97
rete testis 238, 248
retinoblastoma, testicular metastases 248
retroperitoneal tumor 242
rhabdomyosarcoma 109, *110*
  bile duct 162
  diaphragm 346–7
  embryonal of vagina 232
  liver metastases 160
  neck 291
  paratesticular 249
  testicular metastases 248
rheumatoid arthritis 313, 315
rheumatoid factor 316

S

sacral agenesis 298
sacral pit 295
sacrococcygeal teratoma 216, 229, *231*
safety of ultrasound 12
salivary glands 287–8
  leukemia 291
  lymphoma 291
  tumors 288–90
sarcoma botryoides 232
scalp wounds 274
Schwachman syndrome 175, 358
sclerosing cholangitis 338
sclerotherapy 336–7
scrotum
  acutely painful 243–6
  embryology 235–8
  hernia 241–2
  hydrocele 238, *239*, 241–2, 248
  masses 241

normal anatomy 238–9, *240*
trauma 249
ultrasound technique 240–1
sedation 4
seminal vesicle 236
seminiferous tubules 238
seminoma 241
Sertoli cells 219, 235
sex, genetic 219
sickle cell disease 169, *170*
situs inversus 134, 166, 358
skeletal abnormalities, congenital 33–4
skeletal dysplasias 25
skin, angioma 295
skull
　fracture 274, 275
　lemon-shaped 24, *25*
　see also cranium
slipped capital femoral epiphysis 313, 316
small for gestational age babies 20
sodium tetradecyl sulfate sclerotherapy 336
soft tissue masses 317, *318–19*
　ultrasound technique 301–2
spermatic cord 239
　hydrocele 238, *239*
　rotation 244
　twisted 243, 244
sphincter of Oddi 189
spina bifida 23–4, *25*, 291, *292*, 295
spinal canal, dilation 297
spinal cord 291, *293*, 294
　closure 291, *292*
　tethering 297
　traumatic lesions in newborn 298
　ultrasound examination 294
spinal dysraphism 295
　occult 295–7
spine 291
　abnormalities 216, 343
　anatomy 291, 293–5
　caudal regression syndrome 25, 297–8
　congenital anomalies 22–5, *26*
　embryology 291
　fetal ultrasound 18–19, *21*, 22–5, *26*
　lipoma 296
　meningocele/myelomeningocele 297
　neuropore closure 291, *292*
　ultrasound
　　indications 295
　　technique 291, 293–5
spleen
　abscess 167–8

accessory 164
cardiac abnormalities 165–6
congenital variants 164–6
cysts 167
development 163
diffuse abnormalities 168–9, *170*
focal lesions 167–9, *170*
hemangioma 167
hematoma 170
hydatid infections 167
infarction 169, *170*
leukemia 168, 169
lymphangioma 167
lymphoma 168–9
neoplasia 168–9
normal 163, *165*
peliosis 169
small 167, *170*
storage disorders 169
trauma 170
wandering 165
splenic artery 169, 173
splenogonadal fusion 164
splenomegaly 167
splenosis 170
splenunculi 164, *165*
Staphylococcus aureus
　adrenal abscess 116
　central venous access infection 329
　osteomyelitis 311
　parotitis 288
steatorrhea 154, 174
sternocleidomastoid muscle 283, 285
steroids
　peliosis therapy 169
　systemic 316
Still disease 316
stomach abnormalities/tumors 188–9
storage disorders 169
struvite renal stones 85
subarachnoid hemorrhage 261, 263, 264
　traumatic 274
subclavian vein puncture 324, *325*, 326
subdural hemorrhage 261, 263, 264
　neonates 268
　traumatic 274
subfertility, testicular calcification 246
sublingual gland 287–8
submandibular gland 287–8
sylvian fissure 257
synovitis, transient 312–13, *314*, 315

aspiration technique 315
ultrasound technique 313, *314*, 315

T

Tamm–Horsfall proteinuria 88, 358
teleradiology 10
tendon abnormalities/tendinitis 317
teratodermoid 189
teratoma 216, 247, 248
　liver metastases 160
　ovarian 228
　pelvic *230*
　sacrococcygeal 216, 229, *231*
testes
　abscess 248
　benign masses 248
　calcification 246, 247
　congenital anomalies 241–3
　cysts 248
　dermoid *247*
　descent 236–7
　echogenic mass 248
　ectopic 237–8
　ectopic adrenal tissue 248
　embryology 235–8
　extratesticular masses 248–9
　fractured 249
　growth arrest 243
　hematocele 249
　hematoma 248, 249
　metastases 248
　microlithiasis 246, *247*, 248
　normal anatomy 238–9, *240*
　position abnormalities 237–8
　retractile 238
　torsion 242, 243–6
　　diagnostic accuracy 245
　　Doppler examination 245–6
　　testicular calcification 246
　　ultrasound technique 244–5
　tumors 247–8
　　extratesticular mass 249
　　primary 248
　　risk 237
　　risk with cryptorchidism 241
　　secondary 248
　ultrasound technique 240–1
　undescended 237, 241
　volume 243
　see also appendix testis
testicular artery 238–9
　normal *244*
　testicular torsion 246
testicular cells 219

testicular feminization 208
testicular veins 239–40
testosterone 219, 235
thalamostriate vessels 272, *273*
thalamus 255
   echogenicity 272, *273*
   hemorrhage 260
thelarche, isolated premature 223, 227
thorax, fetal ultrasound 18, *20*
three-dimensional fetal echocardiography 26
three-dimensional ultrasound 11
thrombophlebitis 329
thymoma 347
thymus 286–7, 347–8
   cysts 286–7
   malignancy 347–8
   mass 286, *287*
thyroglossal duct cysts 281, *282*, 283
thyroid gland 276–80
   accessory tissue 277
   benign nodule adenoma *281*
   carcinoma 280, *281*
   congenital anomalies 277
   cysts *281*
   diffuse enlargement 278–80
   ectopic 277
   embryology 277
   lymphoma *278*
   malignancy 280, *281*
   normal anatomy 276–7
thyroid inferno 279
thyroidectomy, total 280
thyroiditis 278–9
tissue harmonic imaging (THI) 10–11
torticollis
   congenital 284, *285*
   neonatal 303
tracheo-esophageal fistula 28
tracheobronchial tree 344, 345, 350
transducer 359
   high-frequency linear 5
transhepatic biopsy 329, *332*
transposition of the great arteries 26
trauma
   cranium 272, 274–5
   kidneys 94
   peritoneal cavity 202
   scrotum 249
   spinal cord lesions in neonates 298
   spleen 170
trichobezoars 189
trisomy 13 359
   holoprosencephaly 272
trisomy 15 272

trisomy 18 22, *24*, 359
trisomy 21 284, 359
tuberculosis
   mediastinum 348
   parotitis 288
   peliosis 169
   peritoneal 202
   testes 248
   urinary tract infection 70
tuberous sclerosis 75–6, *77*, *80*
   glomerulocystic kidneys 78
tunica albuginea 238
   rupture 249
tunica vaginalis 237
   testicular torsion 244
tunica vasculosa 238–9
Turner syndrome 359
   cystic hygroma 284
   puberty delay 224, 225, *228*
   splenic hemangioma 167
two-dimensional ultrasound 11
tyrosinemia 149, 359

U

ultrasound area 3–4
umbilical artery
   Doppler velocimetry 21
   pulsatility index 22
umbilical ring 183
umbilical vein 132
urachal cyst 45
urachus 359
   abnormalities 45
ureteric bud 40, 359
ureterocele *31*, 44, 62, 359
ureters
   anomalies 43–5
   balloon dilation 101
   bifid 43
   dilated 63
   ectopic 44
   stenosis 58, 96
      renal transplantation 100–1
   stents 100, 101
   stones 86, *87*
   urine leaks 101
urethra 236
   abnormalities 46–7
   dilation 60
   fistula 183
   obstruction 59
   posterior 60
urethral valves, posterior 30, 44, 46–7, 59–60, *61*, 62
uric acid renal stones 85, 86
urinary tract

abnormalities/anomalies 41–7
   fetal ultrasound 28–33, *34*
   lower 43–7
   postnatal investigation 52–64
   structural 66
   upper 41–3
Doppler/color Doppler examination 50, 52
embryology 39–41
lower 43–7
normal appearance 47–50, *51*, 52
ultrasound preparation 47
upper 41–3
see also bladder; kidneys; renal *entries*
urinary tract infection
   imaging 65–8
      protocol 68
   incidence 64
   recurrent 65, 68
   renal calculi 66
   renal candidiasis 69–70
   renal damage 66
   tuberculosis 70
   vesicoureteric reflux 66
   xanthogranulomatous pyelonephritis 69
urine leaks in renal transplantation 101
urinoma 59, 60, *61*, 101
urogenital sinus 46, 216, 222
   abnormalities 216
   lower vagina development 208
   persistent 115
   sinography 219, *222*
urogenital tract malformation 298
   diaphragmatic hernia association 345
urological interventions 337
uterine arteries, Doppler velocimetry 22
uterus 212–13, *214*
   congenital abnormalities 214, *215*
   development 208
   double 214, *215*
   length 213, *214*
   prepubertal development 225
   regression 219
   ultrasound use 219
uveitis 316

V

VACTERL association 28, 359
   cross-fused ectopia 42, *43*
   echogenic kidneys 83
   kidney transplantation 96

spectrum 24
see also VATER syndrome
vagina
   atresia 216
   embryonal rhabdomyosarcoma 232
   fistula 183
   fluid-filled 62
   lower 208, 216
   post-micturition filling 50, *52*
   rhabdomyosarcoma 109
   stenosis 216
   ultrasound use 219
   upper 208
varicocele 239–40, 241, 242–3
   testicular calcification 246
   ultrasound technique 241, 242
vas deferens 238
vascular anomalies, sclerotherapy 336–7
vascular lesions *290*
VATER syndrome 33, 359
   anorectal atresia 198
   ectopic pancreas 172
   see also VACTERL association
vein of Galen, aneurysm 275–6
veins
   malformations and sclerotherapy 336
   occluded 325, 327
veno-occlusive disease 151, 153–4
venous access *see* central venous access
ventricles 255, *257–9*
   coarctation 255, *261*

dilation 260, 265–7
width 253, *254*
ventricular index 253
ventriculomegaly 275
ventriculus terminalis 295
vertebral bodies *293*
vesicoureteric junction abnormalities 44
vesicoureteric reflux 12, 44
   anorectal anomalies 198
   cystography 53–4
   duplex kidney 63, *65*
   grades *45*
   hypertension 93
   multicystic kidney association 59
   primary 44–5
   renal pelvis dilation 54
   urinary tract infection 66
virilization 125, 228
vitelline duct persistence 183–4
voiding urosonography 12, *48*
volvulus 189, 190
vomiting
   bilious 189
   projectile 185
von Hippel–Lindau syndrome 171

W

waiting area 2–3
'wandering tumor' 220, *223*
weight
   estimation of fetal 20
   low birth-weight 241
Wilms tumor 102, 103–6, *107, 108*

associated conditions 104–5
bilateral with recurrence 106, *107, 108*
liver metastases 160
metastatic spread 203
nephroblastomatosis 108
neuroblastoma differential diagnosis 121, *122*
screening 105–6
sonographic appearance 103–4
staging 106
testicular metastases 248
varicocele 243
Wolffian ducts *see* mesonephric (Wolffian) ducts
Wolman disease 127

X

xanthogranulomatous pyelonephritis 69
Wilms tumor 103
Yersinia enterocolitica 203

Z

Zellweger syndrome 359
   congenital hepatic fibrosis 145
   glomerulocystic kidneys 78